Medical Radiology

Radiation Oncology

Series editors

Luther W. Brady
Stephanie E. Combs
Jiade J. Lu

For further volumes:
http://www.springer.com/series/4353

Hans Geinitz · Mack Roach III
Nicholas van As
Editors

Radiotherapy in Prostate Cancer

Innovative Techniques and Current Controversies

Springer

Editors
Hans Geinitz
Department of Radiation Oncology
Krankenhaus der Barmherzigen
Schwestern Linz
Medical Faculty, Johannes Kepler University
Linz
Austria

Mack Roach III
Department of Radiation Oncology
University of California
San Francisco, CA
USA

Nicholas van As
The Institute of Cancer Research
Sutton Surrey
UK

ISSN 0942-5373 ISSN 2197-4187 (electronic)
ISBN 978-3-642-37098-4 ISBN 978-3-642-37099-1 (eBook)
DOI 10.1007/978-3-642-37099-1
Springer Heidelberg New York Dordrecht London

Library of Congress Control Number: 2014953516

Printed on acid-free paper

Springer is part of Springer Science+Business Media (www.springer.com)

For Anja, Nora, Thilo and Vera

Hans Geinitz

Acknowledgments

We would like to thank all the authors who contributed enthusiastically to the completion of this book. While editing the volume we ourselves got new insights and different angles on how to see and practice prostate radiation oncology. Beyond its content, the book is a virtuous example for a fruitful international cooperation embracing Europe and North America.

Linz, October 2014 — Hans Geinitz
San Francisco — Mack Roach III
Sutton — Nicholas van As

Contents

Contributors

Nicolaus Andratschke Department of Radiation Oncology, University Hospital Zurich, Zürich, Switzerland

Giorgio Arcangeli Regina Elena National Cancer Institute, Rome, Italy

Stefano Arcangeli Regina Elena National Cancer Institute, Rome, Italy

Claus Belka Department of Radiation Oncology, Ludwig-Maximilians-University (LMU), Munich, Germany

Dirk Böhmer Department of Radiation Oncology, Charité University Medicine, Berlin, Germany

Michel Bolla Clinique Universitaire de Cancérologie-Radiothérapie, Centre Hospitalier Universitaire Albert Michallon, Grenoble, France

Dirk Bottke Department of Radiotherapy and Radiation Oncology, University Hospital Ulm, Ulm, Germany

Violaine Brun Baronnat Clinique Universitaire de Cancérologie-Radiothérapie, Centre Hospitalier Universitaire Albert Michallon, Grenoble, France

Wilfried Budach Medical Faculty, Department of Radiation Oncology, Heinrich Heine University of Düsseldorf, Düsseldorf, Germany

Jürgen Debus Radiologische Universitätsklinik, Strahlenklinik, Heidelberg, Germany

Georges Decker Department of Radiology, University of Bonn, Bonn, Germany

Marciana Nona Duma Department of Radiation Oncology, Klinikum rechts der Isar, Technische Universität München, München, Germany

Ute Ganswindt Department of Radiation Oncology, Ludwig-Maximilians-University (LMU), Munich, Germany

Michael Geier Department of Radiation Oncology, Krankenhaus der Barmherzigen Schwestern Linz, Linz, Austria

Hans Geinitz Department of Radiation Oncology, Krankenhaus der Barmherzigen Schwestern Linz, Medical Faculty, Johannes Kepler University, Linz, Austria

Pirus Ghadjar Department of Radiation Oncology, Inselspital, Bern University Hospital, Bern, Switzerland

Gregor Goldner Klinik für Strahlentherapie, MUW Wien, Allgemeines Krankenhaus, Wien, Austria

A. L. Grosu Department of Radiation Oncology, Medical University of Freiburg, Freiburg, Germany

Arne Grün Department for Radiation Oncology and Cyberknife Cente, Charité—University Medicine Berlin Campus Virchow-Clinic, Berlin, Germany

Jürgen E. Gschwend Department of Urology, Klinikum rechts der Isar, Technische Universität München, Munich, Germany

Matthias Guckenberger Department of Radiation Oncology, University Hospital Zurich (USZ), Zurich, Switzerland

Gregor Habl Radiologische Universitätsklinik, Strahlenklinik, Heidelberg, Germany

Daniel Robert Henderson Clinical Oncology Royal Marsden Hospital London, London, UK

Thomas Horn Department of Urology, Klinikum rechts der Isar, Technische Universität München, Munich, Germany

Mitchell Kamrava Department of Radiation Oncology, University of California Los Angeles, Los Angeles, CA, US

Marisa A. Kollmeier Department of Radiation Oncology, Memorial Sloan-Kettering Cancer Center, New York, NY, USA

Hubert Kübler Department of Urology, Klinikum rechts der Isar, Technische Universität München, Munich, Germany

Patrick Kupelian Department of Radiation Oncology, University of California Los Angeles, Los Angeles, CA, US

Tanja Langsenlehner Department of Therapeutic Radiology and Oncology, Medical University of Graz, Graz, Austria

Wolfgang Lilleby MD Anderson, Norwegian Cancer Consortium (NCC), Oncology, Oslo, Norway

Tobias Maurer Department of Urology, Klinikum rechts der Isar, Technische Universität München, Munich, Germany

Alexandros Papachristofilou Department of Radiation Oncology, University Hospital Basel, Basel, Switzerland

Pascal Pommier Radiotherapy Department, Centre Léon Bérard, Lyon, France

H. C. Rischke Department of Radiation Oncology, Medical University of Freiburg, Freiburg, Germany; Department of Nuclear Medicine, Medical University of Freiburg, Freiburg, Germany

Mack Roach III Department of Radiation Oncology, Helen Diller Family Comprehensive Cancer Center, University of California San Francisco (UCSF), San Francisco, CA, USA

Irina Sackerer Department of Radiation Oncology, Klinikum rechts der Isar, Technische Universität München, Munich, Germany

Ralf A. Schneider Center for Proton Therapy, Paul Scherrer Institute, Villigen, Switzerland

Lidia Strigari Regina Elena National Cancer Institute, Rome, Italy

Martin Stuschke Direktor der Klinik und Poliklinik für Strahlentherapie, Universitätsklinikum Essen, Essen, Germany

Alexandre Tessier Clinique Universitaire de Cancérologie-Radiothérapie, Centre Hospitalier Universitaire Albert Michallon, Grenoble, France

Reinhard Thamm Department of Radiation Oncology, University of Ulm, Ulm, Germany

Frank Träber Department of Radiology, University of Bonn, Bonn, Germany

Klaus-Rüdiger Trott Department of Oncology, University College London, London, UK

Nikolaos Tselis Sana Klinikum Offenbach Strahlenklinik, Offenbach, Germany

Nicholas van As The Royal Marsden Hospital, London, UK

Camille Verry Clinique Universitaire de Cancérologie-Radiothérapie, Centre Hospitalier Universitaire Albert Michallon, Grenoble, France

Thomas Wiegel Klinik für Strahlentherapie und Radioonkologie, Universitätsklinikum Ulm, Ulm, Germany

Winfried A. Willinek Department of Radiology, University of Bonn, Bonn, Germany

Nikolaos Zamboglou Sana Klinikum Offenbach Strahlenklinik, Offenbach, Germany

Michael J. Zelefsky Department of Radiation Oncology, Memorial Sloan-Kettering Cancer Center, New York, NY, USA

Frank Zimmermann Department of Radiation Oncology, University Hospital Basel, Basel, Switzerland

Part I

Imaging, Delineation and Immobilization

MR Imaging and MR Spectroscopy in Prostate Cancer

Winfried A. Willinek, Georges Decker, and Frank Träber

Contents

Abstract

Multiparametric MR Imaging with high resolution T2-weighted imaging (HR-T2WI), diffusion weighted imaging (DWI), dynamic contrast enhanced MRI (DCE-MRI), and MR spectroscopy (MRS) plays a crucial role in the assessment, localization, staging, biopsy planning, and therapy monitoring of prostate cancer (PCa) through delivering unmatched soft tissue contrast as well as functional information especially regarding cell density, vascularization, and metabolism. It also helps identifying tumors missed on PSA testing, DRE, and TRUS-guided biopsy. HR-T2WI provides a clear depiction of the prostate zonal anatomy and is indispensable for PCa detection, localization, and accurate tumor staging. DWI adds information about cellular density by quantifying Brownian motion of interstitial water molecules and thereby enabling the differentiation of benign from malignant tissue. DCE-MRI is another functional imaging technique which allows for characterizing pharmacokinetic features reflecting the prostatic vascularization through a series of high temporal resolution T1-weighted images following the administration of contrast medium. In-vivo proton MRS investigates the biochemical constituents of prostate tissue noninvasively. Metabolic alterations caused by cancerous infiltration can be identified as well as metabolic response in the course of radiotherapy. While in the healthy gland citrate provides the predominant signal in MR spectra, strong accumulation of choline compounds indicates PCa, and the choline/citrate ratio may serve as suitable biomarker for malignancy. MRS allows simultaneous acquisition of spatially localized spectra from a multitude of tissue volumes as small as 1 cm^3 or below, with complete prostate coverage.

W.A. Willinek (✉) · G. Decker · F. Träber
Department of Radiology, University of Bonn, Sigmund-Freud-Str. 25, 53105 Bonn, Germany
e-mail: Winfried.Willinek@ukb.uni-bonn.de

H. Geinitz et al. (eds.), *Radiotherapy in Prostate Cancer*, Medical Radiology. Radiation Oncology,
DOI: 10.1007/174_2014_1034,
Published Online: 4 September 2014

1 The Role of Magnetic Resonance Imaging (MRI) in the Diagnosis and Therapy Monitoring of Prostate Cancer (PCa)

The diagnosis of prostate cancer (PCa) is mainly based on prostate-specific antigen (PSA) testing, digital rectal examination (DRE), and transrectal ultrasonography (TRUS) with optional TRUS-guided biopsy. All these tests have relevant limitations. PSA testing has a low specificity because some conditions such as infections or benign prostatic hyperplasia (BPH) can also induce PSA elevation (Romero Otero et al. 2014). Furthermore, some studies suggest that PSA testing does not provide an accurate surrogate measure of cancer cure or treatment efficacy up to the first 4–5 years after radiation therapy (Vicini et al. 2005). DRE only allows the posterior surface of the gland to be palpated and neither offers high specificity nor sensitivity nor is it suitable for therapy monitoring.

In case of a suspicious PSA or DRE result, initially a TRUS-guided sextant biopsy with acquisition of 12 cores minimum is recommended to be performed. Unfortunately, TRUS biopsy is prone to underestimating the prevalence and aggressiveness of the disease: about 35 % of PCas are missed by the first biopsy (Djavan et al. 2001) and the highest Gleason score is missed in about 46 % of cases (Noguchi et al. 2001). This often leads to insufficient diagnoses, inaccurate risk assessments, and ultimately a less-than-optimal therapy. Furthermore, patients with understaged PCa may undergo radical surgery without prognostic benefits.

About 15 % of PCa patients have normal PSA levels, and no tumor is palpable in DRE. Unfortunately, among these clinically silent tumors, about 15.6 % have a Gleason score ranging from 7 to 9 (Thompson et al. 2004). Recent studies reported a sensitivity and specificity by MRI of 84.2 and 66.6% respectively in the detection of clinically low-risk PCa with Gleason scores less than or equal to 6. In contrast, cancers with higher Gleason grades, i.e., clinically significant tumors, had a detection accuracy of about 90 % (Kim et al. 2014) and a negative predictive value of up to 95 % (Arumainayagam et al. 2013). Other research groups found diffusion-weighted imaging (DWI) at 3 Tesla (T) alone detecting significant PCa with a sensitivity and specificity ranging from 89 to 91 % and 77 to 81 %, respectively (Bains et al. 2014). These data enhance the important role of MRI in detecting those PCas that need more radical treatments.

Among imaging modalities, MRI is unmatched regarding the morphologic and functional evaluation of the prostate gland (Delongchamps et al. 2011). Computed tomography (CT) does not provide sufficient tissue contrast discrimination in the prostate. However, it is valuable in the assessment of pelvic lymph nodes and bone metastases, although MRI has been shown to be superior here too (Dotan 2008). A recent study with 922 patients who received prostate multiparametric MRI (mp-MRI) before radical prostatectomy reported a detection accuracy of 91 % for lymph node metastases with a negative prediction value of 94.5 % (Jeong et al. 2013).

MRI can not only help identifying tumors missed on PSA testing, DRE, and TRUS-guided biopsy but also increases biopsy yields if performed before biopsy through prior localization. This holds true especially in the anterior parts of the prostate gland, which are typically only difficult to reach by standard TRUS.

In the perspective of the above-mentioned limitations of PSA, DRE, and TRUS, MRI represents an attractive imaging modality with high spatial resolution and excellent soft tissue contrast. For many PCa patients, MRI is currently the only modality to delineate potentially malignant foci. In consequence, MRI of the prostate is increasingly used for detection and localization of PCa including consecutive radiation therapy and radiation boost planning.

Assessment of radiation therapy effectiveness, tumor recurrence, and therapy monitoring in PCa is still a challenge. Local recurrence of PCa is actually diagnosed by PSA kinetics. Unfortunately, patterns of PSA kinetics cannot conclusively differentiate between local therapy failure and distant metastasis (Roach et al. 2006). DRE is difficult to interpret during and after radiation therapy, due to associated effects such as induced fibrosis. MRI and especially DWI can reflect cellular changes in malignant tissue under radiotherapy (Song et al. 2010). With the recent technical advancements in MRI, preliminary studies showed that DWI plays an important role in detecting PCa recurrence after radiation therapy (Kim et al. 2009). Mp-MRI can also be useful in the planning of radiation therapy by providing important information for determination of the radiation boost and coverage (Chang et al. 2014).

With the increasing availability of 3T MR systems, MRI of PCa has dramatically improved. Most functional techniques in mp-MRI benefit when moving from 1.5 to 3 T (Lagemaat and Scheenen 2014). The intrinsic signal-to-noise gain at 3 T allows for replacement of the endorectal coil by phased-array coils which enhances patient comfort and compliance. In the future, combined MR-PET may add further molecular targets to the multiparametric information that is provided already today. However, published data are still limited, and further studies are necessary to establish the clinical role of hybrid imaging in PCa.

Over all, according to the authors' opinion, state-of-the-art MR imaging is indispensable in the modern, interdisciplinary work-up of PCa prioritizing T2-weighted and diffusion-weighted sequences.

2 Multiparametric MRI (mp-MRI)

The first prostate MRI was performed in the mid-1980s (Steyn and Smith 1984). Ever since then, prostate MRI developed from a promising tool to a mature imaging modality, gathering not only morphological but also functional information. State-of-the-art mp-MRI preferably performed at 3 T nowadays includes T2- and T1-weighted imaging yielding morphological information as well as DWI, dynamic-contrast-enhanced perfusion (DCE-MRI), and MR spectroscopy (MRS) providing primarily functional information (Table 1).

Bowel motion artefacts can be reduced by administering an antiperistaltic agent such as butylscopolaminbromid. Patients should be instructed about the importance of not moving during image acquisition. An endorectal coil (ERC) is not an absolute requirement at either 1.5 T or 3 T anymore, but strongly recommended for imaging at 1.5 T (Beyersdorff et al. 2003). 3 T MRI scanners and the associated higher signal-to-noise ratio (SNR) provide excellent image quality without ERCs, which in turn translates generally in better patient acceptance. Phased-array coils with multiple receiving channels are currently used in standard clinical practice.

2.1 T2-Weighted Imaging

T2-weighted imaging (T2WI) can provide high spatial resolution and clear depiction of the zonal anatomy of the prostate and therefore is indispensable for PCa detection, localization, and accurate tumor staging. Anatomically, the prostate gland has four distinct glandular regions, the peripheral zone, central zone, transition zone, and the anterior fibromuscular zone.

A healthy peripheral zone has homogeneous high signal intensity (SI) on T2-weighted images, as it consists mostly of glandular structures. The central zone has variable amounts of inhomogeneous intermediate SI. Several studies in the late 1980s established that PCa in the peripheral zone is characterized by low T2 SI. This is due to unrestricted growing of cancer cells that do not preserve the glandular structure of the peripheral zone (Bezzi et al. 1988) (Fig. 1).

In the central and transition zone, an irregular low-SI area without capsule resembling an "erased charcoal" or a SI-disrespecting normal glandular structure, the capsule or the urethra is considered malignant. High-grade cancers usually have a lower SI than low-grade cancers (Wang et al. 2008).

Interpretation of T2WI includes the evaluation of all adjacent structures in the male pelvis, especially capsule, seminal vesicles, and posterior bladder wall for extra-prostatic tumor invasion as well as for lymph nodes and bone structures regarding lymphogenic or haematogenic tumor spread.

Table 1 Landmark studies correlating imaging modalities with histopathological results

mp-MRI	Histopathological correlation	References
HR T2	Glandular morphology	Bezzi et al. (1988)
DWI	Gleason score	Turkbey et al. (2011)
DCE-MRI	Neoangiogenesis	Engelbrecht et al. (2003)
MRS	Cell metabolism	Costello and Franklin (1997)

Sensitivity and specificity for T2WI differ among studies, Turkbey et al. found a sensitivity of 42 % and specificity of 83 % across all prostatic regions (Turkbey et al. 2010).

One drawback of T2WI alone is the limited specificity of low-SI areas. Benign abnormalities such as chronic prostatitis, atrophy, scars, postirradiation or antihormonal treatment effects, hyperplasia, and postbiopsy hemorrhage may mimic a low-SI-resembling tumor tissue (Kirkham et al. 2006).

2.2 Diffusion-Weighted Imaging (DWI) and the Apparent Diffusion Coefficient (ADC)

DWI adds important information about cellular density on a tissue level to the morphological information from high-resolution T2WI.

DWI as noninvasive, functional MR technique quantifies the Brownian motion of water molecules within tissue. Thereby, it enables not only qualitative but also quantitative tumor assessment. Reduced water diffusion in PCa has been attributed to increased cellularity through uncontrolled tumor growth with a consecutive reduction of the extracellular space. Therefore, DWI primarily provides an important quantitative biophysical parameter that can be used to differentiate benign from malignant prostatic tissue that shows the typical pattern of high SI on images with high b-values and low SI on the ADC map (Hosseinzadeh and Schwarz 2004) (Fig. 2a, b).

DWI in combination with T2WI is not only clinically relevant for improved tumor detection and characterization, but also increasingly used for therapy monitoring before, during, and after treatment (Chenevert et al. 2002). There is evidence that DWI allows to reflect cellular changes in malignant tissue, especially under radiation (Song et al. 2010).

DWI acquisition parameters should be optimized according to the respective MR imaging system as well as to the magnetic field strength that is implemented. The acquisition of at least two different b-values, which specify the sensitivity

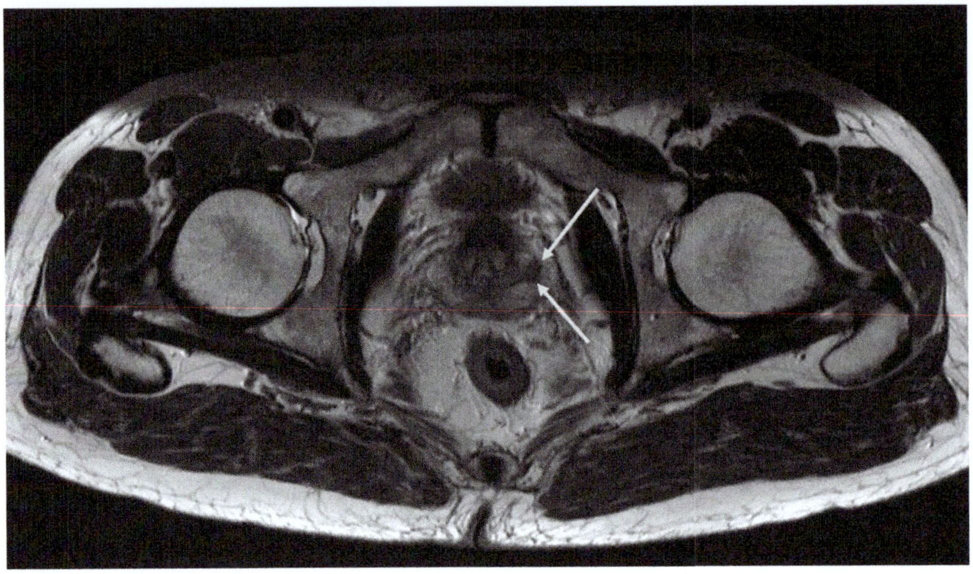

Fig. 1 Axial high resolution T2-weighted TSE showing a PCa lesion in the left peripheral zone (*white arrows*)

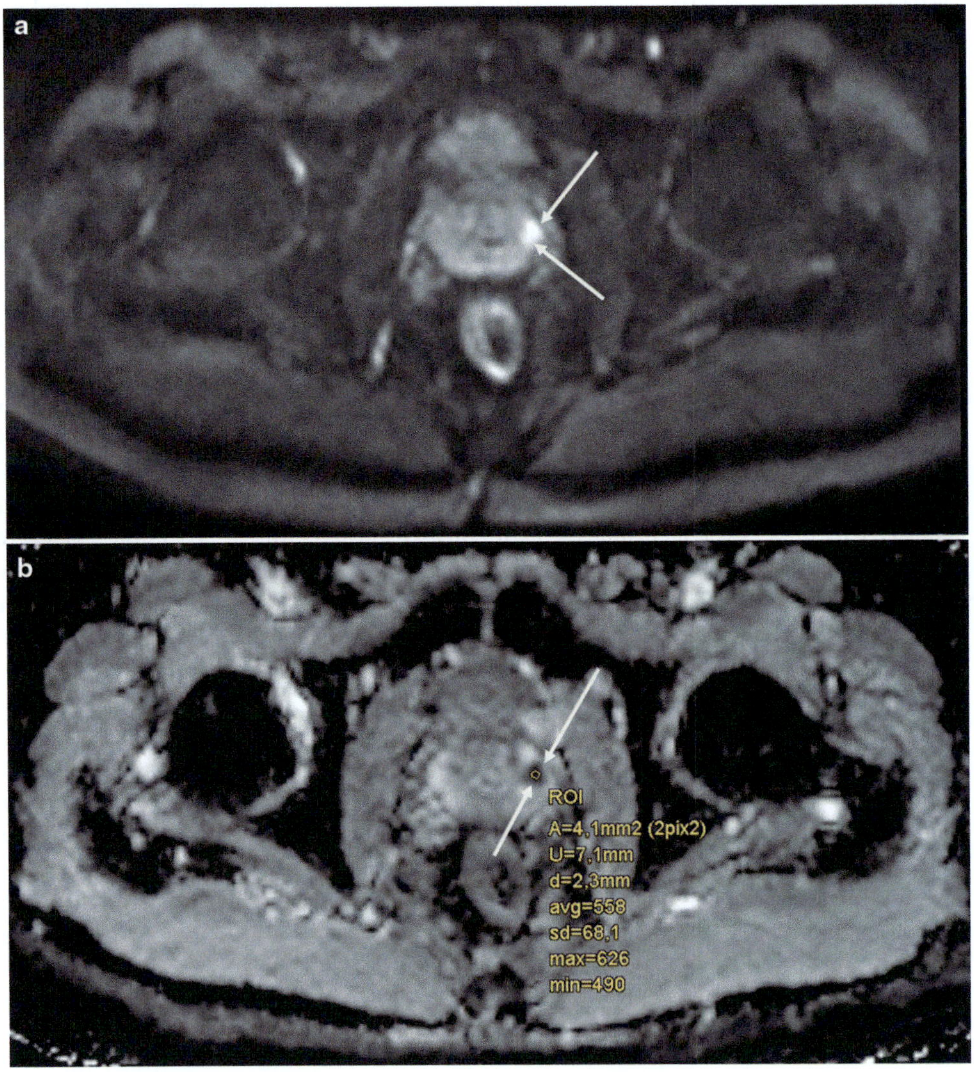

Fig. 2 **a** Axial DWI ($b = 800\ mm^2/s$) highlighting a PCa in the left peripheral zone (*white arrows*) and **b** corresponding axial ADC map

of diffusion weighting, is a prerequisite for the calculation of ADC maps for accurate quantitative analysis. Selection of the appropriate b-values for DWI is crucial because higher b-values increase the sensitivity to detect changes in diffusion, but at the same time impair the signal-to-noise ratio. Benefits of DWI are the relatively short acquisition time and high contrast resolution between tumors and normal tissue that is comparable to positron emission tomography (PET; "PET-like imaging"). A shortcoming of DWI is the vulnerability to susceptibility-induced distortion artefacts due to air/tissue interfaces, for example, at the boundary of the rectal wall.

DWI and the calculated apparent diffusion coefficient (ADC) in particular have initially been used to assess tumor aggressiveness, especially in brain cancers (Sugahara et al. 1999). In the meantime, several groups found out that ADCs obtained from DWI were significantly lower in PCas with higher Gleason scores (Turkbey et al. 2011). This allows for noninvasive assessment of the aggressiveness of PCas that are visible on MR images, which is an important predictor for patient outcome, prognosis, and can also be useful in the planning of radiation therapy.

2.3 Dynamic-Contrast-Enhanced MRI (DCE-MRI, Perfusion Imaging)

DCE-MRI is a functional imaging modality following the intravenous (i.v.) administration of gadolinium-based contrast medium allowing the characterization of pharmacokinetic features reflecting the prostatic vascularization through a series of high temporal resolution axial T1-weighted sequences.

Vascularization and angiogenesis in PCa are mostly induced through the secretion of vascular growth factors in reaction to the presence of local hypoxia or lack of nutrients due to uncontrolled fast growth of malignant cells (Bonekamp and Macura 2008). The resulting changes on a vascular level can be assessed dynamically by DCE-MRI. As the prostate gland is highly vascularized, a simple substraction of images before and after gadolinium administration i.v. is insufficient to properly delineate PCa, and a dynamic imaging series with adequate temporal resolution is required instead to accurately determine the time course of contrast media inflow and washout.

Tumor vessels are generally more permeable and disorganized than normal vessels. Because of the abundance of tumor vessels in PCa and the corresponding vessel walls' vulnerability and permeability, fast contrast arrival and rapid washout are typically observed (Fig. 3a, b). It has been demonstrated that the presence of washout is highly indicative for PCa (Alonzi et al. 2007), even in the absence of low SI in T2WI.

2.4 MR Spectroscopy of Prostate Cancer

2.4.1 ^{1}H-MR Spectrum and Metabolite Signals

While the morphologic and functional properties of normal or neoplastic tissue in the prostate gland can be delineated by MR imaging methods, in vivo proton MR spectroscopy (^{1}H-MRS) and spectroscopic imaging (^{1}H-MRSI) investigate its chemical composition noninvasively and thus yield further insight into prostate metabolism and the metabolic alterations caused by cancerous infiltration. Also, metabolic changes in the course of radiotherapy can be monitored, and the response of PCa to treatment may be assessed by MRS and MRSI. Of the metabolites present in the prostate gland, citrate (Cit), creatine/phosphocreatine (Cr), choline-containing compounds (Cho), and polyamines (PA) have sufficiently high tissue concentrations (above 1 mmol/kg) to be detected by MRS at the magnetic field strengths used for in vivo examinations. Cit is produced by oxidative phosphorylation within the citrate cycle and is extensively stored in healthy prostate tissue mainly in bound form as zinc citrate (Costello et al. 2005). It has a ^{1}H-MRS resonance at 2.65 ppm (chemical shift relative to tetramethylsilane as reference) arising from the non-equivalent methylene protons (CH_2) which are strongly coupled to form two almost overlapping spin doublets. This leads to a characteristic 4-peak spectral pattern at 3 T with two equally high central peaks spaced by 8 Hz and two smaller "outer" satellites each at 16 Hz distance (corresponding to the J coupling constant of Cit) from the central peaks. However, full resolution of all 4 peaks is achieved in vivo only with excellent magnetic field homogeneity, while in many prostate MRS acquisitions at 3 T, the two central constituents appear as a single broadened peak, which is a general issue at the lower field of 1.5 T. Also, the three methyl resonances of Cho, PA, and Cr covering the spectral range of 3.21–3.03 ppm are often not completely resolved, especially at 1.5 T, and therefore, usually the summed intensity (tChoCr) of all peaks in this frequency range is compared to the total area under the citrate components, yielding a metabolite ratio, e.g. called tChoCr/Cit.

Although being itself a complex overlay of several constituents such as glycerol phosphorylcholine (GPC), phosphorylcholine (PC), acetylcholine (ACho), and free choline, the intensity of the Cho peak centered at 3.21 ppm in the proton spectrum of prostate tissue may serve as a biomarker for the detection of malignant disease, just in analogy to the PSA value, with strongly increased Cho level or ratio Cho/Cit being suspicious for PCa (Cornel et al. 1993). As especially the phospholipids GPC and PC are key components released in cell membrane turnover, extensive cell proliferation as it is found in malignant tumors is often accompanied by a characteristic elevation of the choline peak in the ^{1}H-MR spectrum. Simultaneously, the accumulation of

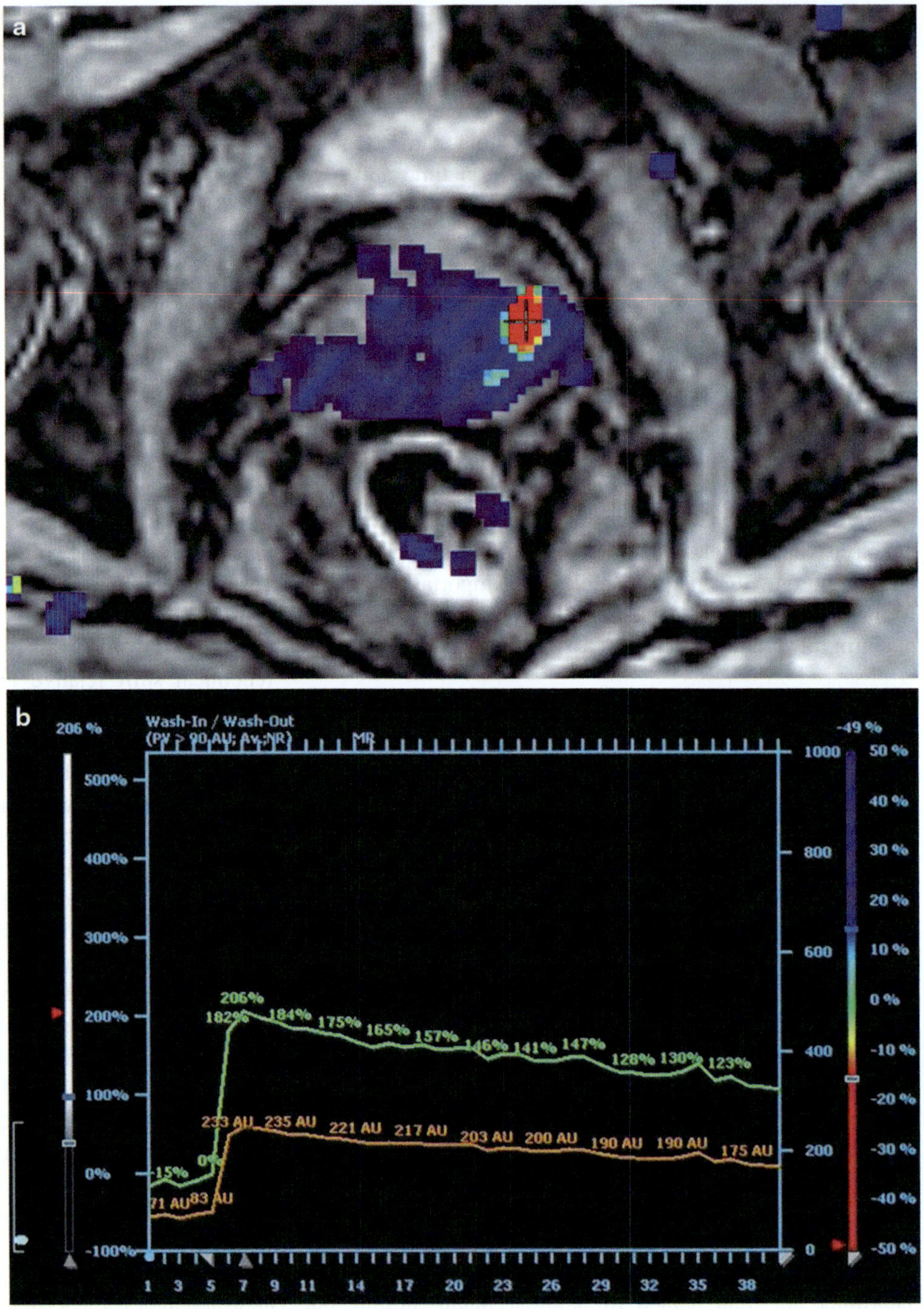

Fig. 3 **a** Axial high temporal resolution DCE-MRI with a PCa lesion in the left peripheral zone (*red spot*). **b** Corresponding enhancement curve with relative (*green curve*) and absolute (*orange curve*) depiction of contrast enhancement arrival and consecutive washout

citrate is inhibited in cancerous prostate tissue, and the MRS intensity of the citrate peaks decreases (Costello and Franklin 1997). Therefore, both effects add up to increase the metabolite ratio Cho/Cit. In contrast, the summed area tChoCr under the Cho, PA, and Cr spectral peaks and its ratio to Cit are less sensitive to indicate PCa, because an elevation in choline levels is at least partly counterbalanced by a reduction of Cr and PA in affected tissue. Nevertheless, in cases or at field strengths with insufficient spectral separation of Cho from the adjacent PA and Cr peaks, the tChoCr/Cit ratio may still serve as a suitable marker to discriminate between benign tissue and PCa, with values <0.8 being considered as normal and tChoCr/Cit >1 as highly suspicious for malignant disease. Correspondingly, a Cho/Cit ratio below 0.5 may indicate benign hyperplasia, while Cho/Cit ratio >0.6 suspects PCa, with borderline assignment for values in between (Crehange et al. 2011). However, such thresholds have to be regarded with care as they may vary depending on the used field strength, the scan parameters (mainly TR and TE) of the MRS acquisition sequence, and the achieved spectral peak resolution. Moreover, the metabolite ratios differ between the prostate zones (with normal Cho/Cit being lower in the peripheral zone), and the cutoff values for discrimination between benign tissue and tumor have to be adjusted to the respective location within the gland.

While ^{1}H-MRS has been shown to be rather specific in the detection of PCa (89–91 % specificity), its sensitivity (75–77 %) is still inferior to other modalities (Manenti et al. 2006). One reason for missing a PCa lesion might be a too small or lacking increase of choline in tumors with only moderate cell proliferation, which is possibly associated with a lower Gleason score. Such a correlation between the Gleason score and the Cho levels in MRS has been found in some, but not in all studies (Zakian et al. 2005; Scheenen et al. 2007; Kobus et al. 2011). Also, PCa with focal size less than 1 cm is prone to be missed by MRS due to its limited spatial resolution, resulting in partial volume averaging with healthy tissue and thus yielding metabolite ratios below the chosen malignancy threshold. On the other hand, false-positive findings may be derived from high Cho signal also occurring in prostatitis, or if an intense narrow spectral peak is observed in MR spectra from the posterior parts in the basal region of the prostate, at the choline frequency of 3.2 ppm. This signal can be assigned to GPC contained in the seminal vesicles, and attention has to be paid not to mistake this "normal" GPC peak from seminal fluid with a pathological elevation of choline levels suspecting prostate cancer in that region.

2.4.2 ^{1}H-MRS Acquisition and Spatial Localization

The achievable spatial resolution for in vivo prostate MRS is one of the major drawbacks of this technique as the size of a tissue volume from which a proton MR spectrum is obtained by far exceeds the spatial dimensions of all other MR imaging methods and of most other imaging modalities. This is a consequence of the more than 10,000-fold lower tissue concentrations of the ^{1}H metabolites of interest (Cho, Cr, Cit) compared to the water protons used in MR imaging. Moreover, the intense spectral peak of water at 4.7 ppm has to be suppressed by suitable prepulses during MRS acquisition (and additionally by filtering algorithms in MRS postprocessing) to allow reliable quantification of the very small metabolite peaks, even when their chemical shift relative to water is quite large. Also, MRS signals from different molecular groups in lipids may overlay and distort the metabolite peaks, particularly of citrate, if the selected MRS volume partially includes fatty tissue. In localized single-volume (SV) ^{1}H-MRS, the metabolite signals are collected from within a brick-shaped tissue volume interactively placed on localizer MR images, which is selected by combining the excitation and refocusing RF pulses with magnetic field gradients for spatial encoding. This volume selection can be performed either with the point-resolved spectroscopy (PRESS) (Bottomley 1987) or the stimulated echo acquisition mode (STEAM) (Frahm et al. 1989) technique. Although the SNR of the metabolite peaks in the acquired MR spectra can strongly be improved by repeating the excitation of the volume of interest (VOI) and accumulating the MRS data ("signal averaging"), this may lead to unacceptably long measurement times if VOI sizes smaller than 2–3 cm^{3} are desired, even at higher magnetic fields with their inherently better SNR. Therefore, in MRS of the prostate, SV techniques are not suited for accurate localization of a tumor within the tissue as the required VOI size would extend over a much too large part of the prostate gland. SV-MRS of prostate cancer might thus only be of interest if the tumor site is already known and the time course of progression or response to therapy is to be investigated in consecutive examinations.

2.4.3 MR Spectroscopic Imaging (MRSI)

By application of the MRSI technique (often also called chemical shift imaging (CSI)), a 2D or 3D grid consisting of a multitude of smaller voxels can be used to collect MR spectra from each of these voxels. To achieve this, similar to the principles of MR imaging, slice selection is performed by gradient switching during RF excitation, and additional phase encoding is applied for in-plane localization. In contrast to the MR imaging of water protons, however, it is not possible to use frequency encoding to acquire a complete row of the image following a single excitation, because the different frequency components of the detected MRS signal are already linked to the spectral information on the metabolites of interest. Therefore, phase encoding for two spatial directions (or even three in 3D-MRSI) has to be used, and as a consequence, $m \times n$ spin excitations spaced by the repetition time TR have to be performed to acquire the desired matrix of $m \times n$ MR spectra from all 2D grid voxels. Fortunately, the SNR in these spectra is not determined by the spin signal only from the corresponding small voxel, but from the total MRSI grid which above all is sampled $m \times n$ times and accumulated. In this way, in-plane voxel sizes around 1 cm^{2} or below can be utilized with sufficient metabolite SNR in 2D-MRSI of the prostate, with typically 10×10–16×16 voxels over a grid extension of 8–12 cm. Because a field of view (FOV) of this size is completely surrounded by body tissue, back-folding of spin signal from outer structures would happen, like in MR imaging with such a small FOV, if only the 2D phase encoding was used for in-plane volume selection. Therefore, additional PRESS or STEAM localization of a VOI smaller than the margins of the phase-encoded FOV but completely covering the prostate gland has to be applied to avoid artificial signal contribution in the spectra of the MRSI voxels, especially from lipids. Suppression of such "outer volume" signals can also be achieved by multiple regional presaturation bars closely

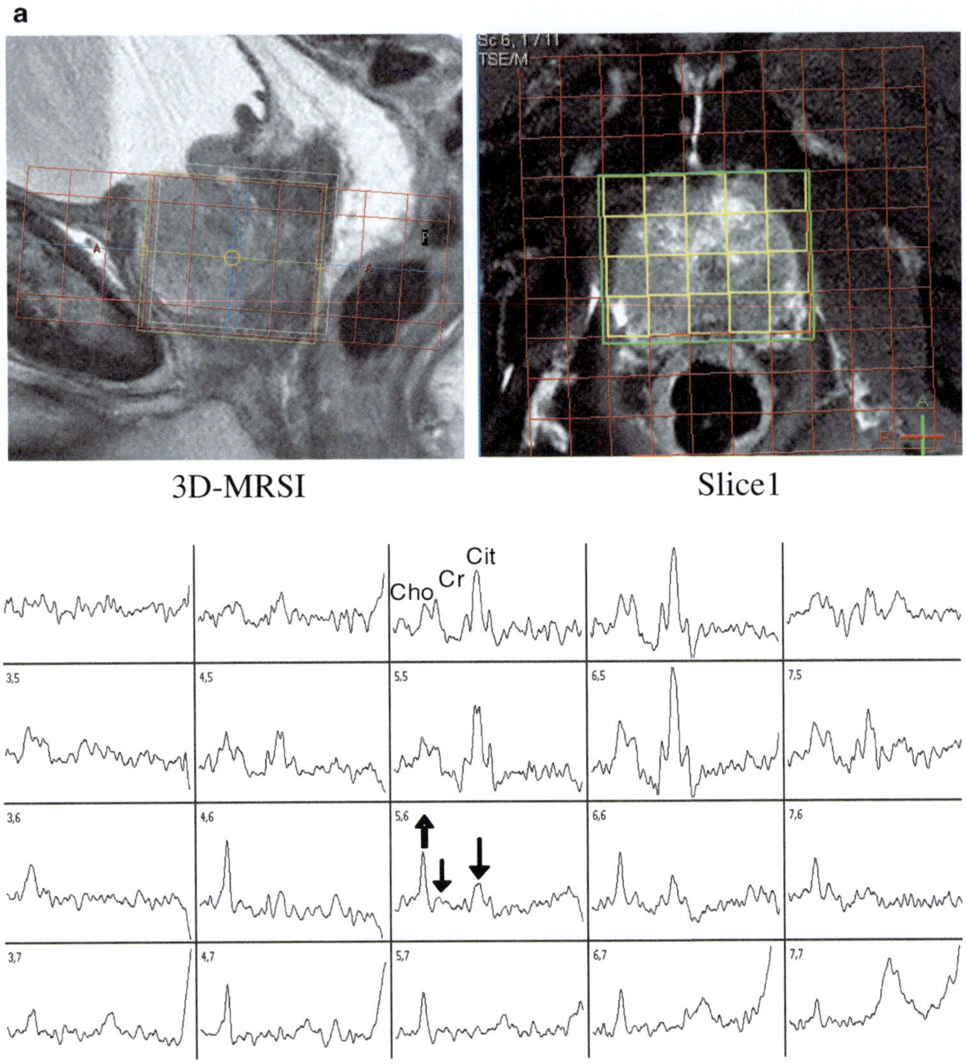

Fig. 4 3D-MRSI (TR/TE 1200/135 ms, acquisition matrix 10 × 10 × 3) of the prostate with external surface coil at 3T in a 74-year-old patient before radiotherapy. Overlay of MRSI grid (*red*) of isotropic 1-cm voxels and PRESS selection volume (*green frame*) on sagittal and transversal T2W MR images, and 2D array of selected MR spectra arranged corresponding to the yellow-framed voxels. **a** Spectra from MRSI slice #1 (at the prostate apex) show normal metabolite levels in the anterior part of the gland and demonstrate prostate cancer focused right posterior, indicated by strongly enlarged choline in association with barely detectable citrate (see up/*down arrows*). **b** Acquired (*red*) and fitted (*blue on green baseline*) spectra from 4 voxels in central MRSI slice (#2) show steep transition from unaffected area (*upper row*) to clearly malignant tissue (*lower row*) in directly adjacent voxels. Vertical scaling of spectra in (**b**) different from (**a**)

adapted to the individual prostate shape. In most cases, the cranio-caudal size of the prostate is too large to be entirely included in a 2D-MRSI acquisition with a slice thickness of 1–2 cm, and a 3D phase encoding scheme with at least three axial slices has to be used then. Fig. 4 shows an example for the image-guided planning of such a 3D-MRSI acquisition (TR/TE 1200/135 ms) with display of the 10 × 10 × 3 voxel grid (red), the PRESS-localized VOI (green frame), and a selection of spectra (yellow-framed voxels) from the peripheral and from the central zone of the prostate within the VOI. In this examination performed before radiotherapy, a high Cho peak and low Cit level indicating extensive tumorous infiltration are present in the spectra from the posterior region of the prostate, with accentuation in the right glandular lobe and apical. Just as the other techniques of multiparametric MR imaging, also MRS and MRSI of the prostate profit from the signal gain achievable by the use of an endorectal RF coil for signal detection, and its application allows to further decrease the minimum voxel size. While at magnetic fields of 2 T or less, the application of ERCs for prostate MRSI is mandatory, at 3 T the inherently higher MR signal and the stronger sensitivity to susceptibility artifacts caused by the endorectal placement might balance out the advantages of such coils. Therefore, also considering the signal increase gained by recent progress in MR detection sensitivity by digital RF chains and coil development, the sole use of external surface coils will at 3 T supply sufficient SNR and spatial resolution for MRSI, combined with more patient comfort.

Corresponding to the cutoff values for the metabolite ratios tChoCr/Cit and Cho/Cit cited before, but on a less stringent scale and thus more considering the dependency of such limits on the location within the prostate gland and on the MRS scan parameters, the new PI-RADS diagnostic grading of prostate lesions has been extended also to assessment by MRS (Barentsz et al. 2012). In the qualitative scoring of MRSI, only the peak heights for Cho and Cit are compared, from PI-RADS 5 corresponding to "Cho>>Cit,

Fig. 4 continued

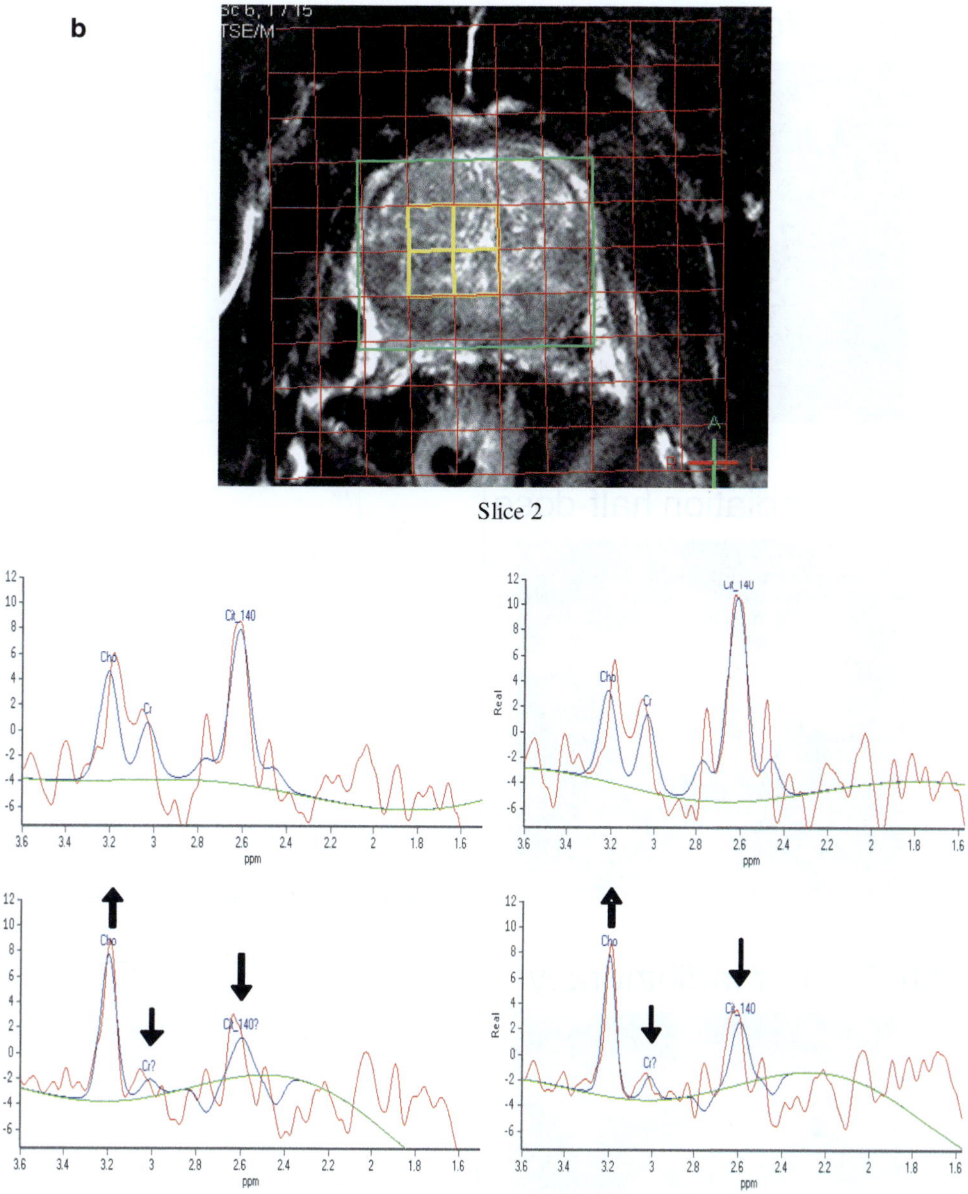

cancer is highly likely to be present" down to PI-RADS 1, assigned when "Cho<<Cit, disease is highly unlikely to be present."

2.4.4 MRSI of the Prostate in Radiotherapy Planning and Follow-Up

While the criteria described above can successfully be applied in the differential diagnosis between malignant disease and benign hyperplasia by MRS and in the localization of tissue with cancerous infiltration to define the target area in radiotherapy planning, a severe problem is encountered when response to therapy or residual/recurrent tumor has to be assessed by MRS in follow-up examinations after or during the course of radiation therapy: The citrate levels in irradiated prostate tissue are strongly decreased due to the metabolic damage induced by the radiation ["metabolic atrophy" (Pickett et al. 2004)], and recovery will not be achieved even years after the end of therapy. Therefore, all metabolite ratios with Cit as denominator will distinctly be elevated almost immediately after the first few radiotherapy fractions even when the tumor responds well and degrades in the course of irradiation. Figure 5 displays the typical alterations of metabolite levels in the course of radiotherapy in a case with prostate cancer located in the left central and peripheral zone, with very low amplitudes of all metabolite signals at therapy cessation demonstrating metabolic atrophy. A similar decline of the citrate levels (and corresponding increase of Cho/Cit and tChoCr/Cit) can also be seen in MRS already before radiotherapy in patients with adjuvant antihormonal therapy (Mueller-Lisse et al. 2007).

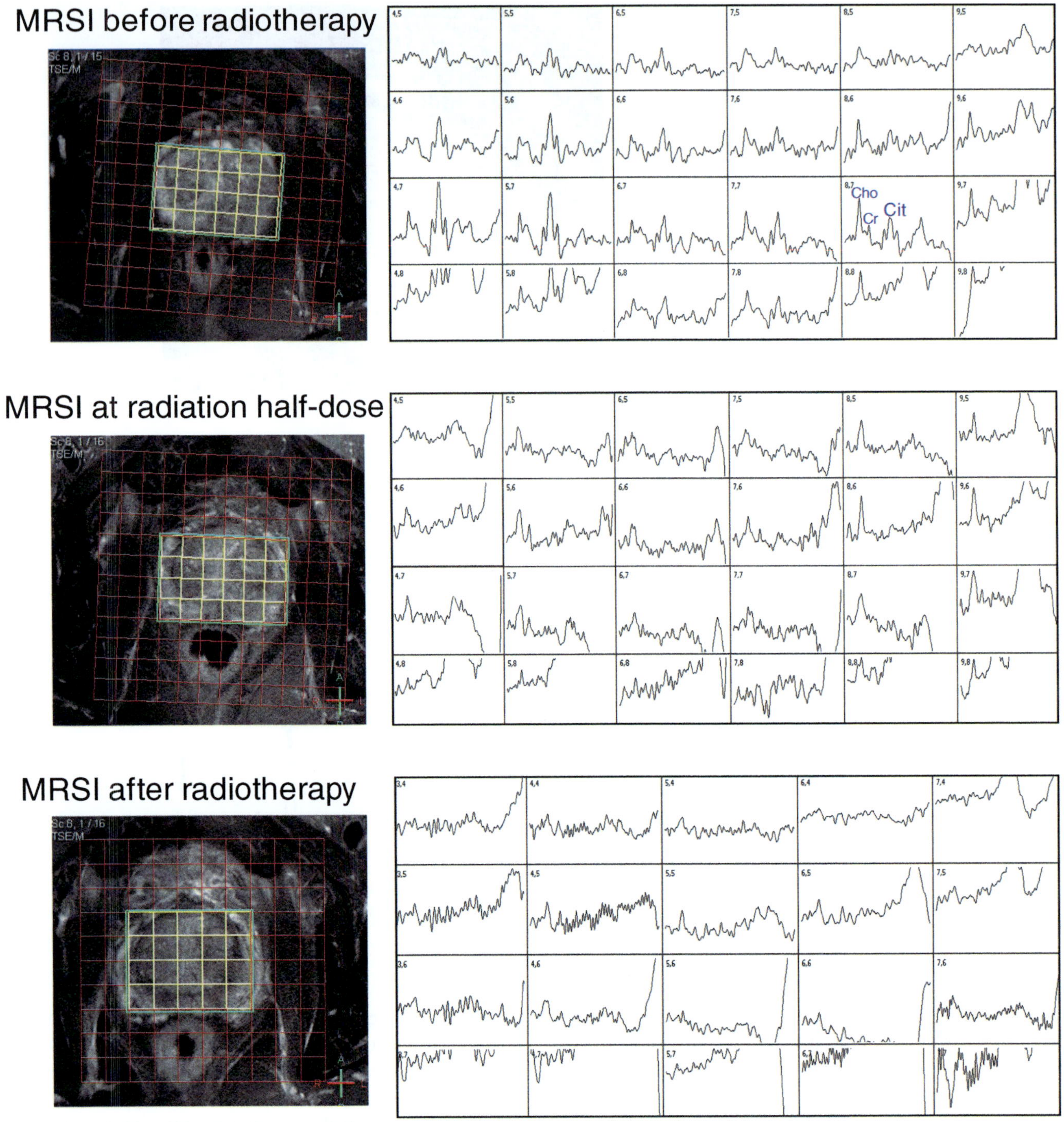

Fig. 5 MRSI at 3 T in the course of radiation therapy of prostate cancer in a 77-year-old patient. Display of MRSI grid and selected voxels within PRESS volume on fat-suppressed TSE and corresponding array of MR spectra acquired before the first therapy session (*upper row*), after reaching half of the total radiation dose (*middle row*) and shortly after the last therapy fraction (*lower row*). Initially, high Cho peak and reduced Cr and Cit signals in almost all spectra from the left glandular lobe indicate the cancerous infiltration. After reaching half of the total dose, citrate is no more detectable anywhere in prostate tissue, but Cho/Cr still remains elevated at the tumor location. In the examination after therapy, only very few MR spectra show metabolite signals above noise level, and this "metabolic atrophy" may be associated with a successful response to radiotherapy

As the ratios Cho/Cr or Cho/(Cr+PA) will not be affected that much by radiation-induced metabolic alterations, strongly increased values or even the mere identification of a distinct Cho peak in certain MRSI voxels may then serve as remaining indicators for tumor residue or recurrence (Westphalen et al. 2010). However, clear cutoff values for these ratios cannot be defined easily, and due to general signal reduction of all metabolites in the course of radiotherapy, an artificial elevation in low-SNR spectra may also be observed. In addition, a final decrease in initially high values for Cho/Cr or Cho/(Cr+PA), indicating metabolic atrophy (and thus a successful response to radiotherapy), may be delayed even for months after therapy cessation. Therefore, in our experience, MR spectroscopy in the radiotherapy of prostate cancer should comprise an MRSI acquisition straight before the beginning of therapy (including antihormonal treatment) to assess tumor location and extension within the gland for a possible definition of target tissue for radiation boosts, and follow-up MRSI not before several months after therapy end to check for focal remaining or newly rising high choline levels. Nevertheless, the relevance of posttherapy choline and citrate levels in irradiated prostate tissue as prognostic factors for relapse-free survival or for tumor recurrence still remains a controversial issue and has to be investigated in further studies.

3 Summary

Multiparametric MR imaging and MR spectroscopy play a pivotal role in the assessment of prostate cancer. Current imaging should include morphology (T2-weighting), diffusion, perfusion, and spectroscopy, preferably at higher field strengths such as 3 T. State-of-the-art imaging allows for tumor detection, local tumor staging, and therapy monitoring. Future studies will provide even more evidence for the value of MR imaging and MR spectroscopy, especially in the context of therapy decision making.

References

Alonzi R, Padhani AR, Allen C (2007) Dynamic contrast enhanced MRI in prostate cancer. Eur J Radiol 63:335–350. doi:10.1016/j.ejrad.2007.06.028

Arumainayagam N, Ahmed HU, Moore CM et al (2013) Multiparametric MR imaging for detection of clinically significant prostate cancer: a validation cohort study with transperineal template prostate mapping as the reference standard. Radiology 268:761–769. doi:10.1148/radiol.13120641

Bains LJ, Studer UE, Froehlich JM et al (2014) Diffusion-weighted magnetic resonance imaging detects significant prostate cancer with a high probability: results of a prospective study with final pathology of prostates with and without cancer as the reference standard. J Urol. doi:10.1016/j.juro.2014.03.039

Barentsz JO, Richenberg J, Clements R et al (2012) ESUR prostate MR guidelines 2012. Eur Radiol 22:746–757. doi:10.1007/s00330-011-2377-y

Beyersdorff D, Darsow U, Stephan C et al (2003) MRI of prostate cancer using three different coil systems: image quality, tumor detection, and staging. RöFo Fortschritte Auf Dem Geb Röntgenstrahlen Nukl 175:799–805. doi:10.1055/s-2003-39929

Bezzi M, Kressel HY, Allen KS et al (1988) Prostatic carcinoma: staging with MR imaging at 1.5 T. Radiology 169:339–346. doi:10.1148/radiology.169.2.3174982

Bonekamp D, Macura KJ (2008) Dynamic contrast-enhanced magnetic resonance imaging in the evaluation of the prostate. Top Magn Reson Imaging TMRI 19:273–284. doi:10.1097/RMR.0b013e3181aacdc2

Bottomley PA (1987) Spatial localization in NMR spectroscopy in vivo. Ann N Y Acad Sci 508:333–348

Chang JH, Lim Joon D, Nguyen BT et al (2014) MRI scans significantly change target coverage decisions in radical radiotherapy for prostate cancer. J Med Imaging Radiat Oncol 58:237–243. doi:10.1111/1754-9485.12107

Chenevert TL, Meyer CR, Moffat BA et al (2002) Diffusion MRI: a new strategy for assessment of cancer therapeutic efficacy. Mol Imaging 1:336–343

Cornel EB, Smits GA, Oosterhof GO et al (1993) Characterization of human prostate cancer, benign prostatic hyperplasia and normal prostate by in vitro 1H and 31P magnetic resonance spectroscopy. J Urol 150:2019–2024

Costello LC, Franklin RB (1997) Citrate metabolism of normal and malignant prostate epithelial cells. Urology 50:3–12. doi:10.1016/S0090-4295(97)00124-6

Costello LC, Franklin RB, Feng P (2005) Mitochondrial function, zinc, and intermediary metabolism relationships in normal prostate and prostate cancer. Mitochondrion 5:143–153. doi:10.1016/j.mito.2005.02.001

Crehange G, Maingon P, Gauthier M et al (2011) Early choline levels from 3-tesla MR spectroscopy after exclusive radiation therapy in patients with clinically localized prostate cancer are predictive of plasmatic levels of PSA at 1 year. Int J Radiat Oncol Biol Phys 81:e407–413. doi:10.1016/j.ijrobp.2011.03.008

Delongchamps NB, Rouanne M, Flam T et al (2011) Multiparametric magnetic resonance imaging for the detection and localization of prostate cancer: combination of T2-weighted, dynamic contrast-enhanced and diffusion-weighted imaging. BJU Int 107:1411–1418. doi:10.1111/j.1464-410X.2010.09808.x

Djavan B, Ravery V, Zlotta A et al (2001) Prospective evaluation of prostate cancer detected on biopsies 1, 2, 3 and 4: when should we stop? J Urol 166:1679–1683

Dotan ZA (2008) Bone imaging in prostate cancer. Nat Clin Pract Urol 5:434–444. doi:10.1038/ncpuro1190

Engelbrecht MR, Huisman HJ, Laheij RJF et al (2003) Discrimination of prostate cancer from normal peripheral zone and central gland tissue by using dynamic contrast-enhanced MR imaging. Radiology 229:248–254. doi:10.1148/radiol.2291020200

Frahm J, Bruhn H, Gyngell ML et al (1989) Localized high-resolution proton NMR spectroscopy using stimulated echoes: initial applications to human brain in vivo. Magn Reson Med Off J Soc Magn Reson Med Soc Magn Reson Med 9:79–93

Hosseinzadeh K, Schwarz SD (2004) Endorectal diffusion-weighted imaging in prostate cancer to differentiate malignant and benign peripheral zone tissue. J Magn Reson Imaging JMRI 20:654–661. doi:10.1002/jmri.20159

Jeong IG, Lim JH, You D et al (2013) Incremental value of magnetic resonance imaging for clinically high risk prostate cancer in 922 radical prostatectomies. J Urol 190:2054–2060. doi:10.1016/j.juro.2013.06.035

Kim CK, Park BK, Lee HM (2009) Prediction of locally recurrent prostate cancer after radiation therapy: Incremental value of 3T diffusion-weighted MRI. J Magn Reson Imaging 29:391–397. doi:10.1002/jmri.21645

Kim JY, Kim SH, Kim YH et al (2014) Low-risk prostate cancer: the accuracy of multiparametric mr imaging for detection. Radiology 130801. doi: 10.1148/radiol.13130801

Kirkham APS, Emberton M, Allen C (2006) How good is MRI at detecting and characterising cancer within the prostate? Eur Urol 50:1163–1174; discussion 1175. doi: 10.1016/j.eururo.2006.06.025

Kobus T, Hambrock T, Hulsbergen-van de Kaa CA et al (2011) In vivo assessment of prostate cancer aggressiveness using magnetic resonance spectroscopic imaging at 3 T with an Endorectal coil. Eur Urol 60:1074–1080. doi:10.1016/j.eururo.2011.03.002

Lagemaat MW, Scheenen TWJ (2014) Role of high-field MR in studies of localized prostate cancer. NMR Biomed 27:67–79. doi:10.1002/nbm.2967

Manenti G, Squillaci E, Carlani M et al (2006) Magnetic resonance imaging of the prostate with spectroscopic imaging using a surface coil initial clinical experience. Radiol Med (Torino) 111:22–32

Mueller-Lisse UG, Swanson MG, Vigneron DB, Kurhanewicz J (2007) Magnetic resonance spectroscopy in patients with locally confined prostate cancer: association of prostatic citrate and metabolic atrophy with time on hormone deprivation therapy, PSA level, and biopsy Gleason score. Eur Radiol 17:371–378. doi:10.1007/s00330-006-0321-3

Noguchi M, Stamey TA, McNeal JE, Yemoto CM (2001) Relationship between systematic biopsies and histological features of 222 radical prostatectomy specimens: lack of prediction of tumor significance for men with nonpalpable prostate cancer. J Urol 166:104–109; discussion 109–110

Pickett B, Ten Haken RK, Kurhanewicz J et al (2004) Time to metabolic atrophy after permanent prostate seed implantation based on magnetic resonance spectroscopic imaging. Int J Radiat Oncol Biol Phys 59:665–673. doi:10.1016/j.ijrobp.2003.11.024

Roach M 3rd, Hanks G, Thames H Jr et al (2006) Defining biochemical failure following radiotherapy with or without hormonal therapy in men with clinically localized prostate cancer: recommendations of the RTOG-ASTRO phoenix consensus conference. Int J Radiat Oncol Biol Phys 65:965–974. doi:10.1016/j.ijrobp.2006.04.029

Romero Otero J, Garcia Gomez B, Campos Juanatey F, Touijer KA (2014) Prostate cancer biomarkers: an update. Urol Oncol. doi:10.1016/j.urolonc.2013.09.017

Scheenen TWJ, Heijmink SWTPJ, Roell SA et al (2007) Three-dimensional proton MR spectroscopy of human prostate at 3 T without Endorectal coil: feasibility. Radiology 245:507–516. doi:10.1148/radiol.2451061444

Song I, Kim CK, Park BK, Park W (2010) Assessment of response to radiotherapy for prostate cancer: value of diffusion-weighted MRI at 3 T. Am J Roentgenol 194:W477–W482. doi:10.2214/AJR.09.3557

Steyn JH, Smith FW (1984) Nuclear magnetic resonance (NMR) imaging of the prostate. Br J Urol 56:679–681

Sugahara T, Korogi Y, Kochi M et al (1999) Usefulness of diffusion-weighted MRI with echo-planar technique in the evaluation of cellularity in gliomas. J Magn Reson Imaging JMRI 9:53–60

Thompson IM, Pauler DK, Goodman PJ et al (2004) Prevalence of prostate cancer among men with a prostate-specific antigen level < or =4.0 ng per milliliter. N Engl J Med 350:2239–2246. doi:10.1056/NEJMoa031918

Turkbey B, Pinto PA, Mani H et al (2010) Prostate cancer: value of multiparametric MR imaging at 3 T for detection-histopathologic correlation. Radiology 255:89–99. doi:10.1148/radiol.09090475

Turkbey B, Shah VP, Pang Y et al (2011) Is apparent diffusion coefficient associated with clinical risk scores for prostate cancers that are visible on 3-T MR images? Radiology 258:488–495

Vicini FA, Vargas C, Abner A et al (2005) Limitations in the use of serum prostate specific antigen levels to monitor patients after treatment for prostate cancer. J Urol 173:1456–1462. doi:10.1097/01.ju.0000157323.55611.23

Wang L, Mazaheri Y, Zhang J et al (2008) Assessment of biologic aggressiveness of prostate cancer: correlation of MR signal intensity with Gleason grade after radical prostatectomy. Radiology 246:168–176. doi:10.1148/radiol.2461070057

Westphalen AC, Coakley FV, Roach M 3rd et al (2010) Locally recurrent prostate cancer after external beam radiation therapy: diagnostic performance of 1.5-T Endorectal MR imaging and MR spectroscopic imaging for detection. Radiology 256:485–492. doi:10.1148/radiol.10092314

Zakian KL, Sircar K, Hricak H et al (2005) Correlation of proton MR spectroscopic imaging with Gleason score based on step-section pathologic analysis after radical prostatectomy. Radiology 234:804–814. doi:10.1148/radiol.2343040363

PET/CT Imaging in Prostate Cancer: Indications and Perspectives for Radiation Therapy

H. C. Rischke and A. L. Grosu

Contents

H. C. Rischke (✉) · A. L. Grosu
Department of Radiation Oncology,
Medical University of Freiburg, Robert Koch Str. 3,
79106 Freiburg, Germany
e-mail: hans.christian.rischke@uniklinik-freiburg.de

H. C. Rischke
Department of Nuclear Medicine,
Medical University of Freiburg, Hugstetter Str. 55,
79106 Freiburg, Germany

Abstract

The goal of prostate cancer therapy is to administer risk-adjusted and patient-specific treatment with maximal cancer control and minimal side effects. Modern radiation techniques such as IMRT and IGRT for example enable application of high dose irradiation to the primary/dominant intraprostatic cancer lesions, to a local recurrent nodule after radical prostatectomy, or to the loco-regional lymph node metastases. Such approaches promise to offer significantly improved long term results but require most accurate imaging tools with the ability to reliably detect not only the primary tumor and nodal involvement but more importantly to precisely indicate their location and extent. In addition presence of distant disease should be reliably detected or excluded. In this review we present a detailed overview over numerous PET/CT-studies, with emphasis on choline-PET/CT, that investigated performance of PET/CT in different clinical scenarios, spanning from the initial presentation to PSA recurrent disease. We discuss benefits and limitations of this imaging device in the primary and salvage setting from the radio-oncologists point of view. In the situation of PSA recurrence, there is increasing evidence that in addition to local salvage RT of the prostate fossa after radical prostatectomy, salvage lymph node therapy seems feasible and advantageous for a significant proportion of patients. The accuracy of choline-PET/CT depends on absolute PSA level, PSA kinetics and the investigation depth level (e.g. lesion based vs. region based vs. patient based). Incorporation of metabolic information from Choline PET/CT or other forthcoming PET-tracers with similar or higher accuracy in the process of RT treatment volume definition appears beneficial for both primary and loco-regional recurrence, when lymph node therapy is indicated.

H. Geinitz et al. (eds.), *Radiotherapy in Prostate Cancer*, Medical Radiology. Radiation Oncology,
DOI: 10.1007/174_2014_1007, © Springer-Verlag Berlin Heidelberg 2014
Published Online: 11 May 2014

1 Introduction

Prostate Cancer (PCa) is currently second to lung cancer the leading cause of cancer death in men (Bernard et al. 2010; Strope and Andriole 2010), and is clinically a heterogeneous disease characterized by an overall long natural course in comparison to the other solid tumors, with a wide spectrum of biologic behavior that ranges from indolent to aggressive (Scher and Heller 2000). Though clinical nomograms based on prostate-specific antigen levels, Gleason score at biopsy and clinical stage at presentation have been developed for probability prediction of lymphatic spread, distant metastasis, and local recurrence (Heidenreich et al. 2008); diagnostic imaging modalities nowadays play an important clinical role in the management of PCa. Due to its biologically and clinically heterogeneous course and appearance evaluation and interpretation of imaging modalities is challenging.

PET/CT has been extensively explored to evaluate the extent of tumor spread both in the primary situation at initial diagnosis and in the state of biochemical recurrence to enable individual therapy concepts, and to assess treatment response (Kelloff et al. 2009).

Different radiotracers have been studied, such as carbon 11 (11C) and fluorine 18 (18F) labeled choline, acetate, and 18F-fluorodeoxyglucose, 18F-fluoro-5-alpha-dihydrotestosterone (18F-FDHT), 11C-methionine and others (Nunez et al. 2002; Albrecht et al. 2007; Dehdashti et al. 2005; Kotzerke et al. 2000; Larson et al. 2004; Toth et al. 2005). To reflect the use of radiopharmaceuticals from the clinicians view only those tracers that have already been evaluated in several clinical studies; and that are widely accepted and in clinical use are discussed in this chapter. 18F and 11C-choline are currently the most used tracer in this respect. Although several studies have evaluated 11C-acetate, 18F-fluorodeoxyglucose, and 18F-fluoride in PCa with interesting and promising results, their potential clinical benefit compared to labeled choline has not been entirely clarified in certain clinical settings. To elucidate the potential value of those tracers they are discussed additionally.

18F-labeled radiotracers, such as 18F-methylcholine or 18F-ethylcholine have a longer half-life than 11C-labeled radiotracers (110 min vs. 19 min). Despite the advantages of image properties of 11C-choline, the short half-life limits utility in the clinical situation as it must be prepared for each imaging study and cannot be transported off-site. 18F-choline can be used in institutions without an on-site cyclotron department and based on physicochemical properties; the short positron range of 18F results in higher spatial resolution and consecutively in better image quality (Bauman et al. 2012). Therefore, it is increasingly used in many institutions in Europe.

2 Radiotracers

2.1 11C-Choline, 18F-Choline

Choline is a quaternary ammonium compound used for phospholipid synthesis in cell membranes and transmembrane signaling (Lawrentschuk et al. 2006). Choline is incorporated into cells via the adenosine-triphosphate (ATP)-dependent choline transporter present in the cell membrane and then phosphorylated to phosphocholine by the choline kinase. Major mechanisms of phosphor-choline accumulation in tumor-cells are the malignancy-induced upregulation of choline kinase including enhanced choline transport, subsequent choline kinase-mediated phosphorylation, and activation of phosphatidylcholine-specific phospholipases (Iorio et al. 2010). Choline is an essential part of cell membrane phospholipids and therefore labeled choline derivates are "trapped" in the form of phosphatidylcholine (lecithin) in the tumor cell membrane (Pieterman et al. 2002; Jadvar 2011). The uptake of choline in tumor-tissue has been shown to be related to the rate of tumor cell proliferation (Bouchelouche et al. 2010). Biodistribution of 11C-choline and 18F-fluorcholine/18F-fluorethylcholine is different. 18F-choline has a longer half-life, but it is characterized by urinary excretion, that is negligible in 11C-choline, and therefore PET/CT-imaging with 18F-choline may interfere in pelvic imaging caused by high tracer accumulation in the bladder (Turkbey et al. 2009; Bouchelouche and Capala 2010). However, normal biodistribution of 18F/11C-choline demonstrates relatively high accumulation in the pancreas, liver, kidneys, and salivary glands, and variable uptake in the bowel (Fig. 1). Before presenting an overview of PET/CT technique and the available studies investigating the value of 11C/18F-choline PET/CT, we briefly discuss the other above-mentioned tracers and their potential.

2.2 11C-Acetate

Acetate is absorbed by cells and converted into acetyl-CoA. In this form, it can be involved into two different metabolic pathways: either anabolic or catabolic. Anabolic means that it can be used to synthesize cholesterol and fatty acids, thus forming cell membrane elements. Catabolic means that it can be oxidized in mitochondria by tricarboxylic acid cycle to CO_2 and H_2O, thus producing energy. Liu (2006) suggested that fatty acid metabolism, more than glycolysis, may be increased in PCa cells. Preclinical studies suggest an extensive involvement of the fatty acids synthesis pathway in acetate uptake in PCa and the upregulation of the key enzyme fatty acid synthase may play a role in genesis of prostate carcinomas (Vavere et al. 2008; Pflug et al. 2003).

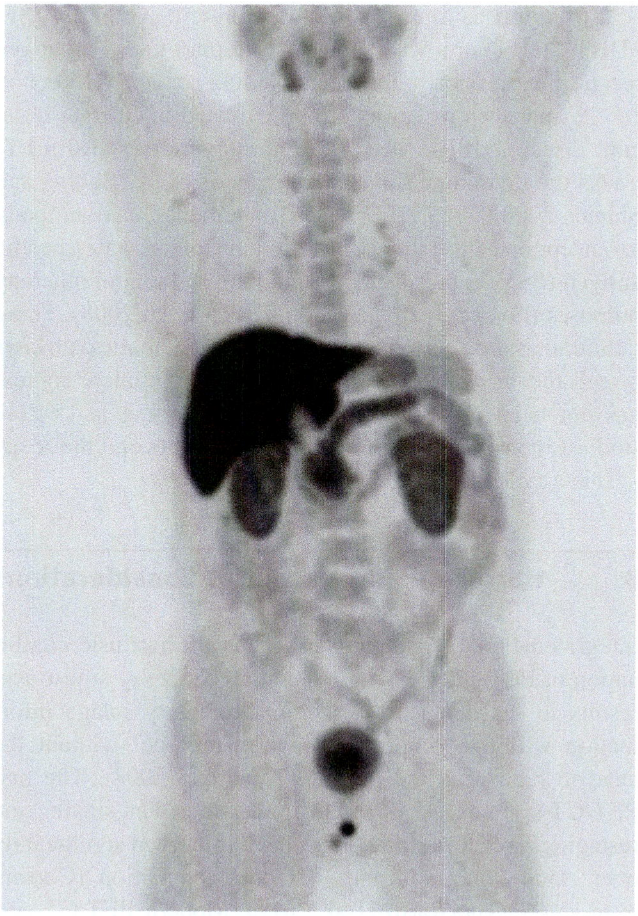

Fig. 1 Normal distribution of 18F-choline

Normal biodistribution of 11C-acetate demonstrates high accumulation in the pancreas, variable uptake in the liver and bowel, and some renal uptake, with little urinary excretion. Therefore, the elimination of 11C-acetate does not interfere with pelvic imaging (Seltzer et al. 2004; Fricke et al. 2003). In general, the biodistribution of 11C-acetate is very similar to 11C-choline. 11C-acetate, as well as the other below-discussed tracers, has been investigated for intra-prostatic primary tumor detection and staging as well as for re-staging of PCa in case of biochemical relapse. As with radiolabeled choline, the use of 11C-acetate for accurate detection of intra-prostatic cancer and the differentiation between cancer and normal prostatic tissue or benign hyperplasia is not feasible (Kato et al. 2002; Castellucci and Jadvar 2012). Kotzerke et al. (2002) found no significant difference between the use of 11C-acetate and 11C-choline in the detection of local recurrence after radical prostatectomy (RP), and Vees et al. (2007) found no significant difference between the detection rate of 11C-acetate and 18F-choline PET/CT. In summary, both 11C-acetate and 11C-choline appear to be equally useful in imaging PCa in individual patients, although more comparative data are eligible. In the era of 18F-choline with its advantage of a relatively long half-life, the potential of being used in centers without on-site cyclotron and at least being commercially available, it remains unclear if these studies will be performed ever. Recently, acetate labeled with a longer lived positron emitter, such as 18F, has been preliminary explored in preclinical studies (Ponde et al. 2007). But 18F-fluoroacetate is not a functional analog of 11C-acetate in normal physiology as it demonstrated prolonged blood retention, rapid clearance from liver, excretion in bile and urine, and high bone uptake due to defluorination (Lindhe et al. 2009). Its potential clinical use in PCa remains to be determined.

2.3 18F-Fluorodeoxyglucose (FDG)

Elevated glucose metabolism in malignant tissue in comparison with the normal tissue is based on increased expression of cellular membrane glucose transporters (Glut-1) and enhanced hexokinase II enzymatic activity in tumors (Gillies et al. 2008; Macheda et al. 2005; Smith 2000). PET-imaging with 18F-FDG, an analog of glucose, tracks the glucose metabolism of tissues. The integral role of FDG PET in oncology has been proven for many different tumors in different clinical situations. However, determination of the exact utility of FDG PET in PCa has not been defined so far and is still evolving (Jadvar 2011). FDG PET/CT showed a sensitivity of 80 % and a positive predictive value of 87 % for detection of prostate tumors with a Gleason score of 7 and greater in men who present with more than an intermediate risk of PCa based on elevated serum PSA level (Minamimoto et al. 2011). It appears that FDG PET may reflect the prostate tumor biology with more accumulation in more aggressive lesions that in less aggressive or indolent lesions (Castellucci and Jadvar 2012). 18F-FDG accumulation may overlap in normal prostate tissue, benign prostatic hyperplasia, and PCa tissues significantly, all of which often coexist (Salminen et al. 2002) and false-positive results may occur with prostatitis (Kao et al. 2008). 18F-FDG PET was less sensitive than 99m Tc-based bone scintigraphy at identifying bone metastases (Shreve et al. 1996). Compared to other tracers 18F-FDG PET/CT seems neither suitable in the diagnosis or loco-regional staging of clinically organ-confined disease nor in the detection of locally recurrent disease because of the relatively similar uptake of 18F-FDG by the post-therapy changes and malignant lesions and because of the high level of excreted radiotracer in the urinary bladder that may mask any lesions in adjacent tissues (Liu et al. 2001). FDG PET/CT may be particularly useful in men with advanced PCa (Fox et al. 2011) as it may distinguish metabolically active osseous lesions from metabolically dormant lesions (Morris et al. 2002). Other studies have also shown a potential prognostic utility for FDG PET with generally higher tumor standardized uptake values (SUV) indicating poorer prognosis than those with lower SUVs, which is similar to the general experience with the other cancer types (Oyama et al. 2002; Meirelles et al. 2010). In summary, although FDG PET/CT is generally limited in the diagnosis and staging of clinically organ-confined disease, it may be able to reflect tumor aggressiveness, potentially detect disease sites in a fraction of men with high serum PSA level at the time of biochemical failure, and be useful in the objective assessment of response to chemotherapy or anti-androgen therapy, and in prognostication (Castellucci and Jadvar 2012).

2.4 18F-Fluoride

18F-Fluoride diffuses through bone capillaries into the bone extracellular fluid. Its plasma clearance is very rapid and its single-passage extraction efficiency is high. The fast blood clearance of 18F-fluoride provides an optimal target to background ratio. 18F-fluoride ions exchange with hydroxyl groups in the hydroxyapatite, at the surface of bone crystals, being particularly active at sites of bone remodeling with high turnover. Therefore, 18F-fluoride uptake represents osteoblastic activity in the neighborhood of osteoblastic, lytic, or marrow-based bone metastases (Jana and Blaufox 2006; Even-Sapir et al. 2007). Recent studies have shown good diagnostic performance of 18F-fluoride, resulting in a sensitivity of 89 % with a specificity of 91 %, but compared to 18F-choline there was no advantage; thus, the specificity of 96 % of 18F-choline was significantly higher with the same sensitivity (Langsteger et al. 2011). Also in the recurrence situation, 18F-fluoride was useful in the detection of occult metastases (Jadvar et al. 2012). Although 18F-fluoride-PET is widely considered superior to classical bone scintigraphy, no prospective studies have yet demonstrated an incremental benefit in staging or patient management. Further experience with 18F-PET/CT is required before it may replace conventional single photon bone scans, which are less expensive and more widely available (Bauman et al. 2012).

2.5 Other Tracers

Other tracers have been or are under current investigation. F18-FACBC (anti-1-amino-3-18F-fluorocyclobutane-1-carboxylic acid) is a synthetic l-leucine analog (Fox et al. 2012) and 11C-methionine is a radiolabeled amino acid. As an essential amino acid, L-methionine plays a central role in the altered metabolism of cancer cells, and the latter has been also studied extensively for brain tumor imaging (Grosu et al. 2005a, b, 2006, 2011); both tracers reflect increasing amino acid transport as a precondition for protein synthesis. 18F-FDHT (18F-fluoro-5α-dihydrotestosterone) tracks androgen receptor expression and reflects binding capacity (Liu et al. 1992); androgen receptors are upregulated in castrate resistant disease. 18F-3′-deoxy-3′-fluorothymidine (18F-FLT) tracks the thymidine salvage pathway of DNA (Bading and Shields 2008). Zr89-DFO-huJ591 is a monoclonal antibody to an epitope on extracellular domain of prostate-specific antigen (PSMA) promising for imaging and immunotherapy purposes (Fox et al. 2012; Pandit-Taskar et al. 2008). These radiotracers are able to visualize specific metabolic pathways or cell receptors. However, their use in the clinical context has not been clarified, thus requiring ongoing and future studies; their potential clinical benefit lies beyond the scope of this article.

3 Hardware and Technical Considerations

Integrated PET/CT imaging based on the intrinsic combination of PET and CT within a combined gantry adjustment results in the acquisition of complementary image information within a single examination protocol without the need to reposition the patient (Townsend 2008). The first PET/CT systems started in 2001, and since then staging and restaging of cancer patients has been improved significantly over stand-alone CT- and PET-data acquisition (Czernin et al. 2007; Thorwarth et al. 2012). Modern PET/CT systems for clinical use combine a whole-body, full ring PET and a multi-slice CT (Thorwarth et al. 2012; Lonsdale and Beyer 2010). Scintillation detectors (typically lutetium oxyorthosilicate (LSO)- or lutetium yttrium oxyorthosilicate (LYSO)-based detectors) are circularly arranged and provide a transverse field-of-view of 60–70 cm with measured isotropic image resolution of around 5 mm, but lesion detectability in PET is not only defined by the spatial resolution of the system, but also by lesion contrast. Thus, lesions that are smaller than the image resolution can still be detected in PET if the contrast between lesion and surrounding tissue is sufficiently high (Thorwarth et al. 2012).

The injected dose depends on the type of radiotracer and is usually in the range of about 3–5 MBq/kg. The uptake phase, the time span after tracer-injection, when the acquisition of the PET-data starts depends on the kind of tracer and on its half-life. Uptake times of 2–120 min are reported in literature (Bauman et al. 2012). For example, delayed imaging after injection of 18F-choline may improve the performance of 18F-choline PET for localizing malignant areas of the prostate, because studies have shown on dual-phase PET of the prostate, areas of malignancy consistently demonstrated stable or increasing 18F-fluorocholine uptake, whereas most areas containing benign tissue demonstrated

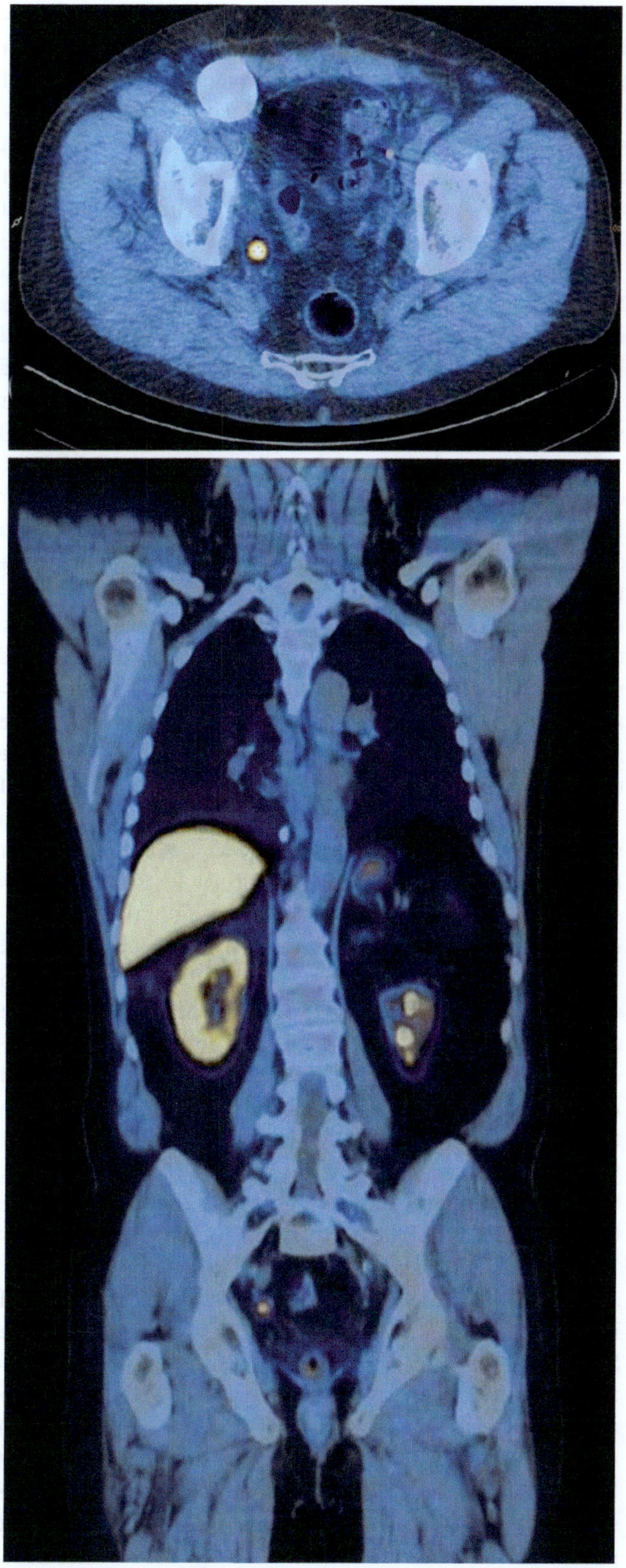

Fig. 2 Patient with isolated lymphnode metastasis in the *right* obturator fossa. PSA level at the time of imaging was 1.18 ng/ml. 26 months before this finding the patient has had already a solitary lymphnode metastasis detected by 18F-choline PET/CT in the *left* obturator fossa, which was consecutively resected and irradiated. PSA level remained <0.2 ng/ml for 12 months after surgery and salvage radiotherapy of pelvic lymphatics, but then slowly increased to 1.18 ng/ml. Because salvage lymphadenectomy and adjuvant radiotherapy was well tolerated 26 months ago with no acute or chronic toxicity, a second salvage lymphadenectomy is considered. At initial diagnosis in 11/2006 this patient presented with a high risk PCa pT3a, pN1 (2/15), cM0, R1, G3, Gleason Score 9 (5 + 4), initial PSA 16 ng/ml. After radical prostatectomy adjuvant irradiation of the prostate fossa (70 Gy) and adjacent lymphatics (45 Gy) was performed until 03/2007. Additionally adjuvant antiandrogen therapy with bicalutamide 150 mg/die was given for 12 months

decreasing uptake (Wurschmidt et al. 2011; Kwee et al. 2006). PET imaging times for a single axial bed position (15–22 cm) are in the range between 1–4 min, resulting in a total emission imaging time for a whole body scan to about 20 min (Thorwarth et al. 2012).

A standard PET/CT examination for whole-body staging contains a CT acquired either for the purpose of attenuation correction (low-dose CT with possibility of anatomical correlation) or acquired for the purpose of full diagnostic information (full dose CT with oral and intravenous contrast-enhancement) followed in any case by a multi-step PET emission scan. It is also possible to acquire both (low dose and full dose multi-phase contrast enhanced CT). Studies have shown that contrast enhanced CT images can also be used for attenuation correction (Thorwarth et al. 2012; Beyer et al. 2004). PET/CT image quality and characteristics depend on the type of examination-protocol, such as patient preparation, administered amount of radiotracer in relation to scan duration, and on the characteristics of the overall system sensitivity, reconstruction method, and settings (Boellaard et al. 2004, 2009). With the new of time-of-flight (TOF) technology and resolution recovery during reconstruction, image quality has been enhanced and consequently the diagnostic quality of the PET images has been improved (Lonsdale and Beyer 2010; Rapisarda et al. 2010; Hoetjes et al. 2010). Consistent and standardized procedures are essential for the expanded use of PET/CT as has been proposed for FDG-PET/CT by the EANM (Boellaard et al. 2010) and are at least desirable for other tracers used in clinical routine. As with the rigorous protocol harmonization efforts by the EANM, every PET/CT center is obliged to ensure high quality assurance to enable best sensitivity and specificity for tumor staging.

4 PET/CT-Imaging of PCa in the primary situation

4.1 Determining T-Stage

PET and PET/CT with 11C- or 18F-labeled choline derivates have been used for detection and determination of local tumor spread at primary PCa diagnosis. Some studies with selected patient groups demonstrated relatively high sensitivities for the detection of primary PCas (Reske et al. 2006; Martorana et al. 2006). Other studies reported lower detection rates. Due to the inability of labeled choline to reliably distinguish between PCa, normal tissue, benign prostatic hypertrophy, or high grade neoplasia, studies showed a high incidence of false-positive findings with consecutively lowered specificity (Farsad et al. 2005; Scher et al. 2007; Giovacchini et al. 2008).

4.1.1 11C-Choline

Studies evaluating visualization of primary prostate carcinomas with 11C-choline PET showed considerable overlap of benign, hyperplastic prostate changes, and PCa (de Jong et al. 2002; Sutinen et al. 2004). Farsad et al. examined the usefulness of 11C-choline PET/CT for primary imaging of PCa by correlating imaging findings and histopathologic sextant analysis of axial step sections in 36 patients. All patients underwent RP and pelvic lymph node dissection after 11C-choline PET/CT. A control group consisted of five patients receiving prostatectomy during surgery for bladder cancer. On a sextant basis, histopathology was used to evaluate 11C-choline uptake with respect to PCa, prostatitis, benign prostatic hyperplasia, and high-grade intraepithelial neoplasia (HGPIN). The sensitivity, specificity, accuracy, positive predictive value, and negative predictive value of PET/CT were 66, 81, 71, 87, and 55 %, respectively. In the 5 control subjects, high-grade prostate intraepithelial neoplasm was detected at histologic examination in 16 of 30 sextants. PET/CT showed increased 11C-choline uptake in 5 of 16 sextants. This study demonstrated the feasibility of using 11C-choline PET/CT to identify cancer foci within the prostate. However, 11C-choline PET/CT had a relative high rate of false-negative results on a sextant basis and prostatic disorders other than cancer may accumulate 11C-choline (Farsad et al. 2005). Reske et al. investigated 26 patients with clinical stage T1, T2, or T3 and biopsy-proven prostate carcinoma, who underwent 11C-choline PET/CT with subsequent radical retropubic prostatovesiculectomy, and standardized prostate tissue sampling. Maximal standardized uptake values (SUVmax) of 11C-choline within 36 segments of the prostate were determined. PET/CT results were correlated with histopathologic results, prostate-specific antigen (PSA), Gleason score, and pT stage. The SUVmax of 11C-choline in PCa tissue was 3.5 ± 1.3 (mean ± SD) and significantly higher than that in prostate tissue with benign histopathologic lesions (2.0 ± 0.6; $P < 0.001$ benign histopathology vs. cancer). Visual and quantitative analyses of segmental 11C-choline uptake of each patient unambiguously located PCa in 26 of 26 patients and 25 of 26 patients, respectively. A threshold SUV of 2.65 yielded an area under the receiver-operating-characteristic (ROC) curve of 0.89 ± 0.01 for correctly locating PCa. The maximal 11C-choline SUVmax did not correlate significantly with PSA or Gleason score, but did correlate with T stage (Reske et al. 2006). In 43 patients with known PCa who had received PET/CT before initial biopsy, Martorana et al. assessed sensitivity of PET/CT for localization of nodules 5 mm or greater (those theoretically large enough for visualization) using RP histopathology as the reference standard. PET/CT demonstrated a sensitivity of 83 % for localization of nodular lesions measuring 5 mm or greater. Logistic regression analysis revealed that only size had an influence on sensitivity. For determination of extraprostatic extension sensitivity of PET/CT was low in comparison with MRI (22 vs. 63 %, $P < 0.001$). The authors concluded PET/CT has good sensitivity for intraprostatic localization of primary PCa nodules 5 mm or greater, but PET/CT does not seem to have any role in staging of extraprostatic extension (Martorana et al. 2006). A study exploring the diagnostic value of 11C-choline PET and PET/CT in a group of 58 patients with suspicion of PCa was conducted by Scher et al. 11C-choline PET and PET/CT demonstrated a sensitivity of 86.5 % and a specificity of 61.9 % in the detection of the primary malignancy. Mean SUVmax for primary malignancy was 4.3 ± 1.7 (2.2–9.8). Mean SUVmax for patients without malignancy was 3.3 ± 0.9 (1.4–4.7) ($P = 0.027$). The authors concluded that a differentiation between benign and malignant lesions is possible in the majority of cases when image interpretation is primarily based on qualitative characteristics. SUVmax may serve as guidance, but false positive findings may occur due to an overlap of 11C-choline uptake between benign and malignant processes (Scher et al. 2007). Giovacchini et al. (2008) performed 11C-choline PET/CT in 19 patients comparing post-prostatectomy histopathologic sextant analysis axial step sections and 11C-choline PET/CT imaging. Based on a sextant analysis with a 11C-choline SUVmax cutoff of 2.5 PET/CT showed a sensitivity, specificity, positive predictive value, negative predictive value, and accuracy of 72, 43, 64, 51, and 60 %, respectively. A retrospective study compared the diagnostic performance of MRI, 3-dimensional MR spectroscopy, combined MRI/MR spectroscopy, and 11C-choline PET/CT for intra-prostatic tumor sextant localization, with histology as the standard of reference in 26 men with biopsy-proved PCa. The sensitivity and specificity were 55 and 86 %, respectively, for PET/CT, 54 and 75 %, respectively, for MRI, and 81 and 67 %, respectively, for MR spectroscopy. Therefore, in this study,

11C-choline PET/CT demonstrated a lower sensitivity relative to MR spectroscopy alone or combined with MRI (Testa et al. 2007). Souvatzoglou et al. evaluated the dependency of the sensitivity of 11C-choline PET/CT for detecting and localizing primary PCa on tumor configuration in the histologic specimen in 43 patients who underwent RP. SUVmax values were calculated in each segment and correlated with histopathology. The authors found that small focal tumors (<5 mm) and rind-like tumors were poorly detected on PET, whereas larger and well-defined tumors were detected by PET; additionally, PCa tissue could not be distinguished from benign pathologies in the prostate as PCa-SUVmax was not significantly different from BPH-SUVmax (benign prostate hyperplasia) and prostatitis-SUVmax (Souvatzoglou et al. 2011).

4.1.2 18F-Choline

PET and PET/CT with 18F-labeled choline derivates have been examined for detection of prostate cancer foci and determination of T-stage. Kwee et al. performed studies with 18F-choline at two different time points to evaluate the efficacy of delayed 18F-choline imaging or imaging at two time points for the localization of primary prostate carcinoma (7 and 60 min) in 26 men. Tracer uptake in the prostate on the initial and delayed images was measured on a sextant basis. Prostate biopsy or whole-prostate histologic examination after RP was used to classify a prostate sextant as a dominant malignant region or probable benign region. The mean SUVmax for malignant findings significantly increased from 7.6 to 8.6 between early and delayed acquisition. The mean SUVmax for presumably benign lesions significantly decreased between the initial and the late image (4.8–3.9). The areas under the receiver operating characteristic curves for distinguishing dominant malignant regions from probable benign regions based on initial SUVmax, delayed SUVmax, and retention index were 0.81, 0.92, and 0.93, respectively (Kwee et al. 2006). In a subsequent study of Kwee et al., all 15 patients who underwent PET with 18F-choline prior to RP histopathologic analysis was performed on step-sectioned whole-mounted prostate specimens. The SUVmax corresponding to prostate sextants on PET was measured by region of interest analysis and compared with histopathologic results. Histopathology demonstrated malignant involvement in 61 of 90 prostate sextants. The mean total tumor volume per specimen was 4.9 ml (range 0.01–28.7 ml). Mean SUVmax was 6.0 ± 2.0 in malignant sextants and 3.8 ± 1.4 in benign sextants ($p < 0.0001$). The area under the receiver operating characteristic curve was 0.82 for sextant detection of malignancy based on SUVmax measurement. Tumor diameter directly correlated with sextant SUVmax in malignant sextants ($r = 0.54$, $p < 0.05$). The authors concluded that 18F-choline PET can serve to localize dominant areas of malignancy in patients with PCa. However, PET with 18F-choline may fail to identify sextants with smaller volumes of malignancy (Kwee et al. 2008). The so far largest series, comprising 130 patients has been published by Beheshti et al. In 111/130 patients, RP with extended pelvic lymph node (LN) dissection was performed. Patients were categorized into groups with intermediate ($n = 47$) or high ($n = 83$) risk of extracapsular extension on the basis of their Gleason scores and prostate specific antigen levels. Significant correlation was found between sections with the highest 18F-choline uptake and sextants with maximal tumor infiltration ($r = 0.68$; $P = 0.0001$) on RP specimens (Beheshti et al. 2010).

4.2 N-Staging

4.2.1 11C-Choline

The first study demonstrating that 11C-choline may be useful for identification of metastatic lymphnodes was published by Kotzerke et al. (2000). They described a per patient sensitivity of 50 % and specificity of 90 % in a series of 23 patients with mixed disease stages.

De Jong et al. prospectively examined 67 consecutive patients with histologically proven PCa with 11C-choline PET. The results of PET were compared with the results of histology of the pelvic lymph nodes and with follow-up data. They reported values of 80, 96, and 93 % for per patient sensitivity, specificity, and accuracy (de Jong et al. 2003). Schiavina et al. included 57 patients in a study with proven PCa and an intermediate or high risk for lymph node metastases. Patients underwent 11C-choline PET/CT prior to prostatectomy and extended pelvic lymph node dissection. Fifteen patients (26 %) had lymphnode metastases, and a total of 41 lymphnode metastases were identified. On a patient analysis, sensitivity, specificity, PPV, NPV, and number of correctly recognized cases at PET/CT were 60.0, 97.6, 90.0, 87.2, and 87.7 %, while on node analysis, these numbers were 41.4, 99.8, 94.4, 97.2, and 97.1 %. The mean diameter (in mm) of the metastatic deposit of true-positive LNs was significantly higher than that of false-negative LNs (9.2 vs. 4.2; $p = 0.001$) (Schiavina et al. 2008).

4.2.2 18F-Choline

Several authors reported about the performance of 18F-choline in detecting metastatic lymphnodes. Husarik et al. (2008) found a per patient sensitivity for nodal detection of 33 % among 43 patients. Beheshti et al. demonstrated in a series of 130 patients a better performance of 18F-choline PET/CT for detecting nodal involvement, particularly among lymph node metastases greater than or equal to 5 mm in size. A total of 912 lymphnodes had been sampled in these patients receiving RP because of high risk and intermediate risk PCa. The reported per lesion sensitivity, specificity, positive, and negative predictive values were 66, 96, 82, and 92 %, respectively (Beheshti et al. 2010). Poulsen et al. (2012) reported among 210 men with intermediate- and high risk PCa undergoing lymphadenectomy and RP a per patient sensitivity, specificity, negative predictive value and positive predictive value of 73 %, 88 %, 59 % and 93 %, while the corresponding values for LN-based analyses were 56 %, 94 %, 40 %, and 97 %, respectively. Both Beheshti and Poulsen focused on men with intermediate- and high-risk PCa, which may account for their findings of better performance of 18F-choline PET/CT in assessing nodal disease.

4.3 M-Staging

In patients suffering from advanced PCa beside locoregional lymphnode metastases frequently distant metastases occur. Typically osseous metastases do appear in large percentage in advanced disease stages. But also soft tissue metastases in lung and liver may be found (Tuncel et al. 2008).

4.3.1 11C-Choline

Tuncel et al. studied the performance of 11C-choline in 45 patients with advanced PCa. Overall, 295 lesions were detected: PET alone, 178 lesions; diagnostic CT, 221 lesions; PET/CT (low-dose CT), 272 lesions; PET/CT (diagnostic CT), 295 lesions. Two thirds of the lesions were located in the bone; one third in the prostate, lymph nodes, periprostatic tissue and soft tissue (lung, liver). The use of diagnostic CT did not result in a statistically significant difference with respect to lesion localization certainty and lesion characterization. PET-negative and PET/CT-positive lesions were mostly localized in the bone (78 %, 91/117) as were PET-positive and CT-negative lesions (72 %, 53/74). Of the latter, 91 % (48/53) represented bone marrow and 9 % (5/53) cortical involvement. The authors concluded that 11C-choline PET/CT improved assessment of metastastic disease including skeletal manifestations, while 11C-PET/CT changed disease management in 24 % of these 45 patients (Tuncel et al. 2008).

4.3.2 18F-Choline

In a preoperative series Beheshti et al. (2010) detected 43 bone metastases in 13/130 patients. Early bone marrow infiltration was detected with only 18F-choline PET in two patients. 18F-choline PET/CT led to a change in therapy in 15 % of all patients and 20 % of high-risk patients. Another study from the same group of investigators correlated the uptake of 18F-choline in bone metastases with the morphologic changes on CT in 70 men with PCa. The standard of reference was other imaging and clinical follow-up. The overall sensitivity and specificity of 18F-choline for the detection of bone metastases were 79 and 97 %, respectively. Lytic lesions demonstrated higher metabolism than blastic lesions. The authors identified 3 correlative PET/CT patterns for bone metastases: lesions with 18F-choline uptake only, probably representing bone marrow infiltration without morphologic changes on CT; lesions with both 18F-choline uptake and CT morphologic changes; and lesions with no 18F-choline uptake, but displaying dense sclerosis on CT (Hounsfield units >825), probably indicating non-viable tumor (Beheshti et al. 2009).

18F-choline and 18F-fluoride have been compared in the detection of bone metastases. Reported sensitivity, specificity, and accuracy was 81, 93, and 86 % for 18F-fluoride, and 74, 99, and 85 for 18F-choline, respectively. This study revealed that 18F-choline might be superior for early detection (i.e., bone marrow involvement) of metastatic bone disease and that in patients with 18F-choline–negative suggestive sclerotic lesions, 18F-fluoride can be helpful, with the limitation that 18F-fluoride PET could also be negative in highly dense sclerotic lesions, presumably reflecting treated disease (Beheshti et al. 2008). Therefore, metabolic and morphologic changes of bone metastases are dynamic processes, and combined imaging is best suited to capture the natural course of these changes to allow for management decisions and accurate assessment of treatment response (Jadvar 2011).

5 PET/CT-Imaging of Recurrent PCa

RP and radiotherapy (RT) are the standard treatment options for clinically localized PCa (Lu-Yao and Yao 1997). However, relapses after initial treatment of localized PCa are not uncommon: the reported rates of biochemical relapse after radical prostatectomy (RP) range from 20 to 53 %, most of them (95 %) occurring in the first 5 years (Han et al. 2003). The reported data after 3D conformal radiation therapy are similar (Chism et al. 2004). Salvage RT is the mainstay therapy in the setting of biochemical relapse after RP that offers the potential of cure. An increase in serum PSA is the most accurate and early index for detecting cancer recurrence or residual disease after RP (Polascik et al. 1999). One of commonly used definitions has been PSA $\geq$ 0.2 ng/ml with one subsequent rise. The American Urological Association and the European Association of Urology put forward a guideline that recommended PSA $\geq$ 0.2 ng/ml with a second confirmatory level of >0.2 ng/ml as the definition of PSA relapse (Choo 2010). After radiation treatment, a rising PSA level 2.0 ng/ml above the nadir value is the most reliable indication of persistent or recurrent disease (Heidenreich et al. 2011). Four different recurrence patterns exist: (1) evidence of only local recurrence in the prostatectomy bed or irradiated prostate gland; (2) evidence of only loco-regional metastases in the pelvic lymph nodes (3) distant metastases (most commonly nodal or osseous), and (4) a combination of local and distant recurrence (Sella et al. 2004).

In patients with biochemical relapse, knowing whether the disease is localized in the prostatectomy bed, irradiated prostate gland, respectively or whether metastasis are present is essential for the treatment planning process. Detection of any distant metastasis obviates the need for local salvage treatment with curative intention. This clinical situation requires a method with a high sensitivity and specificity that allows an early detection of disease localization. In the setting of biochemical relapse with rather low PSA levels, conventional radiological tools, such as ultrasound, including transrectal ultrasound in combination with a TRUS-guided biopsy CT and bone scan proved to have only low sensitivities and has therefore no established role in the diagnostic work up in this clinical scenario (Connolly et al. 1996; Deliveliotis et al. 2007; Naya et al. 2005; Saleem et al. 1998; Scattoni et al. 2004; Shekarriz et al. 1999). Modern functional imaging modalities like PET/CT offer excellent additional information to clinical and therapeutic variables and have shown to provide significant impact in patient management and RT-planning that may translate in consecutive improved disease control and survival rates in different tumor entities (Grosu et al. 2006, 2009, 2011; Nestle et al. 2009; Rischke et al. 2012a).

In the situation of biochemical relapse after primary treatment of localized PCa, studies with choline-PET/CT showed promising results to guide management approaches as these imaging modalities can accurately identify the site of recurrence. PET/CT as a whole body examination allows evaluation of local recurrence and distant metastases in a single step. Most of the studies evaluating patients with PSA-recurrence were performed with labeled choline and we focus on both these tracers. Some data were generated using 11C-acetat; however 11C-acetate and 11C-choline appear to be about equally useful in imaging PCa in individual patients (Kotzerke et al. 2003).

5.1 11C-Choline

Many studies using 11C-choline have demonstrated the value of 11C-choline PET or PET/CT in the situation of PSA relapse. For example Picchio et al. compared 11C-choline to FDG for restaging in 100 patients with biochemical recurrence and a mean PSA of 6.6 ng/ml. Areas with pathologic 11C-choline uptake were found in 47 % of patients and in 27 % of patients using FDG-PET. After 1-year follow-up, 80 % of patients who had a negative 11C-choline PET had an unchanged PSA (Picchio et al. 2003). These results also show, that FDG plays virtually no role in the situation of PSA-recurrence. Rinnab et al. examined 50 patients after primary therapy with 11C-choline PET/CT, most of whom were compared to histopathology. The mean (median, range) PSA level in patients with positive PET/CT was 3.62 (2.42, 0.5–13.1) ng/ml, and that in patients with a negative scan was 0.90 (0.95, 0.41–1.40) ng/ml. The sensitivity at a PSA level of <2.5 ng/ml of PET/CT for detecting recurrence was 91 % (95 % confidence interval, 71–99 %) (Rinnab et al. 2007). Reske et al. studied 49 patients who underwent 11C-choline PET/CT after radical prostatectomy, of whom 36 patients had biochemical evidence and histological evaluation of local recurrence. Thirteen patients had PSA <0.3 ng/ml and no evidence of active disease after 1 year follow-up. Mean PSA of 2.0 ng/ml (0.3–12.1) was found in the group of the 36/49 patients with histologically confirmed local recurrence. 11C-choline PET/CT was true positive in 23/33 patients and true negative in 12/13 controls (Reske et al. 2008).

The relationship between serum PSA value and 11C-choline detection rate was first described by Krause et al. They examined 63 patients with biochemical failure after primary therapy (radiation therapy and radical prostatectomy). Within the whole patient group pathologic lesions were seen in 35/63 patients (56 %). Detection rate for PSA values <1 ng/ml was 36 %, 43 % for a PSA-value 1–<2 ng/ml, 62 % for a PSA-value 2–<3 ng/ml, and 73 % for a PSA-value ≥3 ng/ml (Krause et al. 2008). The linear correlation of the 11C-choline detection rate and PSA value was confirmed by Castellucci in a large cohort of 190 patients. In 106/190 patients data were available for calculation of PSA velocity (vel) doubling time (dt). The detection rate was 12, 34, 42, and 70 %, respectively, in patients with PSAvel < 1 ng/ml/year, 1 < PSAvel ≤2 ng/ml/year, 2 < PSAvel ≤ 5 ng/ml/year, and PSAvel >5 ng/ml/year. The 11C-choline PET/CT detection rate was 20, 40, 48, and 60 %, respectively, in patients with PSAdt >6 months, 4 < PSAdt ≤ 6 months, 2 < PSAdt ≤ 4 months, and PSAdt ≤ 2 months. Trigger PSA level and PSA velocity were found to be independent predictive factors for a PET-positive result ($P = 0.002$; $P = 0.04$) and PSAdt was found to be an independent factor only in patients with trigger PSA less than 2 ng/ml ($P = 0.05$) using multivariate analysis (Castellucci et al. 2009).

Another study conducted by Castellucci et al. with 102 patients 11C-choline PET/CT was able to detect recurrent disease in 28 % of the patients with biochemical relapse characterized by low trigger PSA levels (PSA < 1.5 ng/ml). Very interestingly, 11C-choline PET/CT detected distant unexpected metastases in 21 % of the patients. At multivariate statistical analysis only PSA doubling time and nodal status were shown to be significant and independent predictive factors for positive 11C-choline PET/CT. Therefore, 11C-choline could be suggested to be performed early during initial biochemical relapse in patients presenting with fast PSA kinetics (Castellucci et al. 2011).

Giovacchini calculated PSA doubling time retrospectively in 170 patients and demonstrated that the percentage of patients with positive 11C-choline PET/CT was 27 % for PSADT >6 months, 61 % for PSADT between 3 and 6 months, and 81 % for PSADT <3 months. The percentage of patients who displayed pathological 11C-choline uptake in the skeleton significantly increased ($p < 0.05$) from 3 % for PSADT >6 months to 52 % for PSADT <3 months. Interestingly, patients who displayed pathological 11C-choline uptake in the prostatectomy bed were 0 % for PSADT <3 months and 17 % for PSADT >6 months ($p < 0.05$) (Giovacchini et al. 2010). An additional analysis of these 170 patients showed that in patients with a positive 11C-choline PET/CT have a significantly higher PSA-velocity (PSAvel) than inpatients with negative scans. The percentage of patients with a positive 11C-choline PET/CT was 21 % for PSAvel less than 1 ng/ml per year, 56 % for PSAvel between 1 and 2 ng/ml per year, and 76 % for PSAvel more than 2 ng/ml per year (Giovacchini et al. 2012). 11C-choline-PET/CT has been shown to be a valuable diagnostic tool for the detection of lymph-node metastases of recurrent PCa. Scattoni et al. evaluated 63 nodal sites in 25 patients (median PSA: 1.98 ng/ml) histologically and described a lesion-based sensitivity, specificity, positive predictive value, negative predictive value, and accuracy were 64, 90, 86, 72, and 77 %, respectively. They concluded that the low negative predictive value seems to depend on the limited capability of 11C-choline-PET/CT to detect microscopic lesions, but the high positive predictive value, even with low PSA values, provides a basis for further treatment decisions (Scattoni et al. 2007).

5.2 18F-Choline

Very similar to the published results of 11C-choline, the detection rate obtained by using 18F-choline PET/CT is higher among patients with higher PSA level at the time of recurrence, shorter PSA doubling time, or higher initial Gleason grade. Cimitan et al. described positive 18F-choline scans in 54 patients examined for rising PSA post-radical prostatectomy ($n = 58$), primary RT ($n = 21$), or under anti-androgen therapy ($n = 21$). 18F-choline PET/CT were rarely (3/38) positive among patients with PSA <4 ngml/ml and initial Gleason grade $\leq$7, whereas all patients with a PSA >4 ngml/ml and Gleason score >7 had positive scans. In patients with PSA <4 ngml/ml and Gleason score >7, 18F-choline PET/CT was positive in 54 % of patients (Cimitan et al. 2006). Pelosi et al. found that PET/CT detected disease relapse in 43 % of cases (24/56). PET sensitivity was closely related to serum PSA levels, showing values of 20, 44, and 82 % in the PSA ≤ 1, $1 <$ PSA ≤ 5 and PSA >5 ng/ml subgroups, respectively (Pelosi et al. 2008). Husarik et al. (2008) examined 68 patients for re-staging at biochemical recurrence. They found a good sensitivity of 83–87 % when PSA was >4 ng/ml. When PSA was <4 ng/ml sensitivity decreased about 70–75 %. A total of 71 patients with biochemical failure were studied by Casamassima et al. after PCa treatment: prostatectomy ($n = 28$), RT ($n = 15$), or both ($n = 28$). Detection of local, pelvic, and extra-pelvic nodal and bone metastases was found in 55 % of patients. Median PSA velocity was 0.40 ng/ml/year in PET-negative patients and 2.88 ng/ml/year in PET-positive subjects ($P < 0.05$) (Casamassima et al. 2011). In terms of lymphnode recurrence detection similar to Scattoni et al. (2007) the group of Tilki et al. evaluated the accuracy of combined 18F–choline PET/CT in the detection of lymphnode metastases in PCa patients with rising PSA level after radical prostatectomy. The findings of PET/CT were compared with the histologic results. A lesion-based analysis yielded 18F-cholin PET/CT sensitivity, specificity, positive predictive value and negative predictive value of 40, 96, 76, and 83 %, respectively. A site-based analysis yielded sensitivity, specificity, positive predictive value and negative predictive value of 69, 73, 81, and 58 %, respectively (Tilki et al. 2013).

Jilg et al. (2014) investigated 2,122 resected lymph nodes (with 681 lymph nodes bearing metastases) of 72 patients with positive lymph nodes at choline-PET/CT in the situation of PSA-recurrence. The reported sensitivity, specificity, positive and negative predictive values, and accuracy were region based 92 %, 84 %, 93 %, 82.0 % and 89 %, subregion based 81 %, 94 %, 92 %, 84 % and 87 %, and lesion based 57 %, 98 %, 95 %, 83 % and 85 %, respectively. 71 % of the metastases were in lymph nodes with a less than 10 mm short axis diameter and would have been missed when applying current diagnostic CT-criteria.

6 Summary of Data, Recommendations, and Perspectives

6.1 Primary PCa

Although 11C-choline and 18F-choline have a slightly different biodistribution both tracers are considered to provide similar staging information. Variability in the reported study results reflects the heterogeneity among the type of studies and the variability of the examined patients series: e.g., small versus larger patient cohorts ($n \geq 100$), mixture of different primary tumors, primary versus recurrent and metastatic disease status, variability in Gleason scores and PSA levels at the time of scanning. Scanning protocols differed significantly among the studies, particularly in the timing of scan acquisition after tracer injection and the use of PET versus PET/CT-scanners. In addition to variations in scanning techniques, validation of positive and negative findings was either done by correlation with clinical outcomes or consensus gold standards based on clinical and standard imaging (particularly in determining M-stage), by histopathological results or by biopsy cores, respectively (Bauman et al. 2012).

For the local tumor stage, the distinction between intracapsular (T1–T2) and extracapsular disease (T3–T4) is particularly relevant for treatment decisions. But studies that performed lesion-based or sextant based analysis only showed limited sensitivities between 66 and 87 % and moderate specificities between 43 and 86 % accompanied by, for technical reasons, limited spatial resolution (please see references in paragraph 'Determining T-stage'). In general PET/CT with 11C/18F-choline and 11C-acetate should not be clinically recommended to locally stage primary PCa (Picchio et al. 2011a).

Regarding this restricted value in correctly localizing and defining the extent of the primary tumor within the prostate either using 11C- or 18F-choline, the value of using this technique to guide biopsies in patients with elevated PSA and suspicion of PCa (but repeatedly negative biopsies) is doubtful. Furthermore, it remains to be determined if PET/CT can be successfully used for defining dominant intraprostatic lesions for RT purposes. Histopathologic studies revealed that most patients with PCa have at least one or two dominant intraprostatic tumor lesions, although PCa is a typically multifocal disease (Bott et al. 2010; Karavitakis et al. 2011). For patients scheduled for primary radical RT because of local PCa obtaining high doses is crucial to achieve high biochemical control rates. But risk of toxicity, especially in the rectal mucosa inevitably increases too, thus requiring most precise and accurate radiation techniques (Viani et al. 2009). Local PCa recurrence after primary RT usually originates from the origination of the primary tumor or the initial dominant intraprostatic tumor burden (Cellini et al. 2002). Local dose escalation on dominant intraprostatic tumor burden may result in significant improved disease control without increasing normal tissue complication probability (mainly acute and chronic rectal mucositis/proctitis) as has been calculated by Niyazi et al. in a mathematical model based on different assumptions for responsiveness of PCa to irradiation and different sensitivities and specificities of choline PET (or any other appropriate imaging method). The authors estimated that improved tumor control because of focal dose escalation based on choline PET positive regions has to be considered as realistically low, mainly due to the limited sensitivity of choline PET and the limited specificity, lacking the ability to reliably differentiate between cancer and benign prostate lesions (Niyazi et al. 2010). However, recent studies published by Pinkawa et al. demonstrated that dose escalation using intensity-modulated RT for primary PCa based on 18F-choline is feasible and does not lead to significantly increased toxicity (Pinkawa et al. 2012).

Many studies have shown that Magnetic Resonance Imaging (MRI) using anatomic and functional sequences like Magnetic Resonance Spectroscopy (MRS), Dynamic Contrast Enhanced MRI (DCE-MRI) and Diffusion Weighted Imgaging (DWI) results in high accuracies in detecting primary PCa due to excellent spatial resolution with clear depiction of anatomy/pathoanatomy in combination with visualization of functional properties of prostatic lesions. Combination of anatomic and functional sequences at 3 Tesla results in reported sensitivities and specifcities of 80–88 and 96–100 %, respectively (Yakar et al. 2012). When using functional MRI sequences dose escalation to dominant intraprostatic lesion is feasible with low acute toxicities (Fonteyne et al. 2008) and better sparing of the rectal wall (van Lin et al. 2006). Further studies are needed to elucidate the potential benefits of this dose escalation concept, applying the high sensitivities and specificities of 3 Tesla MRI in the model of Niyazi; and this may result in a potential benefit of this dose escalation strategy on dominant intraprostatic lesions (Niyazi et al. 2010).

The knowledge of nodal involvement and distant disease is crucial to plan the most appropriate treatment, tailored to the patient. Currently, pelvic lymphadenectomy is the gold standard to assess the status of pelvic lymph nodes, being final diagnosis defined by histology (Heidenreich et al. 2008). A diagnostic imaging tool to noninvasively explore patients and to detect metastases would be of particular help in clinical management. In this respect choline-PET/CT is attractive, as it offers maximum staging information in a "single" examination. For detection of lymph node metastasis, 11C-and 18F-choline PET/CT specificity has been reported fairly high. However, its **lesion based** sensitivity is not appropriate. Sensitivities and specificities, reported up-to-date, as described above, are in general about 61 and 96 % (Krause et al. 2013). A negative 11C/18F-choline PET/CT study does not rule out the presence of clinically and prognostic relevant micrometastases in loco-regional or distant lymphnodes. However, when positive, PET/CT is useful for patient management and treatment planning (Picchio et al. 2011a).

11C/18F-choline PET/CT may provide to a significant extent clinically relevant results in selected patients with a higher pre-test probability of metastastic disease in lymphnodes and in the skeleton; these are patients with intermediate to high risk constellation based on established parameters (initial PSA, Gleason-score and clinical T-status). We do recommend performing choline-PET/CT-scanning in patients with primary PCa characterized by high risk features or local advanced disease, because studies and our own experience have shown that therapy management will be changed in 15–24% of patients (Beheshti et al. 2010; Tuncel et al. 2008). Prospective studies are desirable to clearly define the clinical advantage compared to classical staging instruments like bone scintigraphy. However, we recommend choline-PET/CT in patients with PCa treated with primary radiation therapy in order to detect positive lymphnodes in the pelvis and to exclude bone metastases. If lymphnodes in the pelvis are positive, we principally discuss the irradiation of the pelvic lymphatics. IMRT of pelvic lymph node regions is based on the consideration that loco-regional lymph node involvement is a different clinical situation and not a surrogate of distant metastastic spread bearing the potential to prolong the progression free survival or maybe even the chance of cure (Morris et al. 2001; Crehange et al. 2012).

6.2 PSA Recurrence

In the situation of PSA recurrence, post radical prostatectomy or post high dose irradiation of the prostate, there is obvious evidence that PET/CT with 11C/18F-choline is clinically indicated for the detection of lymph nodal and bone metastases. Reported values of sensitivity and specificity for lymph nodal and distant metastases detection are ranging between 64 and 98 % and between 90 and 100 %, respectively (Picchio et al. 2011b).

The strength of 11C/18F-choline PET/CT is represented by its high specificity and positive predictive values. Likewise, Picchio et al. concluded we do recommend performing choline PET/CT, when a lymphnode or distant osseous recurrence is suspected. In this situation 11C/18F-choline PET/CT should be performed as the first procedure in restaging PSA relapse patients to provide individualized therapy strategies as described below (Picchio et al. 2011a).

According to the results of Castellucci and Giovacchini, obtained in relatively large patients series (Castellucci et al. 2011; Giovacchini et al. 2010) there is a clear relationship between PET/CT detection rate and both trigger PSA values and PSA kinetics, represented by PSA doubling time and PSA velocity. Although the PSA value of 1 ng/ml has been suggested as a cut off value in clinical practice, (Picchio et al. 2011b) in fact no definitive cut off PSA-value exists, that can be used as general standard recommendation, when a PET/CT-scan should be performed. Individual risk factors such as PSA doubling time and PSA velocity must be considered. On the other hand for detection of local recurrence at low PSA values ($\ll$1 ng/ml) or when residual disease after radical prostatectomy is suspected by elevated PSA values PET/CT may not be useful. The reported sensitivity at PSA $<$ 1 ng/ml was 20 % in the study of Pelosi et al. and 36 % in the study of Krause et al. (2008) and Pelosi et al. (2008). Interestingly even in patients with PSA recurrence and very short PSA doubling times (<3 months) Giovacchini did not find any local recurrent tumor (Giovacchini et al. 2010).

From the radiation oncologists point of view especially patients who have a low likelihood for distant metastasis, a precise imaging method for local staging is desirable. It remains to be determined whether modern PET-scanners (high resolution PET images with 2 × 2 × 2 mm voxel size) and individual designed scanning protocols (e.g. delayed imaging) may improve sensitivity of choline-PET/CT at low PSA-levels. In principle, PET/CT is attractive for RT-planning purposes as this examination can be carried out in RT-position and used for RT-planning. Nevertheless, for salvage-RT-planning purposes a more accurate imaging method that allows coregistration with the RT-planning CT to define directly a gross target volume (GTV) for local dose escalation is desirable. The reason for this need is that the outcome of salvage RT after radical prostatectomy depends on several different variables and the most consistent variable associated with PSA relapse-free outcome has been PSA level prior to salvage RT (Symon et al. 2006; MacDonald et al. 2004). The lower the PSA level is at the time of salvage RT, the better is the treatment outcome of salvage RT. Another variable is the optimal radiation dose required for local control in patients with biochemical relapse. A recently published regression meta-analysis about the outcome of conventional salvage RT (radiation to the whole prostatic fossa) comprised a total of 3,828 patients (Ohri et al. 2012). In this study, Ohri et al. identified increased salvage RT dose and decreased pre-salvage RT PSA level as independent predictors of improved 5-year biochemical free survival. Salvage RT dose was also identified as an independent predictor of both late gastrointestinal and late genitourinary toxicity.

To lower the total dose to the organs at risk (e.g., rectal mucosa, and bladder) and increase dose to macroscopic tumor nodules modern IMRT (Intensity Modulated Radiation Therapy)-RT-planning for dose escalation to macroscopic nodules of recurrent tumor in the fossa prostatica may be appropriate (Rischke et al. 2012b). MRI using endorectal coils has shown to visualize local recurrence in the prostate fossa at low PSA-levels more accurately than any other technique, the reported sensitivities and specificities were 79 and 100%, respectively (Casciani et al. 2008; Sciarra et al. 2008). Using an endorectal coil leads to distortion of local anatomy; thus, these image data sets cannot be fused to planning CT. A recent study investigating DCE-MRI without endorectal coil in the detection of local recurrent PCa after radical prostatectomy using an appropriate DCE-scanning protocol showed a similar sensitivity at a high specificity (Rischke et al. 2012c). Preliminary experience based on this concept of focal dose escalation based on functional imaging showed promising results without increased acute toxicity (Kirste et al. 2011).

Our recommendations are as follows: in case of moderately elevated PSA-levels (e.g. ≤1.0 ng/ml), but rather short PSA-doubling time (<6 months) a pre-salvage RT diagnostic work up with choline-PET/CT should be considered to rule out possible lymphnode or osseous metastasis. If PSA is >1.0 ng/ml, we recommend independently from PSA-kinetics a choline-PET/CT. Though it is obvious that with the current PET/CT-scanner technique these recommendations will not produce positive findings in every patient; it is definitely clear that any detection of distant metastases has a major impact on patient management, e.g., local ablative concept versus palliative concept.

For evaluation of the prostate fossa in the situation of PSA-relapse, whether there is local recurrence or not, we advocate DCE-MRI even at low PSA levels (PSA ≤ 0.5–1 ng/ml) as has been shown, that all patients had positive MRI finding with a PSA >0.54 ng/ml (Rischke et al. 2012c).

6.3 Perspectives in the Situation of Relapse with Locoregional Lymphnode Metastases

PSA relapse may occur not only as local recurrence, but may also represent metastastic disease. The treatment of only local recurrence with salvage RT has been investigated extensively and general recommendations have been given (Mottet et al. 2011).

Choline PET/CT may offer acceptable sensitivity and specificity in the situation of locoregional lymphnode relapse. Especially the finding of high **regional sensitivity** of 92 % in conjunction with high specificity suggests whole lymph node regions as a target in the absence of distant metastases (Jilg et al. 2014). An example for 18F-Choline-PET/CT-scan showing a nodal metastases is given in Fig. 2. It has been discussed, that there may be a different outcome between patients with bone metastases and patients with solitary or few pelvic lymphnode metastases (Briganti et al. 2009). Two recent published studies included a relevant number of patients and evaluated the benefit of extended lymphadenectomy of patients with evidence of nodal metastasis detected and guided by 11C/18F-choline PET/CT (Rigatti et al. 2011; Jilg et al. 2012). Rigatti et al. described a prolonged biochemical free survival and clinical progression free survival at 5-year follow-up in 35 % of patients (n = 72) receiving 11C-choline PET/CT guided surgery. Jilg et al. evaluated the impact of salvage lymph node dissection with adjuvant RT in patients with nodal recurrence of PCa guided by 11C/18F-choline PET/CT. Of 52 patients treated with salvage lymph node dissections, 24 resulted in complete biochemical response followed by 1-year biochemical recurrence-free survival of 71.8 %. Clinical progression-free survival was 25.6 % and cancer specific survival was 77.7 % at 5 years. These results show that 11C/18F-choline guided salvage lymph node dissection is feasible for the treatment of nodal recurrence of PCa and that a specific population has a lasting complete PSA response (Jilg et al. 2012). The rationale of this therapy concept was the consideration that nodal/adjacent lymphatics may not be addressed solely by lymphadenectomy. Therefore further adjuvant salvage RT of involved lymph node regions may eradicate areas for high risk of microscopic disease.

Others used 18F-choline PET for gross-tumor-volume (GTV) definition in 71 patients with limited nodal recurrence after external beam radiation therapy. With stereotactic body radiation therapy, reduction of gastrointestinal toxicity was achieved and the 3-year disease control was 90 % (Casamassima et al. 2011). According to those encouraging results of choline-PET/CT guided salvage therapy in locoregional relapse further randomized studies are needed to investigate whether salvage lymphonodectomy alone, in combination with adjuvant RT or RT alone results in the best clinical and biochemical disease control.

6.4 Therapy Monitoring

PET/CT may offer a new instrument for therapy monitoring and to predict earlier and more precise the outcome of a certain therapy strategy, because conventional imaging modalities like bone scintigraphy or CT may lag behind tumor response. FDG-PET/CT may be useful for monitoring metabolic response in aggressive PCa (Jadvar 2011). The findings in the study of Beheshti et al. (2009) indicated the potential of 18F-choline to detect early metabolic response in patients under antiandrogen therapy. However, further studies regarding therapy monitoring with PET/CT of patients with metastastic disease are essential to elucidate its potential benefit in palliative situations.

6.5 Closing Remarks

The main advantage of PET/CT is its capability to noninvasively detect and localize recurrent disease as well as detect distant metastasis in local advanced/high risk PCa in one single step, with relevant consequences for patient management. Very recently published, highly interesting results of a study on 37 patients with biochemical recurrence of PCa with head to head comparison of the performance of Choline PET/CT vs. 68Ga-PSMA PET/CT showed significant improved detection rates using the 68Ga-PSMA tracer. 68Ga-PSMA showed higher lesion to background contrast than Choline PET/CT and was more sensitive at low PSA levels with detection of small lymph node metastases and bone marrow metastases. PSMA is a cell surface protein that is significantly overexpressed in PCa cells and therefore provides a promising target for PCa-specific imaging and therapy. Another striking aspect is the fact that no cyclotron is required. 68Ga can be extracted from a commercially available 68Ge/68Ga radionuclide generator. In contrast, radiolabelling choline tracers require isotopes produced by a cost-intensive cyclotron (Afshar-Oromieh et al. 2014).

Prospective clinical imaging trials using various PET tracers, rigorously controlled for clinical state, therapy, and well defined clinical endpoints are needed to further establish the optimal role of PET/CT in the management of PCa patients. However, incorporation of metabolic information from Choline PET/CT or other forthcoming tracers with similar or higher accuracy in the process of RT treatment volume definition appears beneficial for both primary and loco-regional recurrence, when lymph node therapy is indicated.

References

Albrecht S et al (2007) (11)C-acetate PET in the early evaluation of prostate cancer recurrence. Eur J Nucl Med Mol Imaging 34(2): 185–196

Bading JR, Shields AF (2008) Imaging of cell proliferation: status and prospects. J Nucl Med 49(2):64S–80S

Bauman G et al (2012) 18F-fluorocholine for prostate cancer imaging: a systematic review of the literature. Prostate Cancer Prostatic Dis 15(1):45–55

Beheshti M et al (2008) Detection of bone metastases in patients with prostate cancer by 18F fluorocholine and 18F fluoride PET-CT: a comparative study. Eur J Nucl Med Mol Imaging 35(10):1766–1774

Beheshti M et al (2009) The use of F-18 choline PET in the assessment of bone metastases in prostate cancer: correlation with morphological changes on CT. Mol Imaging Biol 11(6):446–454

Beheshti M et al (2010) 18F choline PET/CT in the preoperative staging of prostate cancer in patients with intermediate or high risk of extracapsular disease: a prospective study of 130 patients. Radiology 254(3):925–933

Bernard JR Jr et al (2010) Salvage radiotherapy for rising prostate-specific antigen levels after radical prostatectomy for prostate cancer: dose-response analysis. Int J Radiat Oncol Biol Phys 76(3):735–740

Beyer T et al (2004) Acquisition protocol considerations for combined PET/CT imaging. J Nucl Med 45(1):25S–35S

Boellaard R (2009) Standards for PET image acquisition and quantitative data analysis. J Nucl Med 50(1):11S–20S

Boellaard R et al (2004) Effects of noise, image resolution, and ROI definition on the accuracy of standard uptake values: a simulation study. J Nucl Med 45(9):1519–1527

Boellaard R et al (2010) FDG PET and PET/CT: EANM procedure guidelines for tumour PET imaging: version 1.0. Eur J Nucl Med Mol Imaging 37(1):181–200

Bott SR et al (2010) The index lesion and focal therapy: an analysis of the pathological characteristics of prostate cancer. BJU Int 106(11):1607–1611

Bouchelouche K, Capala J (2010) Image and treat1: an individualized approach to urological tumors. Curr Opin Oncol 22(3):274–280

Bouchelouche K et al (2010) Imaging prostate cancer: an update on positron emission tomography and magnetic resonance imaging. Curr Urol Rep 11(3):180–190

Briganti A et al (2009) Two positive nodes represent a significant cut-off value for cancer specific survival in patients with node positive prostate cancer. A new proposal based on a two-institution experience on 703 consecutive N + patients treated with radical prostatectomy, extended pelvic lymph node dissection and adjuvant therapy. Eur Urol 55(2):261–270

Casamassima F et al (2011) Efficacy of eradicative radiotherapy for limited nodal metastases detected with choline PET scan in prostate cancer patients. Tumori 97(1):49–55

Casciani E et al (2008) Endorectal and dynamic contrast-enhanced MRI for detection of local recurrence after radical prostatectomy. AJR Am J Roentgenol 190(5):1187–1192

Castellucci P, Jadvar H (2012) PET/CT in prostate cancer: non-choline radiopharmaceuticals. Q J Nucl Med Mol Imaging 56(4):367–374

Castellucci P et al (2009) Influence of trigger PSA and PSA kinetics on 11C-Choline PET/CT detection rate in patients with biochemical relapse after radical prostatectomy. J Nucl Med 50(9):1394–1400

Castellucci P et al (2011) Is there a role for (1)(1)C-choline PET/CT in the early detection of metastatic disease in surgically treated prostate cancer patients with a mild PSA increase <1.5 ng/ml? Eur J Nucl Med Mol Imaging 38(1):55–63

Cellini N et al (2002) Analysis of intraprostatic failures in patients treated with hormonal therapy and radiotherapy: implications for conformal therapy planning. Int J Radiat Oncol Biol Phys 53(3): 595–599

Chism DB et al (2004) A comparison of the single and double factor high-risk models for risk assignment of prostate cancer treated with 3D conformal radiotherapy. Int J Radiat Oncol Biol Phys 59(2):380–385

Choo R (2010) Salvage radiotherapy for patients with PSA relapse following radical prostatectomy: issues and challenges. Cancer Res Treat 42(1):1–11

Cimitan M et al (2006) [18F]fluorocholine PET/CT imaging for the detection of recurrent prostate cancer at PSA relapse: experience in 100 consecutive patients. Eur J Nucl Med Mol Imaging 33(12): 1387–1398

Connolly JA et al (1996) Local recurrence after radical prostatectomy: characteristics in size, location, and relationship to prostate-specific antigen and surgical margins. Urology 47(2):225–231

Crehange et al (2012) Management of prostate cancer patients with lymph node involvement: a rapidly evolving paradigm. Cancer Treat Rev 38(8):956–967

Czernin J, Allen-Auerbach M, Schelbert HR (2007) Improvements in cancer staging with PET/CT: literature-based evidence as of September 2006. J Nucl Med 48(1):78S–88S

de Jong IJ et al (2002) Visualization of prostate cancer with 11C-choline positron emission tomography. Eur Urol 42(1):18–23

de Jong IJ et al (2003) Preoperative staging of pelvic lymph nodes in prostate cancer by 11C-choline PET. J Nucl Med 44(3):331–335

Dehdashti F et al (2005) Positron tomographic assessment of androgen receptors in prostatic carcinoma. Eur J Nucl Med Mol Imaging 32(3):344–350

Deliveliotis C et al (2007) Diagnostic efficacy of transrectal ultrasound-guided biopsy of the prostatic fossa in patients with rising PSA following radical prostatectomy. World J Urol 25(3):309–313

Even-Sapir E et al (2007) 18F-Fluoride positron emission tomography and positron emission tomography/computed tomography. Semin Nucl Med 37(6):462–469

Farsad M et al (2005) Detection and localization of prostate cancer: correlation of (11)C-choline PET/CT with histopathologic step-section analysis. J Nucl Med 46(10):1642–1649

Fonteyne V et al (2008) Intensity-modulated radiotherapy as primary therapy for prostate cancer: report on acute toxicity after dose escalation with simultaneous integrated boost to intraprostatic lesion. Int J Radiat Oncol Biol Phys 72(3):799–807

Fox JJ, Schoder H, Larson SM (2012) Molecular imaging of prostate cancer. Curr Opin Urol 22(4):320–327

Fox JJ et al (2011) Developing imaging strategies for castration resistant prostate cancer. Acta Oncol 50(1):39–48

Fricke E et al (2003) Positron emission tomography with 11C-acetate and 18F-FDG in prostate cancer patients. Eur J Nucl Med Mol Imaging 30(4):607–611

Gillies RJ, Robey I, Gatenby RA (2008) Causes and consequences of increased glucose metabolism of cancers. J Nucl Med 49(2):24S–42S

Giovacchini G et al (2008) [(11)C]choline uptake with PET/CT for the initial diagnosis of prostate cancer: relation to PSA levels, tumour stage and anti-androgenic therapy. Eur J Nucl Med Mol Imaging 35(6):1065–1073

Giovacchini G et al (2010) PSA doubling time for prediction of [(11)C]choline PET/CT findings in prostate cancer patients with biochemical failure after radical prostatectomy. Eur J Nucl Med Mol Imaging 37(6):1106–1116

Giovacchini G et al (2012) Prostate-specific antigen velocity versus prostate-specific antigen doubling time for prediction of 11C choline PET/CT in prostate cancer patients with biochemical failure after radical prostatectomy. Clin Nucl Med 37(4):325–331

Grosu AL, Nestle U, Weber WA (2009) How to use functional imaging information for radiotherapy planning. Eur J Cancer 45(1):461–463

Grosu AL, Wiedenmann N, Molls M (2005a) Biological imaging in radiation oncology. Z Med Phys 15(3):141–145

Grosu AL et al (2005b) L-(methyl-11C) methionine positron emission tomography for target delineation in resected high-grade gliomas before radiotherapy. Int J Radiat Oncol Biol Phys 63(1):64–74

Grosu AL et al (2006) 11C-methionine PET improves the target volume delineation of meningiomas treated with stereotactic fractionated radiotherapy. Int J Radiat Oncol Biol Phys 66(2):339–344

Grosu AL et al (2011) An interindividual comparison of O-(2-[18F]fluoroethyl)-L-tyrosine (FET)- and L-[methyl-11C]methionine (MET)-PET in patients with brain gliomas and metastases. Int J Radiat Oncol Biol Phys 81(4):1049–1058

Han M et al (2003) Biochemical (prostate specific antigen) recurrence probability following radical prostatectomy for clinically localized prostate cancer. J Urol 169(2):517–523

Heidenreich A et al (2008) EAU guidelines on prostate cancer. Eur Urol 53(1):68–80

Heidenreich A et al (2011) EAU guidelines on prostate cancer. Part I: screening, diagnosis, and treatment of clinically localised disease. Actas Urol Esp 35(9):501–514

Hoetjes NJ et al (2010) Partial volume correction strategies for quantitative FDG PET in oncology. Eur J Nucl Med Mol Imaging 37(9):1679–1687

Husarik DB et al (2008) Evaluation of [(18)F]-choline PET/CT for staging and restaging of prostate cancer. Eur J Nucl Med Mol Imaging 35(2):253–263

Iorio E et al (2010) Activation of phosphatidylcholine cycle enzymes in human epithelial ovarian cancer cells. Cancer Res 70(5):2126–2135

Jadvar H (2011) Prostate cancer: PET with 18F-FDG, 18F- or 11C-acetate, and 18F- or 11C-choline. J Nucl Med 52(1):81–89

Jadvar H et al (2012) Prospective evaluation of 18F-NaF and 18F-FDG PET/CT in detection of occult metastatic disease in biochemical recurrence of prostate cancer. Clin Nucl Med 37(7):637–643

Jana S, Blaufox MD (2006) Nuclear medicine studies of the prostate, testes, and bladder. Semin Nucl Med 36(1):51–72

Jilg CA et al (2012) Salvage lymph node dissection with adjuvant radiotherapy for nodal recurrence of prostate cancer. J Urol 188(6):2190–2197

Jilg CA et al (2014) Detection of lymph node metastasis in patients with nodal prostate cancer relapse using 18F/11C-choline positron emission tomography/computerized tomography: influence of size of nodal tumor infiltration and accuracy related to lymph node regions. J Urol 192

Kao PF, Chou YH, Lai CW (2008) Diffuse FDG uptake in acute prostatitis. Clin Nucl Med 33(4):308–310

Karavitakis M et al (2011) Tumor focality in prostate cancer: implications for focal therapy. Nat Rev Clin Oncol 8(1):48–55

Kato T et al (2002) Accumulation of [11C] acetate in normal prostate and benign prostatic hyperplasia: comparison with prostate cancer. Eur J Nucl Med Mol Imaging 29(11):1492–1495

Kelloff GJ, Choyke P, Coffey DS (2009) Challenges in clinical prostate cancer: role of imaging. AJR Am J Roentgenol 192(6): 1455–1470

Kirste S, Volegova-Neher N, Henne K, Knippen S, Rischke HC, Schäfer AO (2011) Dose escalated radiotherapy of macroscopic local recurrence after radiacal prostatectomy. Strahlenther Onkol 187(1):112

Kotzerke J et al (2000) Experience with carbon-11 choline positron emission tomography in prostate carcinoma. Eur J Nucl Med 27(9):1415–1419

Kotzerke J et al (2002) Carbon-11 acetate positron emission tomography can detect local recurrence of prostate cancer. Eur J Nucl Med Mol Imaging 29(10):1380–1384

Kotzerke J et al (2003) Intraindividual comparison of [11C]acetate and [11C]choline PET for detection of metastases of prostate cancer. Nuklearmedizin 42(1):25–30

Krause BJ, Souvatzoglou M, Treiber U (2013) Imaging of prostate cancer with PET/CT and radioactively labeled choline derivates. Urol Oncol 31(4):427–435

Krause BJ et al (2008) The detection rate of [11C]choline-PET/CT depends on the serum PSA-value in patients with biochemical recurrence of prostate cancer. Eur J Nucl Med Mol Imaging 35(1): 18–23

Kwee SA et al (2006) Localization of primary prostate cancer with dual-phase 18F-fluorocholine PET. J Nucl Med 47(2): 262–269

Kwee SA et al (2008) Use of step-section histopathology to evaluate 18F-fluorocholine PET sextant localization of prostate cancer. Mol Imaging 7(1):12–20

Langsteger W et al (2011) Fluorocholine (18F) and sodium fluoride (18F) PET/CT in the detection of prostate cancer: prospective comparison of diagnostic performance determined by masked reading. Q J Nucl Med Mol Imaging 55(4):448–457

Larson SM et al (2004) Tumor localization of 16beta-18F-fluoro-5alpha-dihydrotestosterone versus 18F-FDG in patients with progressive, metastatic prostate cancer. J Nucl Med 45(3):366–373

Lawrentschuk N et al (2006) Positron emission tomography and molecular imaging of the prostate: an update. BJU Int 97(5): 923–931

Lindhe O et al (2009) [(18)F]Fluoroacetate is not a functional analogue of [(11)C]acetate in normal physiology. Eur J Nucl Med Mol Imaging 36(9):1453–1459

Liu Y (2006) Fatty acid oxidation is a dominant bioenergetic pathway in prostate cancer. Prostate Cancer Prostatic Dis 9(3):230–234

Liu A et al (1992) Fluorine-18-labeled androgens: radiochemical synthesis and tissue distribution studies on six fluorine-substituted androgens, potential imaging agents for prostatic cancer. J Nucl Med 33(5):724–734

Liu IJ et al (2001) Fluorodeoxyglucose positron emission tomography studies in diagnosis and staging of clinically organ-confined prostate cancer. Urology 57(1):108–111

Lonsdale MN, Beyer T (2010) Dual-modality PET/CT instrumentation-today and tomorrow. Eur J Radiol 73(3):452–460

Lu-Yao GL, Yao SL (1997) Population-based study of long-term survival in patients with clinically localised prostate cancer. Lancet 349(9056):906–910
MacDonald OK et al (2004) Salvage radiotherapy for men with isolated rising PSA or locally palpable recurrence after radical prostatectomy: do outcomes differ? Urology 64(4):760–764
Macheda ML, Rogers S, Best JD (2005) Molecular and cellular regulation of glucose transporter (GLUT) proteins in cancer. J Cell Physiol 202(3):654–662
Martorana G et al (2006) 11C-choline positron emission tomography/computerized tomography for tumor localization of primary prostate cancer in comparison with 12-core biopsy. J Urol 176(3): 954–960 (discussion)
Meirelles GS et al (2010) Prognostic value of baseline [18F] fluorodeoxyglucose positron emission tomography and 99mTc-MDP bone scan in progressing metastatic prostate cancer. Clin Cancer Res 16(24):6093–6099
Minamimoto R et al (2011) The potential of FDG-PET/CT for detecting prostate cancer in patients with an elevated serum PSA level. Ann Nucl Med 25(1):21–27
Morris AD et al (2001) The value of external beam radiation of nodal positive prostate cancer: a multivariate analysis. Urol Oncol 6(6):255–260
Morris MJ et al (2002) Fluorinated deoxyglucose positron emission tomography imaging in progressive metastatic prostate cancer. Urology 59(6):913–918
Mottet N et al (2011) EAU guidelines on prostate cancer. Part II: treatment of advanced, relapsing, and castration-resistant prostate cancer. Actas Urol Esp 35(10):565–579
Naya Y et al (2005) Efficacy of prostatic fossa biopsy in detecting local recurrence after radical prostatectomy. Urology 66(2): 350–355
Nestle U et al (2009) Biological imaging in radiation therapy: role of positron emission tomography. Phys Med Biol 54(1):R1–R25
Niyazi M et al (2010) Choline PET based dose-painting in prostate cancer–modelling of dose effects. Radiat Oncol 5:23
Nunez R et al (2002) Combined 18F-FDG and 11C-methionine PET scans in patients with newly progressive metastatic prostate cancer. J Nucl Med 43(1):46–55
Ohri N et al (2012) Can early implementation of salvage radiotherapy for prostate cancer improve the therapeutic ratio? A systematic review and regression meta-analysis with radiobiological modelling. Eur J Cancer 48(6):837–844
Oyama N et al (2002) Prognostic value of 2-deoxy-2-[F-18]fluoro-D-glucose positron emission tomography imaging for patients with prostate cancer. Mol Imaging Biol 4(1):99–104
Pandit-Taskar N et al (2008) Antibody mass escalation study in patients with castration-resistant prostate cancer using 111In-J591: lesion detectability and dosimetric projections for 90Y radioimmunotherapy. J Nucl Med 49(7):1066–1074
Pelosi E et al (2008) Role of whole-body 18F-choline PET/CT in disease detection in patients with biochemical relapse after radical treatment for prostate cancer. Radiol Med 113(6):895–904
Pflug BR et al (2003) Increased fatty acid synthase expression and activity during progression of prostate cancer in the TRAMP model. Prostate 57(3):245–254
Picchio M, Giovannini E, Messa C (2011a) The role of PET/computed tomography scan in the management of prostate cancer. Curr Opin Urol 21(3):230–236
Picchio M et al (2003) Value of [11C]choline-positron emission tomography for re-staging prostate cancer: a comparison with [18F]fluorodeoxyglucose-positron emission tomography. J Urol 169(4):1337–1340
Picchio M et al (2011b) The role of choline positron emission tomography/computed tomography in the management of patients with prostate-specific antigen progression after radical treatment of prostate cancer. Eur Urol 59(1):51–60
Pieterman RM et al (2002) Comparison of (11)C-choline and (18)F-FDG PET in primary diagnosis and staging of patients with thoracic cancer. J Nucl Med 43(2):167–172
Pinkawa M et al (2012) Dose-escalation using intensity-modulated radiotherapy for prostate cancer—evaluation of quality of life with and without (18)F-choline PET-CT detected simultaneous integrated boost. Radiat Oncol 7:14
Polascik TJ, Oesterling JE, Partin AW (1999) Prostate specific antigen: a decade of discovery–what we have learned and where we are going. J Urol 162(2):293–306
Ponde DE et al (2007) 18F-fluoroacetate: a potential acetate analog for prostate tumor imaging–in vivo evaluation of 18F-fluoroacetate versus 11C-acetate. J Nucl Med 48(3):420–428
Poulsen MH et al (2012) [18F]fluoromethylcholine (FCH) positron emission tomography/computed tomography (PET/CT) for lymph node staging of prostate cancer: a prospective study of 210 patients. BJU Int 110(11):1666–1671
Rapisarda E et al (2010) Image-based point spread function implementation in a fully 3D OSEM reconstruction algorithm for PET. Phys Med Biol 55(14):4131–4151
Reske SN, Blumstein NM, Glatting G (2008) [11C]choline PET/CT imaging in occult local relapse of prostate cancer after radical prostatectomy. Eur J Nucl Med Mol Imaging 35(1):9–17
Reske SN et al (2006) Imaging prostate cancer with 11C-choline PET/CT. J Nucl Med 47(8):1249–1254
Rigatti P et al (2011) Pelvic/retroperitoneal salvage lymph node dissection for patients treated with radical prostatectomy with biochemical recurrence and nodal recurrence detected by [11C]choline positron emission tomography/computed tomography. Eur Urol 60(5):935–943
Rinnab L et al (2007) Evaluation of [11C]-choline positron-emission/computed tomography in patients with increasing prostate-specific antigen levels after primary treatment for prostate cancer. BJU Int 100(4):786–793
Rischke HC et al (2012a) Correlation of the genotype of paragangliomas and pheochromocytomas with their metabolic phenotype on 3,4-dihydroxy-6-18F-fluoro-L-phenylalanin PET. J Nucl Med 53(9):1352–1358
Rischke HC et al (2012b) Treatment of recurrent prostate cancer following radical prostatectomy: the radiation-oncologists point of view. Q J Nucl Med Mol Imaging 56(5):409–420
Rischke HC et al (2012c) Detection of local recurrent prostate cancer after radical prostatectomy in terms of salvage radiotherapy using dynamic contrast enhanced-MRI without Endorectal coil. Radiat Oncol 7(1):185
Saleem MD et al (1998) Factors predicting cancer detection in biopsy of the prostatic fossa after radical prostatectomy. Urology 51(2): 283–286
Salminen E et al (2002) Investigations with FDG-PET scanning in prostate cancer show limited value for clinical practice. Acta Oncol 41(5):425–429
Scattoni V et al (2004) Diagnosis of local recurrence after radical prostatectomy. BJU Int 93(5):680–688
Scattoni V et al (2007) Detection of lymph-node metastases with integrated [11C]choline PET/CT in patients with PSA failure after radical retropubic prostatectomy: results confirmed by open pelvic-retroperitoneal lymphadenectomy. Eur Urol 52(2):423–429
Scher HI, Heller G (2000) Clinical states in prostate cancer: toward a dynamic model of disease progression. Urology 55(3):323–327

Scher B et al (2007) Value of 11C-choline PET and PET/CT in patients with suspected prostate cancer. Eur J Nucl Med Mol Imaging 34(1):45–53

Schiavina R et al (2008) 11C-choline positron emission tomography/computerized tomography for preoperative lymph-node staging in intermediate-risk and high-risk prostate cancer: comparison with clinical staging nomograms. Eur Urol 54(2):392–401

Sciarra A et al (2008) Role of dynamic contrast-enhanced magnetic resonance (MR) imaging and proton MR spectroscopic imaging in the detection of local recurrence after radical prostatectomy for prostate cancer. Eur Urol 54(3):589–600

Sella T et al (2004) Suspected local recurrence after radical prostatectomy: endorectal coil MR imaging. Radiology 231(2):379–385

Seltzer MA et al (2004) Radiation dose estimates in humans for (11)C-acetate whole-body PET. J Nucl Med 45(7):1233–1236

Shekarriz B et al (1999) Vesicourethral anastomosis biopsy after radical prostatectomy: predictive value of prostate-specific antigen and pathologic stage. Urology 54(6):1044–1048

Shreve PD et al (1996) Metastatic prostate cancer: initial findings of PET with 2-deoxy-2-[F-18]fluoro-D-glucose. Radiology 199(3):751–756

Smith TA (2000) Mammalian hexokinases and their abnormal expression in cancer. Br J Biomed Sci 57(2):170–178

Souvatzoglou M et al (2011) The sensitivity of [11C]choline PET/CT to localize prostate cancer depends on the tumor configuration. Clin Cancer Res 17(11):3751–3759

Strope SA, Andriole GL (2010) Prostate cancer screening: current status and future perspectives. Nat Rev Urol 7(9):487–493

Sutinen E et al (2004) Kinetics of [(11)C]choline uptake in prostate cancer: a PET study. Eur J Nucl Med Mol Imaging 31(3):317–324

Symon Z et al (2006) Radiation rescue for biochemical failure after surgery for prostate cancer: predictive parameters and an assessment of contemporary predictive models. Am J Clin Oncol 29(5):446–450

Testa C et al (2007) Prostate cancer: sextant localization with MR imaging, MR spectroscopy, and 11C-choline PET/CT. Radiology 244(3):797–806

Thorwarth D et al (2012) Integration of FDG-PET/CT into external beam radiation therapy planning: technical aspects and recommendations on methodological approaches. Nuklearmedizin 51(4):140–153

Tilki D et al (2013) 18F-Fluoroethylcholine PET/CT identifies lymph node metastasis in patients with prostate-specific antigen failure after radical prostatectomy, but underestimates its extent. Eur Urol 63:792–796

Toth G et al (2005) Detection of prostate cancer with 11C-methionine positron emission tomography. J Urol 173(1):66–69 (discussion)

Townsend DW (2008) Multimodality imaging of structure and function. Phys Med Biol 53(4):R1–R39

Tuncel M et al (2008) [(11)C]Choline positron emission tomography/computed tomography for staging and restaging of patients with advanced prostate cancer. Nucl Med Biol 35(6):689–695

Turkbey B et al (2009) Imaging localized prostate cancer: current approaches and new developments. AJR Am J Roentgenol 192(6):1471–1480

van Lin EN et al (2006) IMRT boost dose planning on dominant intraprostatic lesions: gold marker-based three-dimensional fusion of CT with dynamic contrast-enhanced and 1H-spectroscopic MRI. Int J Radiat Oncol Biol Phys 65(1):291–303

Vavere AL et al (2008) 1-11C-acetate as a PET radiopharmaceutical for imaging fatty acid synthase expression in prostate cancer. J Nucl Med 49(2):327–334

Vees H et al (2007) 18F-choline and/or 11C-acetate positron emission tomography: detection of residual or progressive subclinical disease at very low prostate-specific antigen values (<1 ng/ml) after radical prostatectomy. BJU Int 99(6):1415–1420

Viani GA, Stefano EJ, Afonso SL (2009) Higher-than-conventional radiation doses in localized prostate cancer treatment: a meta-analysis of randomized, controlled trials. Int J Radiat Oncol Biol Phys 74(5):1405–1418

Wurschmidt F et al (2011) [18F]fluoroethylcholine-PET/CT imaging for radiation treatment planning of recurrent and primary prostate cancer with dose escalation to PET/CT-positive lymph nodes. Radiat Oncol 6:44

Yakar D et al (2012) Predictive value of MRI in the localization, staging, volume estimation, assessment of aggressiveness, and guidance of radiotherapy and biopsies in prostate cancer. J Magn Reson Imaging 35(1):20–31

Target Volume Definition in Primary Prostate Cancer Radiotherapy

Dirk Böhmer

Contents

Abstract

The organ contouring section of this book provides a summary of the available evidence on prostate cancer target volume definition. The reader will find comprehensive data supporting the extension of the clinical target volume beyond the prostate for patients with risk factors such as a high pre-treatment PSA value or a high Gleason score. Furthermore the necessity to adapt planning target volume margins according to the applied treatment technique and verification method is elaborated.

1 Introduction

In general target delineation is not depending on radiotherapy technique, whether 3D-conformal, IMRT or rotation techniques are used. Tumor related risk factors such as transcapsular tumor spread or tumor grading rather determine the extent of target volume delineation. Regarding prostate cancer delineation the determining factors are clinical tumor extension according to the UICC tumor stage, the Gleason score as well as the number of positive biopsies defined by random prostate biopsy and the PSA level. The European Organization for Research and Treatment of Cancer (EORTC) radiation oncology group (ROG) developed the first comprehensive guideline on target volume definition for primary radiotherapy in prostate cancer which was published in 2006. They provide thorough information on target and organ at risk volume definition, imaging, patient set-up and treatment verification (Boehmer et al. 2006). This chapter refers to clinical or prognostic risk factors which are the commonly known factors as defined according to the National Comprehensive Cancer Network (NCCN) and Anthony D'Amico.

Table 1 summarizes the risk group classification.

D. Böhmer (✉)
Department of Radiation Oncology, Charité University Medicine, Campus Virchow Klinikum, Augustenburger Platz 1, 13353 Berlin, Germany
e-mail: dirk.boehmer@charite.de

H. Geinitz et al. (eds.), *Radiotherapy in Prostate Cancer*, Medical Radiology. Radiation Oncology,
DOI: 10.1007/174_2014_958,
Published Online: 13 February 2014

Table 1 Risk group definition according to D'Amico and NCCN

Risk group	Low	Intermediate	High
NCCN			
T-Stage	cT1c + cT2a and	cT2b – 2c and/or	cT3 or
PSA	<10 ng/ml and	>10–20 ng/ml and/or	>20 ng/ml or
Gleason sum	<7	=7	8–10
D'Amico et al. (1997a, 1998, 1999)			
T-Stage	cT1c – 2a and	cT2b and/or	cT2c – cT3 or
PSA	<10 ng/ml and	>10–20 ng/ml and/or	>20 ng/ml or
Gleason sum	<7	=7	8–10

Note that the two classifications differ only by clinical stage in intermediate and high risk tumors

2 International Commission on Radiation Units and Measurement (ICRU) Volumes Definition

ICRU 50, ICRU 62 and ICRU 82 provide a comprehensive definition of target volumes and organs at risk (OAR) in radiotherapy. The ICRU 50, published in 1993, presented the first concept of standardizing definitions of target volume delineation and organs at risk (International Commission on Radiation Units and Measurements 1993). The 1999 supplement (ICRU 62) introduced additional volumes that would change the extension of target volumes based on published data on internal organ motion and positioning uncertainties(International Commission on Radiation Units and Measurements 1999). In its latest modification from 2010 the ICRU report 83 takes into consideration new developments in imaging modalities as well as new radiation techniques and their influence on target volume definition(International Commission on Radiation Units and Measurements 2010).

The Gross Tumor Volume (GTV) comprises the macroscopic tumor extension. These are all tumor manifestations that are visible clinically as defined by the TNM system. Additional information is derived from imaging techniques such as ultrasound, computed tomography (CT), magnetic resonance imaging (MRI), functional MRI or position emission tomography (PET), respectively. It may not only include the primary tumor but also lymph node metastases or distant tumor manifestations.

The Clinical Target Volume (CTV) is defined as the GTV plus a volume that is considered at risk of containing subclinical or microscopic disease. The extent of this margin differs widely among different tumor locations or different tumor histologies. Until now there is no consensus on how the risk of subclinical disease is defined but typically a probability of occult disease of 5–10 % is assumed to require treatment. The consideration of the consequences of failure, and the expected feasibility of salvage treatment furthermore influence the clinical judgment(International Commission on Radiation Units and Measurements 2010).

The Planning Target Volume (PTV) comprises the CTV with an additional margin derived from internal organ movement and patient set-up error. The PTV is the only target structure of which the size changes depending on the precision of the applied radiotherapy technique. Without any measures to determine the exact position of the prostate before or during the treatment fraction the CTV-PTV margin should cover the mentioned errors to provide a high probability of CTV coverage of the applied radiotherapy.

The Internal Target Volume (ITV) was introduced first in the ICRU report 62. The aim was to take into account possible changes of the CTV in terms of size shape and position. In prostate cancer these changes may be attributed to varying volumes of adjacent organs, namely rectum and bladder, which may cause altering CTV volumes.

The planning organ-at-risk volume (PRV) is directly associated with the ITV. Due to varying filling states of organs at risk the ITV allows for an improved determination of doses received by organs at risk during a treatment course. As volumes may vary substantially a precise measurement of these doses is not possible as the volume of an OAR may change not only between treatment fractions but also within a single fraction (inter- and intrafraction deviation). Furthermore a larger OAR volume may be advantageous as well as a distinct disadvantage in certain clinical situations. The rectum for instance may receive a significantly lower dose when fully extended by the use of an endrectal balloon, as the PTV positioned anteriorly will be treated in a constant position. In a systematic review a reduction of the rectal wall dose was shown in planning studies when an endorectal balloon was used. Yet there are no clinical studies to confirm whether rectal toxicities are reduced as well. (Smeenk et al. 2010). Furthermore an extended rectum may shift the prostate anteriorly and thus may result in an increased rectal dose when no image guided radiotherapy is applied.

Current randomized trials have used a variety of target delineations. Table 2 gives an overview of the available randomized trials on hypofractionation and dose escalation in primary prostate cancer radiotherapy. Obviously the target volume definition is different in each trial although prostate plus seminal vesicles were used as the CTV in most trials. The definitions of the PTV margins are variable as well, ranging from 3 to 20 mm.

The following paragraphs will collect and sum up the available evidence on target volume definition.

Table 2 Summary of target volume definitions in the published Phase III trials

Phase III trials	CTV-definition	CTV-PTV margin
Arcangeli et al. (2012)	prostate + SV	10 mm uniform
Lukka et al. (2005)	prostate	15, 10 mm at PRI
Pollack et al. (2006)	prostate + 9 mm inferiorly + proximal SV (intermediate risk); whole SV + LN (high risk)	conv. IMRT: 8, 5 mm at PRI hypo. IMRT: 7, 3 mm at PRI
Norkus et al. (2009)	prostate + base of SV	8–10 mm
Yeoh et al. (2011)	prostate	2D-RT: 15, 20 mm superior + inferior 3D-RT: 15 mm uniform
MD Anderson (Kuban et al. 2008)	prostate + SV	ant. + inf.: 12.5–15 mm post. + sup.: 7.5–10 mm
Dutch trial (Al-Mamgani et al. 2011)	prostate ± SV	Arm A: 10 mm (68 Gy) Arm B: 10 mm (68 Gy) Arm B: 5 mm (last 10 Gy)
PROG96-09 (Zietman et al. 2005)	prostate + 5 mm	7–10 mm
GETUG 06 (Beckendorf et al. 2011)	46 Gy: prostate + SV Arm A: prostate (24 Gy) Arm B: prostate (34 Gy)	10 mm (5 mm posteriorly)
MRC RT01 (Dearnaley et al. 2007)	low-risk: prostate + base of SV + 5 mm intermediate + high-risk: prostate + SV + 5 mm	5–10 mm

Hypo-*FX* hypofractionation; *SV* seminal vesicles; *LN* lymph nodes; *IMRT* intensity modulated radiotherapy; *RT* radiotherapy; *PRI* prostate rectum interface

3 Pathological Considerations for Prostate Cancer Clinical Target Volume Delineation

3.1 CTV Delineation in Low-Risk Prostate Cancer

Knowledge of the natural spread of prostate cancer is crucial for determination of reasonable clinical target volumes. The most comprehensive data on this issue can be derived from pathological studies. The tumor related bottleneck factors for CTV definitions are (a) the presence of extracapsular extension (ECE) and (b) seminal vesicle invasion (SVI).

In 1997 D'Amico et al. found in a retrospective analysis of 749 prostatectomy specimens that the risk of pathologic SVI as well as macroscopic extracapsular tumor extension is only 2 % in low risk patients. They furthermore found that the risk of PSA relapse is similar in patients undergoing radical prostatectomy or radiotherapy when patients without clinical risk factors were included (D'Amico et al. 1997b). These factors were defined as PSA <10 ng/ml, clinical stage <T2c and Gleason score <7, respectively. Further pathological studies confirmed these results (Kestin et al. 2002). Taking these findings into account there is no sensible reason to include the seminal vesicles into the CTV in patients with low risk prostate cancer. As the risk of ECE is similarly low it is obvious to delineate the prostate only as CTV defined by the visible boundaries on planning computed tomography or magnetic resonance imaging. An example of CTV delineation is shown in Fig. 1b.

Does this hold true for patients *with* clinical risk factors?

3.2 CTV Delineation in Intermediate- and High-Risk Prostate Cancer

To shed light on this question it is useful to focus on the two most relevant factors of tumor recurrence after definitive therapy; namely extracapsular tumor extension and seminal vesicle involvement. It is well understood that the risk for these factors rises with increasing clinical risk factors. The question whether the degree of extracapsular extension may influence treatment outcome has been addressed by many author. Just recently van Veggel published an outcome study after radical prostatectomy focusing on the associated pathological ECE evaluation. Evaluation of the biochemical relapse rate of 134 patients according to different definitions of ECE revealed a significant association of the extent of ECE with the rate of biochemical relapse rates (van Veggel et al. 2011). Their results confirmed studies from various other authors (Epstein et al. 1993; Wheeler et al. 1998; Davis et al. 1999). To be able to apply these results to target volume definition in prostate cancer radiotherapy it is necessary to evaluate the specific amount of extracapsular tumor extension. In the largest published series The et al. found that among all prostatectomy specimens with extracapsular tumor extension only 2.8 % show an extension of more than 5 mm from the capsule (Teh et al. 2003). Several pathological studies have confirmed that more than 90 % of all patients who present with ECE have a radial tumor extension from the capsule of less than 4–5 mm (Davis et al. 1999; Schwartz et al. 2007; Sohayda et al. 2000).

CTV definition of the prostate gland plus an additional circumferential margin of 5 mm would thus cover more than 90 % of tumor extensions outside the prostate. At the prostate rectum interface the anterior rectal wall represents

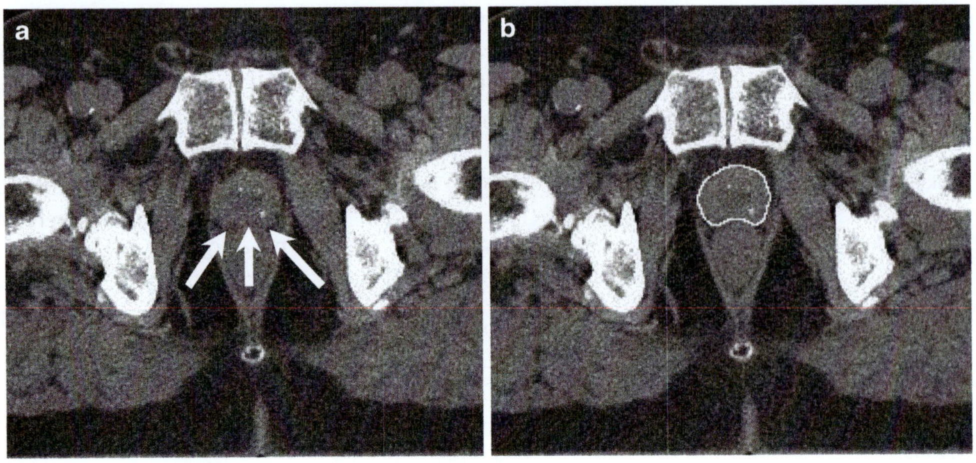

Fig. 1 Typical CT slice in the mid-gland region. *Arrows* indicate the fat layer at the prostate rectum interface (**a**). CTV contour of the same CT slice (**b**)

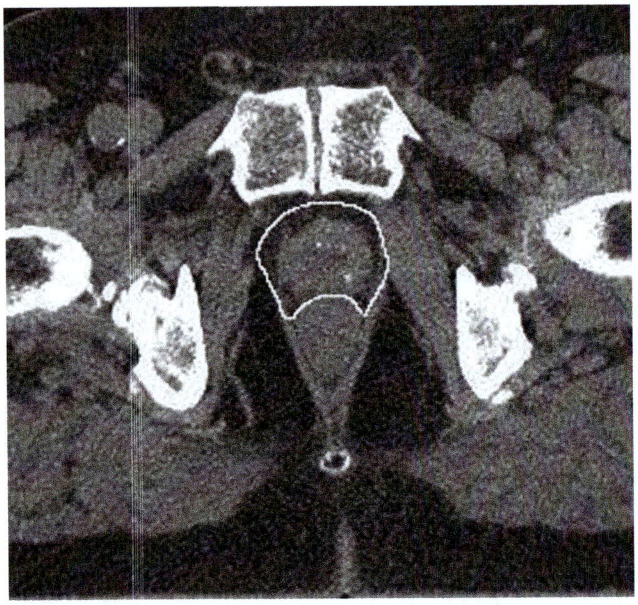

Fig. 2 Contouring of the prostate plus a 5 mm margin to include the possible periprostatic extension in patients with risk factors

a solid boundary for tumor cells so that the CTV can be reduced posteriorly. An example is shown in Fig. 2.

Kestin and colleagues reviewed 344 prostatectomy specimens with regard to SVI. They found that the tumor never involves the whole SV; the most distant cancer found was 1.5 cm apart from the SV tip. Including the proximal 2 cm of the SV into the CTV would include 90 % of pathological involved seminal vesicles. In terms of certainty of CT definitions of the seminal vesicle compared to pathological measurements they furthermore found that the two methods are in well agreement (Kestin et al. 2002). Given that 38 % of all patients showed at least one high risk feature it seems advisable to include the proximal 2.0–2.5 cm of the seminal vesicles into CTV in order to cover more than 90 % of all SVI. Finally only 1 % of low-risk patients had a SVI which confirms not to include SVs into CTV in this patient group. With each prognostic high risk factor the rate of SVI rises from 15 % with one high risk factor, 28 % with two and 58 % with three high risk factors respectively.

With regard to CTV definition it may be reasonable to include the base of the seminal vesicles (proximal 2–2.5 cm) into the CTV for all patients with high risk features. Yet one must be aware that with only one high risk factor the number of patients who are treated with a larger CTV without having a SVI is considerably high. The treating physician must refer to the available data to gain informed consent with the patient.

4 CT/MRI and Target Delineation

CT scans are still considered standard for target delineation. There are two main reasons indicating that this will not change thoroughgoing within the next 10 years. Firstly CT scanners are available at the disposal of all radiotherapy units and are mainly used as dedicated imaging systems. Secondly treatment planning systems are nowadays continuing to calculate tissue specific doses based on Hounsfield units. Just recently the Department of Oncology of the University Hospital in Helsinki, Finland commissioned an MRI-only based treatment planning procedure for external beam radiotherapy of prostate cancer (Kapanen et al. 2012). Yet the use of MRI based systems across the board will not be realistic within the next decade.

Using CT scans for prostate cancer treatment planning is known to contain inaccuracies. An analysis of the pathologic prostate volume and the CTV delineated in 10 patients whose preoperative CT scans were available showed an almost twofold increase of the respective volumes (Teh et al. 2003). Although the significance of this result is limited due to the small number of analyzed CT scans the issue of volume overestimation must be scrutinized.

It is a well-known fact that CT scans overestimate the "true" prostate volume by 20–60 % when compared with MRI scans. Yet there is a lack of precise information on the exact regions of overestimation. In a multiobserver study on CT-MRI prostate delineation the volume overestimation was 40 % favoring the CT scans. The authors point out that the CT volume did not encompass the whole MRI volume indicating that the differences in size between CT and MRI are not evenly distributed around the delineated prostate (Rasch et al. 1999). The largest differences are seen at the apex of the prostate where the MRI is able to clearly distinguish between apex, the urogenital diaphragm and the plexus Santorini. The soft tissue contrast in MRI allows for an easily visible boundary layer just as well at the prostate base, with the higher signal intensity of the seminal vesicles compared to the prostatic tissue. These two regions showed the largest CT-MRI volume differences among the observers.

These findings are of crucial relevance in terms of target volume definition. Whereas the risk of transcapsular extension is very small in the anterior or anterolateral parts of the gland, it is highest in the posterior and posterolateral parts. Thus the periprostatic region at the prostate-rectum interface is at the highest risk of tumor recurrence when underdosed by radiotherapy.

That implies that we have to focus on the CT based overestimation in these anatomic areas. To our knowledge there is no study or paper giving details about this special issue throughout the literature. But we do know that CT can often discriminate precisely the posterolateral area cranially of the apex region where there is usually a thin fatty layer between the posterior surface of the prostate and the rectal wall. Figure 1a shows an example of this area. Figure 1b shows the prostate contour of this CT slice.

Considering a patient with intermediate or high risk factors who has a substantial risk of transcapsular spread and furthermore assuming the extracapsular extension to be in most cases not larger than 5 mm the resulting contour for the CTV is shown in Fig. 2. Note that any anatomic boundary such as rectal wall, bone or muscle represents a demarcation line which is usually not crossed by tumor cells except in locally advanced T4 tumors. Thus the CTV contour should include this boundary but should not include the given organ.

5 CTV-PTV Margin

The PTV represents a security margin encompassing the CTV that considers daily set-up errors of the patient and the individual internal organ motion (see "CTV Delineation in Intermediate-and High-Risk Prostate Cancer"). This margin may be defined uniformly or may be smaller towards the prostate–rectum interface.

There is consensus that the PTV is being contoured by a computer planning system as an automatically generated margin. The PTV must not be generated by hand as for an individual observer it is not possible to draw a three-dimensional margin encompassing the CTV.

The CTV-PTV margin is depending on the type and precision of the verification method of the patients' daily treatment as well as intrafractional motion but not on the type of therapy, e. g. 3D-conformal or IMRT. Obviously a daily online set-up verification and correction requires smaller PTV margins compared to an offline verification protocol that is performed once or twice weekly. Recently image guided radiotherapy has emerged as a tool to verify and if necessary correct the patients' position before each treatment by using cone beam CT, ultrasound, intraprostatic fiducial markers or implanted electronic devices. These systems are able to minimize interfraction motion to a great extent.

There are numerous studies that tried to define the CTV-PTV margin based on analyses of the number of verifications performed per week. The largest study with regard to image guidance and inter- as well as intrafraction motion was performed by Kotte et al. (2007). They analyzed more than 11.000 measurements of online set-up verifications of 427 patients who were treated with a 5-field IMRT. All patients had implanted fiducial gold markers and verification was performed before each treatment session and before each treated field. They found that there is substantial intrafraction motion with 66 % of all measurements with a motion outside a range of 2 mm and 28 % outside a range of 3 mm. The authors where able to demonstrate that with a daily set-up correction systematic and random set-up error were smaller than 1 mm. In conclusion they recommend a minimum CTV-PTV margin of 2 mm when a daily set-up verification of the prostate position is performed before each treatment session.

Graf et al. conducted a study on 23 prostate cancer patients with implanted gold markers and calculated the necessary CTV-PTV margin relative to the frequency of set-up verifications and corrections (Graf et al. 2009). Table 3 shows their main results.

Margins were calculated using a formula developed by van Herk (2004). The key message of this analysis states that with daily set-up corrections a CTV-PTV margin of 5 mm is appropriate whereas once weekly or no correction requires 10 mm margins (Graf et al. 2009).

The relevance of a constant or reproducible filling status of the rectum and/or the bladder has not been of major concern for decades. In 2005 De Crevoisier published a landmark study of an increased risk of biochemical relapse after prostate radiotherapy if the rectum had been distended (filled) during planning CT. The authors found on multivariate analysis that rectal distension was an

Table 3 PTV margins calculated from the frequency of set-up corrections

Random σ and systematic Σ error [mm]							PTV-Margin [mm]		
Direction	LR		SI		AP		LR	SI	AP
	Σ	σ	Σ	σ	Σ	σ			
No correction	2.0	2.9	2.7	3.9	2.6	4.3	**7.0**	**9.5**	**9.5**
Correction 1x/week	1.9	2.8	2.3	3.5	2.4	3.9	**6.7**	**8.2**	**8.7**
Correction 3x/week	1.6	2.5	1.8	3.0	1.7	3.3	**5.8**	**6.6**	**7.7**
Correction 5x/week	1.4	2.0	1.4	2.3	1.3	2.2	**4.9**	**5.1**	**4.8**

LR left–right; *SI* superior–inferior; *AP* anterior–posterior; adapted from (Graf et al. 2009)

independent risk factor for biochemical failure with a hazard ratio of 3.89 (95 % C.I. 1.58–9.56, p = 0.003) (de Crevoisier et al. 2005). This was confirmed in a subgroup analysis of the Dutch dose escalation trial. The authors found an increased risk of failure in patients with a 25 % risk of seminal vesicle involvement and a risk of geometric miss defined by anorectal volume >90 cm^3 and symptoms of diarrhea at least 25 % of the treatment time (Heemsbergen et al. 2007).

Results from these studies provide evidence that an empty rectum during planning CT provides improved biochemical control in patients undergoing definitive radiotherapy for prostate cancer. This involves only patients who are treated with conventional verification techniques, e. g. offline correction-protocols. In case of image guided radiotherapy the risk of a geographic miss is reduced substantially because the image guidance positions the prostate irrespective of the distension of the rectum.

The relevance of patient instructions with regard to constant filling status of the rectum and bladder was explored in a study to evaluate whether this patient preparation yields an improvement of target stability. The authors where able to demonstrate that with proper patient instructions the calculated CTV-PTV margins would be as low as with image guided radiotherapy (Graf et al. 2012).

In summary CTV-PTV margins must be adapted to the type of patient set-up verification and the frequency of these verifications. With regard to treatment precision in prostate cancer radiotherapy radiation oncologists may select from a variety of verification options, namely implanted fiducial markers or electronic devices, cone beam or MV-CT or ultrasound However, these procedures are not yet available throughout the radiotherapy community.

The significance of bladder and rectal filling status is important and may help to reduce deviations in position and shape of the prostate.

References

Al-Mamgani A, van Putten WL, van der Wielen GJ, Levendag PC, Incrocci L (2011) Dose escalation and quality of life in patients with localized prostate cancer treated with radiotherapy: long-term results of the Dutch randomized dose-escalation trial (CKTO 96–10 trial). Int J Radiat Oncol Biol Phys 79(4):1004–1012. doi:10.1016/j.ijrobp.2009.12.039

Arcangeli S, Strigari L, Gomellini S, Saracino B, Petrongari MG, Pinnaro P, Pinzi V, Arcangeli G (2012) Updated results and patterns of failure in a randomized hypofractionation trial for high-risk prostate cancer. Int J Radiat Oncol Biol Phys 84(5):1172–1178. doi:10.1016/j.ijrobp.2012.02.049

Beckendorf V, Guerif S, Le Prise E, Cosset JM, Bougnoux A, Chauvet B, Salem N, Chapet O, Bourdain S, Bachaud JM, Maingon P, Hannoun-Levi JM, Malissard L, Simon JM, Pommier P, Hay M, Dubray B, Lagrange JL, Luporsi E, Bey P (2011) 70 Gy versus 80 Gy in localized prostate cancer: 5-year results of GETUG 06 randomized trial. Int J Radiat Oncol Biol Phys 80(4):1056–1063. doi:10.1016/j.ijrobp.2010.03.049

Boehmer D, Maingon P, Poortmans P, Baron MH, Miralbell R, Remouchamps V, Scrase C, Bossi A, Bolla M (2006) Guidelines for primary radiotherapy of patients with prostate cancer. Radiother Oncol: J Eur Soc Ther Radiol Oncol 79(3):259–269. doi:10.1016/j.radonc.2006.05.012

D'Amico AV, Whittington R, Kaplan I, Beard C, Schultz D, Malkowicz SB, Tomaszewski JE, Wein A, Coleman CN (1997b) Equivalent 5-year bNED in select prostate cancer patients managed with surgery or radiation therapy despite exclusion of the seminal vesicles from the CTV. Int J Radiat Oncol Biol Phys 39(2):335–340

D'Amico AV, Whittington R, Schultz D, Malkowicz SB, Tomaszewski JE, Wein A (1997a) Outcome based staging for clinically localized adenocarcinoma of the prostate. J urol 158(4):1422–1426

D'Amico AV, Whittington R, Malkowicz SB, Fondurulia J, Chen MH, Kaplan I, Beard CJ, Tomaszewski JE, Renshaw AA, Wein A, Coleman CN (1999) Pretreatment nomogram for prostate-specific antigen recurrence after radical prostatectomy or external-beam radiation therapy for clinically localized prostate cancer. J Clin Oncol: Off J Am Soc Clin Oncol 17(1):168–172

D'Amico AV, Whittington R, Malkowicz SB, Schultz D, Blank K, Broderick GA, Tomaszewski JE, Renshaw AA, Kaplan I, Beard CJ, Wein A (1998) Biochemical outcome after radical prostatectomy, external beam radiation therapy, or interstitial radiation therapy for clinically localized prostate cancer. JAMA J Am Med Assoc 280(11):969–974

Davis BJ, Pisansky TM, Wilson TM, Rothenberg HJ, Pacelli A, Hillman DW, Sargent DJ, Bostwick DG (1999) The radial distance of extraprostatic extension of prostate carcinoma: implications for prostate brachytherapy. Cancer 85(12):2630–2637

de Crevoisier R, Tucker SL, Dong L, Mohan R, Cheung R, Cox JD, Kuban DA (2005) Increased risk of biochemical and local failure in patients with distended rectum on the planning CT for prostate cancer radiotherapy. Int J Radiat Oncol Biol Phys 62(4):965–973. doi:10.1016/j.ijrobp.2004.11.032

Dearnaley DP, Sydes MR, Graham JD, Aird EG, Bottomley D, Cowan RA, Huddart RA, Jose CC, Matthews JH, Millar J, Moore AR, Morgan RC, Russell JM, Scrase CD, Stephens RJ, Syndikus I, Parmar MK (2007) Escalated-dose versus standard-dose conformal radiotherapy in prostate cancer: first results from the MRC RT01 randomised controlled trial. Lancet Oncol 8(6):475–487. doi:10.1016/S1470-2045(07)70143-2

Epstein JI, Carmichael MJ, Pizov G, Walsh PC (1993) Influence of capsular penetration on progression following radical prostatectomy: a study of 196 cases with long-term followup. J urol 150(1):135–141

Graf R, Wust P, Budach V, Boehmer D (2009) Potentials of on-line repositioning based on implanted fiducial markers and electronic portal imaging in prostate cancer radiotherapy. Radiat Oncol 4:13. doi:10.1186/1748-717X-4-13

Graf R, Boehmer D, Nadobny J, Budach V, Wust P (2012) Appropriate patient instructions can reduce prostate motion. Radiat Oncol 7:125. doi:10.1186/1748-717X-7-125

Heemsbergen WD, Hoogeman MS, Witte MG, Peeters ST, Incrocci L, Lebesque JV (2007) Increased risk of biochemical and clinical failure for prostate patients with a large rectum at radiotherapy planning: results from the Dutch trial of 68 GY versus 78 Gy. Int J Radiat Oncol Biol Phys 67(5):1418–1424. doi:10.1016/j.ijrobp.2006.11.014

International Commission on Radiation Units and Measurements (1993) Prescribing, recording, and reporting photon beam therapy. ICRU report 50, Oxford University Press

International Commission on Radiation Units and Measurements (1999) Prescribing, recording, and reporting photon beam therapy (Supplement to ICRU report 50). ICRU Report 62, Oxford University Press

International Commission on Radiation Units and Measurements (2010) Prescribing, recording, and reporting photon-beam intensity-modulated radiation therapy (IMRT). ICRU report 83, Oxford University Press vol 10(1). doi:10.1093/jicru/ndq002

Kapanen M, Collan J, Beule A, Seppala T, Saarilahti K, Tenhunen M (2012) Commissioning of MRI-only based treatment planning procedure for external beam radiotherapy of prostate. Magn Reson Med: Off j Soc Magn Reson Med/Soc Mag Reson Med. doi:10.1002/mrm.24459

Kotte AN, Hofman P, Lagendijk JJ, van Vulpen M, van der Heide UA (2007) Intrafraction motion of the prostate during external-beam radiation therapy: analysis of 427 patients with implanted fiducial markers. Int J Radiat Oncol Biol Phys 69(2):419–425. doi:10.1016/j.ijrobp.2007.03.029

Kestin L, Goldstein N, Vicini F, Yan D, Korman H, Martinez A (2002) Treatment of prostate cancer with radiotherapy: should the entire seminal vesicles be included in the clinical target volume? Int J Radiat Oncol Biol Phys 54(3):686–697

Kuban DA, Tucker SL, Dong L, Starkschall G, Huang EH, Cheung MR, Lee AK, Pollack A (2008) Long-term results of the M. D. Anderson randomized dose-escalation trial for prostate cancer. Int J Radiat Oncol Biol Phys 70(1):67–74. doi:10.1016/j.ijrobp.2007.06.054

Lukka H, Hayter C, Julian JA, Warde P, Morris WJ, Gospodarowicz M, Levine M, Sathya J, Choo R, Prichard H, Brundage M, Kwan W (2005) Randomized trial comparing two fractionation schedules for patients with localized prostate cancer. J Clin Oncol: Off J Am Soc Clin Oncol 23(25):6132–6138. doi:10.1200/JCO.2005.06.153

Norkus D, Miller A, Kurtinaitis J, Haverkamp U, Popov S, Prott FJ, Valuckas KP (2009) A randomized trial comparing hypofractionated and conventionally fractionated three-dimensional external-beam radiotherapy for localized prostate adenocarcinoma : a report on acute toxicity. Strahlenther Onkol 185(11):715–721. doi:10.1007/s00066-009-1982-z

Pollack A, Hanlon AL, Horwitz EM, Feigenberg SJ, Konski AA, Movsas B, Greenberg RE, Uzzo RG, Ma CM, McNeeley SW, Buyyounouski MK, Price RA Jr (2006) Dosimetry and preliminary acute toxicity in the first 100 men treated for prostate cancer on a randomized hypofractionation dose escalation trial. Int J Radiat Oncol Biol Phys 64(2):518–526. doi:10.1016/j.ijrobp.2005.07.970

Rasch C, Barillot I, Remeijer P, Touw A, van Herk M, Lebesque JV (1999) Definition of the prostate in CT and MRI: a multi-observer study. Int J Radiat Oncol Biol Phys 43(1):57–66

Schwartz DJ, Sengupta S, Hillman DW, Sargent DJ, Cheville JC, Wilson TM, Mynderse LA, Choo R, Davis BJ (2007) Prediction of radial distance of extraprostatic extension from pretherapy factors. Int J Radiat Oncol Biol Phys 69(2):411–418. doi:10.1016/j.ijrobp.2007.03.016

Smeenk RJ, Teh BS, Butler EB, van Lin EN, Kaanders JH (2010) Is there a role for endorectal balloons in prostate radiotherapy? A systematic review. Radiother Oncol: J Eur Soc Ther Radiol Oncol 95(3):277–282. doi:10.1016/j.radonc.2010.04.016

Sohayda C, Kupelian PA, Levin HS, Klein EA (2000) Extent of extracapsular extension in localized prostate cancer. Urology 55(3):382–386

Teh BS, Bastasch MD, Wheeler TM, Mai WY, Frolov A, Uhl BM, Lu HH, Carpenter LS, Chiu JK, McGary J, Woo SY, Grant WH 3rd, Butler EB (2003) IMRT for prostate cancer: defining target volume based on correlated pathologic volume of disease. Int J Radiat Oncol Biol Phys 56(1):184–191

van Herk M (2004) Errors and margins in radiotherapy. Semin Radiat Oncol 14(1):52–64. doi:10.1053/j.semradonc.2003.10.003

van Veggel BA, van Oort IM, Witjes JA, Kiemeney LA, Hulsbergen-van de Kaa CA (2011) Quantification of extraprostatic extension in prostate cancer: different parameters correlated to biochemical recurrence after radical prostatectomy. Histopathology 59(4):692–702. doi:10.1111/j.1365-2559.2011.03986.x

Wheeler TM, Dillioglugil O, Kattan MW, Arakawa A, Soh S, Suyama K, Ohori M, Scardino PT (1998) Clinical and pathological significance of the level and extent of capsular invasion in clinical stage T1–2 prostate cancer. Hum Pathol 29(8):856–862

Yeoh EE, Botten RJ, Butters J, Di Matteo AC, Holloway RH, Fowler J (2011) Hypofractionated versus conventionally fractionated radiotherapy for prostate carcinoma: final results of phase III randomized trial. Int J Radiat Oncol Biol Phys 81(5):1271–1278. doi:10.1016/j.ijrobp.2010.07.1984

Zietman AL, DeSilvio ML, Slater JD, Rossi CJ Jr, Miller DW, Adams JA, Shipley WU (2005) Comparison of conventional-dose vs high-dose conformal radiation therapy in clinically localized adenocarcinoma of the prostate: a randomized controlled trial. JAMA J Am Med Assoc 294(10):1233–1239. doi:10.1001/jama.294.10.1233

Value of Patient Immobilization in External Beam Radiotherapy for Prostate Cancer

Matthias Guckenberger

Contents

Abstract

Recent developments in external beam radiotherapy for prostate cancer (dose escalation, hypo fractionation) require more accurate treatment delivery. This chapter summarizes the value of external patient positioning devices as well as diets to reduce prostate position variability.

1 Introduction

The practice of external beam radiotherapy (EBRT) for localized prostate cancer has undergone substantial changes in the recent years. Several prospective trials consistently demonstrated improved biochemical control after treatment with escalated irradiation doses of 74–78 Gy. Studies with long-term follow-up suggest that this improved biochemical control transfers into improved freedom from distant metastases (Zelefsky et al. 2011) and cancer-specific survival (Kuban et al. 2011). The low alpha/beta ratio of prostate cancer was confirmed in a recent study based on almost 6,000 patients and was independent of the risk stratification and treatment with androgen deprivation (Miralbell et al. 2012). This further supports evaluation of hypo-fractionated protocol and early results are promising (Arcangeli et al. 2012; Dearnaley et al. 2012). The role of prophylactic pelvic irradiation remains controversial after two randomized trials. However, despite the lack of high-level evidence, pelvic irradiation is practiced by many centers based on surgical practice of extended lymph node dissection and experiences from other cancer types (Morikawa and Roach 2011), where prophylactic lymph node irradiation is standard of care.

All these recent developments—escalation of the irradiation dose, hypo-fractionation and pelvic irradiation—bear the risk of increased rates of toxicity. As a consequence, an improved accuracy of external beam radiotherapy (EBRT) is warranted to counterbalance all these

M. Guckenberger (✉)
Department of Radiation Oncology, University Hospital Zurich (USZ), Rämistrasse 100, CH-8091, Zurich, Switzerland
e-mail: Matthias.Guckenberger@usz.ch

H. Geinitz et al. (eds.), *Radiotherapy in Prostate Cancer*, Medical Radiology. Radiation Oncology,
DOI: 10.1007/174_2014_1008, © Springer-Verlag Berlin Heidelberg 2014
Published Online: 11 May 2014

potential detrimental effects. In principle, two technological strategies are currently explored in EBRT of prostate cancer: (1) reduction of inter-fractional and intra-fractional target position uncertainties to subsequently reduce safety margins and improve sparing of critical Organs-At-Risk (OAR); (2) improved conformity of the irradiation doses to the complex shaped target volumes in prostate cancer to minimize incidental irradiation of OARs.

2 Patient Positioning and External Patient Immobilization

Four randomized trials have been conducted, all addressing the issue of patient positioning and immobilization in prostate cancer.

Nuttling et al. (2000) compared a "conventional treatment position" (supine with a foam head pad and the ankles immobilized in ankle stocks) and an immobilization system, where a customized cushion supported the pelvis from the iliac crest to the upper thigh; a foam head pad and ankle stocks were used in analogy to conventional positioning. Thirty patients were randomly assigned to these two positioning systems and patient setup errors detected in electronic portal images (EPI) were the primary endpoints of this study. Based on a total of 1,600 EPIs, no statistically significant difference in systematic and random patient positioning errors were detected. Radiographers reported that patients found the immobilization device more comfortable, but when using the immobilization device, they noticed greater difficulty in patient positioning and alignment to skin tattoos. Based on the results of this study, the authors stopped the use of the immobilization device in their clinical practice.

Kneebone et al. (2003) randomly assigned 100 prostate or bladder cancer patients to either prone positioning with no immobilization devices or prone positioning using a customized Uvex cast of the pelvis as well as ankle- and shoulder-stabilizing devices. Patient setup errors based on the pelvic bony structures were evaluated in weekly acquired EPIs. The more rigid immobilization method significantly decreased setup error uncertainties: major deviations >10 mm were reduced from 31 to 11 %. Systematic errors especially in anterior-posterior direction were reduced by the more rigid immobilization (from 2.4 to 0.8 mm). No differences in patient comfort and total treatment time were reported between the two positioning procedures.

Bayley et al. (2004) asked the important question of supine versus prone patient positioning in prostate cancer. Twenty eight patients acted as their own controls: they were randomly assigned to start treatment in either supine position (immobilization in a customized Vac-Loc) or prone position (immobilization in a customized Hip-Fix); after midpoint of the irradiation course, treatment was re-planned and finished in the other position. In contrast to the previous two studies, prostate motion was analyzed via lateral EPIs of prostate implanted fiducial markers. The study clearly demonstrated that prostate motion in the anterior-posterior direction was significantly smaller in the supine position. Larger safety margins were required in prone position to account for this increased prostate motion, which then resulted in increased dose exposure of the OARs bladder, small bowel and rectum. Additionally, supine position was significantly more comfortable for the patients and setup was significantly easier for the radiation therapists.

Rosewall et al. (2008) evaluated inter- and intra-fraction prostate motion in a standard VacLok immobilization device or in the BodyFix system incorporating an abdominal compression element, which may reduce abdominal movement. Prostate motion was analyzed via daily pre and posttreatment assessment of prostate implanted markers in EPIs. In summary, immobilization in the BodyFix system with abdominal compression did not influence inter-fractional or inter-fractional prostate motion compared to a standard VacLok.

These four studies suggest that patients should be treated in supine position: advantages are reduced intra-fractional prostate motion, best patient comfort, and simultaneously easiest patient setup by the RTTs. No clear advantage of more advanced immobilization devices compared to a standard knee and ankle support could be demonstrated.

A potential benefit of any external patient positioning or immobilization device is limited by internal prostate motion independently from the bony anatomy of the pelvis. O'Daniel et al. (2006) calculated safety margins for patient setup based on skin marks and based on bone anatomy: prostate position errors were evaluated in CT re-simulations acquired 3 times per week. Safety margins calculated with the van Herk formula were 12.2 and 10.4 mm in anterior-posterior direction with the skin marks alignment and bone alignment technique, respectively. Similar results were reported by Beltran et al. (2008) in 40 prostate cancer patients: safety margins for compensation of inter-fractional prostate position errors were 9.8 and 10.7 mm for tattoo alignment and bone alignment, respectively.

All these results show limited value of external patient positioning and immobilization devices and clearly indicate the need for image guidance with direct verification of the prostate position to improve the accuracy of EBRT delivery.

Steenbakkers et al. (2004) however conducted an interesting study where supine patient positioning was evaluated with either legs flat on the treatment couch or with a knee support. The study was conducted in 10 male volunteers with MRI scans in the different treatment positions. The knee support shifted both the rectum and prostate dorsally but the shift was larger for the rectum resulting in an increased distance between the target and the OAR. This reduced dose exposure of the rectum.

The study by Steenbakkers et al. also demonstrated the impact of external patient positioning on the internal position and geometry of the target and OARs. Even in the era of IGRT, patient positioning should therefore be performed with care to avoid complex changes of the patient's anatomy, which cannot be corrected with a single couch shift.

3 Internal Prostate Immobilization Strategies

This chapter will not discuss active internal prostate immobilization strategies like the endorectal balloon, which will be addressed in another section of the book ("Internal immobilization—from rectal balloon to hyaluronic acid").

Diets and/or anti-flatulent medications have been analyzed by several groups: it is the hypothesis that diets and/or magnesia laxatives achieve a more regular bowel motion and reduce rectal gas and thereby reduce inter-fractional and intra-fractional prostate motion.

Initial promising results were reported by Smitsmans et al. (2008), where feces and (moving) gas occurrence in the cone-beam CT (CBCT) scans, the success rate of automatic software-based CT—CBCT image registration, and the statistics of prostate motion were assessed. A dietary protocol combined with magnesium oxide tablets was practiced in 26 patients and compared to a reference cohort of 23 patients without these interventions. Feces, gas, and moving gas was significantly decreased in the diet group, which also improved the feasibility of CBCT-based image guidance. However, inter-fractional prostate motion was not influenced by dietary intervention.

Further studies failed to demonstrate a reduction of inter-fractional (Lips et al. 2011; McNair et al. 2011) or intra-fractional (Nichol et al. 2010) prostate motion by diets and/or magnesia laxative. The largest study by Lips et al. (2011) evaluated dietary guidelines to obtain regular bowel movements and to reduce intestinal gas by avoiding certain foods and air swallowing. Intra-fractional prostate motion was assessed in 739 patients treated without the diet and 105 patients were treated with radiotherapy after introduction of the diet. No data about the compliance of the patients were available. Contrary to the hypothesis of the study, the median intra-fraction prostate motion per patient was increased after the introduction of the diet from 2.5 to 3.0 mm with the diet; the percentage of patients with clinically relevant intra-fraction motion increased significantly from 19.1 % without diet to 42.9 % with diet.

The same group of Lips et al. (Abdollah et al. 2012) conducted a double-blind placebo-controlled randomized clinical trial with magnesium oxide to reduce intra-fraction prostate motion. Ninety two patients were randomly assigned to either magnesium oxide (500 mg twice a day) or placebo during the course of radiotherapy. The primary outcome was intra-fraction prostate motion and quality of life and acute toxicity were secondary outcome measures. Intra-fractional prostate motion (treatment time 5–7 min) was assessed daily via imaging of implanted fiducial markers. The results confirmed previous retrospective studies: none of the primary or secondary endpoints showed a significant difference between the two study arms and the authors therefore concluded that there is no indication to use magnesium oxide in clinical practice. Again, the authors discussed either non-compliance or inefficacy of the magnesium oxide as reasons for the negative results of this study.

4 Conclusions

In conclusion, internal motion of the prostate independently of the pelvic bones is the major component of prostate position uncertainties. This issue cannot be addressed with rigid external positioning and immobilization devices. The current literature therefore suggests supine patient positioning with a knee and ankle support for improved patient comfort and reproducible patient setup by the RTTs. Diets and/or anti-flatulent medications did not result in decreased inter-fractional or intra-fractional prostate motion and cannot be recommended for routine clinical practice. However, even in the era of IGRT, patient positioning should be performed with care to avoid complex changes of the patients' internal anatomy.

References

Abdollah F, Suardi N, Cozzarini C, Gallina A, Capitanio U, Bianchi M, Sun M, Fossati N, Passoni NM, Fiorino C et al (2012) Selecting the optimal candidate for adjuvant radiotherapy after radical prostatectomy for prostate cancer: a long-term survival analysis. Eur Urol 63(6):998–1008

Arcangeli S, Strigari L, Gomellini S, Saracino B, Petrongari MG, Pinnaro P, Pinzi V, Arcangeli G (2012) Updated results and patterns of failure in a randomized hypofractionation trial for high-risk prostate cancer. Int J Radiat Oncol Biol Phys 84(5):1172–1178

Bayley AJ, Catton CN, Haycocks T, Kelly V, Alasti H, Bristow R, Catton P, Crook J, Gospodarowicz MK, McLean M et al (2004) A randomized trial of supine vs. prone positioning in patients undergoing escalated dose conformal radiotherapy for prostate cancer. Radiot Oncol J Eur Soc Ther Radiol Oncol 70(1):37–44

Beltran C, Herman MG, Davis BJ (2008) Planning target margin calculations for prostate radiotherapy based on intrafraction and interfraction motion using four localization methods. Int J Radiat Oncol Biol Phys 70(1):289–295

Dearnaley D, Syndikus I, Sumo G, Bidmead M, Bloomfield D, Clark C, Gao A, Hassan S, Horwich A, Huddart R et al (2012) Conventional versus hypofractionated high-dose intensity-modulated radiotherapy for prostate cancer: preliminary safety results from the CHHiP randomised controlled trial. Lancet Oncol 13(1):43–54

Kneebone A, Gebski V, Hogendoorn N, Turner S (2003) A randomized trial evaluating rigid immobilization for pelvic irradiation. Int J Radiat Oncol Biol Phys 56(4):1105–1111

Kuban DA, Levy LB, Cheung MR, Lee AK, Choi S, Frank S, Pollack A (2011) Long-term failure patterns and survival in a randomized dose-escalation trial for prostate cancer. Who dies of disease? Int J Radiat Oncol Biol Phys 79(5):1310–1317

Lips IM, Kotte AN, van Gils CH, van Leerdam ME, van der Heide UA, van Vulpen M (2011) Influence of antiflatulent dietary advice on intrafraction motion for prostate cancer radiotherapy. Int J Radiat Oncol Biol Phys 81(4):e401–e406

McNair HA, Wedlake L, McVey GP, Thomas K, Andreyev J, Dearnaley DP (2011) Can diet combined with treatment scheduling achieve consistency of rectal filling in patients receiving radiotherapy to the prostate? Radiot Oncol 101(3):471–478

Miralbell R, Roberts SA, Zubizarreta E, Hendry JH (2012) Dose-fractionation sensitivity of prostate cancer deduced from radiotherapy outcomes of 5,969 patients in seven international institutional datasets: alpha/beta = 1.4 (0.9-2.2) Gy. Int J Radiat Oncol Biol Phys 82(1):e17–e24

Morikawa LK, Roach M 3rd (2011) Pelvic nodal radiotherapy in patients with unfavorable intermediate and high-risk prostate cancer: evidence, rationale, and future directions. Int J Radiat Oncol Biol Phys 80(1):6–16

Nichol AM, Warde PR, Lockwood GA, Kirilova AK, Bayley A, Bristow R, Crook J, Gospodarowicz M, McLean M, Milosevic M et al (2010) A cinematic magnetic resonance imaging study of milk of magnesia laxative and an antiflatulent diet to reduce intrafraction prostate motion. Int J Radiat Oncol Biol Phys 77(4):1072–1078

Nutting CM, Khoo VS, Walker V, McNair H, Beardmore C, Norman A, Dearnaley DP (2000) A randomized study of the use of a customized immobilization system in the treatment of prostate cancer with conformal radiotherapy. Radiot Oncol J Eur Soc Ther Radiol Oncol 54(1):1–9

O'Daniel JC, Dong L, Zhang L, de Crevoisier R, Wang H, Lee AK, Cheung R, Tucker SL, Kudchadker RJ, Bonnen MD et al (2006) Dosimetric comparison of four target alignment methods for prostate cancer radiotherapy. Int J Radiat Oncol Biol Phys 66(3):883–891

Rosewall T, Chung P, Bayley A, Lockwood G, Alasti H, Bristow R, Kong V, Milosevic M, Catton C (2008) A randomized comparison of interfraction and intrafraction prostate motion with and without abdominal compression. Radiot Oncol J Eur Soc Ther Radiol Oncol 88(1):88–94

Smitsmans MH, Pos FJ, de Bois J, Heemsbergen WD, Sonke JJ, Lebesque JV, van Herk M (2008) The influence of a dietary protocol on cone beam CT-guided radiotherapy for prostate cancer patients. Int J Radiat Oncol Biol Phys 71(4):1279–1286

Steenbakkers RJ, Duppen JC, Betgen A, Lotz HT, Remeijer P, Fitton I, Nowak PJ, van Herk M, Rasch CR (2004) Impact of knee support and shape of tabletop on rectum and prostate position. Int J Radiat Oncol Biol Phys 60(5):1364–1372

Zelefsky MJ, Pei X, Chou JF, Schechter M, Kollmeier M, Cox B, Yamada Y, Fidaleo A, Sperling D, Happersett L et al (2011) Dose escalation for prostate cancer radiotherapy: predictors of long-term biochemical tumor control and distant metastases-free survival outcomes. Eur Urol 60(6):1133–1139

Internal Immobilization: From Rectal Balloon to Hyaluronic Acid

Gregor Goldner

Contents

Abstract

Within the last decades, numerous adoptions in prostate cancer radiotherapy were implemented. Advanced techniques such as image-guided radiotherapy and (volumetric) intensity-modulated radiotherapy (VMAT/IMRT) allowed to escalate dose resulting in local doses applied of ~80 Gy and more. However, dose escalation is limited by toxicity of normal tissues, especially anorectal toxicity and as a consequence various efforts to protect the rectum such as the use of an endorectal balloon or injection/insertion of a rectal spacer (hyaluronic acid, gel, biodegradable balloon) are performed.

1 Introduction

Within the last decades, numerous adoptions in prostate cancer radiotherapy were implemented. Advanced techniques such as image-guided radiotherapy and (volumetric) intensity-modulated radiotherapy (VMAT/IMRT) allowed to escalate dose resulting in local doses applied of ~80 Gy and more. However, dose escalation is limited by toxicity of normal tissues, especially anorectal toxicity and as a consequence various efforts to protect the rectum such as the use of an endorectal balloon or injection/insertion of a rectal spacer (hyaluronic acid, gel, biodegradable balloon) are performed.

2 Endorectal Balloon

Endorectal balloons (erB) are applied in external prostate radiotherapy since many years resulting in numerous articles addressing its issue. Smeenk et al. recently published a systematic review on the role of erB in prostate cancer radiotherapy (Smeenk et al. 2010). The main goal is to achieve immobilization of the prostate by reducing intrafractional and interfractional motion. Furthermore, due to

G. Goldner (✉)
Klinik für Strahlentherapie, MUW Wien, Allgemeines Krankenhaus, Währinger Gürtel 18–20, Wien 1090, Austria
e-mail: Gregor.Goldner@akhwien.at

H. Geinitz et al. (eds.), *Radiotherapy in Prostate Cancer*, Medical Radiology. Radiation Oncology,
DOI: 10.1007/174_2013_917, © Springer-Verlag Berlin Heidelberg 2013
Published Online: 7 September 2013

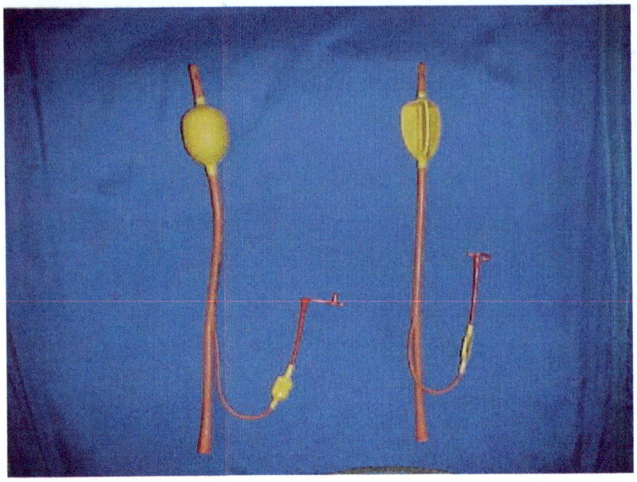

Fig. 1 Endorectal balloon filled with 40 ml air (*left*) and deflated (*right*)

distension of the rectum, the dose at the posterior rectal wall might be minimized; in addition radioprotection is discussed due to stretching of the rectal wall leading to hypoxia and due to lower dose at the air–rectum interface. However patients' tolerance, daily application, and reproducibility of position, impact on toxicity are topics being discussed.

2.1 Products

- Nordmann®, Rüsch AG, Germany (Fig. 1): is made of rubber coated by silkolatex, filled with 40–60 cc of air resulting in a diameter up to 4 cm. The balloon is 5 cm long and fixed on a 30 cm rectal tube
- QLrad B.V.®, Netherland: is made of silicon, filled with 80 cc of air resulting in a diameter up to 6 cm. The balloon is 3 cm long and fixed on a 20 cm shaft with stopper
- E-Z-EM®, USA: is made of silicon, filled with 60–100 cc of air resulting in a diameter of up to 6 cm. The balloon is 4–5 cm long and fixed on a 15 cm shaft
- Medrad®, USA: is made of latex, filled with 60–100 cc of air resulting in a diameter up to 4 cm. The balloon is 9 cm long and fixed on a 33 cm shaft.

2.2 Application and Patient's Tolerance

The erB is enveloped with a condom sheath and the condom is lubricated, the ensheathed erB is carefully inserted into the anorectum and then inflated with air for the daily treatment. In case of proton therapy the balloon is filled with water. The balloon catheter is then pulled back, such that the balloon seats itself against the anorectal junction to ensure reproducible position and, in case a stopper is available, the stopper is adjusted. To minimize patients discomfort during erB application local anaestetic gel might be used. After radiotherapy is finished the erB is deflated and gently removed. The whole workload needs about 2–3 min setup time (Van Lin et al. 2005; Patel et al. 2003) per fractionation.

Within an Austrian–German multicenter trial, patients acceptance of the erB was analyzed in 429 patients. No major complaints were reported in 79 % of the patients and erB application had to be stopped due to pain in 4 % of patients only. Patients reporting acute rectal side effects experienced significantly more erB discomfort (Goldner et al. 2006). In another study, the number of treatments in which the erB was tolerated was recorded. 3,561 patients received proton irradiation of the prostate and seminal vesicles with or without X-ray treatment of the pelvis. Only 2.4 % of patients refused the erB for 1 or more treatments. A significant tolerance advantage (99.5 % vs. 95.7 %.) in those who received protons alone (= local) compared with combination treatment (local + pelvic) could be detected (Ronson et al. 2006).

2.3 Immobilization

It is expected that erBs reduce intrafraction and interfraction motion of the prostate and as a consequence CTV—PTV margins might be minimized. Intrafraction motion was investigated by (Wang et al. 2012) measuring real-time prostate motion in 29 non-erB patients and 30 erB patients. Large motion up to 1 cm was only detected in the non-erB group. Prostate motion increased as a function of treatment time for displacements >2–8 mm for the non-erB group and >2–4 mm for the erB-group. The symmetrical internal margin could be reduced from 5 to 3 mm for 6 min treatment time and beyond 6 min treatment time this margin could be reduced from 9 to 5 mm. They concluded that the erB reduced internal margin in almost all directions, especially in the anterior-posterior direction. Likewise (Smeenk et al. 2012) observed a significant treatment time-related reduction of intrafraction motion with the erB. Prostate motion for 15 patients with erB was tracked in real time using an electronic tracking system and compared to 15 patients without erB. Within the first 2.5 min prostate displacements were negligible. After 10-min treatment time, intrafraction motion of >5 and >7 mm was found in 0.7 and 0.3 % in the erB-group compared to 4.6 and 1.4 % in the non-erB-group. Again the largest reduction of displacement was found in the anterior-posterior direction. Analyzing repeated CT-images with one minute intervals (D'Amico et al. 2001) found a reduced maximum prostate displacement in any direction from 4 to ≤1 mm by the use of a erB. With regard to interfractional motion Wachter et al. (2002) were able to demonstrate that maximum displacements of the prostate larger than 5 mm in the anterior-posterior direction was reduced from 80 to 20 % by the use of an erB. However, other studies were not able to confirm that interfraction motion can be reduced by the application of an erB (Van Lin et al. 2005; El-Bassiouni et al. 2006). Van Lin et al. (2005) found no differences in systematic and random prostate motion and concluded that erB application did not reduce interfraction prostate motion.

2.4 Reproducibility

Several reports addressed the question of the reproducibility of the erB position and its impact on the dose distribution within the treatment volume as well as the organs at risk. During radiation therapy for the treatment of prostate cancer erB position and the impact position interventions was investigated. Manual adjustment of the erB based on information of cone-beam CT resulted in increased dose coverage (D95) from 94 to 98 % and increased the similarity in shape of the prostate to the radiotherapy plan (Jones et al. 2012). The authors concluded that image-guided interventions in erB volume and/or position during prostate radiotherapy are necessary to ensure the delivery of the dose distribution as planned (Jones et al. 2012). High variations in erB position are found mainly in the superior—inferior direction (Ahmad et al. 2005; Ciernik et al. 2003). Using an erB with a stopper on the shaft might minimize this setup variations. Due to potential setup variations reduced dose at the prostate and or seminal vesicles might be caused. Image guidance (Cone-beam CT or portal imaging verification) should be performed to verify and if necessary adjust erB position. In case erB application has to be stopped a new treatment plan has to be performed.

2.5 Radioprotection of the Rectum/Rectal Wall

Beside immobilization the erB might as well serve for radioprotection of the rectum. Within external beam radiotherapy, dose reduction up to 15 % at 1–2 mm depth might be produced due to the tissue–air interface (The et al. 2005, 2002) and as a consequence dose at the rectal wall might decrease. (Van Lin et al. 2007) were able to demonstrate that the rectal mucosal regions receiving a dose >40 Gy showed less severe teleangiectasia when an erB was applied. This might be caused due to the tissue–air interface and/or due to hypoxia within the rectal wall caused by stretching and therefore resulting in radioresistance. The dosimetric consequences and rectal wall sparing effect of an erB in prostate cancer radiotherapy was investigated in several studies. The anterior part of the rectal wall, adjacent the peripheral zone of the prostate, will inevitably be in the high-dose region due to the safety margin needed regardless of treatment technique. However due to distension of the rectum, at least the posterior part of the rectal wall can be pushed away from the prostate and the high-dose region (Figs. 2, 3). A comparative study of three types of erBs was performed by van (Van Lin et al. 2005). A significant reduction of rectal wall volumes exposed to >50 Gy and >70 Gy could be detected with all types of erBs in case of 3D-CRT (four-field-box technique). The larger the volume of the balloon, the more reduction of rectal wall exposure could be achieved. However, in case of the use of IMRT technique no significant difference could be detected. A significant reduction of relative rectal wall volume at the posterior wall could also be detected by Wachter et al. using a 40 cc air filled balloon (Wachter et al. 2002) within

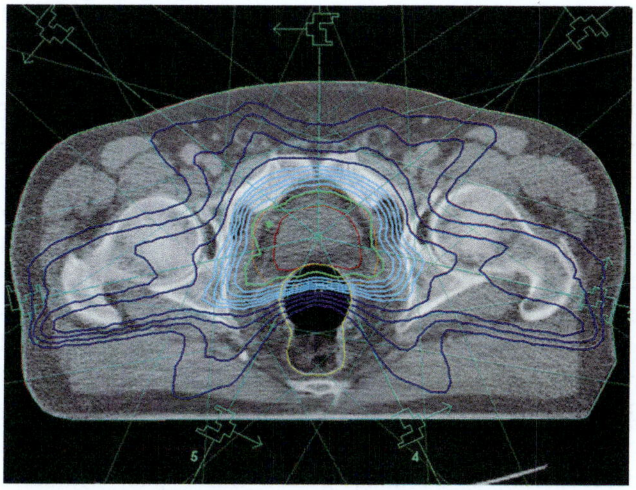

Fig. 2 Treatment plan: IMRT with endorectal balloon

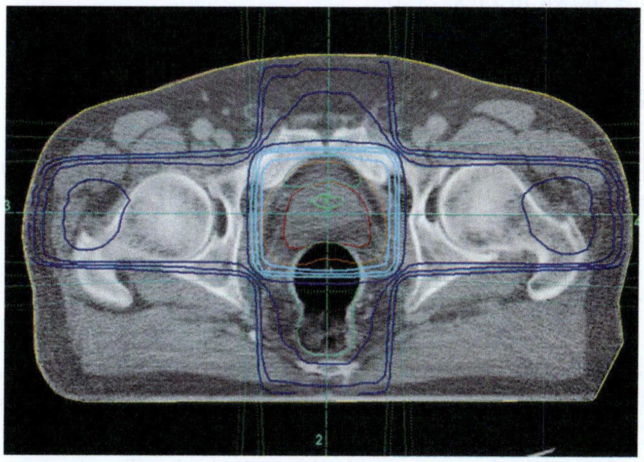

Fig. 3 Treatment plan: four-field box technique with endorectal balloon

patients treated by a four-field box technique for localized prostate cancer. Whereas, no statistically significant difference was observed at the anterior rectum wall, and in case the PTV included also the seminal vesicles the advantage of posterior rectal wall sparing was lost. Using a 60 cc air filled balloon, a significant reduction of rectal wall volume exposed to >60 Gy was also found by Patel et al. including the seminal vesicles into the CTV (Patel et al. 2003). Patel et al. analyzed dose-volume histograms with an inflated or deflated balloon with both three-dimensional (3D)-conformal and intensity-modulated radiation therapy. The erB resulted in a mean fractional high-dose rectal sparing of 39 %. In addition they could demonstrate that the use of an erB with a 3D-CRT plan produced about as much rectal dose sparing as an image-guided IMRT plan without a balloon, and inclusion of a balloon with IMRT produced further rectal sparing (treatment plans with an erB in place are shown in Figs. 2, 3).

2.6 Impact on Rectal Toxicity

Only one comparative study evaluating the impact of erB in regard of toxicity has been performed until now. Analyzing toxicity rates and endoscopic verified mucosal changes of the rectum (Van Lin et al. 2007) compared 24 patients with erB to 24 patients without erB within a prospective study treating patients up to 67,5 Gy. The acute urinary and rectal side effects were similar for the erB and non-erB group. Late urinary toxicity in both groups was mild with no Grade $\geq$3 and was comparable for both groups. Late rectal toxicity (Grade $\geq$1) was significantly higher for the non-erB group (5/24 vs 14/24 patients; $p = 0.003$) and rectal bleeding was detected in 13 % in the erB group compared to 33 % in the non-erB group (p = 0.17). A total of 146 endoscopies and 2,336 mucosal areas were investigated. Significantly, less high-grade telangiectasia was observed in the erB group at the lateral and posterior part of the rectal wall. However, Van Lin et al. concluded that longer follow-up and more comparative studies are necessary.

Toxicity data on dose escalation for localized prostate cancer patients compared 66–70 Gy and 74 Gy within one single institution. All patients were treated by four-field box technique using an erB. Including a total of 398 patients they reported on low rates of grade 3 rectal and urogenital toxicity (1, 5 and 3, 3 %) after a median follow-up of 64 months (Goldner et al. 2009). The same group reported on 178 primary prostate cancer patients treated within an Austrian–German multicenter trial by three-dimensional radiotherapy up to a local dose of 70 Gy or 74 Gy using an erB. After a median follow-up of 74 months the 5-year actuarial incidence rates for GI/GU grade $\geq$2 side effects were 19 and 23 % (Schmid et al. 2012).

2.7 Summary

The erB is used within daily prostate cancer radiotherapy in various departments. Intrafractional prostate motion seems to be reduced by the use of an erB. With regard to interfractional prostate motion not all reports were able to confirm a displacement reduction. However, position verification and correction protocols have still to be performed to avoid large variations. Radioprotection is discussed due to distension of the rectum, due to stretching of the rectal wall leading to hypoxia and due to the tissue–air interface. Endorectal balloons may therefore lead to reduced rectal toxicity. But further clinical comparative studies are necessary to confirm this hypothesis.

3 Rectal Spacer: Hyaluronic Acid (HA), Space OAR Gel, Biodegradable Balloon

Within the last years, different tools have been tested and implemented to reduce radiation of the rectum by increasing the spatial separation toward the prostate in order to reduce radiation dose even at the anterior rectal wall and as a consequence rectal toxicity. Morancy et al. reported within a small pilot study including three patients about injection of patient's blood between the rectum and the prostate. However, only moderate separation was achieved and stability of distance lasted just for one week (Morancy et al. 2008). Hyaluronic acid, Space OAR gel, or biodegradable balloons are used to create a longer lasting protective distance to the rectal wall resulting in lower doses applied during the whole treatment course within external radiotherapy. The number of reports is limited but steadily rising. Most of these articles are dealing about applicability, stability, reduction of rectal dose-volume exposure, and impact on acute toxicity.

3.1 Products

- Space OAR™ System, Augmenix, USA: is a polyethylene glycol based gel consisting of two components which are simultaneously injected and then polymerize within 10 s into a soft hydrogel.
- Hyaluronic Acid, Hyalgan, Sanofi Aventis USA/Synvisc Genzyme Corporation, USA: is a modified degradable polysaccharide.

- ProSpace® (BioProtect Ltd, Israel) is a biodegradable and inflatable interstitial balloon made of a polymer called poly (lactide-co-ecaprolactone).

3.2 Application

The application has to be performed under local, spinal, or light general anesthesia into the perirectal space between Denonvilliers fascia and the anterior rectal wall under transrectal ultrasound (TRUS) guidance in lithotomy position. Care has to be taken to avoid injection into the rectal wall. A needle is advanced transperineally and following hydrodissection with a saline solution the gel is injected. In case of hydrogel application procedure is limited by the short time of chemical reaction of the two components. In case a biodegradable balloon is used ,an introducer is placed and 5–10 cc saline is injected to create space for subsequent balloon inflation. The inflated balloon might be deflated and replaced if misspositioned.

3.3 Reproducibility/Stability and Radioprotection of the Rectum/ Rectal Wall

Clinical reports about the biodegradable balloon are limited so far (Kovacs et al. 2010; Levy et al. 2009; Melchert et al. 2013). Levy et al. (2009) reported about the proper functionality of the insertion-mounting device as well as the balloon capability to retain its inflated form. Within a multicenter study Melchert et al. were able to demonstrate a remarkable reduction of rectal volume exposed to higher radiation dose comparing dose-volume histograms prior and after insertion of the biodegradable balloon in 26 patients (Melchert et al. 2013).

Already in 2007 (Prada et al. 2009) reported on 27 patients receiving external and HDR-brachytherapy boost. Before the second HDR fraction 6 mL of hyaluronic acid (HA) was injected under TRUS guidance in the perirectal fat creating a space between the rectum and prostate of 2.0 cm. For the HDR boost dose of 1150 cGy, the mean Dmax at the rectum was reduced from 708 to 507 cGy ($p<0.001$). The hyaluronic acid did not migrate or change in mass/shape for close to 1 year. In 2009 the same group compared 36 prostate cancer patients receiving permanent interstitial brachytherapy with HA to 33 patients without (Prada et al. 2009). After a median follow-up of 18 months 5 % of patients with HA vs 36 % of patients without showed endoscopic verified rectal mucosal changes, and rectal bleeding was found in 0 vs 12 % of patients. Recently, the same group reported on 40 patients receiving HDR-monotherapy with 19 Gy after transperineal HA injection experiencing no acute toxicity Grade ≥2 was observed (Prada et al. 2012).

Wilder et al. (2010) measured in 10 patients the anteroposterior dimensions of cross-linked hyaluronan gel during high-dose rate brachytherapy (22 Gy) combined with intensity-modulated radiation therapy (50, 4 Gy). The mean distance at the start was 13 mm compared to 10 mm at the end. None of the 10 patients reported acute diarrhea according to the National Cancer Institute Common Terminology Criteria for Adverse Events (NCI CTCAE v 3.0.) Whereas, a control group of 239 patients receiving the same treatment without rectal spacer reported 2.5 % Grade ≥2 acute diarrhea. The mean rectal IMRT doses per fraction were reduced from 1.05 to 0.74 Gy with hyalform (Wilder et al. 2011).

Hatiboglu et al. (2012) analyzed 27 patients receiving hydrogel injection with regard to space creation, stability of spacer, duration of procedure, and reduction of rectal dose for prostate cancer patients receiving IMRT up to 78 Gy. Before hydrogel insertion the mean space between prostate and rectum was about 5 mm compared to about 15 mm after insertion, resulting in a space creation of 10 mm. The hydrogel stayed stable for 3 months and was absorbed after 6 months. The injection procedure time from TRUS insertion to removal was 16 min. The mean rectal V70 was reduced from 14.6 to 5.8 %. Evaluating 15 patients (Pinkawa et al. 2013) found a stable distance between the prostate and anterior rectal wall during the radiotherapy course (before/end) after injection of the hydrogel spacer with a mean distance of 1.6/1.5 cm at the base; 1.2/1.3 cm in the middle and 1.0/1.1 cm at the apex. Furthermore, dosimetric comparisons based on CT scans prior and after injection of hydrogel were also performed by Pinkawa et al. (2011) treating 18 patients up to 78 Gy. Regardless of treatment technique (3D-CRT four-field technique or IMRT), a significant reduction of rectal dose could be achieved. Relative rectum volumes within the 50–76 Gy isodoses were reduced by 30–67 % in 3D-CRT and by 22–89 % in IMRT treatment plans, respectively.

The impact of such spacer with regard to quality of life was analyzed in two papers. (Pinkawa et al. 2012) performed a match pair comparison of patients treated by either 3D conformal radiotherapy (70.2 Gy) alone, intensity-modulated radiotherapy (76 Gy) alone, or hydrogel spacer with intensity-modulated radiotherapy (76–78 Gy) with 28 patients in each subgroup. Using a validated questionnaire (Expanded Prostate Cancer Index Composite) patients were surveyed before, at the last day and 2–3 months after radiotherapy. Bowel bother scores were only significantly different in comparison to baseline levels in the spacer group. However more patients in the spacer group were bothered by uncontrolled bowel movements, which might be caused due to irritation of the anal sphincter. (Wilder et al. 2011) were able to demonstrate decreased bowel bother scores in patients receiving hyalform spacer in 35 patients receiving intensity-modulated radiotherapy and high-dose rate brachytherapy compared to a control group of 5 patients without hyalform. Within a multi-institutional phase II trial 52 patients received IMRT (78 Gy) after injection of an absorbable hydrogel (Uhl et al. 2013). The authors reported that 12 % of the patients (6/48) had acute Grade 2 intestinal side effects. Within a first analysis regarding "early" late toxicity after 12-month follow-up none of the 27 evaluated patients suffered from $\geq$ grade 2 gastrointestinal side effects.

3.4 Summary

Absorbable spacers placed between the prostate and the rectum prior to prostate cancer radiotherapy offer the possibility to reduce dose at the rectum. In contrast to the endorectal balloon this reduction of dose is also involving the anterior rectal wall. It could be demonstrated that these spacers are sufficiently long stable to maintain the space during the whole course of radiotherapy. Application has to be performed under anesthesia due to its invasive character. The aim of such spacer is to minimize rectal toxicity and/or to escalate dose further. However, dose escalation is not only limited by the rectum but also by other normal tissues within or surrounding the PTV (e.g., urethra, bladder, and anal sphincter). Patients receiving external radiotherapy and/or brachytherapy showed favorable rectal dose-volume parameters after implantation of such temporary spacers. Acute rectal toxicity rates could be minimized however data on late rectal toxicity have to follow.

References

Ahmad S, Vlachaki MT, Teslow TN et al (2005) Impact of setup uncertainty in the dosimetry of prostate and surrounding tissues in prostate cancer patients treated with Peacock/IMRT. Med Dosim 30:1–7

Ciernik IF, Baumert BG, Egil P et al (2003) Online correction of beam portals in the treatment of prostate cancer using an endorectal balloon device. Radiother Oncol 67:285–294

D'Amico AV, Manola J, Loffredo M et al (2001) A practical method to achieve prostate gland immobilization and target verification for daily treatment. Int J Radiat Oncol Biol Phys 51:1431–1436

El-Bassiouni M, Davis JB, El-Attar I et al (2006) Target motion variability and on-line positioning accuracy during external-beam radiation therapy of prostate cancer with an endorectal balloon device. Strahlenther Onkol 182:531–536

Goldner G, Geinitz H, Wachter S et al (2006) 3D-conformal radiotherapy of localized prostate cancer within an Austrian-German multicenter trial: a prospective study of patients' acceptance of the rectal balloon during treatment. Wien Klin Wochenschr 118:224–229

Goldner G, Dimopoulos J, Kirisits C et al (2009) Moderate dose escalation in three-dimensional conformal localized prostate cancer radiotherapy single-institutional experience in 398 patients comparing 66 Gy versus 70 Gy versus 74 Gy. Strahlenther Onkol 185:438–445

Hatiboglu G, Pinkawa M, Vallee JP et al (2012) Application technique: placement of a prostate-rectum spacer in men undergoing prostate radiation therapy. BJU Int 110:E647–E652

Jones BL, GAn G, Diot Q et al (2012) Dosimetric and deformation effects of image-guided interventions during stereotactic body radiation therapy of the prostate using an endorectal balloon. Med Phys 39:3080–3088

Kovacs G, Scarzello G, Koiziol I et al (2010) Significant rectal dose reduction during prostate cancer radiotherapy using novel biodegradeable inflatable balloon system: interim results of a prospective multi center study. Int J Radiat Oncol Biol Phys 78:S77

Levy Y, Paz A, Yosef RB et al (2009) Biodegradable inflatable balloon for reducingradiation adverse effects in prostate cancer. J Biomed Mater Res B Appl Biomater 91:855–867

Melchert C, Gez E, Bohlen G et al (2013) Interstitial biodegradable balloon for reduced rectal dose during prostate radiotherapy: results of a virtual planning investigation based on the pre- and post-implant imaging data of an international multicenter study. Radiother Oncol 106:210–214

Morancy TJ, Winkfield KM, Karasiewicz CA et al (2008) Use of a blood-patch technique to reduce rectal dose during cesium-131 prostate brachytherapy. Int J Radiat Oncol Biol Phys 72:331–332

Patel RR, Orton N, Tomé WA et al (2003) Rectal dose sparing with a balloon catheter and ultrasound localization in conformal radiation therapy for prostate cancer. Radiother Oncol 67:285–294

Pinkawa M, Corral NE, Caffaro M et al (2011) Application of a spacer gel to optimize three-dimensional conformal and intensity modulated radiotherapy for prostate cancer. Radiother Oncol 100:436–441

Pinkawa M, Piroth MD, Holy R et al (2012) Quality of life after intensity-modulated radiotherapy for prostate cancer with a hydrogel. Strahlenther Onkol 188:917–925

Pinkawa M, Piroth MD, Holy R et al (2013) Spacer stability and prostate position variability during radiotherapy for prostate cancer applying a hydrogel to protect the rectal wall. Radiother Oncol 106:220–224

Prada PJ, Fernandez J, Martinez AA et al (2007) Transperineal injection of hyaluronic acid in anterior perirectal fat to decrease rectal toxicity from radiation delivered with intensity modulated brachytherapy or EBRT for prostate cancer patients. Int J Radiat Oncol Biol Phys 69:95–102

Prada PJ, Gonzalez H, Menendez C et al (2009) Transperineal injection of hyaluronic acid in anterior perirectal fat to decrease rectal toxicity from radiation delivered with low-dose-rate brachytherapy for prostate cancer patients. Brachytherapy 8:210–217

Prada PJ, Jiminez I, Gonzalez-Suarez H et al (2012) High dose rate interstitial brachytherapy as monotherapy in one fraction and transperineal hyaluronic acid injection into the perirectal fat for the treatment of favourable stage prostate cancer: treatment description and preliminary results. Brachytherapy 11:105–110

Ronson BB, Yonemoto LT, Rossi CJ et al (2006) Patient tolerance of rectal balloons in conformal radiation treatment of prostate cancer. Int J Radiat Oncol Biol Phys 64:1367–1370

Schmid MP, Pötter R, Bombosch V et al (2012) Late gastrointestinal and urogenital side-effects after radiotherapy—Incidence and prevalence. Subgroup-analysis within the prospective Austrian–German phase II multicenter trial for localized prostate cancer. Radiother Oncol 104:114–118

Smeenk RJ, Teh BS, Butler EB et al (2010) Is there a role for endorectal balloons in prostate radiotherapy? A syst rev Radiother Oncol 95:277–282

Smeenk RJ, Louwe RJW, Langen KM et al (2012) An endorectal balloon reduces intrafraction prostate motion during radiotherapy. Int J Radiat Oncol Biol Phys 83:661–669

The BS, McGary JE, Dong L et al (2002) The use of rectal balloon during the delivery of intensity modulated radiation therapy (IMRT) for prostate cancer: more than just aprostate gland immobilization device? Cancer J 8:476–483

The BS, Dong L, McGary JE et al (2005) Rectal wall sparing by dosimetric effect of rectal balloon used during intensity-modulated radiation therapy (IMRT) for prostate cancer. Med Dosim 30:25–30

Uhl M, van Triest B, Eble MJ et al (2013) Low rectal toxicity after dose escalated IMRT treatment of prostate cancer using absorbable hydrogel for increasing and maintaining space between the rectum and prostate: results of a multi-institutional phase II trial. Radiother Oncol 106:215–219

Van Lin EN, van der Vight LP, Witjes JA et al (2005a) The effect of an endorectal balloon and off-line correction on the interfraction systematic and random prostate position variations: a comparative study. Int J Radiat Oncol Biol Phys 61:278–288

Van Lin EN, Hoffmann AL, van Kollenburg P et al (2005b) Rectal wall sparing effect of three different endorectal balloons in 3D conformal and IMRT prostate radiotherapy. Int J Radiat Oncol Biol Phys 63:565–576

Van Lin EN, Kristinsson J, Philippens ME et al (2007) Reduced late rectal mucosal changes after prostate three-dimensional conformal radiotherapy with endorectal balloon as observed in repeated endoscopy. Int J Radiat Oncol Biol Phys 67:799–811

Wachter S, Gerstner N, Dorner D et al (2002) The influence of a rectal balloon tube as internal immobilization device on variations of volumes and dose volume histograms during treatment course of conformal radiotherapy for prostate cancer. Int J Radiat Oncol Biol Phys 52:91–100

Wang KK, Vapiwala N, Deville C et al (2012) A study to quantify the effectiveness of daily endorectal balloon for prostate intrafraction motion management. Int J Radiat Oncol Biol Phys 83:1055–1063

Wilder RB, Barme GA, Gilbert RF et al (2010) Cross-linked hyaluronan gel reduces the acute rectal toxicity of radiotherapy for prostate cancer. Int J Radiat Oncol Biol Phys 77:824–830

Wilder RB, Barme GA, Gilbert RF et al (2011) Cross-linked hyaluronan gel improves the quality of life of prostate cancer patients undergoing radiotherapy. Brachytherapy 10:44–50

Part II

Clinical Endpoints

Biochemical Recurrence: A Valuable Endpoint?

Tanja Langsenlehner

Contents

T. Langsenlehner (✉)
Department of Therapeutic Radiology and Oncology, Medical University of Graz, Auenbruggerplatz 32, 8036 Graz, Austria
e-mail: tanja.langsenlehner@medunigraz.at

Abstract

Clinically relevant outcomes such as distant metastases and death from prostate cancer do not occur for many years after definitive treatment for localized prostate cancer. In view of the long natural history of prostate cancer, the identification and validation of surrogate endpoints that can be measured earlier and correlate with clinical progression or survival are of great utility in clinical cancer research. With the introduction of prostate-specific antigen (PSA) as a marker in the mid-1980s, PSA has become an important tool for monitoring disease progression following definitve treatment of localized prostate cancer and the concept of "biochemical" recurrence, an event that precedes clinical recurrence by many years, has been developed. Biochemical failure has become widely accepted to evaluate the effectiveness of definitive local therapies and is used for both research and clinical purposes. Biochemical recurrence has been investigated as a prognostic factor and as a potential surrogate endpoint in different stages of disease; however, on the basis of conflicting results from previous studies, a consensus on the ability of biochemical failure to act as a reliable surrogate endpoint for clinical progression and survival has not yet been reached.

1 Definition of Biochemical Failure

Depending on the type of therapy, the level of PSA which would be defined as indicating disease recurrence varies. Many investigators have examined the appropriate definition of biochemical recurrence for clinical purposes and a large number of different definitions of biochemical recurrence have been published (Cookson et al. 2007; Stephenson et al. 2006). However, strict definitions for biochemical recurrence are necessary to identify men at risk for disease progression and to allow comparisons among patients treated similarly.

H. Geinitz et al. (eds.), *Radiotherapy in Prostate Cancer*, Medical Radiology. Radiation Oncology,
DOI: 10.1007/174_2013_904,

Published Online: 8 August 2013

1.1 Biochemical Recurrence After Radical Prostatectomy

The most useful definition of biochemical recurrence provides a close correlation of biochemical recurrence with clinical endpoints such as prostate cancer metastasis or death from prostate cancer and should thus lead to a suitable balance between early detection and treatment of prostate cancer patients otherwise destined to experience clinical disease progression (i.e., high sensitivity) and avoidance of unnecessary treatment of men who would not develop disease recurrence (i.e., good specificity) (Cookson et al. 2007; Nielsen and Partin 2007).

Following radical prostatectomy, the serum PSA level should become undetectable within 6 weeks of surgery as its source of production has been removed. Thus, a detectable PSA following radical prostatectomy implies residual prostate tissue and most likely residual or recurrent prostate cancer.

Several cutpoints for determining PSA recurrence after radical prostatectomy have been investigated (Freedland et al. 2003). For patients with postoperative PSA levels between 0.01 and 0.1 ng/mL, Freedland and colleagues have shown that the risk of developing a PSA value higher than 0.1 ng/mL was 36 % at 1 year and 67 % at 3 years. Among patients with postoperative PSA levels of 0.2–0.3 ng/mL, the 1- and 3-year risks of additional PSA progression were 86 and 100 %, respectively. This led to their conclusion that 0.2 ng/mL represents the most reliable cutpoint to define PSA recurrence after radical prostatectomy.

In contrast, Amling and colleagues found 3-year rates of PSA progression in only 49 % of patients with a PSA level of 0.2 ng/mL and a PSA progression rate of 72 % in patients with PSA levels above 0.4 ng/mL (Amling et al. 2001). These findings have shown that men with low but detectable postoperative PSA values may not develop additional increases in PSA.

Stephenson and colleagues performed multivariate regression analyses on a series of 10 candidate definitions of biochemical failure after prostatectomy, testing their associations with the subsequent development of distant metastases (Stephenson et al. 2006). They demonstrated that a PSA level of 0.4 ng/mL and rising after prostatectomy best correlated with the development of distant metastases.

Given the high degree of variability that exists in the prostate cancer literature, in 2007, the American Urological Association (AUA) Prostate Cancer Guidelines Update Panel has recommended a standard definition for biochemical recurrence after radical prostatectomy based on a literature review of studies published from 1991 to 2004. Based on its clinical utility as a sensitive and portable marker for disease recurrence, the Panel selected a value of PSA for defining recurrence and recommended that biochemical (PSA) recurrence following radical prostatectomy should be defined as a serum PSA of $\geq$0.2 ng/mL, with a second confirmatory level of PSA of $\geq$0.2 ng/mL. The first postoperative PSA should be obtained between 6 weeks and 3 months following therapy (Cookson et al. 2007).

1.2 Biochemical Recurrence After Radiotherapy

With radiation, the prostate remains intact and still produces at least a small amount of PSA which can vary with conditions such as prostatitis, the "bounce" phenomenon, gland size, and length of time from treatment.

In a Consensus Conference sponsored by the American Society for Therapeutic Radiology and Oncology (ASTRO) in 1996 to establish a definition of biochemical failure after external beam radiotherapy (EBRT), biochemical failure was defined as three consecutive PSA rises after a nadir with the date of failure as the point halfway between the nadir date and the first rise or any rise great enough to prompt initiation of secondary (salvage) treatment (American Society for Therapeutic Radiology and Oncology Consensus Panel 1997).

Subsequent studies illuminated a number of fundamental methodological limitations of this definition, and several alternative candidate definitions of failure have been presented in the literature (Horwitz et al. 2005; Kuban et al. 2005). The Consensus Panel's requirement for 3 consecutive rises in PSA made the ASTRO definition highly sensitive to the duration and frequency of follow-up. Indeed, the Panel later recommended a minimum period of observation of 2 years, with PSA measurements quarterly for the first 2 years and semi-annually thereafter. Furthermore, the ASTRO definition was not linked to clinical progression or survival and developed to address EBRT monotherapy only. Another shortcoming was the potential for false positives secondary to "benign PSA bounces".

In January 2005, a second Consensus Conference was sponsored by ASTRO and the Radiation Therapy Oncology Group (RTOG) in Phoenix, Arizona in order to address the above-mentioned shortcomings of the ASTRO definition including, most importantly, the lack of correlation with clinical endpoints. The expert panel reviewed numerous candidate definitions of failure using data from multiple institutions in which patients were treated with brachytherapy and/or external beam radiation with or without hormonal treatment, with priority on their specificity for predicting subsequent clinical outcomes (local failure, distant failure, initiation of hormonal therapy or PSA >25 ng/mL).

On the basis of this strategy, the panel recommended definition of biochemical recurrence as "(1) a rise by 2 ng/mL or more above the nadir PSA be considered the standard definition for biochemical failure after EBRT with or without

HT; (2) the date of failure be determined "at call" (not backdated)" (Roach et al. 2006). Patients undergoing salvage therapies such as androgen deprivation therapy, radical prostatectomy, brachytherapy, or cryosurgery not meeting these PSA criteria for failure were also recommended to be declared as failures at the time a positive biopsy is obtained or salvage therapy is administered.

The panel also recommended that investigators be allowed to use the ASTRO Consensus Definition after EBRT alone (no hormonal therapy) with strict adherence to guidelines including "adequate follow-up" but recommended the use of the ASTRO consensus definition to be considered inappropriate when comparing patients treated with radiotherapy and hormonal therapy to those treated without hormonal therapy.

2 Biochemical Recurrence as a Surrogate Marker of Prostate Cancer Disease Progression in Clinical Trials

Due to the long survival time of prostate cancer patients, clinical trials of prostate cancer, especially those evaluating treatments for clinically localized disease that are designed with primary endpoints of overall or prostate cancer—specific survival, require long follow-up periods. Biochemical progression can be measured after a shorter follow-up time. In recent years, an increasing number of randomized clinical studies investigating modern local therapies for localized prostate cancer has been reported using freedom from biochemical failure as primary endpoint, however, data on clinical outcomes or survival are limited.

2.1 Biochemical Recurrence After Dose-Escalated Radiotherapy

A number of studies provide evidence for the efficacy of dose-escalation in prostate cancer, and mature results from randomized trials show that disease control using a PSA end point improves with increasing radiation dose (Kuban et al. 2008; Peeters et al. 2006; Sathya et al. 2005; Zietman et al. 2010). To date, no randomized trial has documented a survival advantage attributable to escalated radiation doses.

In 2011, Kuban and colleagues reported long-term failure patterns as well as survival rates using data from the M.D. Anderson randomized dose-escalation trial for prostate cancer (Kuban et al. 2011). They observed that higher pretreatment PSA (>10 ng/mL) and high-risk patients who were treated to the lower 70 Gy dose had nearly twice as many PSA failures and more than four times as many distant failures. These patients also had a significantly higher risk of dying from prostate cancer. For overall survival, no significant difference was found between patients treated with 70 Gy and those treated with 78 Gy, even in case of high-risk disease or pretreatment PSA >10 ng/mL.

PSA failure increased the risk of death for the population as a whole, however, PSA recurrence alone did not equate to disease-related death within 10 years for the majority of patients. The authors observed that patients at highest risk of dying from prostate cancer were characterized by a shorter median interval from treatment to biochemical failure, and a more rapid PSA doubling time during that interval, furthermore, they had high Gleason scores (9–10), and a PSA >10.5 ng/mL at diagnosis.

2.2 PSA Recurrence and Hypofractionation

Data from prospective randomized trials to investigate moderate hypofractionation have already been published and doses used in these trials ranged from 75.6 to 80 Gy (1.8–2 Gy per fraction) in the conventionally fractionated arm versus 62–72 Gy with 2.4–3.1 Gy per fraction in the hypofractionated treatment arm (Arcangeli et al. 2010; Kuban et al. 2010; Pollack et al. 2011). In two trials, no difference in freedom from biochemical failures was reported after median follow-up times of about 5 years. In contrast, the early results by Arcangeli and colleagues who compared hypofractionation with a conventionally fractionated dose-escalated (80 Gy) schedule showed a significant improvement in freedom from biochemical failures at 3 years in the hypofractionation arm (Arcangeli et al. 2010).

In an update of the results, the increase in the freedom from biochemical failure became insignificant, furthermore, a difference in freedom from local failure and freedom from distant failure was not observed. Only for patients with a pretreatment PSA level of 20 ng/mL or less, an increase in the 5-year rates of freedom from biochemical failure, freedom from local failure and freedom from distant failure was found in subgroup analysis (Arcangeli et al. 2012).

The use of biochemical failure as an endpoint in hypofractionation trials has been discussed controversially. Improvement of biochemical control does not necessarily mean better local tumor control because PSA failure does not indicate whether failure is local or distant. It has therefore been suggested that the α/β ratio should more appropriately be evaluated by long-term results of freedom from local failure as freedom from biochemical failure can be affected, particularly in high-risk disease, by the presence of occult metastases before treatment (Arcangeli et al. 2012).

2.3 Radiotherapy for Biochemical Recurrence After Radical Prostatectomy

Accumulating evidence indicates that postoperative radiotherapy to the prostate bed favorably influences the course of disease in men with adverse pathologic features. To date, three phase 3 randomized trials of adjuvant radiotherapy versus observation have reported improved freedom from biochemical recurrence and local control (Bolla et al. 2005; Thompson et al. 2009; Wiegel et al. 2009). In SWOG 8794, adjuvant radiotherapy has been associated with improved metastasis-free survival and overall survival whereas in EORTC 22911, an impact on these end points has not been demonstrated.

However, prostate cancer differs from most other malignancies because of its slowly developing nature and even resection of prostate cancer with positive surgical margins is not always followed by rapid biochemical recurrence.

With the use of salvage RT, therapy- and treatment-related complications are limited to patients who have evidence of biochemical recurrence. In contrast to adjuvant radiotherapy, no evidence from prospective randomized trials currently shows that salvage radiotherapy improves freedom from biochemical recurrence, local failure, distant metastasis, cancer-specific survival, or overall survival but several observational studies have reported durable responses to salvage radiotherapy in a substantial proportion of high-risk patients and reduced prostate cancer-specific mortality.

The optimal PSA cut point at which to administer salvage radiotherapy is poorly defined, although it appears salvage RT should be given at the earliest signs of PSA recurrence, once the clinician is convinced a rising PSA trend represents recurrent cancer. Currently, it is recommended to offer salvage radiotherapy before the postoperative PSA reaches 0.5 ng/ml (Stephenson et al. 2012).

However, previous findings have shown that men with low but detectable postoperative PSA values may not have additional increases in PSA, additionally the majority of patients with biochemical recurrence will not develop a local recurrence or distant disease. Therefore, a thorough patient and physician discussion regarding risks and benefits is strongly recommended and clinical decision to initiate treatment should be individualized based on overall patient risk factors and the use of other prognostic tools such as nomograms considering tumor Gleason grade, pathological stage, and PSA kinetics (Amling et al. 2001; Stephenson et al. 2006, 2012).

2.4 Comparison of Local Therapies using a PSA Endpoint

Given the absence of randomized clinical trials that directly compare different treatment modalities, physicians and patients have to rely largely upon the use of retrospective studies to compare treatment results. The comparison of outcomes from studies involving surgery (radical prostatectomy or robotic radical prostatectomy), external beam radiotherapy (3-dimensional conformal radiotherapy, intensity modulated radiotherapy, protons), brachytherapy, cryotherapy or high intensity focused ultrasound remains problematic due to the nonuniformity of reporting results. Furthermore, technical advances in these treatments have made long-term comparisons difficult.

Endpoints other than PSA based such as survival are subject to variables including patient age, comorbidities, aggressive nature of the disease, etc., may be completely independent of the treatment given and lead to false conclusions about a treatment's efficacy to eradicate all of the disease. By some investigators, biochemical progression-free survival has been suggested to be less dependent on confounding variables and to more appropriately reflect the efficacy of the treatment in eradicating disease (Grimm et al. 2012).

Recently, a comparative analysis of PSA relaps-free survival outcomes was performed by Grimm and colleagues to evaluate the effectiveness of different local treatment approaches including surgery, external beam radiation (conformal, intensity modulated radiotherapy, protons), brachytherapy, cryotherapy, or high intensity focused ultrasound (Grimm et al. 2012). The authors reported that in terms of biochemical progression-free survival, brachytherapy provided superior outcome in patients with low-risk disease. For intermediate-risk disease, the combination of EBRT and brachytherapy appeared equivalent to brachytherapy alone. For high-risk patients, combination therapies involving EBRT and brachytherapy plus or minus androgen deprivation therapy appeared superior to seed implant alone, surgery alone, or EBRT.

Major limitations of such an approach that have to be taken into account include differences in the PSA kinetics and differences in accepted standards of biochemical success or failure following the different modalities of primary local therapy. Given these limitations, findings from studies comparing biochemical recurrence-free survival outcomes following surgery and radiation for clinically localized prostate cancer have to be interpreted very cautiously.

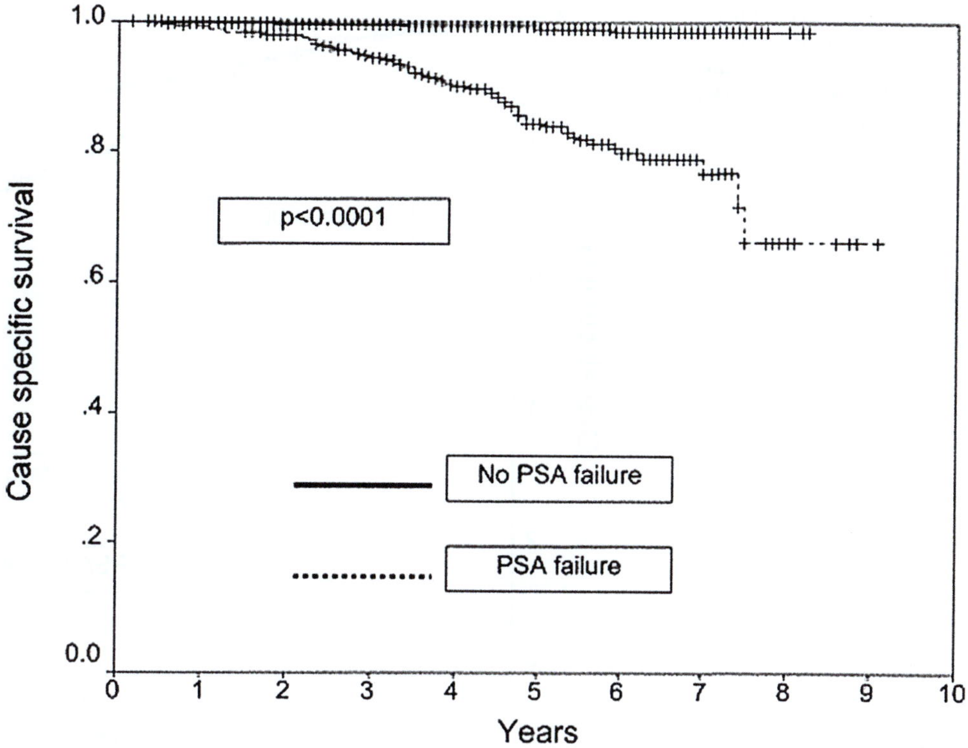

Fig. 1 Cause-specific survival in patients with and without prostate- specific antigen failure (adopted from Kwan et al. (Kwan et al. 2004))

3 Biochemical Failure as a Prognostic Factor for Clinical Failure and Survival

Since the purpose of measuring post-treatment PSA is to provide an early surrogate for clinical failure and disease-specific survival, the relationship between the biochemical and clinical parameters is critically important.

Patients who fail biochemically have been shown to be more likely to die from prostate cancer compared to those who do not experience biochemical relaps. Without PSA failure, relapse of prostate cancer and deaths from prostate cancer are extremely rare. However, disease-specific survival may only have a small impact on overall survival as prostate cancer generally occurs in an elderly population with many competing causes of death.

To date, the influence of biochemical failure on overall survival has been the subject of only a few studies and the results on the relationship between biochemical failure and overall survival are conflicting with some reports failing to demonstrate a relationship and others showing that biochemical failure can predict overall survival (Kupelian et al. 2002; Kwan et al. 2004; Pollack et al. 2003; Sandler et al. 2000; Williams et al. 2004).

Kupelian and colleagues reported in 2002 their observations on the impact of biochemical relapse and confounding factors on overall survival rates during the first 10 years after definitive radiation therapy for localized prostate cancer in a retrospective analysis on 936 cases. In their study sample, biochemical failure after definitive radiotherapy for localized prostate cancer was not significantly associated with increased mortality within the first 10 years after initial therapy, although for patients displaying biochemical relapse, a trend toward worse outcome was observed at 10 years. The authors suggested that longer follow-up from initial therapy would be needed to fully understand the impact of biochemical failure on overall survival and that significant differences might be observed at 15 or 20 years after therapy (Kupelian et al. 2002).

Kwan and colleagues examined the relationship between PSA failure and both overall survival and cause-specific survival using data from 1786 patients who were treated with radical radiotherapy for prostate cancer and prospectively followed at the B.C. Cancer Agency (BCCA). The authors found that biochemical failure was not only associated with a poorer prostate cancer-specific survival but also with overall survival leading to 5-year overall survival rates of 79.5 % among patients who had PSA failure versus 87.5 % among those who had not failed (Figs. 1 and 2). In contrast to the Kupelian series, the proportion of patients with more advanced stage of disease was much higher, a fact that might have contributed to the different results. Examination of the effect of PSA failure in different subgroups revealed a poorer overall survival only in biochemically failed patients younger than age 75 with high-risk disease (Kwan et al. 2004).

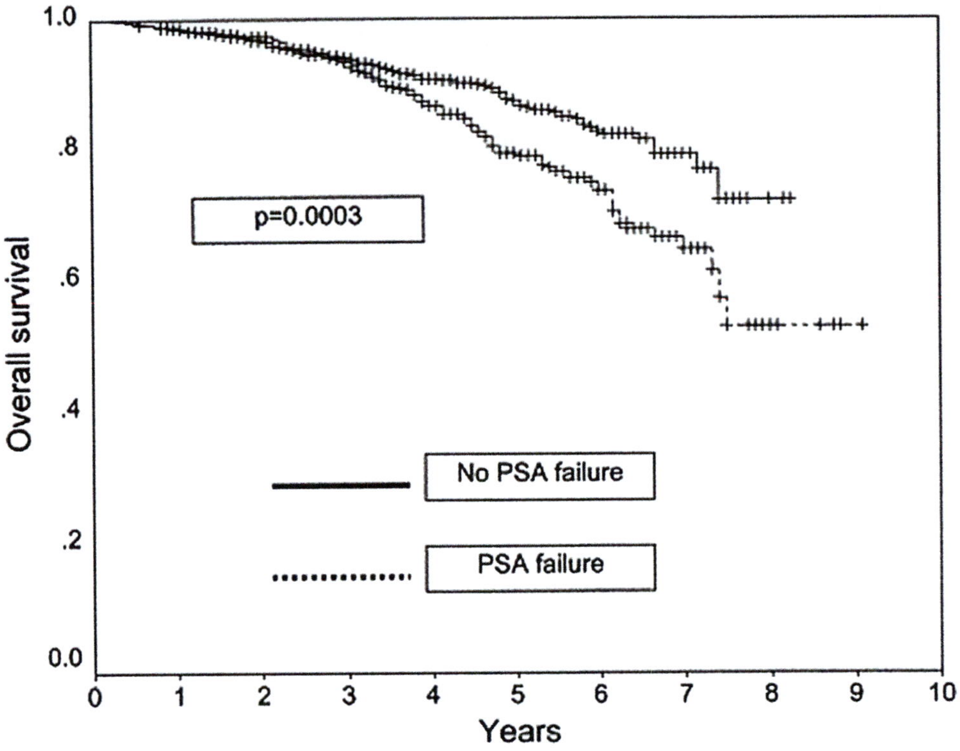

Fig. 2 Overall survival in patients with and without prostate- specific antigen failure (adopted from Kwan et al. (Kwan et al. 2004))

Previously, Soto and coworkers showed significantly better overall survival rates in biochemically failed patients with low-risk features and a pretreatment PSA velocity of ≤2 ng/mL/year compared to high-risk patients in biochemical recurrence (Soto et al. 2008). This emphasizes the idea that not all biochemical recurrence events are equivalent in terms of survival, and the need to determine whether biochemical recurrences are clinically significant and as such warrant further therapy. Thus, an increasing interest in analyzing the ability of additional prognostic factors such as the pretreatment initial prostate-specific antigen PSA, T stage, and Gleason score as well as PSA kinetics to predict for inferior prostate treatment outcomes, including survival has been generated.

4 PSA Recurrence: A Valuable Surrogate Marker in Clinical Trials?

The identification and rigorous validation of surrogate endpoints for overall or disease-specific survival are of great utility in clinical cancer research because the use of surrogate endpoints substantially decreases the size and duration of clinical trials allowing more rapid prospective testing of hypotheses and potentially accelerating the development of improvements in cancer treatment.

Established prognostic factors do not necessarily make valid surrogate end points. Surrogate endpoints used in clinical trials to evaluate the efficacy of new developmental therapies should be associated with a clinically meaningful outcome. To confirm surrogacy in patients treated with new versus standard interventions, there must be a strong correlation between the relative effect of the treatment on the surrogate and the relative effect on the true endpoint (Collette 2008; Collette et al. 2006; Johnson et al. 2003).

In recent years, biochemical recurrence by itself as well as PSA kinetics have been analyzed as surrogate endpoints to predict of prostate treatment outcomes in clinical studies. Most commonly, the "Prentice Criteria" have been used to demonstrate the validity of a putative surrogate endpoint (e. g. PSA) as a replacement endpoint for a true endpoint (e. g. survival). The Prentice Criteria require four conditions to be fulfilled (Prentice 1989):

(a) There must be a statistically significant treatment effect on the PSA endpoint (in univariate analysis)
(b) There must be a statistically significant treatment effect on survival (univariate analysis)
(c) The PSA endpoint must be a statistically significant prognostic factor for survival (univariate analysis)
(d) The treatment effect on survival must completely vanish in a survival model with both the treatment and the PSA endpoint as explanatory variables (multivariate analysis).

More recently, a methodology known as the "meta-analytic validation" has been developed. This method consists in deriving a model to predict in new trials the treatment effect on survival from the observed treatment effect on the PSA end point using survival and PSA data from several randomized trials (Collette 2008; Collette et al. 2006).

One of the first studies addressing the surrogacy issue was reported by D'Amico and colleagues in 2003 who studied PSA doubling time as a potential surrogate for prostate cancer mortality in a non-randomized cohort of 5918 men treated with surgery and 2751 with radiation (D'Amico et al. 2003). They showed that the Prentice criteria were fulfilled when using PSA doubling time less than 3 months. However, the applicability of the results was limited by the use of data from a community treatment outcomes database, which were not collected prospectively and the fact that only few patients actually had a PSA doubling time shorter than 3 months. Nevertheless, PSA doubling time at a cutpoint of less than 3 months emerged as a promising surrogate endpoint candidate for prostate cancer-specific mortality, and the place of PSA doubling time in future surrogacy analyses was established.

Using data from the RTOG trial 92-02 that compared short-term versus long-term androgen deprivation in addition to irradiation for T2c-T4 prostate cancer, Sandler and colleagues showed that time to biochemical recurrence (defined according to the ASTRO definition) was not a surrogate for cancer-specific survival (Sandler et al. 2003). Time to PSA failure was longer in the long-term androgen deprivation arm but the survival time after PSA failure was shorter. This was thought to be due to the finding that secondary therapy was more successful in men failing short-term androgen deprivation who survived longer than men who failed long-term androgen deprivation.

Valicenti and colleagues reported from the same study that post-treatment PSA doubling times of less than 6, 9, and 12 months were statistically significantly associated with prostate cancer—specific survival, but did not meet all of Prentice's requirements for a surrogate endpoint of cancer-specific survival. Thus, the authors concluded that the risk of dying of prostate cancer cannot fully be explained by PSA doubling time (Valicenti et al. 2006).

Denham and colleagues studied the value of both PSA doubling time and time to biochemical failure (defined according to the Phoenix criteria) as surrogate candidates for prostate cancer-specific mortality after primary therapy using data from the Trans-Tasman Radiation Oncology Group (TROG) trial 96.01 (Denham et al. 2008). In this trial, 802 patients receiving radiotherapy for locally advanced, non-metastatic prostate cancer were randomly assigned to 0, 3, or 6 months neoadjuvant short-term androgen deprivation. The authors reported that all four Prentice criteria were fulfilled and that prostate cancer-specific mortality was successfully predicted at all time to biochemical failure cutpoints between 1.5 and 2.5 years, and by PSA doubling time at the less than 12 and less than 15- month cutpoints. Best fits to prostate cancer-specific mortality were provided by time to biochemical failure at the less than 1.5 and less than 2 year cutpoints and at the PSA doubling time cutpoint of less than 12 months. The predictive value of the surrogate endpoints, time to biochemical failure less than 2 years and PSA doubling time less than 12 months, is shown in the cancer-specific survival plots (Fig. 3). The authors concluded that time to biochemical failure and PSA doubling time were prognostic variables potent enough to act as surrogate endpoint candidates for prostate cancer-specific mortality.

In the same dataset, Denham and colleagues also determined how the occurrence of biochemical failure itself related to prostate cancer-specific mortality and demonstrated that the occurrence of biochemical failure was a far weaker predictor of cancer death than time to biochemical failure (Denham et al. 2009). It was also shown that prognostic factors for early cancer death changed dramatically at biochemical recurrence. Highly prognostic factors at randomization, such as high Gleason score grouping and T classification, lost their prognostic importance, whereas factors such as shorter time to biochemical failure and PSA doubling time became powerful predictors of prostate cancer death at this time point.

In two meta-analytic validations using data from the bicalutamide trials, biochemical progression-free survival as surrogate for clinical progression-free survival in nonmetastatic disease and for overall survival in metastatic disease was studied. In patients with metastatic disease, two definitions of time to PSA progression (TTPP) were assessed: (1) For TTPP-1, PSA progression was defined as a PSA value above normal (4 ng/mL), representing a first increase 20 % above the nadir. (2) For TTPP-2, PSA progression was defined as a PSA value 2.5 times the normal range (10 ng/mL), representing a first increase 50 % above the moving average (based on three consecutive measurements) nadir. In the analyses, only a moderate correlation between the treatment effects on the PSA end point and on the clinical end point was observed. The authors concluded that a treatment benefit for the PSA end point is not sufficient to guarantee a benefit for the clinical end point but may help in decision making to prematurely stop a phase 3 trial, as in the absence of a clear benefit for the PSA end point, any benefit on clinical relapse or survival is very unlikely (Collette et al. 2005, 2006; Newling et al. 2004).

D'Amico and colleagues assessed whether two metrics of PSA (PSA value after completion of therapy (PSA end) and PSA nadir) could act as surrogates for prostate cancer-specific mortality (D'Amico et al. 2012). Their analysis included individual patients' data from two randomized controlled trials—the Dana Farber Cancer Institute (DFCI) 95-096 trial (D'Amico et al. 2008) and the TROG 9601 trial (Denham et al. 2008) that showed a statistically and clinically significant reduction in prostate cancer-specific mortality when 6 months of androgen suppression was added to radiotherapy compared to radiotherapy alone. The cutoff values were chosen on the basis of reports suggesting that a

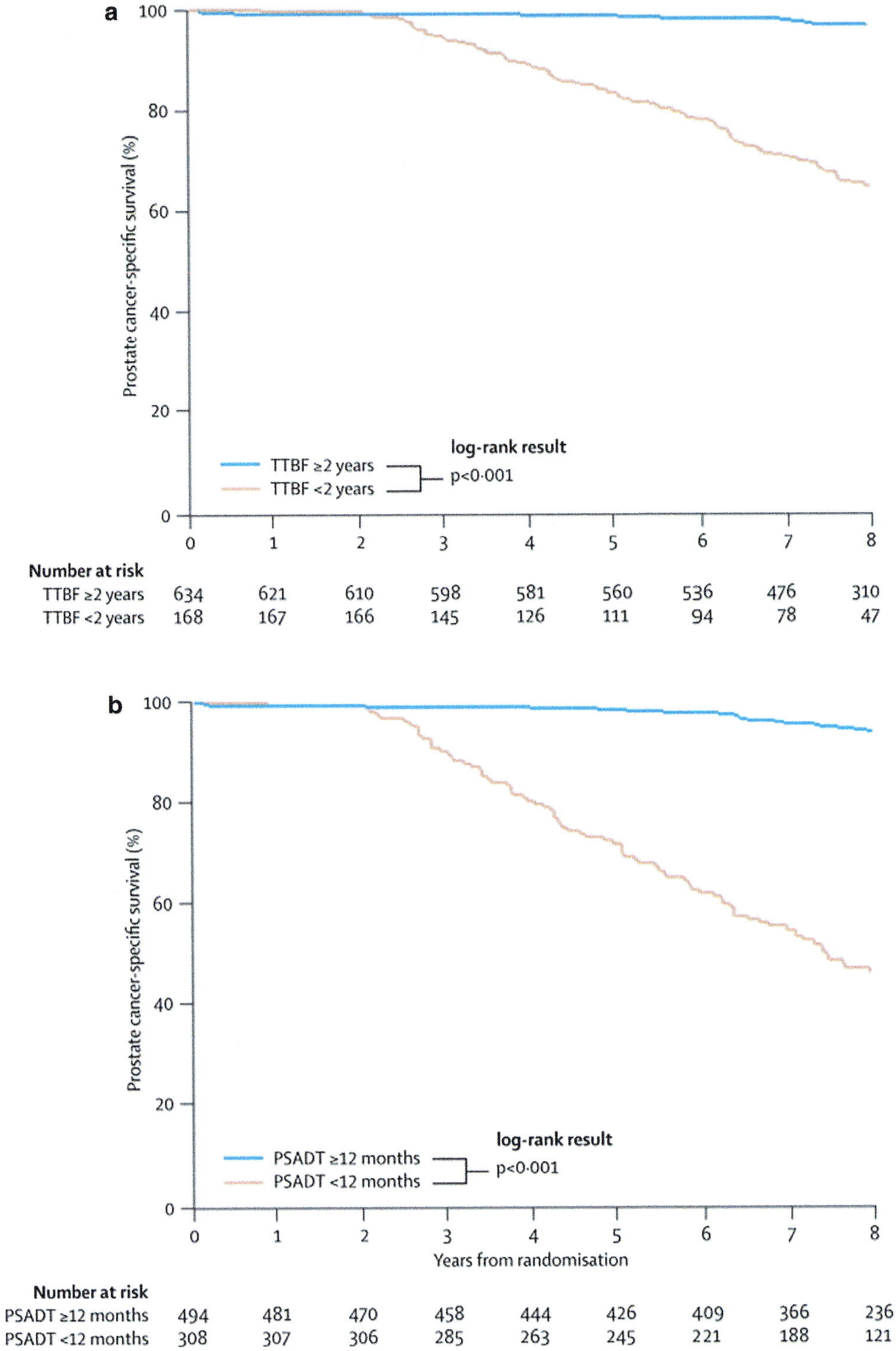

Fig. 3 Time to prostate cancer death from randomisation, stratified by **a** time to biochemical failure (TTBF; <2 vs ≥2 years) and **b** prostate-specific antigen doubling time (PSADT; <12 months vs ≥12 months); adopted from Denham et al. (Denham et al. 2008)

PSA nadir of more than 0.5 ng/mL after radiotherapy and short-course androgen suppression was associated with an increased risk of recurrence (Benchikh El Fegoun et al. 2008; Lamb et al. 2011; Zelefsky et al. 1998). The authors found that both PSA nadir and PSA end concentrations of more than 0.5 ng/mL were surrogates for prostate cancer-specific mortality, permitting early identification of men in whom radiotherapy and 6 months of androgen suppression is insufficient for cure. The authors suggested that men with PSA end values exceeding 0.5 ng/mL following radiotherapy and 6 months of androgen suppression should be considered for long-term androgen suppression. Additionally, clinical researchers could use the PSA nadir of more than 0.5 ng/mL as an eligibility criteria for an early (at time of PSA nadir) versus delayed (at time of PSA failure) intervention with salvage androgen suppression (D'Amico et al. 2012).

5 Conclusion

PSA is an important tool for monitoring disease progression following treatment of definitive localized prostate cancer allowing for early measure of treatment failure, long before clinical disease becomes evident or survival is affected.

However, a consensus on the ability of biochemical failure to act as a surrogate endpoint for survival has not yet been reached. Although most agree that biochemical failure is a useful surrogate for treatment efficacy, the relationship and timeline between PSA failure, clinical failure, and survival is less well documented.

The value of biochemical recurrence by itself as a predictor of prostate cancer-specific mortality has been questioned lately because survival after biochemical recurrence is highly variable. Thus, in recent years an interest in analyzing the PSA kinetics has been generated to help refine the ability to predict of prostate treatment outcomes. Several studies to identify a PSA endpoint as a surrogate endpoint for prostate cancer-specific survival have focused on the kinetics of increasing post-treatment serum PSA levels and have found that rapid PSA increases, or short post-treatment PSA doubling times, after local therapy are associated with the development of metastatic disease and prostate cancer—specific mortality.

In studies, evaluating advances in local therapy for prostate cancer, clinical failure has less frequently been reported, mainly due to the fact that long-term follow-up is necessary to measure this end point. However, as it is the clinical recurrence that will impact survival, in clinical trials, distant metastasis, and general clinical treatment failure should be evaluated thoroughly along with overall and prostate cancer–specific survival endpoints.

References

American Society for Therapeutic Radiology and Oncology Consensus Panel (1997) Consensus statement: guidelines for PSA following radiation therapy. Int J Radiat Oncol Biol Phys 37:1035–1041

Amling CL, Bergstralh EJ, Blute ML et al (2001) Defining prostate specific antigen progression after radical prostatectomy: what is the most appropriate cut point? J Urol 165:1146–1151

Arcangeli G, Saracino B, Gomellini S et al (2010) A prospective phase III randomized trial of hypofractionation versus conventional fractionation in patients with high-risk prostate cancer. Int J Radiat Oncol Biol Phys 78:11–18

Arcangeli S, Strigari L, Gomellini S et al (2012) Updated results and patterns of failure in a randomized hypofractionation trial for high-risk prostate cancer. Int J Radiat Oncol Biol Phys 84:1172–1178

Benchikh El Fegoun A, Villers A et al (2008) PSA and follow-up after treatment of prostate cancer. Prog Urol 18:137–144

Bolla M, van Poppel H, Collette L et al (2005) European Organization for Research and Treatment of Cancer. Postoperative radiotherapy after radical prostatectomy: a randomised controlled trial (EORTC trial 22911). Lancet 366:572–578

Collette L (2008) Prostate-specific antigen (PSA) as a surrogate end point for survival in prostate cancer clinical trials. Eur Urol 53:6–9

Collette L, Burzykowski T, Caroll KJ et al (2005) PSA is not a valid surrogate endpoint for overall survival in patients with metastatic prostate cancer. A joint research of the European Organisation for Research and Treatment of Cancer, the Limburgs Universitair Centrum and AstraZeneca Pharmaceuticals. J Clin Oncol 23:6139–6148

Collette L, Burzykowski T, Schröder FH (2006) Prostate-specific antigen (PSA) alone is not an appropriate surrogate marker of long-term therapeutic benefit in prostate cancer trials. Eur J Cancer 42:1344–1350

Cookson MS, Aus G, Burnett AL et al (2007) Variation in the definition of biochemical recurrence in patients treated for localized prostate cancer: the American Urological Association Prostate Guidelines for Localized Prostate Cancer Update Panel report and recommendations for a standard in the reporting of surgical outcomes. J Urol 177:540–545

D'Amico AV, Chen M, Renshaw AA et al (2008) Androgen suppression and radiation vs radiation alone for prostate cancer: a randomized trial. JAMA 299:289–295

D'Amico AV, Chen M-H, de Castro M et al (2012) Surrogate endpoints for prostate cancer-specific mortality after radiotherapy and androgen suppression therapy in men with localised or locally advanced prostate cancer: an analysis of two randomised trials. Lancet Oncol 13:189–195

D'Amico AV, Moul JW, Carroll PR et al (2003) Surrogate end point for prostate cancer specific mortality after radical prostatectomy or radiation therapy. J Natl Canc Inst 95:1376–1383

Denham JW, Steigler A, Wilcox C et al (2008) Time to biochemical failure and prostate-specific antigen doubling time as surrogates for prostate cancer specific mortality: evidence from the TROG 96.01 randomised controlled trial. Lancet Oncol 9:1058–1068

Denham JW, Steigler A, Wilcox C et al (2009) Why are pretreatment prostate-specific antigen levels and biochemical recurrence poor predictors of prostate cancer survival? Cancer 115:4477–4487

Freedland SJ, Sutter ME, Dorey F et al (2003) Defining the ideal cutpoint for determining PSA recurrence after radical prostatectomy. Prostate-specific antigen. Urology 61:365–369

Grimm P, Billiet I, Bostwick D et al (2012) Comparative analysis of prostate-specific antigen free survival outcomes for patients with low, intermediate and high-risk prostate cancer treatment by radical therapy. Results from the Prostate Cancer Results Study Group. BJU Int 109(Suppl 1):22–29

Horwitz EM, Thames HD, Kuban DA et al (2005) Definitions of biochemical failure that best predict clinical failure in patients with prostate cancer treated with external beam radiation alone: a multi-institutional pooled analysis. J Urol 173:797–802

Johnson JR, Williams G, Pazdur R (2003) Endpoints and United States Food and Drug Administration approval of oncology drugs. J Clin Oncol 21:1401–1411

Kuban D, Thames H, Levy L et al (2005) Failure definition-dependent differences in outcome following radiation for localized prostate cancer: can one size fit all? Int J Radiat Oncol Biol Phys 61:409–414

Kuban DA, Levy LB, Cheung MR et al (2011) Long-term failure patterns and survival in a randomized dose escalation trial for prostate cancer. Who dies of disease? Int J Radiat Oncol Biol Phys 79:1310–1317

Kuban DA, Nogueras-Gonzalez NG, Hamblin L et al (2010) Preliminary report of a randomized dose escalation trial for prostate cancer using hypofractionation. Int J Radiat Oncol Biol Phys 78(suppl):S58

Kuban DA, Tucker SL, Dong L et al (2008) Long-term results of the M. D. Anderson randomized dose-escalation trial for prostate cancer. Int J Radiat Oncol Biol Phys 70:67–74

Kupelian PA, Buchsbaum JC, Patel C et al (2002) Impact of biochemical failure on overall survival after radiation therapy for localized prostate cancer in the PSA era. Int J Radiat Oncol Biol Phys 52:704–711

Kwan W, Pickles T, Duncan G et al (2004) PSA failure and the risk of death in prostate cancer patients treated with radiotherapy. Int J Radiat Oncol Biol Phys 60:1040–1046

Lamb DS, Denham JW, Joseph D et al (2011) A comparison of the prognostic value of early PSA test-based variables following external beam radiotherapy, with or without preceding androgen deprivation: analysis of data from the Trog96.01 randomized trial. Int J Radiat Oncol Biol Phys 79:385–391

Newling D, Carroll K, Morris T (2004) Is prostate-specific antigen progression a surrogate for objective clinical progression in early prostate cancer? J Clin Oncol 22:4652

Nielsen ME, Partin AW (2007) The impact of definitions of failure on the interpretation of biochemical recurrence following treatment of clinically localized prostate cancer. Rev Urol 9:57–62

Peeters ST, Heemsbergen WD, Koper PC et al (2006) Dose-response in radiotherapy for localized prostate cancer: Results of the Dutch multicenter randomized phase III trial comparing 68 Gy of radiotherapy with 78 Gy. J Clin Oncol 24:1990–1996

Pollack A, Hanlon AL, Movsas B et al (2003) Biochemical failure as a determinant of distant metastasis and death in prostate cancertreated with radiotherapy. Int J Radiat Oncol Biol Phys 57:19–23

Pollack AW, Buyyounouski M, Horwitz E et al (2011) Five year results of a randomized external beam radiotherapy hypofractionation trial for prostate cancer. Int J Radiat Oncol Biol Phys 81(suppl):S1

Prentice RL (1989) Surrogate endpoints in clinical trials: definitions and operational criteria. Stat Med 8:431–440

Roach M III, Hanks G, Thames H Jr et al (2006) Defining biochemical failure following radiotherapy with or without hormonal therapy in men with clinically localized prostate cancer: recommendations of the RTOG-ASTRO Phoenix Consensus Conference. Int J Radiat Oncol Biol Phys 65:965–974

Sandler HM, Dunn RL, McLaughlin PW et al (2000) Overall survival after prostate-specific-antigen-detected recurrence following conformal radiation therapy. Int J Radiat Oncol Biol Phys 48:629–633

Sandler HM, Pajak TF, Hanks GE et al (2003) Can biochemical failure (ASTRO definition) be used as a surrogate endpoint for prostate cancer survival in phase III localized prostate cancer clinical trials? Analysis of RTOG protocol 92–02. J Clin Oncol 22:381

Sathya JR, Davis IR, Julian JA et al (2005) Randomized trial comparing iridium implant plus external-beam radiation therapy with external-beam radiation therapy alone in node-negative locally advanced cancer of the prostate. J Clin Oncol 23: 1192–1199

Soto DE, Andridge RR, Pan CC et al (2008) In patients experiencing biochemical failure after radiotherapy, pretreatment risk group and PSA velocity predict differences in overall survival and biochemical failure-free interval. Int J Radiat Oncol Biol Phys 71: 1295–1301

Stephenson AJ, Bolla M, Briganti A et al (2012) Postoperative radiation therapy for pathologically advanced prostate cancer after radical prostatectomy. Eur Urol 61:443–451

Stephenson AJ, Kattan MW, Eastham JA et al (2006) Defining biochemical recurrence of prostate cancer after radical prostatectomy: a proposal for a standardized definition. J Clin Oncol 24:3973–3978

Thompson IM, Tangen CM, Paradelo J et al (2009) Adjuvant radiotherapy for pathological T3N0M0 prostate cancer significantly reduces risk of metastases and improves survival: long-term followup of a randomized clinical trial. J Urol 181:956–962

Valicenti RK, DeSilvio M, Hanks GE et al (2006) Posttreatment prostatic-specific antigen doubling time as a surrogate endpoint for prostate cancer-specific survival: an analysis of Radiation Therapy Oncology Group Protocol 92-02. Int J Radiat Oncol Biol Phys 66:1064–1071

Wiegel T, Bottke D, Steiner U et al (2009) Phase III postoperative adjuvant radiotherapy after radical prostatectomy compared with radical prostatectomy alone in pT3 prostate cancer with postoperative undetectable prostate-specific antigen: ARO 96-02/AUO AP 09/95. J Clin Oncol 27:2924–2930

Williams SG, Duchesne GM, Millar JL et al (2004) Both pretreatment prostate-specific antigen level and posttreatment biochemical failure are independent predictors of overall survival after radiotherapy for prostate cancer. Int J Radiat Oncol Biol Phys 60:1082–1087

Zelefsky MJ, Lyass O, Fuks Z et al (1998) Predictors of improved outcome for patients with localized prostate cancer treated with neoadjuvant androgen ablation therapy and three-dimensional conformal radiotherapy. J Clin Oncol 16:3380–3385

Zietman AL, Bae K, Slater JD et al (2010) Randomized trial comparing conventional-dose with high-dose conformal radiation therapy in early-stage adenocarcinoma of the prostate: Long-term results from Proton Radiation Oncology Group/American College of Radiology 95-09. J Clin Oncol 28:1106–1111

Overall- and Disease-Specific Survival in Prostata Cancer: Too Long to Wait?

Wolfgang Lilleby

Contents

Abstract

There is a substantial body of evidence supporting the efficacy of primary radiotherapy in men with prostate cancer. Unfortuantely, and especially men with prognostic high risk prostate cancer will experience undertreatment with fatal consequences in this population. On the other hand, low risk patients should benefit from diagnostic breakthroughs achieved by modern staging techniques and optimised treatment developments, sparing these men for unnecessary side effects and harms. It is up to the uro-oncologic community to encourage clinical randomised trials comparing radiotherapy with surgery to improve the disease-specific survival and overall outcome in these patients.

1 Introduction

Prostate cancer (PCa) is among the most commonly occurring malignancies in the world and is one of the few that continues to show an increasing incidence. Today, PCa is the second leading cause of cancer-related deaths after lung cancer in developed countries and major risk factors include age, family, history, and ethnicity (Jemal et al. 2011). One man in six will develop PCa during his lifetime, and one man in 34 will die of the disease (Bray et al. 2010). The probability of developing PCa sharply increases in the sixth decade of life and further increases after the age of 70 years (Kvale et al. 2010). The aging of the current population means that the disease will become an even greater public health issue in the near future.

For the concept of radiotherapy added to androgen deprivation, an increased long-term survival, both prostate cancer-specific survival (PCSS) and overall survival (OS), has been shown in prospectively randomized trials for patients with locally advanced or high-risk local PCa (Warde et al. 2011; Bolla et al. 2009; Widmark et al. 2009).

W. Lilleby (✉)
MD Anderson, Norwegian Cancer Consortium—NCC, Oncology, Oslo, Norway
e-mail: wolfgang.lilleby@ous-hf.no

H. Geinitz et al. (eds.), *Radiotherapy in Prostate Cancer*, Medical Radiology. Radiation Oncology, DOI: 10.1007/174_2013_941,

Published Online: 3 December 2013

For the opposite concept, i.e., adjuvant androgen deprivation therapy (ADT) added to external beam radiotherapy (EBRT), the RTOG trial 85-31 showed improved 5-year-disease-free survival (DFS) for patients with Gleason score 8–10 (Pilepich et al. 2005).

Still, life-expectancy of men in Western countries and the biological course of PCa demands long-term follow-up data to answer the challenges linked to this potentially threatening disease in a satisfactory way.

What are the current lessons from large prospectively randomized trials and how can we implement the increasing insight into tumor biology to the daily decision-making process? The necessary debate of PCa once raised by Whithmore posing the famous questions about PCa—"Is cure possible for those in whom it is necessary? Is cure necessary in those for whom it is possible?"—has still its appealing actuality. Moreover, are the clinical results from pre-PSA trials or selected single-institution cohorts reflecting overall and disease-specific disease satisfactory enough and are these results transferable to today's clinical cohorts? There is an increasing awareness for unsustainable health costs and long-lasting side effects in overtreated men. Obviously, issues of survivorship related to treatment-induced morbidity become more important in the near future.

Confronted with these challenges, will the future further inspire patiently constructed randomized prospective trials and wait for final overall survival rates to prove right or wrong for modern treatment approaches in the end? These questions are not trivial. The declining mortality in PCa also depicted in countries without a population-based screening program challenges the present paradigm (Center et al. 2012). In the past a number of randomized trials have demonstrated a significantly improved patient outcome both in surgical and radiotherapeutical series (Warde et al. 2011; Widmark et al. 2009; Pilepich et al. 2001, 2005; Bill-Axelson et al. 2011; Bolla et al. 1997; Hanks et al. 2003; Zelefsky et al. 2008). The trend is likely attributed to advances in curative treatment, such as surgical techniques, more effective oncologic treatment especially in locally advanced disease, and general technical improvements. There is a preceding shift in daily practice to continuously more skilled methods introduced in radiotherapy (intensity-modulated-, proton beam-, or stereotactic treatment) and also in surgery (robot-assisted) over the last decade. However, the verdict of recent years' efforts in increasing early detection of PCa is at present unclear. Still, there is no doubt about the psychological distress for the patient having a cancer diagnosis.

OS is the gold standard in reporting the treatment efficacy for men treated with radiotherapy (RT) or prostatectomy (PRECT). However, in an often slow progressing disease such as PCa mainly manifested in an elderly population the task to gain unconfounded OS data can be precluded. These hurdles, the tumor biology, age, and comorbidity, make a rational approach to this cancer entity demanding. Often, a surrogate endpoint is introduced as a substitute for a clinically meaningful endpoint that measures directly how a patient feels, functions, or survives (Fleming and DeMets 1996). The National Institutes of Health in USA define a surrogate marker as a biomarker intended to substitute for a clinical endpoint. Consequently, it is tempting to use the serum prostate-specific antigen (PSA) level as a surrogate marker in PCa. In a retrospective data analysis of the RTOG 92-02 trial, Ray et al. using Prentice's criteria (Prentice 2009; Ray et al. 2009) found that both distant metastasis and general clinical failure at 3 years were possible candidate surrogate endpoints for PCSS at 10 years. Notably, biochemical relapse expressed by various PSA definitions is not a robust surrogate endpoint for PCSS since increasing PSA may pose little threat to longevity in many patients (Stephenson et al. 2012).

In this chapter, we will mainly overview RT combined with or without hormonal treatment in relation to the outcome parameter OS, and expand the review on prospectively randomized trials evaluating the effectiveness of RT to PCSS.

In addition, recognizing surgery as an equal approach in localized PCa and often the favored management in young men with localized PCa, we will mention pivotal surgical randomized prospectively trials as appropriate in the text.

The general risk evaluation of a patient with PCa is done by the established risk factors serum PSA, histologically by grading (Gleason score) and assessment of the tumor size (T-category). These factors are included to form risk groups allocating patients to low-, intermediate-, and high-risk.

Currently, patients with PCa are classified into the following risk categories (Heidenreich et al. 2011):

Low-risk:
PSA $<$ 10 ng/ml and biopsy Gleason score 6 and T-category cT1c–cT2a.

Intermediate-risk:
PSA $=$ 10.1–20 ng/ml or biopsy Gleason score 7 or T-category cT2b–c.

High-risk:
PSA $>$ 20 ng/ml or biopsy Gleason score 8–10 or T-category $\geq$ cT3a.

2 Is Cure Necessary in Those for Whom it is Possible? Localized Low-Risk PCa

The term localized carcinoma of the prostate refers to a tumor that is clinically confined within the prostatic capsule and with no evidence of metastatic spread.

Currently, unfortunately there exists no molecular marker or any staging device that can distinguish between clinically significant localized tumors from those that will remain indolent throughout the patient's life.

In the European Rotterdam Screening Prostate Cancer study (ERSPC) a significant number of the detected cancers (48 %) were regarded as indolent (Schroder et al. 2012). Draisma et al. estimated that PSA testing introduced lead time bias advancing the date of diagnosis by 12 years for men ≤55 years and by 6 years for men >55 years (Draisma et al. 2009).

Removing the prostate by radical prostatectomy provides the best opportunity of pathologic staging thereby confirming early PCa and the chance of long-term cure. A life expectancy >10 years is the most frequently used benchmark for definitive therapy for patients with localized PCa. The overall 15 years PCSS for men with clinically localized disease treated with radical prostatectomy is 93 %, for Gleason scores 2–4, 5–7, and for 8–10 it is 98, 91, and 76 %, respectively (Eggener et al. 2011).

In the pre-PSA era a randomized study from Sweden (SPCG-4) retrieved 695 patients with localized PCa (cT1a–cT2) between 1989 and 1999 to either radical prostatectomy or watchful waiting. After a median follow-up of 8.2 years, surgery decreased prostate cancer-related death by 44 % and overall mortality by 26 % when compared with watchful waiting (Bill-Axelson et al. 2011). The number needed to avert one death was 15 overall and 7 for men under 65 years of age and there was no significant reduction in death from other causes, PCa death, or risk of distant metastases in those above 65 years. Because in that trial the total number of deaths from PCa was high ($n = 136$ men), it would require 20 men to undergo prostatectomy to save one man from death. In contrast to that data from the pre-PSA era the 15-year prostate cancer-specific mortality of localized disease for men aged 55–74 years with a Gleason score <7 was 1 % when postponing active treatment. To avoid overtreatment, in the PSA era, active surveillance is more often recommended in men with localized disease (Dall'Era et al. 2012).

Looking toward the PSA era one should be sensitized that major events such as stage migration have occurred. Pound and colleagues calculated the average time to metastatic disease after biochemical relapse to be 8 years after local therapy, and an additional 5-year survival for those patients who ultimately died of PCa (Pound et al. 1999).

The lead time and overdetection associated with PSA screening make PCa outcome studies from the pre-PSA era difficult to interpret in a contemporary setting. Parker et al. estimated that the 15-year PCa survival benefit of radical treatment in screened detected PCa was strongest in men with high-grade disease, whereas current clinical practice preferentially targets radical treatment to patients with low-grade PCa (Parker et al. 2006).

Taking into account the risk of upgrading of contemporary Gleason grades, the mortality rates from the pre-PSA era are likely to be biased by an artifact due to the Will Roger phenomenon (Albertsen et al. 2005). The Will Roger phenomenon refers to improvement in a factor mainly due to change in observation, in case of PCa the Gleason grading. In former studies Gleason score =< 6 was quite often found (SPCG-4 72 %), but due to the introduction of pathological upgrading in prostatectomies there has been a Gleason score shift attributing to higher grades in biopsy material (Epstein et al. 2012). The practical implication of this phenomenon is a worse prognosis in a patient with a Gleason score evaluated in the pre-PSA era compared to a patient with a Gleason score assessed in the PSA era.

Acknowledging the moderate survival benefits of treatment with curative intent, the prostate, lung, colorectal, and ovarian trial (PLCO) assessed also comorbidity as factor influencing mortality effect of screening (Andriole et al. 2009). In this study the modified Charlson comorbidity score (0 = none comorbidity, >= 1 = one or more comorbid conditions) included a vast range of medical conditions. No statistically significant interaction with respect to PCa mortality and comorbidity was observed after 13 years of follow-up (Andriole et al. 2012). In other words, not even the discrimination between patients with or without comorbidity was a helpful tool to select patients for active treatment.

There is a paucity of clinical trials comparing surgery to other treatment modalities. Due to very poor accrual the attempt to compare outcome in low-risk men between brachytherapy (BT) and PRECT, the SPIRIT trial, was stopped (Wallace et al. 2006). Nevertheless, in a publication using the SPIRIT data, patients receiving BT scored better in the urinary and sexual domains, and in patient satisfaction (Crook et al. 2011). In another recent attempt to compare PRECT with BT, the SPARE trial was also abandoned due to low accrual (Dall'Era et al. 2012; Eccles et al. 2013).

In the debate on active surveillance compared to actively intervening in localized PCa issues of treatment-induced morbidity should not be missed. A considerable number of patients will be harmed by treatment-induced side effects including erectile dysfunction, urinary leakage, and rectal discomfort after primary treatment (Sanda et al. 2008; Steinsvik et al. 2010; Stensvold et al. 2012). The overall survival benefit for men treated with RT combined with ADT for localized PCa comes with a price to be paid regarding chronic fatigue after irradiation, cognitive impairment, and a slightly increased risk of secondary neoplasia (Brenner et al. 2005; Kyrdalen et al. 2010; Lilleby et al. 2013; Morris et al. 2013).

3 Is Cure Possible for Those in Whom it is Necessary? Local and Locally Advanced Intermediate to High-Risk PCa

Improvements in the field of radiation oncology such as conformal radiation therapy, the use of intensity-modulated radiotherapy (IMRT), and the use of fiducial markers to employ image-guided techniques have optimized delivery and cancer control but also reduced treatment-related damage to surrounding tissues.

Supported by findings of residual cancer in post-radiation biopsies the concept of dose escalation using higher doses of radiation for organ-confined disease has been consecutively implemented in modern radiation schedules. In other words, the dose–response relationship has been established for PCa in RT (Kuban and Dong 2004). In regard to retrospective analyses of intermediate to high-risk PCa high doses were needed to achieve tumor control.

At least four randomized trials investigated the effectiveness of dose escalation in conformal RT (Zelefsky et al. 2008; Martinez et al. 2003; Peeters et al. 2006; Valicenti et al. 2000). All demonstrated a 10–20 % improvement in biochemical control with doses =>74 Gy. Multiple trials have demonstrated that doses of 78–81 Gy are needed to obtain sustained control in localized high-risk PCa. If doses greater than 81 Gy are needed, it remains controversial. Furthermore, hypofractionation either delivered by IMRT or brachytherapy techniques added interesting insights into successful radiation schemes in the last decade (Kovacs et al. 2005). But importantly, none of these studies have so far reached significance for PCSS or OS. In a recently published article by Viani et al., only biochemical DFS in five randomized, controlled trials with a total of 2,812 were reported for dose escalated studies evaluated by meta-analysis (Viani et al. 2009).

Six trials, including the Dutch and MRC RT01 study (Dearnaley et al. 2007), evaluated PCSS with at least median 5-year follow-up. The pooled results from these trials showed a statistical benefit for high-dose RT in terms of biochemical freedom of disease (BFS), for all low-, intermediate-, and high-risk patients. There was no difference in the OS rate or PCSS, respectively ($p = 0.38$ and $p = 0.45$) in the groups receiving dose-escalated RT or conventional RT.

Thus, the role of dose escalation with RT appears promising in all risk groups. However, none of the randomized dose escalation trials demonstrated a disease-specific or overall survival benefit. So far only external radiotherapy (EBRT) combined with ADT applying conventional doses has shown improved overall and PCSS rates.

Recently, more medical evidence for the beneficial side of active radiotherapeutic intervention in patients with prognostic unfavorably intermediate to high-risk profiles became available. In a newly published report from the MD Anderson Cancer Center patients with low- and intermediate-risk treated with definitive RT were unlikely to die of PCa (Kim et al. 2012). Men with high-risk disease had the highest risk of dying from PCa following RT. Treatment with ADT nearly halved the risk of PCa mortality.

Increasing dose of RT also led to a significant eradication of tumor cells. In a recent report by Solberg et al., as many as 22 % of prostate biopsies taken after radiotherapy in the SPCG study showed evidence of residual cancer (Solberg et al. 2011). Residual cancer was also associated with PSA recurrence, local tumor progression, clinical recurrence, and cancer-specific death. Similar figures have been presented from the RTOG 94-08 data (ASCO-GU 2011 abstract #6).

In light of these results the outcome in prostate cancer-specific mortality and published radiation doses from previous trials in high-risk and locally advanced PCa must be regarded as suboptimal compared to today's standards. Nevertheless, various questions addressing the duration and sequency of ADT in men with intermediate and high-risk disease are still a matter of debate. Two recent meta-analyses confirmed the inferiority of short-term ADT to 3-year suppression for PCSS and OS at 5-year in prognostically high-risk PCa (Kim et al. 2012; Bria et al. 2009; Shelley et al. 2009).

3.1 Combined ADT and RT with Regard to Outcome

The RTOG 85-31 randomized trial was designed to evaluate the effectiveness of ADT, using goserelin, in locally advanced PCa treated with EBRT (Pilepich et al. 2005). Eligible patients were those with palpable primary tumors extending beyond the prostatic gland or those with regional lymph node involvement. In addition, patients with positive margins and/or seminal vesicle affection after prostatectomy could be included. From 1987 to 1991, 977 patients were enrolled. Median follow-up was 7.6 years for the entire group and the 10-year absolute survival rates were 49 % for the combined arm versus 39 % for EBRT alone ($p = 0.002$, see Table 1). The disease-specific mortality was 16 % versus 22 % in favor of the adjuvant ADT group.

RTOG 86-10 assessed the impact of ADT before and concurrent with RT (Pilepich et al. 2001). In that study, 471 men were randomly assigned to EBRT with or without ADT plus flutamide between 1987 and 1991. ADT was administered for 2 months before and 2 months during EBRT. Patients with bulky tumors with or without lymph node affection and no sign of M+ disease were eligible. At a median follow-up of 12.5 years, 456 patients were evaluated. The median survival time was increased from 7.7 to 8.7 years. ADT significantly decreased the rates of disease-specific mortality (35 % vs. 47 %, $p = 0.006$), increased

Table 1 Large randomized trials combining radiotherapy with androgen suppression

Trial	Eligibility	Arms	DFS (%)	OS (%)
RTOG 85-31	T3 or T1-2, N+ or pT3	RT versus RT + ADT	10 years 23 versus 37 ($P < 0.0001$)	10 years 39 versus 49 ($P = 0.002$)
RTOG 86-10	T2b-4, N+	RT versus RT + NHT	10 years 3 versus 11 ($P < 0.001$)	10 years 34 versus 43 ($P = 0.12$)
RTOG 92-02	T2c-4, N+ sPSA < 150 ng/mL	RT + NHT versus RT + NHT + ADT	5 years 28.1 versus 46.4 ($P < 0.001$)	5-years 78.5 versus 80 ($P = 0.73$)
RTOG 94-13	T2c-4, N+ risk > 15 %	WP + NHT WP + ADT PO + NHT	4 years 59.6 48.9	4 years 84.7 versus 84.3 ($P = 0.73$)
T94-0110	T3	ADT + RT versus ADT		7 years 74 versus 66 $p = 0.0033$
EORTC 22,863	T3-4 or T1-2 WHO 3	RT versus RT + ADT	5 years 45 versus 74 ($P < 0.001$)	5 years 62 versus 78 ($P = 0$ .002)
SPCG-7	T2-3, pN0 PSA < 70 ng/mL	AA versus RT + AA		10 years 29.6 versus 39.4

DFS disease-free survival, *OS* overall survival, *RTOG* Radiation Oncology Group, *ADT* adjuvant androgen deprivation therapy, *AA* antiandrogen hormone treatment, *EORTC* European Organisation for Research and Treatment of Cancer, *WHO* World Health Organization, *PSA* prostate-specific antigen, *WP* whole pelvis, *PO* prostate only, *SPCAG* Scandinavian Prostate Cancer Group

disease-free survival (11 % vs. 3 %), and overall survival (43 % vs. 34 %, Table 1).

Still, the clinical benefit was seen in Gleason score 2–6 tumors only, and not in patients diagnosed with a Gleason score of 7–10.

In the EORTC 22,863, Bolla et al. assessed the role of adjuvant ADT in high-risk patients (Bolla et al. 1997). Patients in the adjuvant ADT arm received androgen suppression on the first day of EBRT, and continued for 3 years. Follow-up was 66 months and 484 patients were included. At 5 years the disease-free survival was 74 % versus 40 % with ADT and without ADT and overall survival 78 % versus 62 % in the combined arm versus EBRT alone ($p = 0.001$).

In the post-PSA era, several randomized trials have been conducted by the RTOG. RTOG 92-02 investigated the impact of neoadjuvant and concomitant ADT (4 months totally) and the same radiotherapy in addition to 2 years of adjuvant ADT (Hanks et al. 2003). Median follow-up was 5.8 years, patients with long-term ADT experienced a statistically significant improvement for all endpoints compared to short-term ADT. Overall, a 10 % overall survival advantage for those patients with a high Gleason score 8–10 and a longer course of ADT versus short-term course of ADT was reported.

RTOG 94-13 compared two different sequencing regimes of adjuvant ADT as well as the role of whole pelvic EBRT (Lawton et al. 2007). This study was designed to investigate if whole pelvis EBRT followed by a boost to the prostate achieves a progression-free survival of at least 10 % compared to ADT and EBRT to the prostate only. Due to unsuspected hormone/radiation interactions the verdict is still not settled.

The EORTC 22,961 enrolled 970 patients with locally advanced PCa to either 6 months of ADT and 70 Gy or 3 years of ADT plus 70 Gy (Bolla et al. 2009). Despite improved progression-free survival in the long course ADT arm, there were no overall survival differences so far.

In the SPCG-7 phase III trial the effect of endocrine therapy alone compared to endocrine therapy combined with EBRT (range 70–74 Gy) was assessed (Widmark et al. 2009). From 1996 to 2002, 875 patients with locally advanced PCa (T3; 78 %) were randomized to endocrine treatment alone (3 months of total androgen blockage followed by continuous endocrine treatment using flutamide or to endocrine treatment combined with EBRT). The primary endpoint was PCSS. At a median follow-up of 7.6 years, this study showed an absolute 12 % difference in mortality in favor of the combined arm (23.9 % vs. 11.9 %, CI 4.9–19.1, relative risk = 0.44). The overall mortality was halved at 10 years for prostate cancer-specific death.

The National Cancer Institute of Canada-Clinical Trials Group/Southwest Oncology Group T94-0110 trial showed a significant reduction in the mortality risks with the addition of RT to ADT after median follow-up of 7 years (overall survival 74 % with ADT + EBRT compared to 66 % to ADT, $p = 0.0033$) (Warde et al. 2011). This trial included 1,205 patients and provides convincing evidence that local

Table 2 Comparison of outcome in patients treated with high-dose-rate-brachytherapy boost actuarial 5-year estimates

Reference	Risk group	No. of patients	bNED (%)	DFS (%)	PCSS (%)	OS (%)	Period (months)
Åstrøm et al.	All	214	82	91	97	89	48[a]
	High	47	56	80	86	74	
	Intermediate	87	87	93	100	92	
	Low	80	92	94	100	94	
Galalae et al.	All	588	77	67	96	85	60[b]
	High	354	69	61	95	85	
	Intermediate	188	88	75	99	86	
	Low	46	96	83	100	88	
Martinez et al.	All	207	74	68	98	92	58[b]
	High	35	50	41	97	91	
	Intermediate	75	75	72	97	93	
	Low	97	85	77	100	92	
Lilleby et al.	All	275	98.5	95.6	99.3	96.3	42[a]
	High	256	98.8	95.2	99.6	96.8	
	Intermediate	19	100	100	96	92	
Phan et al.	All	309	86				59[a]
	High	67	78				
	Intermediate	109	90				
	Low	133	98				
Viani et al.	All	131	81				62.8[a]
	High	66	71				
	Intermediate	65	87				

Observation period [a] median and [b] mean

bNED biochemical non-evidence of disease, *DFS* disease-free survival, *PCSS* Prostate cancer-specific survival, *OS* overall survival

control disease in the prostate improves survival in patients with locally advanced PCa. Interestingly, treatment-induced morbidity was not substantially different from the toxicity seen in the ADT-only cohort.

Also, in earlier stage of PCa the influence of ADT was investigated. D'Amico et al. designed a study testing 70 Gy plus 6 months of ADT versus EBRT alone for patients with intermediate risk (D'Amico et al. 2008). At a median follow-up of 4.5 years they found an overall survival advantage at 5 years for the combined group (88 % vs. 78 %, $p = 0.04$).

The results of seven published prospective randomized trials are acknowledged in Table 1.

3.2 HDR-Brachytherapy and LDR-Brachytherapy Outcome

For intermediate and high-risk disease there are concerns that BT alone may not adequately treat the periprostatic tissues and micrometastic spread nearby, and therefore, it may be used optimally as a boost in combination with EBRT and ADT in prognostically high-risk patients. It also has a potential biological advantage through the delivery of high doses per fraction. Dose escalation is feasible by combining RT with high-dose rate after loading BT, which provides optimal intensity-modulated conformal radiation dose delivery (Morris et al. 2013; Kuban and Dong 2004; Martinez et al. 2003). Hoskins' group recently published their findings applying neoadjuvant ADT to 76 % of their patients and adjuvant ADT to almost all high-risk patients, and they could demonstrate a significant dose–response relationship in the HDR-BT/EBRT arm (EBRT 35.75 Gy + HDR-BT 8.5 Gy × 2) resulting in improved 31 % reduction in the risk of recurrence compared to RT alone after a median observation time of 7.1 years (Hoskin et al. 2012). Trimodality therapy, a concept including ADT, RT, and a brachytherapy boost technique, administered in one recent population showed a favorable 5-year OS estimate (96 %) in comparison with published reports on OS in similar series employing only EBRT ± ADT (Lilleby et al. 2012). Lilleby et al. found a high rate of PCSS (99.3 %, see Table 2) compared with other series, conducted in a group of high-risk patients after a median follow-up of 44.2 months (Lilleby et al. 2012). The rigorous surgical staging procedures confirming pN0 status in most of the treated patients may have contributed to these excellent results. Still, only prospectively randomized trials can clarify the beneficial role of long-term ADT with HDR-BT + EBRT compared to ADT + EBRT in high-risk patients.

Conformal LDR-brachytherapy has shown acceptable late side effects and especially low frequency of clinically relevant rectal damage (Martinez et al. 2003; Yoshioka 2009).

In a long-term follow-up study by Zelefsky et al. comparing LDR-BT versus EBRT using IMRT in 729 patients, Grade 2 GI side effects were reported in 5.1 and 1.4 %, respectively (Zelefsky et al. 2011). Grade 2 GU treatment-related toxicity was more often described in the LDR-BT group 15.6 versus 4.3 % for the EBRT group ($p < 0.0001$). There was no difference in Grade 3 GI toxicity for both treatment modalities. The overall side effects are mild with low risk of developing incontinence and loss of potency (Hinnen et al. 2010).

So far, only one small randomized study has been performed (Giberti et al. 2009) comparing LDR-BT to PRECT and others had been stopped prematurely due to insufficient accrual (Crook et al. 2011; Eccles et al. 2013). However, the results from multi-center collaborations (Morris et al. 2013; Dickinson et al. 2013) show comparable biochemical disease-free intervals to PRECT and EBRT and add to the growing body of evidence that LDR-BT is an effective and durable treatment option for men with low-risk PCa. This modality may be especially valuable for men unfit for active surveillance or in those who wish active intervention.

4 Conclusion

PCa is a heterogeneous disease with indolent as well as aggressive courses leading to overtreatment with significant side effects in early small tumor volume PCa (Stamey et al. 1999) and undertreatment with substantial morbidity and fatal outcome due to progressive disease in cases with locally advanced cancers. As patients with an aggressive course succumb to PCa, the right treatment decision demands evidence-based facts on objective and consented parameters to support it.

Due to improved outcome issues related to long survivorship in PCa, adverse effects and quality of life should be a fundamental integral part in each patient's counselling. Thus, there is considerable risk of being sidetracked by randomization methodology when looking for small gains in large groups. Instead, relevant healthcare breakthroughs in terms of PCCS will presumably only be achieved by identifying and including high-risk patients into randomized trials in whom it is clinically necessary to improve cure with acceptable morbidity. Modern staging and improvements in diagnostic markers will presumably spare low-risk patients from unnecessary intervention with the risk of treatment-induced morbidity in the future.

This is not the beginning of the end. The next generation of trials in PCa has to take into account the changing landscape in PCa, integrating new achievements in molecular diagnostics, and patient's preferences leading to personalized medicine with modern radiotherapy as one major treatment cornerstone.

References

Albertsen PC, Hanley JA, Barrows GH, Penson DF, Kowalczyk PD, Sanders MM, Fine J (2005) Prostate cancer and the Will Rogers phenomenon. J Natl Cancer Inst 97(17):1248–1253

Andriole GL, Crawford ED, Grubb RL III, Buys SS, Chia D, Church TR, Fouad MN, Gelmann EP, Kvale PA, Reding DJ, Weissfeld JL, Yokochi LA et al (2009) Mortality results from a randomized prostate-cancer screening trial. N Engl J Med 360(13):1310–1319

Andriole GL, Crawford ED, Grubb RL III, Buys SS, Chia D, Church TR, Fouad MN, Isaacs C, Kvale PA, Reding DJ, Weissfeld JL, Yokochi LA et al (2012) Prostate cancer screening in the randomized prostate, lung, colorectal, and ovarian cancer screening trial: mortality results after 13 years of follow-up. J Natl Cancer Inst 104(2):125–132

Bill-Axelson A, Holmberg L, Ruutu M, Garmo H, Stark JR, Busch C, Nordling S, Haggman M, Andersson SO, Bratell S, Spangberg A, Palmgren J et al (2011) Radical prostatectomy versus watchful waiting in early prostate cancer. N Engl J Med 364(18):1708–1717

Bolla M, de Reijke TM, Van TG, Van den Bergh AC, Oddens J, Poortmans PM, Gez E, Kil P, Akdas A, Soete G, Kariakine O, van der Steen-Banasik EM et al (2009) Duration of androgen suppression in the treatment of prostate cancer. N Engl J Med 360(24):2516–2527

Bolla M, Gonzalez D, Warde P, Dubois JB, Mirimanoff RO, Storme G, Bernier J, Kuten A, Sternberg C, Gil T, Collette L, Pierart M (1997) Improved survival in patients with locally advanced prostate cancer treated with radiotherapy and goserelin. N Engl J Med 337(5):295–300

Bray F, Lortet-Tieulent J, Ferlay J, Forman D, Auvinen A (2010) Prostate cancer incidence and mortality trends in 37 European countries: an overview. Eur J Cancer 46(17):3040–3052

Brenner DJ, Hall EJ, Curtis RE, Ron E (2005) Prostate radiotherapy is associated with second cancers in many organs, not just the colorectum. Gastroenterology 129(2):773–774

Bria E, Cuppone F, Giannarelli D, Milella M, Ruggeri EM, Sperduti I, Pinnaro P, Terzoli E, Cognetti F, Carlini P (2009) Does hormone treatment added to radiotherapy improve outcome in locally advanced prostate cancer? Meta-analysis of randomized trials. Cancer 115(15):3446–3456

Center MM, Jemal A, Lortet-Tieulent J, Ward E, Ferlay J, Brawley O, Bray F (2012) International variation in prostate cancer incidence and mortality rates. Eur Urol 61(6):1079–1092

Crook JM, Gomez-Iturriaga A, Wallace K, Ma C, Fung S, Alibhai S, Jewett M, Fleshner N (2011) Comparison of health-related quality of life 5 years after SPIRIT: surgical prostatectomy versus interstitial radiation intervention trial. J Clin Oncol 29(4):362–368

Dall'Era MA, Albertsen PC, Bangma C, Carroll PR, Carter HB, Cooperberg MR, Freedland SJ, Klotz LH, Parker C, Soloway MS (2012) Active surveillance for prostate cancer: a systematic review of the literature. Eur Urol 62(6):976–983

D'Amico AV, Chen MH, Renshaw AA, Loffredo M, Kantoff PW (2008) Androgen suppression and radiation vs radiation alone for prostate cancer: a randomized trial. JAMA 299(3):289–295

Dearnaley DP, Sydes MR, Graham JD, Aird EG, Bottomley D, Cowan RA, Huddart RA, Jose CC, Matthews JH, Millar J, Moore AR, Morgan RC et al (2007) Escalated-dose versus standard-dose conformal radiotherapy in prostate cancer: first results from the MRC RT01 randomised controlled trial. Lancet Oncol 8(6):475–487

Dickinson P, Malik J, Mandall P, Swindell R, Bottomley D, Hoskin P, Logue J, Wylie J (2013) Five year outcomes following I-125 seed brachytherapy for low risk prostate cancer at three United Kingdom cancer centres. BJU Int. doi: 10.1111/bju.12358

Draisma G, Etzioni R, Tsodikov A, Mariotto A, Wever E, Gulati R, Feuer E, de KH (2009) Lead time and overdiagnosis in prostate-specific antigen screening: importance of methods and context. J Natl Cancer Inst 101(6):374–383

Eccles BK, Cross W, Rosario DJ, Doble A, Parker C, Logue J, Little L, Stanton L, Bottomley D (2013) SABRE 1 (Surgery Against Brachytherapy—a Randomised Evaluation): feasibility randomised controlled trial (RCT) of brachytherapy vs radical prostatectomy in low-intermediate risk clinically localised prostate cancer. BJU Int 112(3):330–337

Eggener SE, Scardino PT, Walsh PC, Han M, Partin AW, Trock BJ, Feng Z, Wood DP, Eastham JA, Yossepowitch O, Rabah DM, Kattan MW et al (2011) Predicting 15-year prostate cancer specific mortality after radical prostatectomy. J Urol 185(3):869–875

Epstein JI, Feng Z, Trock BJ, Pierorazio PM (2012) Upgrading and downgrading of prostate cancer from biopsy to radical prostatectomy: incidence and predictive factors using the modified Gleason grading system and factoring in tertiary grades. Eur Urol 61(5): 1019–1024

Fleming TR, DeMets DL (1996) Surrogate end points in clinical trials: are we being misled? Ann Intern Med 125(7):605–613

Giberti C, Chiono L, Gallo F, Schenone M, Gastaldi E (2009) Radical retropubic prostatectomy versus brachytherapy for low-risk prostatic cancer: a prospective study. World J Urol 27(5):607–612

Hanks GE, Pajak TF, Porter A, Grignon D, Brereton H, Venkatesan V, Horwitz EM, Lawton C, Rosenthal SA, Sandler HM, Shipley WU (2003) Phase III trial of long-term adjuvant androgen deprivation after neoadjuvant hormonal cytoreduction and radiotherapy in locally advanced carcinoma of the prostate: the radiation therapy oncology group protocol 92–02. J Clin Oncol 21(21):3972–3978

Heidenreich A, Bellmunt J, Bolla M, Joniau S, Mason M, Matveev V, Mottet N (2011) Schmid HP, van der KT, Wiegel T, Zattoni F. [EAU guidelines on prostate cancer. Part I: screening, diagnosis, and treatment of clinically localised disease]. Actas Urol Esp 35(9):501–514

Hinnen KA, Battermann JJ, van Roermund JG, Moerland MA, Jurgenliemk-Schulz IM, Frank SJ, van VM (2010) Long-term biochemical and survival outcome of 921 patients treated with I-125 permanent prostate brachytherapy. Int J Radiat Oncol Biol Phys 76(5):1433–1438

Hoskin PJ, Rojas AM, Bownes PJ, Lowe GJ, Ostler PJ, Bryant L (2012) Randomised trial of external beam radiotherapy alone or combined with high-dose-rate brachytherapy boost for localised prostate cancer. Radiother Oncol 103(2):217–222

Jemal A, Bray F, Center MM, Ferlay J, Ward E, Forman D (2011) Global cancer statistics. CA Cancer J Clin 61(2):69–90

Kim MM, Hoffman KE, Levy LB, Frank SJ, Pugh TJ, Choi S, Nguyen QN, McGuire SE, Lee AK, Kuban DA (2012) Prostate cancer-specific mortality after definitive radiation therapy: who dies of disease? Eur J Cancer 48(11):1664–1671

Kovacs G, Potter R, Loch T, Hammer J, Kolkman-Deurloo IK, de la Rosette JJ, Bertermann H (2005) GEC/ESTRO-EAU recommendations on temporary brachytherapy using stepping sources for localised prostate cancer. Radiother Oncol 74(2):137–148

Kuban DA, Dong L (2004) High-dose intensity modulated radiation therapy for prostate cancer. Curr Urol Rep 5(3):197–202

Kvale R, Moller B, Angelsen A, Dahl O, Fossa SD, Halvorsen OJ, Hoem L, Solberg A, Wahlqvist R, Bray F (2010) Regional trends in prostate cancer incidence, treatment with curative intent and mortality in Norway 1980–2007. Cancer Epidemiol 34(4):359–367

Kyrdalen AE, Dahl AA, Hernes E, Hem E, Fossa SD (2010) Fatigue in prostate cancer survivors treated with definitive radiotherapy and LHRH analogs. Prostate 70(13):1480–1489

Lawton CA, DeSilvio M, Roach M III, Uhl V, Kirsch R, Seider M, Rotman M, Jones C, Asbell S, Valicenti R, Hahn S, Thomas CR Jr (2007) An update of the phase III trial comparing whole pelvic to prostate only radiotherapy and neoadjuvant to adjuvant total androgen suppression: updated analysis of RTOG 94–13, with emphasis on unexpected hormone/radiation interactions. Int J Radiat Oncol Biol Phys 69(3):646–655

Lilleby W, Stensvold A, Dahl AA (2013) Intensity-modulated radiotherapy to the pelvis and androgen deprivation in men with locally advanced prostate cancer: a study of adverse effects and their relation to quality of life. Prostate 73(10):1038–1047

Lilleby W, Tafjord G, Raabe NK (2012) Implementation of high-dose-rate brachytherapy and androgen deprivation in patients with prostate cancer. Int J Radiat Oncol Biol Phys 83(3):933–939

Martinez A, Gonzalez J, Spencer W, Gustafson G, Kestin L, Kearney D, Vicini FA (2003) Conformal high dose rate brachytherapy improves biochemical control and cause specific survival in patients with prostate cancer and poor prognostic factors. J Urol 169(3):974–979

Morris WJ, Keyes M, Spadinger I, Kwan W, Liu M, McKenzie M, Pai H, Pickles T, Tyldesley S (2013) Population-based 10-year oncologic outcomes after low-dose-rate brachytherapy for low-risk and intermediate-risk prostate cancer. Cancer 119(8):1537–1546

Parker C, Muston D, Melia J, Moss S, Dearnaley D (2006) A model of the natural history of screen-detected prostate cancer, and the effect of radical treatment on overall survival. Br J Cancer 94(10):1361–1368

Peeters ST, Heemsbergen WD, Koper PC, van Putten WL, Slot A, Dielwart MF, Bonfrer JM, Incrocci L, Lebesque JV (2006) Dose-response in radiotherapy for localized prostate cancer: results of the Dutch multicenter randomized phase III trial comparing 68 Gy of radiotherapy with 78 Gy. J Clin Oncol 24(13):1990–1996

Pilepich MV, Winter K, John MJ, Mesic JB, Sause W, Rubin P, Lawton C, Machtay M, Grignon D (2001) Phase III radiation therapy oncology group (RTOG) trial 86–10 of androgen deprivation adjuvant to definitive radiotherapy in locally advanced carcinoma of the prostate. Int J Radiat Oncol Biol Phys 50(5): 1243–1252

Pilepich MV, Winter K, Lawton CA, Krisch RE, Wolkov HB, Movsas B, Hug EB, Asbell SO, Grignon D (2005) Androgen suppression adjuvant to definitive radiotherapy in prostate carcinoma–long-term results of phase III RTOG 85-31. Int J Radiat Oncol Biol Phys 61(5):1285–1290

Pound CR, Partin AW, Eisenberger MA, Chan DW, Pearson JD, Walsh PC (1999) Natural history of progression after PSA elevation following radical prostatectomy. JAMA 281(17):1591–1597

Prentice RL (2009) Surrogate and mediating endpoints: current status and future directions. J Natl Cancer Inst 101(4):216–217

Ray ME, Bae K, Hussain MH, Hanks GE, Shipley WU, Sandler HM (2009) Potential surrogate endpoints for prostate cancer survival: analysis of a phase III randomized trial. J Natl Cancer Inst 101(4):228–236

Sanda MG, Dunn RL, Michalski J, Sandler HM, Northouse L, Hembroff L, Lin X, Greenfield TK, Litwin MS, Saigal CS, Mahadevan A, Klein E et al (2008) Quality of life and satisfaction with outcome among prostate-cancer survivors. N Engl J Med 358(12):1250–1261

Schroder FH, Hugosson J, Roobol MJ, Tammela TL, Ciatto S, Nelen V, Kwiatkowski M, Lujan M, Lilja H, Zappa M, Denis LJ, Recker F et al (2012) Prostate-cancer mortality at 11 years of follow-up. N Engl J Med 366(11):981–990

Shelley MD, Kumar S, Coles B, Wilt T, Staffurth J, Mason MD (2009) Adjuvant hormone therapy for localised and locally advanced prostate carcinoma: a systematic review and meta-analysis of randomised trials. Cancer Treat Rev 35(7):540–546

Solberg A, Haugen OA, Viset T, Bergh A, Tasdemir I, Ahlgren G, Widmark A, Angelsen A (2011) Residual prostate cancer in patients treated with endocrine therapy with or without radical radiotherapy: a side study of the SPCG-7 randomized trial. Int J Radiat Oncol Biol Phys 80(1):55–61

Stamey TA, McNeal JE, Yemoto CM, Sigal BM, Johnstone IM (1999) Biological determinants of cancer progression in men with prostate cancer. JAMA 281(15):1395–1400

Steinsvik EA, Fossa SD, Axcrona K, Fransson P, Widmark A, Dahl AA (2010) Do perceptions of adverse events differ between patients and physicians? Findings from a randomized, controlled trial of radical treatment for prostate cancer. J Urol 184(2):525–531

Stensvold A, Dahl AA, Brennhovd B, Cvancarova M, Fossa SD, Lilleby W, Axcrona K, Smeland S (2012) Methods for prospective studies of adverse effects as applied to prostate cancer patients treated with surgery or radiotherapy without hormones. Prostate 72(6):668–676

Stephenson AJ, Bolla M, Briganti A, Cozzarini C, Moul JW, Roach M III, van Poppel H, Zietman A (2012) Postoperative radiation therapy for pathologically advanced prostate cancer after radical prostatectomy. Eur Urol 61(3):443–451

Valicenti R, Lu J, Pilepich M, Asbell S, Grignon D (2000) Survival advantage from higher-dose radiation therapy for clinically localized prostate cancer treated on the radiation therapy oncology group trials. J Clin Oncol 18(14):2740–2746

Viani GA, Stefano EJ, Afonso SL (2009) Higher-than-conventional radiation doses in localized prostate cancer treatment: a meta-analysis of randomized, controlled trials. Int J Radiat Oncol Biol Phys 74(5):1405–1418

Wallace K, Fleshner N, Jewett M, Basiuk J, Crook J (2006) Impact of a multi-disciplinary patient education session on accrual to a difficult clinical trial: the Toronto experience with the surgical prostatectomy versus interstitial radiation intervention trial. J Clin Oncol 24(25):4158–4162

Warde P, Mason M, Ding K, Kirkbride P, Brundage M, Cowan R, Gospodarowicz M, Sanders K, Kostashuk E, Swanson G, Barber J, Hiltz A et al (2011) Combined androgen deprivation therapy and radiation therapy for locally advanced prostate cancer: a randomised, phase 3 trial. Lancet 378(9809):2104–2111

Widmark A, Klepp O, Solberg A, Damber JE, Angelsen A, Fransson P, Lund JA, Tasdemir I, Hoyer M, Wiklund F, Fossa SD (2009) Endocrine treatment, with or without radiotherapy, in locally advanced prostate cancer (SPCG-7/SFUO-3): an open randomised phase III trial. Lancet 373(9660):301–308

Yoshioka Y (2009) Current status and perspectives of brachytherapy for prostate cancer. Int J Clin Oncol 14(1):31–36

Zelefsky MJ, Pei X, Chou JF, Schechter M, Kollmeier M, Cox B, Yamada Y, Fidaleo A, Sperling D, Happersett L, Zhang Z (2011) Dose escalation for prostate cancer radiotherapy: predictors of long-term biochemical tumor control and distant metastases-free survival outcomes. Eur Urol 60(6):1133–1139

Zelefsky MJ, Yamada Y, Fuks Z, Zhang Z, Hunt M, Cahlon O, Park J, Shippy A (2008) Long-term results of conformal radiotherapy for prostate cancer: impact of dose escalation on biochemical tumor control and distant metastases-free survival outcomes. Int J Radiat Oncol Biol Phys 71(4):1028–1033

Late Toxicity and Quality of Life

Michael Geier and Hans Geinitz

Contents

M. Geier (✉) · H. Geinitz
Department of Radiation Oncology,
Krankenhaus der Barmherzigen Schwestern Linz,
Seilerstätte 4, 4020 Linz, Austria
e-mail: Michael.Geier@bhs.at

Abstract

As there seems to be no perceptible impact of treatment choice on overall survival of patients with localized prostate cancer, other criteria have to be taken into consideration choosing the appropriate treatment option for the individual patient. There is increasing awareness that predicted functional outcomes, including quality of life, alongside objective measures of late adverse genitourinary and gastrointestinal toxicity are essential components of the decision-making process in the management of patients with prostate cancer. Assessing the impact of available treatment modalities on health-related quality of life (HRQOL) therefore is gaining further importance. This chapter gives an overview of the main toxicity scoring instruments and HRQOL measures. It furthermore summarizes pathophysiological mechanisms of the mainly reported late toxicities after radiotherapy and gives a short overview of their possible treatment options. Due to the large amount of studies on side effects and HRQOL in prostate cancer patients it is beyond the scope of this chapter to give a comprehensive review on this issue. Instead, general aspects as well as particular problems and obstacles regarding the assessment and interpretation of HRQOL-Data will be highlighted.

1 Introduction

Patients with clinically localized prostate cancer have a favorable long-term overall and cancer-specific rate of survival regardless of treatment choice. By now, there are only a few completed prospective, randomized trials that evaluate differences in survival outcomes between radical prostatectomy and external beam radiation therapy (Alicikus et al. 2011; Birkhahn et al. 2011; D'amico et al. 1998). As there seems to be no perceptible impact on overall survival, other criteria have to be taken into consideration choosing the appropriate treatment option for the individual patient. There

H. Geinitz et al. (eds.), *Radiotherapy in Prostate Cancer*, Medical Radiology. Radiation Oncology,
DOI: 10.1007/174_2014_1035,

Published Online: 22 August 2014

is increasing awareness that predicted functional outcomes including quality of life alongside with objective measures of late adverse genitourinary and gastrointestinal toxicity are essential components of the decision-making process in the management of patients with prostate cancer. In this regard, it has to be mentioned that even acute and late side effects in published data are not easily comparable, mostly due to the large variety of adapted toxicity scales (Hoeller et al. 2003). In contrast to these more or less exactly and objectively measurable treatment-related issues, the evaluation of health-related quality of life (HRQOL) comprises even more uncertainties and difficulties especially when comparing current available data on HRQL for patients with surgery versus radiotherapy or when comparing the results of different radiotherapy concepts. Besides to HRQOL inherent issues, associated with the multifactorial and complex quality of life (QOL) concept, there are also study-related methodical and statistical uncertainties, making it hard drawing a clear conclusion how and to what extent HRQOL is influenced by prostate cancer treatment.

This chapter gives an overview on the main toxicity and HRQOL scoring instruments. It furthermore focuses on reported late toxicity after definitive radiotherapy for prostate cancer and its impact on the patients' HRQOL. Due to the vast amount of studies on side effects as well as on HRQOL in prostate cancer patients, it is beyond the scope of this chapter to give a comprehensive review. Instead, general aspects as well as particular problems and obstacles, which to our opinion represent important issues, will be highlighted.

2 Late Toxicity Scoring

2.1 RTOG/EORTC Late Morbidity System

The necessity of quantifying and scoring late effects has always been a concern of radiation oncologists. Therefore, a grading system was encouraged by the Radiation Therapy Oncology Group (RTOG) and the European Organization for Research and Treatment of Cancer (EORTC), called Late Effects Morbidity Scales in the late 1970s. The Acute Radiation Morbidity Scoring Criteria were developed in 1985 as complimentary to the Late Effects Scoring Criteria. The RTOG/EORTC Late Radiation Morbidity Scoring Scheme grades severity of reactions from 0 to 5. The categories can be summarized in the following manner. Zero means the absence of radiation effects and 1, 2, 3 describing mild, moderate to severe side effects. For grade 4, toxicities usually are local necrosis or the loss of function concerning the specific organ or tissue characteristic, whereas grade 5 effects lead to death. In most RTOG publications, major toxicities have been reported as grades 3, 4, and 5 taken together. Cumulative probabilities of "major" toxicities are often presented as risk estimates at discrete intervals, such as 1 year and 2 year. These probabilities are also presented graphically to show the propensity for continued increases with time (Cox et al. 1995).

2.2 LENT-SOMA

The National Cancer Institute (NCI) consensus conferences have led to the introduction of SOMA classification for late toxicity: *subjective*, *objective*, *management* criteria with *analytic* laboratory and imaging procedures. These scales, specific for each organ, form a scaffold for understanding the expression of later injury because their contents are the substance of late effects in normal tissue (LENT) expression (LENT-SOMA tables, Radiother Oncol. 1995; 35:17–60).

2.3 CTCAE

As reported by Trotti et al. (Trotti et al. 2003), the (NCI) Common Toxicity Criteria system (CTC version 1.0) was first created in 1983 to aid in the recognition and grading adverse effects of chemotherapy. It was updated and expanded in 1998 (CTC version 2.0) but remained focused on acute effects. In an effort to create a single grading platform incorporating full surgical side effects as well as late effects and pediatric criteria, the NCI has guided the development of a significant revision of the CTC (CTCAE version 3.0) in 2006. Nevertheless, it does not clearly and consistently distinguish between early and late effects. Since the third version, the CTC has been renamed the Common Terminology Criteria for Adverse Events version 3.0 (CTCAE version 3.0) and was again updated in 2010 (CTCAE v4.0). Like the aforementioned scoring systems, the CTCAE divides severity of adverse events into 5 graduations. Grade 1 effects are minimal and usually asymptomatic and do not interfere with functional endpoints. Interventions or medications are generally not indicated for these minor effects. Grade 2 effects are considered moderate and are usually symptomatic, and interventions such as local treatment or medications may be indicated. They may or may not interfere with specific functions but not enough to impair activities of daily living. Grade 3 effects are considered severe and very undesirable. There are usually multiple, disruptive symptoms. More serious interventions, including surgery or hospitalization, may be indicated. Grade 4 effects are potentially life threatening, catastrophic, disabling, or result in loss of organ, organ function, or limb. A grade 5 event is specified as death related to an AE.

3 Quality of Life Measures

In contrast to the mostly physician-reported toxicity data, evaluation of HRQOL is usually patient-reported. In this regard, survey instrument measuring HRQOL in prostate cancer as reported by Sommers and Ramsey (1999) should be valid, reliable, responsive, and feasible. This means a valid instrument is able to measure what it is intended for. Reliability describes the ability of an instrument to yield the same results on separate occasions at stable disease. A reliable instrument therefore can distinguish between real "intergroup" differences and statistical noise. A responsive instrument further has the ability to find small differences between analyzed groups. Currently, there is a wide range of HRQOL questionnaires available more or less meeting these criteria, and their use should be based on the purpose of the assessment.

In general, the instruments used in HRQOL assessment can be divided into generic or specific measures. The first mentioned assess overall well-being by addressing general health perceptions and social, emotional as well as physical function. Furthermore, they allow comparing, e.g., health states in prostate cancer with the general population and other conditions. The specific measures predominantly aim on domains and issues that are specific to a certain disease or treatment. They focus on how dysfunction in a single organ or disease affects overall HRQOL. By assessing what is likely to be most relevant to an individual with the specific disease, e.g., urinary dysfunction after prostate cancer treatment or anxiety about recurrence of a malignancy, they usually are able to detect HRQOL changes more often than generic instruments. Nevertheless, there is an overlap of generic and disease-specific instruments, and so their interplay must be considered when using HRQOL outcomes for research or in clinical practice (Fossa et al. 1997). In the section below, we review the most frequently used instruments in the prostate literature.

3.1 Generic Health-Related Quality of Life (HRQOL) Instruments

The RAND (Research and Development)-Organization Medical Outcomes Study 36-Item Health Survey (SF-36) and its shorter counterpart (SF-12) are the most commonly applied generic instruments for men with prostate cancer (Ware and Sherbourne 1992). The 36-item questionnaire takes about 10 min to complete and includes eight domains of health: physical function, role limitation owing to physical problems, bodily pain, general health perception, social function, emotional well-being, role limitation resulting from emotional problems, fatigue and energy. The SF-36 further summarizes HRQOL into two domains, physical and mental, which are most readily accessible to clinicians. The SF-12 includes only the two summary domains, but is similar to SF-36 in clinical and research utility (Gandhi et al. 2001; Jenkinson et al. 2001; Lim and Fisher 1999; Resnick and Nahm 2001; Salyers et al. 2000). Due to the fact that both do not specifically yield on bowel, sexual, and urinary function, prostate cancer patients with a significantly decreased function in these issues may have comparable scores to age-matched men without prostate cancer (Litwin et al. 1995; Schlenk et al. 1998).

3.2 Cancer-Specific HRQOL Instruments

General cancer-specific instruments offer a bit more nuanced view of HRQOL in men with prostate cancer compared to a generic measure.

The European Organization for the Research and Treatment of Cancer Quality of Life Questionnaire (EORTC QLQ-C30) is a generic core questionnaire developed 1988, with the current version 3.0 of the QLQ-C30 available. It measures broader aspects of cancer-specific HRQOL in five functional domains (physical, role, cognitive, emotional, and social functioning), a global health status scale, three symptom scales (fatigue, nausea/vomiting, and pain), and six single items (dyspnea, insomnia, appetite loss, constipation, diarrhea, and financial difficulties due to disease or treatment) (Aaronson et al. 1993; Holzner et al. 2006). Modules specific for diseases including cancers of the prostate (Vachalec et al. 2002), breast (Sprangers et al. 1996), lung (Bergman et al. 1994), head and neck (Bjordal et al. 1994) as well as other sites have been developed. These modules can be used separately or in conjunction with the core instrument.

The Functional Assessment of Cancer Therapy (FACT) instrument contains the FACT-G a general, self-administered, 28-item survey which builds 5 domains/scales measuring physical, social/family, emotional "well-being" and the relationship with the physicians (Holzner et al. 2006). It also can be paired with a set of items specific to different tumor sites.

3.3 Prostate Cancer-Specific HRQOL Instruments

There are several instruments specific to prostate cancer available which can be used on their own or in conjunction with generic HRQOL tools to assess quality of life in men with prostate cancer.

Like aforementioned is it possible to the extend the EORTC QLQ-CQ30 core questionnaire with the 25-item EORTC QLQ-PR25 supplementary module that assesses aspects of HRQOL specific to prostate cancer (van Andel et al. 2008). The EORTC QLQ-PR25 has four domains focusing on sexual activity and functioning, urinary symptoms, bowel symptoms, and treatment-related symptoms during the past 1 and 4 weeks.

The FACT-G instrument also can be enhanced using the disease-specific FACT-Prostate (FACT-P) modifier (Esper et al. 1997). It contains a 12-item prostate cancer subscale focused on pain, erectile and urinary habits, and sense of "manhood".

The 20-item UCLA-PCI is a "stand-alone" disease-specific HRQOL instrument that besides to sexual, urinary, and bowel function also evaluates bother, which reflects any distress caused by dysfunction, obviously an important issue in HRQOL as this describes the degree to which symptoms are interfering with an individual's life. The UCLA-PCI has been widely validated in men with and without prostate cancer from several ethnicities and countries and has been translated into and validated in Chinese, Dutch, French, German, Icelandic, Italian, Japanese, Portuguese, and Spanish.

The 50-item EPIC (Expanded Prostate Cancer Index Composite) is a comprehensive instrument (Wei et al. 2000) also designed to evaluate function and bother after prostate cancer treatment. It was developed using parts from the UCLA-PCI enhanced with items in part addressing more radiotherapy-related voiding and storage symptoms, hematuria and hormonal symptoms. Several versions of the EPIC have been validated, including a short form and an instrument containing only hormonal domains (Szymanski et al. 2010).

4 Prostate-Specific Late Toxicity

4.1 Genitourinary Late Toxicity

In general, main acute genitourinary symptoms in prostate cancer patients treated with radiotherapy comprise alguria and increase in frequency, especially nocturia, urgency, obstruction, hematuria, and more uncommon urinary incontinence. These symptoms can appear usually during the second half or the last third of therapy and mostly resolve within 3 months after treatment spontaneously. Severe side effects as fistulas or obstruction are rarely reported and normally related to tumor infiltration rather than to radiotherapy effects.

The development of late bladder injury is most likely primarily manifested in a bladder wall fibrosis with resultant loss of bladder wall compliance and contraction. The underlying pathophysiology behind these changes is supposed to be a radiation-induced damage to the vascular endothelial cells with subsequent vascular hyperplasia, perivascular fibrosis and in the end vascular occlusion that occur months to years after exposition to radiation. The resultant vascular ischemia leads to fibrosis and degeneration of the bladder wall, which in turn causes the clinical bladder dysfunction (Antonakopoulos et al. 1984; Stewart 1985, 1986). Stewart furthermore could show that acute epithelial cell damage is not associated with late bladder dysfunction, but together with the resulting inflammation of the bladder wall, it is supposed to be one possible pathophysiological mechanism for acute urogenital side effects.

Though the mechanisms of radiation-induced injury differing from acute to late toxicity, the latter mainly shows similar symptoms, regarding frequency including nocturia and urgency. Urinary incontinence, hematuria, and reduced uroflow, caused by urethral stenosis, are observed to a lesser extent.

Whether genitourinary acute and late side effects in general are rather caused by radiation-induced changes of the bladder itself or changes in the bladder neck including the prostatic urethra is not clearly understood by now, since a discrimination of the genitourinary symptoms regarding their origin in clinical studies is probably not feasible, because of their very similar irritative nature. However, there is indirect evidence coming from data in the post-prostatectomy setting where significantly less GU toxicity is observed (Grade 2: 2–5 % versus 15–30 %) (Wiegel et al. 2009; Zelefsky et al. 1997) at a similar to slightly lower dose range as compared to the primary radiotherapy setting. Thus, it might be hypothesized that clinically significant GU toxicity at least to some extent may rather be caused by inflammatoric processes of the prostate or the prostatic urethra than by changes comprising the bladder. Most likely due to these uncertainties regarding the exact topographical or functional origin of late urogenital toxicities no clear correlations between the dose distribution and side effects could be found by now, though, for example, there are already some considerations that higher dose peaks to the bladder neck including the prostatic urethra are associated with stronger voiding symptoms.

At least a characteristic pattern of complaints of the two up-to-date most common radiotherapy modalities (EBRT versus brachytherapy) could be identified and should be incorporated into an individual treatment recommendation, considering the patient-specific pretreatment symptoms. Therefore, low dose rate brachytherapy, for example, is usually not recommended to patients showing an elevated pretreatment IPSS due to its possible higher obstructive and irritative GU side effects.

4.2 Gastrointestinal Late Toxicity

4.2.1 Symptoms/Endpoints

The late gastrointestinal toxicity in prostate cancer patients treated with radiotherapy is mainly generated by radiation-induced rectal injury. Chronic proctitis occurs usually about 8–13 months after radiotherapy (Tagkalidis and Tjandra 2001), but late side effects can take up to 3 years to develop (Fiorino et al. 2009). The main reported symptom is late rectal bleeding, which is easy to assess and due to its low pre-treatment incidence easy to be detected as a radiation-induced side effect. Further symptoms of chronic rectal toxicity comprise elevated stool frequency, diarrhea and urge as well as mucous discharge and pain. Rare late complications are deep ulcerations and fistulas which are mainly associated with unnecessary biopsies to the anterior rectal wall due to rectal bleeding after prostate brachytherapy (Gelblum and Potters 2000; Theodorescu et al. 2000; Tran et al. 2005). Late fecal incontinence is also rarely reported after prostate radiotherapy, but might be underreported due to the patient´s embarrassment reporting fecal incontinence as well as due to the fact that the most prospective studies do not properly asses incontinence as a specific clinical endpoint (Putta and Andreyev 2005). Nevertheless, even when it is rarely reported fecal incontinence can profoundly affect the patients' quality of life. On the other hand, low to intermediate grade rectal bleeding does typically not compromise the patients' daily activities to a greater extend. Furthermore, concerning gastrointestinal late toxicity many symptoms and especially late rectal bleeding can subside with further follow-up of more than 4–5 years as it has been shown by Goldner et al. (Goldner et al. 2011) and others. Therefore, studies evaluating late radiation-induced gastrointestinal toxicity should consider the incidence and prevalence of side effects with a sufficient follow-up.

4.2.2 Pathophysiological Changes

Rectal bleeding With regard to rectal bleeding chronic radiation-induced rectal injury on the cellular level is characterized by a progressive vasculitis with subsequent thrombosis of small arteries and arterioles. This in turn can lead to a bowel wall ischemia of varying severity. Serious ischemia can consecutively cause necrosis with following deep ulceration and fistula formation. Due to the forming of small collateral vessels, longer-term changes are manifested in the development of teleangiectasis and neovascularization. These superficial small vessels are fragile and therefore susceptible for trauma and subsequent mucosal bleeding (Donner 1998). Moreover, the lamina propria can become fibrotic, and collagen can be deposited under the superficial epithelium. This again implies the risk of ulceration, mucosal sloughing, and fistulization (Buchi and Dixon 1987). In addition, the rectal mucosa is more vulnerable based on the reduced ability to regenerate which further results a thin mucosa built of atypical endothelial cells. On histopathological specimens of the rectal wall, small abscesses can be seen in the deep crypts, and beneath the intima, large foam cells can be found which are considered to be evidence of radiation-induced vascular injury. In the thickened and fibrotic submucosa, an infiltration by large actiniforme fibroblasts is often observed, and the muscularis propria also shows focal areas of fibrosis or penetrating ulcers. In the serosa, similarly diffuse hyaline modifications with immigration of fibroblasts as well as development of teleangiectasia and ischemic changes in larger vessels are observed. This ischemia results in the development of an opaque and thickened tissue surrounding the rectal wall (Zimmermann and Feldmann 1998).

Fecal Incontinence In contrast to rectal bleeding, the exact pathophysiology of radiation-induced fecal incontinence is not clearly understood by now. Due to the fact that in several patients with clinical measurable incontinence, no relevant morphologic changes of the anal sphincter complex —regarding thickness, etc,—were detected (Petersen et al. 2007; Yeoh et al. 1998). A group of other factors is hypothesized to build clinical correlates of incontinence. Besides the core factor of a reduced sphincter tone, several clinical signs are considered to be associated with radiation-induced incontinence, like a reduced rectal compliance and squeeze pressure (Berndtsson et al. 2002; Petersen et al. 2007; Yeoh et al. 1998). In this context, connective tissue remodeling of the rectum, including smooth muscle cell hypertrophy as well as decreased neural function due to damages in the myenteric plexus controlling the continence-related muscles, seems to be very important regarding the development of fecal incontinence after radiotherapy. These two processes are supposed to play a part in the reduction of rectal volumes at sensory threshold, the reduction of maximal rectal tolerance, and the reduction of compliance after pelvic radiation (Varma and Smith 1986; Varma et al. 1985, 1986). Moreover, a lumbosacral plexopathy was considered to influence fecal continence after radiotherapy (Georgiou et al. 1993; Iglicki et al. 1996). This presumable impact of a nerve damage as a basic cause was confirmed by several studies. For example, a significant decline in nerve density of the internal anal sphincter about 6–12 months after radiotherapy was reported by da Silva and interpreted as a myenteric plexus injury (Dasilva et al. 2003). In addition, a remarkable decreased electrosensitivity of the rectal wall was observed after pelvic radiotherapy (Kushwaha et al. 2003). Taken together, anorectal dysfunction after pelvic radiotherapy seems to be caused by a variety of pathophysiological changes in different morphological and functional structures responsible for fecal incontinence.

4.2.3 Predictors of Late Toxicity

Risk factors Patient-related risk factors for a higher incidence of radiation-induced proctitis in general were found to be a younger age, history of previous abdominal surgery, hypertension, vasculopathy, diabetes and hemorrhoids as well as acute radiation-induced proctitis, inflammatoric bowel diseases, connective tissue diseases, and a mutation in the ataxia–teleangiectasia gene (Garg et al. 2006; Gilinsky et al. 1983; Lanciano et al. 1992; Potish et al. 1979; Tagkalidis and Tjandra 2001).

Dose volume histogram (DVH) parameters Since late rectal complications are one of the main findings limiting dose escalation in prostate radiotherapy and as they are shown to be consistently correlated with DVH parameters, a big interest of radiation oncologists in that issue is obvious. This manifests in the enormous amount of data published in the literature regarding the correlation of DVH parameters with radiation-induced rectal acute and late toxicity.

Significant correlations of various dose volume parameters especially with the endpoint of rectal bleeding were found by numerous studies using EBRT for prostate cancer. Unfortunately, endpoints as well as follow-up differed between studies. Moreover, cutoff values for distinct dose volume parameters extracted from single patient populations are rarely prospectively verified in a second population. Also, different dose volume parameters are rarely combined and evaluated jointly; thus, a great part of dose volume histogram information is discharged, when only single parameters are evaluated. Nevertheless, QUANTEC (Quantitative Analysis of Normal Tissue Effects in the Clinic) and other initiatives took an effort to define cutoff values that are regarded to be clinically safe when using EBRT for prostate cancer patients. Data of selected studies as well as the QUANTEC recommendations are listed below.

Analyzing patients of an Italian intergroup study that were treated to doses between 70 and 78 Gy Fiorino et al. (2002, 2003) stated the following recommendations for rectal dose constraints with regard to the incidence of RTOG grade 2 late rectal bleeding: fractional volume of the rectum receiving ≥50Gy (V50) < 60, V60 < 45 , and V70 < 25 %. The last mentioned cutoff value, e.g., V70 < 25 % was confirmed by another study with the same RTOG endpoint, in patients treated at the William Beaumont Hospital with adaptive image guided 3D-CRT to total doses in the range from 70.2 to 79.2 Gy (Vargas et al. 2005). The V70 recommendation was furthermore confirmed by Fiorino et al. later analyzing patients of a multicenter study treated at 70–80 Gy. Rectal late bleeding ≥ grade 2 was evaluated according to the LENT-SOMA scale, and the DVH cutoff values in addition to the V70 recommendation were comparable to the constraints stated above, e.g., V75 < 5, V60 < 40, and V50 < 55 % (Fellin et al. 2009; Fiorino et al. 2008).

The proposed rectal constraints considering overall late toxicity instead of rectal bleeding as a single clinical endpoint are very similar to the already mentioned. Huang et al., for example, published data from the MD Anderson Center analyzing 163 patients with regard to the incidence of late GI toxicity 6 years after radiotherapy (total dose 74–78 Gy). The overall late 61 toxicity RTOG grade 2 or higher was about 25 %. Correlating rectal DVH data with the incidence of late toxicity they found that the percentage of the rectum receiving a certain dose was more predictive of late rectal side effects than the absolute volume and further recommended to keep the rectal V60 below 40 %, the V70 below 25 %, the V75.6 below 15 %, and the V78 below 5 %, respectively (Huang et al. 2002). On the other hand, Cahlon et al. reported a grade 2 or higher late rectal toxicity (CTCAE) of about 4 % even with a V75.6 < 30 % and a V47 < 53 %, evaluating the data of 478 patients treated to a total dose of 86.4 Gy using IMRT (Cahlon et al. 2008).

DVH data and fecal incontinence With a risk of less than 1 % severe fecal incontinence characterized as the need of multiple pad use per week, it is a rare late radiation side effect. Although the development of this condition is supposed to be a multifactorial process, a significant correlation of rectal DVH parameters with the incidence of fecal incontinence could be demonstrated by some studies (Fiorino et al. 2008; Peeters et al. 2006). In contrast to rectal bleeding where predominantly the higher dose regions are most predictive, late fecal incontinence rather was associated with intermediate doses to larger volumes of the rectum. Two large studies recommended a V40 of the rectum below 65 % as a predictor for a low incontinence risk about 1–2 % (Fiorino et al. 2008; Peeters et al. 2006).

In 2010, the RTOG published the QUANTEC data aiming to develop a general dose constraint recommendation for every organ site, by taking the main individual publications into consideration. With regard to rectal toxicity, data were summarized by Michalski et al. (2010) and they recommended the following rectal dose constraints to limit grade ≥2 late rectal toxicity to <15 % and the probability of grade ≥3 late rectal toxicity to <10 %, when patients were treated to a total dose of about 80 Gy using 1.8–2 Gy per fraction: V50 < 50 %, V60 < 35, V65 < 25, V70 < 20, and V75 < 15 %.

However, looking at these recommendations, some limitations and several other aspects have to be considered. First to mention is the fact that a planning CT scan is not necessary reflecting the anatomical situation during the whole course of treatment. Moreover, uncertainties in contouring (e.g., inter- and intraobserver variability) have to be regarded as further possible variables, when using the recommended dose constraints.

Beyond the plain DVH data also spatial dose distribution, i.e., the anatomical localization of radiation dose, seems to be relevant for the prediction of rectal late effects, as some authors found that doses to larger volumes of the distal rectum are associated with a higher risk of late fecal incontinence and rectal bleeding (Al-Abany et al. 2004; Heemsbergen et al. 2005; Vordermark et al. 2003). Furthermore, higher doses to the posterior rectal wall and upper parts of the rectum are shown to be predictive for higher late toxicity (Fiorino et al. 2002; Heemsbergen et al. 2005; Munbodh et al. 2008; Peeters et al. 2006; Skwarchuk et al. 2000). In contrast to these data, there is good evidence that very small volumes of the rectum can tolerate very high radiation doses when using prostate brachytherapy. Albert et al. (2008), for example, reported DVH constraints from LDR seed brachytherapy at UCSF and that the absolute volume of the rectum receiving 100 Gy was predictive for late proctitis needing argon laser treatment. Patients with a V100 of more than 8 ccm had a 20 % incidence for the above-mentioned toxicity, whereas none was seen in patients with a V100 below 8 ccm. Furthermore, Waterman and Dicker found the maximum point dose to the rectum also predictive for RTOG $\geq$ 2 rectal bleeding reporting a 0.4 % rate for a dose of 150 Gy, 1.2 % for 200 Gy, and 4.7 % for 300 Gy in their patient sample (Waterman and Dicker 2003).

4.2.4 New Radiation Techniques

The introduction of IMRT and IGRT techniques was supposed to open the field for dose escalation without significantly increasing rectal side effects. Due to an adequate reduction of safety margins applying IGRT and due to the higher dose conformity to the prostate by IMRT, rectal doses should be reduced, which in turn should lead to lower rectal side effects at equal or higher doses in the PTV. Indeed, several studies—although not randomized—could observe this positive effect (Cahlon et al. 2008; Zelefsky et al. 2002) and were incorporated in the QUANTEC review (Michalski et al. 2010). Zelefsky et al. (2008) compared the long-term late rectal toxicity after IMRT and 3D-CRT and demonstrated a significant lower incidence of late rectal grade 2 or higher toxicity in the high-dose IMRT arm as compared to the lower dose 3D-CRT arm (5 % vs. 13 %). However, acute toxicity was somewhat more pronounced in the high-dose IMRT arm.

Furthermore, several studies found reduced late rectal mucosal changes after IMRT or 3D-CRT using endorectal balloons (D'amico et al. 2006; Teh et al. 2005; van Lin et al. 2007), as they can reduce the rectal wall volumes receiving higher doses than 40 Gy (van Lin et al. 2007). (See also chapter "Internal immobilization—from rectal balloon to hyaluronic acid").

4.2.5 Treatment of Radiation-Induced Proctitis

Probably, due to the quite low incidence of late rectal side effects that require treatment, there are only a few more or less effective treatment options tested in prospective studies. In a randomized double-blind study by Clarke et al., 30 sessions of hyperbaric oxygen at 2.0 atmospheres absolute showed an improved healing response compared to the same treatment with 1.1 atmospheres according to an absolute risk reduction of 32 % (Clarke et al. 2008). The benefit of sucralfate orally as well as rectally applied in the treatment of radiation-induced proctitis could be shown in small retrospective studies (Kochhar et al. 1999; Sasai et al. 1998). Kennedy et al. (2001) found a combination of vitamin E and vitamin C significantly effective in reducing symptom indices for bleeding, diarrhea, and urgency, analyzing 20 patients prospectively, that developed symptoms after radiotherapy for prostate cancer or gynecological malignancies. The by now most effective symptomatic treatment for rectal bleeding in patients suffering from proctitis is an argon laser therapy (Kaassis et al. 2000; Taieb et al. 2001; Taylor et al. 2000; Viggiano et al. 1993).

5 Impact of Radiotherapy on Quality of Life of Prostate Cancer Patients

For several reasons, assessing the impact of available treatment modalities especially on health-related quality of life (HRQOL) is gaining importance for patients with localized prostate cancer: At first in the PSA era, most patients are asymptomatic, due to the early diagnosis after detecting elevated PSA levels, thus "harming" the patients with side effects is not counterbalanced by improving symptoms. Furthermore, even without treatment, survival of many patients with prostate cancer is good and might in early stages not differ much from those actively treated. Active surveillance strategies are presently gaining in popularity among patients and physicians. Thus, the QOL impact of not having (immediate) treatment-related side effects has to be weighed against the effect of eventual symptomatic disease progression and the issues of leaving the tumor untreated. In the presence of several presumably equally effective treatment options, data on the time course of side effects as well as on HRQOL are essential components to facilitate decision making by both patients and clinicians.

Within the last decades, an evolution of HRQOL assessment took place from not considering HRQOL in general at all to meanwhile excessively sampling "HRQOL data" using multiple often institutional and not validated questionnaires in a retrospective manner. In the last years, HRQOL studies started to became more conformal using with increased frequency established and validated questionnaires within prospective studies and—in a few cases—even in the randomized setting (Al-Mamgani et al. 2011; Hoskin et al. 2013). Nevertheless, due to the large variations within the published literature regarding the endpoints, study design, treatment details, and modalities as well as the used measures and toxicity scores, it would go beyond the scope of this chapter to give a comprehensive summary on this topic. Rather, we like to focus on some crucial issues and discuss selected studies.

5.1 Global HRQOL

Already in 1999, Lilleby et al. stated that in spite of considerable malignancy and/or treatment-related morbidity, global HRQOL was not or only slightly impaired in the majority of patients with localized prostate cancer after definitive radiotherapy or radical prostatectomy with no significant difference as compared to an age-matched normal population. In their cross-sectional study, they evaluated morbidity, side effects, and quality of life of 154 patients who had undergone definitive radiotherapy and 108 patients with radical prostatectomy at the Norwegian Radium Hospital during 1987–1995. Using the EORTC-C30 core questionnaire to assess the general HRQOL and furthermore several disease-specific symptom scores like the IPSS, to their point of view, general HRQOL dimensions (physical function, emotional function, fatigue) are as a rule of greater significance for HRQOL than sexuality and lower urinary tract symptoms (Lilleby et al. 1999).

The finding that—independently of the used generic score—global HRQOL is mostly not significantly or relevantly affected by radiotherapy side effects also was reported by the majority of recent published prospective and/or longitudinal studies using 3D-CRT, IMRT, or brachytherapy (BT) alone or in combination with EBRT (Geinitz et al. 2010; Goineau et al. 2013; Huang et al. 2010; Lips et al. 2009; Pardo et al. 2010; Roeloffzen et al. 2010; Schaake et al. 2013), even after dose escalation (Goineau et al. 2013; Lips et al. 2009; Marchand et al. 2010), when comparing baseline global HRQOL scales with the changes during follow-up. Though some studies have the limitation of a short follow, there is a growing number of long-term studies. Hoskin et al., for example, reported on their randomized study applying combined hypofractionated 3D-CRT and HDR brachytherapy (Hoskin et al. 2013) and described no significant or clinically relevant global HRQOL impairments after a follow-up of 10.5 years. Another published randomized trial treating patients with normofractionated 3D-CRT to total doses of 68 Gy versus 78 Gy found clinically relevant deterioration of HRQOL scales only in the high-dose arm with regard to role and physical functioning, whereas there was no significant or clinically relevant deterioration in the corresponding scales of the low-dose arm (Al-Mamgani et al. 2011). However, the follow-up of about 36 months in this study is still short. Some of the aforementioned trials moreover compared the course of HRQOL in their patient samples to an age-matched normative cohort (Schaake et al. 2013). Though some significant HRQOL impairments compared to the baseline and the normative cohort were found, all changes showed no or only borderline clinical relevance. Fossa et al. reported a significant correlation of late RTOG/EORTC genitourinary or gastrointestinal toxicity with global health status (Jereczek-Fossa et al. 2013) and (Hoskin et al. 2013) reported it for genitourinary late effects, not evaluating the impact of gastrointestinal effects.

Until 2014, no prospective data were published that could demonstrate a clinically significant impact of specific treatment-related side effects on HRQOL. In 2014, however, Schaake et al. published the first study that demonstrated a clinically significant effect for two specific treatment-related adverse effects—e.g., urinary incontinence and rectal discomfort—in a prospectively evaluated cohort of 227 patients treated with external beam radiotherapy (Schaake et al. 2014). According to the authors, one explanation for the fact that this association had not been demonstrated may originate in the circumstance that the more recent criteria from Cocks et al. (2011, 2012) were used to assess the clinical relevance of QOL changes. In contrast, the aforementioned earlier studies used the criteria from Osoba et al. (1998) to define clinical relevance. The Cocks criteria have the advantage that for every single functional or symptom scale, a specific graduation into categories was created, whereas according to Osoba et al., changes in all scales were classified using the same graduation scheme, suggesting changes clinically relevant, if scales increase or decrease to the amount of at least 10 absolute points or 10 % of the total scale range. The Cocks criteria additionally distinguish between cross-sectional and longitudinal differences.

5.2 Disease-Specific HRQOL

Due to the fact that severe impairment of global health-related QOL is rare in patients receiving primary radiotherapy for prostate cancer, disease-specific health-related quality of life events seem to be primary determinants of outcome (Hoskin et al. 2013). In the last decade, disease-specific health-related quality of life also was intensively evaluated by numerous studies including some of the previously cited. Large variations with regard to the used study designs, treatment parameters, treatment modalities, and follow-up are making it very challenging to compare the published results. However, some general patterns regarding the time course of HRQOL after definitive radiotherapy may be derived from the published data.

In general, the incidence of severe late disease-related impairments of HRQOL is low, even if disease-specific measures are used to assess HRQOL. In terms of EBRT, the mean impairments of disease-specific HRQOL are mostly reported to be slight or moderate. With regard to urinary symptom and bother scales, the most pronounced deterioration was consistently reported during the first months after treatment, with a recovery of specific HRQOL scales 1–2 years after treatment (Geinitz et al. 2010; Gore et al. 2009; Huang et al. 2010). The further course beyond this time was reported inconsistently, with a second slight and gradual deterioration around 5 years after therapy observed in some studies (Pardo et al. 2010). In contrast to that others showed no further significant impairment (Goineau et al. 2013; Huang et al. 2010), including one study following patients up to 10.5 years after treatment using combined

EBRT and BT (Hoskin et al. 2013). In terms of bowel symptoms and bother, a bit more pronounced impairments with similar courses over time were reported. In this context, often complete recovery from bowel bother was reported up to 36 months after treatment (Pardo et al. 2010), whereas some studies using predominantly IMRT showed not even a significant deterioration of specific HRQOL scales after the immediate first months after treatment or even during the whole follow-up, comprising follow-up times up to 54 months (Geinitz et al. 2010; Goineau et al. 2013; Lips et al. 2007; Marchand et al. 2010). With regard to IMRT, there is growing information that in general, it seems to be possible to carrying out dose-escalated radiotherapy without producing further specific treatment-related HRQOL impairments (Goineau et al. 2013; Jereczek-Fossa et al. 2013; Lips et al. 2007; Marchand et al. 2010; Shinohara et al. 2013).

For low dose rate brachytherapy, only slight to moderate impairments are reported after an initial pronounced deterioration of urinary bother scales up to 1 year after treatment with either a slow recovery not reaching baseline levels as compared to EBRT arms (Huang et al. 2010) or a complete recovery to baseline levels (Gore et al. 2009). In terms of bowel functioning and bother scores or gastrointestinal HRQOL, respectively, most studies reported no or only slight impairments after brachytherapy.

5.3 Risk Factors

With regard to the reviewed literature, we found no risk factor that consistently correlated with HRQOL changes in all studies. Nevertheless, some treatment or patient-related factors at least might be considered as potential risk factors for HRQOL impairment such as hormonal therapy (Huang et al. 2010; Marchand et al. 2010; Sanda et al. 2008), late toxicity (Hoskin et al. 2013; Jereczek-Fossa et al. 2013; Schaake et al. 2014), comorbidity (Schaake et al. 2013), and age (Huang et al. 2010; Schaake et al. 2014).

5.4 Limitations and Issues Confounding HRQOL Data

When interpreting HRQOL data in general several methodical as well as statistical issues and uncertainties have to be considered, some of which are listed below.

The inherent subjective nature of QOL assessment has to be regarded as a general methodical issue making it difficult in QOL studies to gain significant and comparable data that is equivalent to the evaluation of clinical outcome and toxicity in patients. For example, by now, it is nearly impossible to predict the impact of personal capacity, resources, and personality traits, as well as coping strategies or response shift, on the course of the HRQOL after therapy. A response shift describes the patient's ability to adapt their internal standards, values, and the conceptualization of QOL. It can lead to an improved HRQOL in spite of stable or even increasing side effects (Schwartz et al. 2006). In addition, there are a lot more patient-related factors which have not been clearly understood by now. Beyond patient-related traits, selection biases as a consequence of missing data in case of low response rates have to be regarded as methodical issues in QOL assessment. This potential bias is hard to quantify as it is not possible to identify whether patients did not return the questionnaires by random or due to health-related problems. A further issue is more prostate cancer specific, as most patients are elderly men and a decreasing QOL in these populations is not uncommon even without a cancer treatment, inter alia due to increasing comorbidities (Goineau et al. 2013). Furthermore, the interpretation of properly assessed data also might involve some uncertainties, due to the fact that also the development of appropriate instruments for data interpretation to some extent is still an ongoing process. As discussed above, new definitions of clinically relevant QOL changes lead to an identification of previously not appreciated interferences of EBRT-related adverse events with HRQOL (Schaake et al. 2014). A more statistical issue comprises the effect that due to the low incidence and prevalence of severe late effects in definitive radiotherapy for patients with localized prostate cancer, studies often might not have the statistical power to detect a significant influence of late effects on HRQOL. This was stressed by Schaake et al. (2014) in their study as (high grade) fecal incontinence, a symptom that interferes with the patient's daily activities, did not correlate with HRQOL, most likely due to its low incidence in that study.

6 Summary

The lack of prospective randomized studies with sufficient follow-up comparing the impact of surgery, recent radiotherapy techniques (IGRT/IMRT/conformal brachytherapy) as well as active surveillance on toxicity and especially HRQOL leaves many questions unanswered. Due to the median life expectancy of 13.8 years after treatment (Walz et al. 2007), an accurate prospective evaluation of HRQOL and symptoms with a follow-up of about 10 years seems to be necessary to understand the comprehensive experience of men living with a diagnosis of prostate cancer. Nevertheless, the possible risks of complications as well as the deterioration of HRQOL must be carefully weighed against the risk of relapse during the patient's expected life span. For high-dose radiotherapy, IMRT techniques should be used, as it could be consistently shown that by means of IMRT dose escalation most likely can be carried out without significantly increasing late effects or deteriorating the patients' HRQOL. With regard to quality of life research, further understanding of patient-related traits and attitudes and their impact on post-treatment HRQOL as well as new instruments rating HRQOL perception appear to be worth studied.

References

Aaronson NK, Ahmedzai S, Bergman B et al (1993) The European Organization for Research and Treatment of Cancer QLQ-C30: a quality-of-life instrument for use in international clinical trials in oncology. J Natl Cancer Inst 85:365–376

Al-Abany M, Helgason AR, Cronqvist AK et al (2004) Dose to the anal sphincter region and risk of fecal leakage. Acta Oncol 43:117–118

Al-Mamgani A, van Putten WL, van der Wielen GJ et al (2011) Dose escalation and quality of life in patients with localized prostate cancer treated with radiotherapy: long-term results of the Dutch randomized dose-escalation trial (CKTO 96-10 trial). Int J Radiat Oncol Biol Phys 79:1004–1012

Albert M, Song JS, Schultz D et al (2008) Defining the rectal dose constraint for permanent radioactive seed implantation of the prostate. Urol oncol 26:147–152

Alicikus ZA, Yamada Y, Zhang Z et al (2011) Ten-year outcomes of high-dose, intensity-modulated radiotherapy for localized prostate cancer. Cancer 117:1429–1437

Antonakopoulos GN, Hicks RM, Berry RJ (1984) The subcellular basis of damage to the human urinary bladder induced by irradiation. J Pathol 143:103–116

Bergman B, Aaronson NK, Ahmedzai S et al (1994) The EORTC QLQ-LC13: a modular supplement to the EORTC Core Quality of Life Questionnaire (QLQ-C30) for use in lung cancer clinical trials. EORTC study group on quality of life. Eur J Cancer 30A:635–642

Berndtsson I, Lennernas B, Hulten L (2002) Anorectal function after modern conformal radiation therapy for prostate cancer: a pilot study. Tech coloproctol 6:101–104

Birkhahn M, Penson DF, Cai J et al (2011) Long-term outcome in patients with a Gleason score ≤6 prostate cancer treated by radical prostatectomy. BJU Int 108:660–664

Bjordal K, Ahlner-Elmqvist M, Tollesson E et al (1994) Development of a European Organization for Research and Treatment of Cancer (EORTC) questionnaire module to be used in quality of life assessments in head and neck cancer patients. EORTC quality of life study group. Acta Oncol 33:879–885

Buchi KN, Dixon JA (1987) Argon laser treatment of hemorrhagic radiation proctitis. Gastrointest endosc 33:27–30

Cahlon O, Zelefsky MJ, Shippy A et al (2008) Ultra-high dose (86.4 Gy) IMRT for localized prostate cancer: toxicity and biochemical outcomes. Int J Radiat Oncol Biol Phys 71:330–337

Clarke RE, Tenorio LM, Hussey JR et al (2008) Hyperbaric oxygen treatment of chronic refractory radiation proctitis: a randomized and controlled double-blind crossover trial with long-term follow-up. Int J Radiat Oncol Biol Phys 72:134–143

Cocks K, King MT, Velikova G et al (2012) Evidence-based guidelines for interpreting change scores for the European Organisation for the Research and Treatment of Cancer Quality of life questionnaire core 30. Eur J Cancer 48:1713–1721

Cocks K, King MT, Velikova G et al (2011) Evidence-based guidelines for determination of sample size and interpretation of the European organisation for the research and treatment of cancer quality of life questionnaire core 30. J Clin Oncol 29:89–96

Cox JD, Stetz J, Pajak TF (1995) Toxicity criteria of the Radiation Therapy Oncology Group (RTOG) and the European Organization for Research and Treatment of Cancer (EORTC). Int J Radiat Oncol Biol Phys 31:1341–1346

D'amico AV, Manola J, Mcmahon E et al (2006) A prospective evaluation of rectal bleeding after dose-escalated three-dimensional conformal radiation therapy using an intrarectal balloon for prostate gland localization and immobilization. Urology 67:780–784

D'amico AV, Whittington R, Malkowicz SB et al (1998) Biochemical outcome after radical prostatectomy, external beam radiation therapy, or interstitial radiation therapy for clinically localized prostate cancer. JAMA 280:969–974

Dasilva AF, Tuch DS, Wiegell MR et al (2003) A primer on diffusion tensor imaging of anatomical substructures. Neurosurg Focus 15:E4

Donner CS (1998) Pathophysiology and therapy of chronic radiation-induced injury to the colon. Dig Dis 16:253–261

Esper P, Mo F, Chodak G et al (1997) Measuring quality of life in men with prostate cancer using the functional assessment of cancer therapy-prostate instrument. Urology 50:920–928

Fellin G, Fiorino C, Rancati T et al (2009) Clinical and dosimetric predictors of late rectal toxicity after conformal radiation for localized prostate cancer: results of a large multicenter observational study. Radiother Oncol 93:197–202

Fiorino C, Cozzarini C, Vavassori V et al (2002) Relationships between DVHs and late rectal bleeding after radiotherapy for prostate cancer: analysis of a large group of patients pooled from three institutions. Radiother Oncol 64:1–12

Fiorino C, Fellin G, Rancati T et al (2008) Clinical and dosimetric predictors of late rectal syndrome after 3D-CRT for localized prostate cancer: preliminary results of a multicenter prospective study. Int J Radiat Oncol Biol Phys 70:1130–1137

Fiorino C, Rancati T, Valdagni R (2009) Predictive models of toxicity in external radiotherapy: dosimetric issues. Cancer 115:3135–3140

Fiorino C, Sanguineti G, Cozzarini C et al (2003) Rectal dose-volume constraints in high-dose radiotherapy of localized prostate cancer. Int J Radiat Oncol Biol Phys 57:953–962

Fossa SD, Woehre H, Kurth KH et al (1997) Influence of urological morbidity on quality of life in patients with prostate cancer. Eur Urol 31(Suppl 3):3–8

Gandhi SK, Salmon JW, Zhao SZ et al (2001) Psychometric evaluation of the 12-item short-form health survey (SF-12) in osteoarthritis and rheumatoid arthritis clinical trials. Clin Ther 23:1080–1098

Garg AK, Mai WY, Mcgary JE et al (2006) Radiation proctopathy in the treatment of prostate cancer. Int J Radiat Oncol Biol Phys 66:1294–1305

Geinitz H, Thamm R, Scholz C et al (2010) Longitudinal analysis of quality of life in patients receiving conformal radiation therapy for prostate cancer. Strahlenther Onkol 186:46–52

Gelblum DY, Potters L (2000) Rectal complications associated with transperineal interstitial brachytherapy for prostate cancer. Int J Radiat Oncol Biol Phys 48:119–124

Georgiou A, Grigsby PW, Perez CA (1993) Radiation induced lumbosacral plexopathy in gynecologic tumors: clinical findings and dosimetric analysis. Int J Radiat Oncol Biol Phys 26:479–482

Gilinsky NH, Burns DG, Barbezat GO et al (1983) The natural history of radiation-induced proctosigmoiditis: an analysis of 88 patients. Q J Med 52:40–53

Goineau A, Marchand V, Rigaud J et al (2013) Prospective evaluation of quality of life 54 months after high-dose intensity-modulated radiotherapy for localized prostate cancer. Radiat Oncol 8:53

Goldner G, Potter R, Kranz A et al (2011) Healing of late endoscopic changes in the rectum between 12 and 65 months after external beam radiotherapy. Strahlenther Onkol 187:202–205

Gore JL, Kwan L, Lee SP et al (2009) Survivorship beyond convalescence: 48-month quality-of-life outcomes after treatment for localized prostate cancer. J Natl Cancer Inst 101:888–892

Heemsbergen WD, Hoogeman MS, Hart GA et al (2005) Gastrointestinal toxicity and its relation to dose distributions in the anorectal region of prostate cancer patients treated with radiotherapy. Int J Radiat Oncol Biol Phys 61:1011–1018

Hoeller U, Tribius S, Kuhlmey A et al (2003) Increasing the rate of late toxicity by changing the score? A comparison of RTOG/EORTC and LENT/SOMA scores. Int J Radiat Oncol Biol Phys 55:1013–1018

Holzner B, Bode RK, Hahn EA et al (2006) Equating EORTC QLQ-C30 and FACT-G scores and its use in oncological research. Eur J Cancer 42:3169–3177

Hoskin PJ, Rojas AM, Ostler PJ et al (2013) Quality of life after radical radiotherapy for prostate cancer: longitudinal study from a randomised trial of external beam radiotherapy alone or in combination with high dose rate brachytherapy. Clin Oncol (R Coll Radiol) 25: 321–327

Huang EH, Pollack A, Levy L et al (2002) Late rectal toxicity: dose-volume effects of conformal radiotherapy for prostate cancer. Int J Radiat Oncol Biol Phys 54:1314–1321

Huang GJ, Sadetsky N, Penson DF (2010) Health related quality of life for men treated for localized prostate cancer with long-term followup. J Urol 183:2206–2212

Iglicki F, Coffin B, Ille O et al (1996) Fecal incontinence after pelvic radiotherapy: evidences for a lumbosacral plexopathy. Report of a case. Dis Colon Rectum 39:465–467

Jenkinson C, Chandola T, Coulter A et al (2001) An assessment of the construct validity of the SF-12 summary scores across ethnic groups. J Publ Health Med 23:187–194

Jereczek-Fossa BA, Santoro L, Zerini D et al (2013) Image guided hypofractionated radiotherapy and quality of life for localized prostate cancer: prospective longitudinal study in 337 patients. J Urol 189:2099–2103

Kaassis M, Oberti E, Burtin P et al (2000) Argon plasma coagulation for the treatment of hemorrhagic radiation proctitis. Endoscopy 32:673–676

Kennedy M, Bruninga K, Mutlu EA et al (2001) Successful and sustained treatment of chronic radiation proctitis with antioxidant vitamins E and C. Am J Gastroenterol 96:1080–1084

Kochhar R, Sriram PV, Sharma SC et al (1999) Natural history of late radiation proctosigmoiditis treated with topical sucralfate suspension. Dig Dis Sci 44:973–978

Kushwaha RS, Hayne D, Vaizey CJ et al (2003) Physiologic changes of the anorectum after pelvic radiotherapy for the treatment of prostate and bladder cancer. Dis Colon Rectum 46:1182–1188

Lanciano RM, Martz K, Montana GS et al (1992) Influence of age, prior abdominal surgery, fraction size, and dose on complications after radiation therapy for squamous cell cancer of the uterine cervix. A Patterns Care Study Cancer 69:2124–2130

Lilleby W, Fossa SD, Waehre HR et al (1999) Long-term morbidity and quality of life in patients with localized prostate cancer undergoing definitive radiotherapy or radical prostatectomy. Int J Radiat Oncol Biol Phys 43:735–743

Lim LL, Fisher JD (1999) Use of the 12-item short-form (SF-12) health survey in an Australian heart and stroke population. Qual Life Res Int J Qual Life Aspects of Treat, Care Rehabil 8:1–8

Lips I, Dehnad H, Kruger AB et al (2007) Health-related quality of life in patients with locally advanced prostate cancer after 76 Gy intensity-modulated radiotherapy versus 70 Gy conformal radiotherapy in a prospective and longitudinal study. Int J Radiat Oncol Biol Phys 69:656–661

Lips IM, van Gils CH, van der Heide UA et al (2009) Health-related quality of life 3 years after high-dose intensity-modulated radiotherapy with gold fiducial marker-based position verification. BJU Int 103:762–767

Litwin MS, Hays RD, Fink A et al (1995) Quality-of-life outcomes in men treated for localized prostate cancer. JAMA 273:129–135

Marchand V, Bourdin S, Charbonnel C et al (2010) No impairment of quality of life 18 months after high-dose intensity-modulated radiotherapy for localized prostate cancer: a prospective study. Int J Radiat Oncol Biol Phys 77:1053–1059

Michalski JM, Gay H, Jackson A et al (2010) Radiation dose-volume effects in radiation-induced rectal injury. Int J Radiat Oncol Biol Phys 76:S123–S129

Munbodh R, Jackson A, Bauer J et al (2008) Dosimetric and anatomic indicators of late rectal toxicity after high-dose intensity modulated radiation therapy for prostate cancer. Med Phys 35:2137–2150

Osoba D, Rodrigues G, Myles J et al (1998) Interpreting the significance of changes in health-related quality-of-life scores. J Clin Oncol 16:139–144

Pardo Y, Guedea F, Aguilo F et al (2010) Quality-of-life impact of primary treatments for localized prostate cancer in patients without hormonal treatment. J Clin Oncol 28:4687–4696

Peeters ST, Heemsbergen WD, Koper PC et al (2006a) Dose-response in radiotherapy for localized prostate cancer: results of the Dutch multicenter randomized phase III trial comparing 68 Gy of radiotherapy with 78 Gy. J Clin Oncol 24:1990–1996

Peeters ST, Hoogeman MS, Heemsbergen WD et al (2006b) Rectal bleeding, fecal incontinence, and high stool frequency after conformal radiotherapy for prostate cancer: normal tissue complication probability modeling. Int J Radiat Oncol Biol Phys 66:11–19

Petersen S, Jongen J, Petersen C et al (2007) Radiation-induced sequelae affecting the continence organ: incidence, pathogenesis, and treatment. Dis Colon Rectum 50:1466–1474

Potish RA, Jones TK Jr, Levitt SH (1979) Factors predisposing to radiation-related small-bowel damage. Radiology 132:479–482

Putta S, Andreyev HJ (2005) Faecal incontinence: a late side-effect of pelvic radiotherapy. Clin Oncol (R Coll Radiol) 17:469–477

Resnick B, Nahm ES (2001) Reliability and validity testing of the revised 12-item short-form health survey in older adults. J Nurs Meas 9:151–161

Roeloffzen EM, Lips IM, van Gellekom MP et al (2010) Health-related quality of life up to six years after (125) I brachytherapy for early-stage prostate cancer. Int J Radiat Oncol Biol Phys 76:1054–1060

Salyers MP, Bosworth HB, Swanson JW et al (2000) Reliability and validity of the SF-12 health survey among people with severe mental illness. Med Care 38:1141–1150

Sanda MG, Dunn RL, Michalski J et al (2008) Quality of life and satisfaction with outcome among prostate-cancer survivors. N Engl J Med 358:1250–1261

Sasai T, Hiraishi H, Suzuki Y et al (1998) Treatment of chronic post-radiation proctitis with oral administration of sucralfate. Am J Gastroenterol 93:1593–1595

Schaake W, De Groot M, Krijnen WP et al (2013) Quality of life among prostate cancer patients: a prospective longitudinal population-based study. Radiother Oncol 108:299–305

Schaake W, Wiegman EM, De Groot M et al (2014) The impact of gastrointestinal and genitourinary toxicity on health related quality of life among irradiated prostate cancer patients. Radiother Oncol 110:284–290

Schlenk EA, Erlen JA, Dunbar-Jacob J et al (1998) Health-related quality of life in chronic disorders: a comparison across studies using the MOS SF-36. Qual Life Res Int J Qual Life Aspects Treat, Care Rehabil 7:57–65

Schwartz CE, Bode R, Repucci N et al (2006) The clinical significance of adaptation to changing health: a meta-analysis of response shift. Qual Life Res Int J Qual Life Aspects Treat, Care Rehabil 15:1533–1550

Shinohara N, Maruyama S, Shimizu S et al (2013) Longitudinal comparison of quality of life after real-time tumor-tracking intensity-modulated radiation therapy and radical prostatectomy in patients with localized prostate cancer. J Radiat Res 54:1095–1101

Skwarchuk MW, Jackson A, Zelefsky MJ et al (2000) Late rectal toxicity after conformal radiotherapy of prostate cancer (I): multivariate analysis and dose-response. Int J Radiat Oncol Biol Phys 47:103–113

Sommers SD, Ramsey SD (1999) A review of quality-of-life evaluations in prostate cancer. Pharmaco Econ 16:127–140

Sprangers MA, Groenvold M, Arraras JI et al (1996) The European Organization for Research and Treatment of Cancer breast cancer-specific quality-of-life questionnaire module: first results from a three-country field study. J Clin Oncol 14:2756–2768

Stewart FA (1986) Mechanism of bladder damage and repair after treatment with radiation and cytostatic drugs. Br J Cancer Suppl 7:280–291

Stewart FA (1985) The proliferative and functional response of mouse bladder to treatment with radiation and cyclophosphamide. Radiother Oncol 4:353–362

Szymanski KM, Wei JT, Dunn RL et al (2010) Development and validation of an abbreviated version of the expanded prostate cancer index composite instrument for measuring health-related quality of life among prostate cancer survivors. Urology 76:1245–1250

Tagkalidis PP, Tjandra JJ (2001) Chronic radiation proctitis. ANZ J Surg 71:230–237

Taieb S, Rolachon A, Cenni JC et al (2001) Effective use of argon plasma coagulation in the treatment of severe radiation proctitis. Dis Colon Rectum 44:1766–1771

Taylor JG, Disario JA, Bjorkman DJ (2000) KTP laser therapy for bleeding from chronic radiation proctopathy. Gastrointest Endosc 52:353–357

Teh BS, Dong L, Mcgary JE et al (2005) Rectal wall sparing by dosimetric effect of rectal balloon used during intensity-modulated radiation therapy (IMRT) for prostate cancer. Med Dosim 30:25–30

Theodorescu D, Gillenwater JY, Koutrouvelis PG (2000) Prostatourethral-rectal fistula after prostate brachytherapy. Cancer 89:2085–2091

Tran A, Wallner K, Merrick G et al (2005) Rectal fistulas after prostate brachytherapy. Int J Radiat Oncol Biol Phys 63:150–154

Trotti A, Colevas AD, Setser A et al (2003) CTCAE v3.0: development of a comprehensive grading system for the adverse effects of cancer treatment. Semin Radiat Oncol 13:176–181

Vachalec S, Bottomley A, Aaronson N et al (2002) Confusion about European Organisation for research and treatment of cancer quality of life prostate module (EORTC QLQ-PR25): a response. Expert Rev Pharmacoeconomics Outcomes Res 2:6

van Andel G, Bottomley A, Fossa SD et al (2008) An international field study of the EORTC QLQ-PR25: a questionnaire for assessing the health-related quality of life of patients with prostate cancer. Eur J Cancer 44:2418–2424

van Lin EN, Kristinsson J, Philippens ME et al (2007) Reduced late rectal mucosal changes after prostate three-dimensional conformal radiotherapy with endorectal balloon as observed in repeated endoscopy. Int J Radiat Oncol Biol Phys 67:799–811

Vargas C, Martinez A, Kestin LL et al (2005) Dose-volume analysis of predictors for chronic rectal toxicity after treatment of prostate cancer with adaptive image-guided radiotherapy. Int J Radiat Oncol Biol Phys 62:1297–1308

Varma JS, Smith AN (1986) Anorectal function following colo-anal sleeve anastomosis for chronic radiation injury to the rectum. Br J Surg 73:285–289

Varma JS, Smith AN, Busuttil A (1985) Correlation of clinical and manometric abnormalities of rectal function following chronic radiation injury. Br J Surg 72:875–878

Varma JS, Smith AN, Busuttil A (1986) Function of the anal sphincters after chronic radiation injury. Gut 27:528–533

Viggiano TR, Zighelboim J, Ahlquist DA et al (1993) Endoscopic Nd: YAG laser coagulation of bleeding from radiation proctopathy. Gastrointest Endosc 39:513–517

Vordermark D, Schwab M, Ness-Dourdoumas R et al (2003) Association of anorectal dose-volume histograms and impaired fecal continence after 3D conformal radiotherapy for carcinoma of the prostate. Radiother Oncol 69:209–214

Walz J, Gallina A, Saad F et al (2007) A nomogram predicting 10-year life expectancy in candidates for radical prostatectomy or radiotherapy for prostate cancer. J Clin Oncol 25:3576–3581

Ware JE Jr, Sherbourne CD (1992) The MOS 36-item short-form health survey (SF-36). I. conceptual framework and item selection. Med Care 30:473–483

Waterman FM, Dicker AP (2003) Probability of late rectal morbidity in 125I prostate brachytherapy. Int J Radiat Oncol Biol Phys 55: 342–353

Wei JT, Dunn RL, Litwin MS et al (2000) Development and validation of the expanded prostate cancer index composite (EPIC) for comprehensive assessment of health-related quality of life in men with prostate cancer. Urology 56:899–905

Wiegel T, Bottke D, Steiner U et al (2009) Phase III postoperative adjuvant radiotherapy after radical prostatectomy compared with radical prostatectomy alone in pT3 prostate cancer with postoperative undetectable prostate-specific antigen: ARO 96-02/AUO AP 09/95. J Clin Oncol 27:2924–2930

Yeoh EK, Russo A, Botten R et al (1998) Acute effects of therapeutic irradiation for prostatic carcinoma on anorectal function. Gut 43:123–127

Zelefsky MJ, Aschkenasy E, Kelsen S et al (1997) Tolerance and early outcome results of postprostatectomy three-dimensional conformal radiotherapy. Int J Radiat Oncol Biol Phys 39:327–333

Zelefsky MJ, Fuks Z, Hunt M et al (2002) High-dose intensity modulated radiation therapy for prostate cancer: early toxicity and biochemical outcome in 772 patients. Int J Radiat Oncol Biol Phys 53:1111–1116

Zelefsky MJ, Levin EJ, Hunt M et al (2008) Incidence of late rectal and urinary toxicities after three-dimensional conformal radiotherapy and intensity-modulated radiotherapy for localized prostate cancer. Int J Radiat Oncol Biol Phys 70:1124–1129

Zimmermann FB, Feldmann HJ (1998) Radiation proctitis. Clinical and pathological manifestations, therapy and prophylaxis of acute and late injurious effects of radiation on the rectal mucosa. Strahlenther Onkol 174(3):85–89

Part III

Dose Escalation and New Radiation Techniques

Dose Escalation: An Update on Randomised Clinical Trials

Wilfried Budach and Irina Sackerer

Contents

Abstract

Many studies have investigated the relationship between dose and treatment outcome with regard to clinical or biochemical disease free-survival. The relationship to other endpoints such as overall survival and disease-specific survival is still unclear, with different dose-correlations detected in different studies. Currently, several phase III randomised trials published in the recent years provided their long-term results with high level of evidence.

1 Introduction

In the last decade, the incidence of prostate cancer increased in all industrialised countries. External beam radiation therapy is decidedly one of the curative treatment options. Several single institution and cohort studies published in the last decade found a dose-response relationship in clinical and biochemical disease-free survival as well as in treatment-associated genitourinary and gastrointestinal toxicity. Some trials also observed a dose-response in overall survival.

Rapid employment of modern technology in conformal radiotherapy using 3D conformal techniques, intensity-modulated radiotherapy, and image guidance has enabled more precise and accurately treatment approach that allows the delivery of higher radiation dose and improved disease control with an acceptable level of side effects.

However, even better outcomes have been reported in patients treated with modern techniques that allow the radiotherapy doses in the prostate gland to be escalated safely above 74 Gy. Nonetheless, although many studies have investigated the relationship between dose and treatment outcome with regard to clinical and biochemical disease-free survival, the relationship with other endpoints

Conflict of interest: none.

W. Budach
Medical Faculty, Department of Radiation Oncology, Heinrich Heine University of Düsseldorf, Moorenstraße 5, 40225 Düsseldorf, Germany

I. Sackerer (✉)
Department of Radiation Oncology, Medical Faculty, Technical University of Munich, Klinikum rechts der Isar, Ismaninger Str 22, 81675 Munich, Germany
e-mail: irina.sackerer@mri.tum.de

H. Geinitz et al. (eds.), *Radiotherapy in Prostate Cancer*, Medical Radiology. Radiation Oncology,
DOI: 10.1007/174_2014_1032,
Published Online: 15 July 2014

Table 1 Published randomised dose escalation trials using external beam percutaneous radiotherapy

Trial/update	*n*	Risk	Groups (%)	Dose	Treatment modality	End point	Hormonal therapy
Boston Zietman et al. (2010)	393	Low Intermediate High	58 37 5	70.2 Gy vs 79.2 Gy	3D 50.4 Gy/1.8 Gy + proton boost	FFF 10 y BF ASTRO Phoenix	no
MD Anderson Kuban et al. (2008)	301	Low Intermediate High	20 46 34	70 Gy vs 78 Gy	3D 46 Gy/2.0 Gy + boost	FFF 8 y. BF ASTRO	no
Dutch Al-Mamgani et al. (2011)	669	Low Intermediate High	18 27 55	68 Gy vs 78 Gy	3D 50/Gy2.0 Gy + boost	FFF 7 y. BF ASTRO Phoenix	6 months –3 years
MRC Dearnaley et al. (2007)	843	Low Intermediate High	24 32 44	64 Gy vs 74 Gy	3D 64 Gy/2.0 Gy + boost	FFF 5y. BF nadir + 2 ng/ml	~6 months
RMH Dearnaley et al. (2005)	126	Low Intermediate High	18 72 10	64 Gy vs 74 Gy	3D 64 Gy/2.0 Gy + boost	FFF 5y. BF nadir + 2 ng/ml	~6 months

FFF freedom from biochemical or clinical failure, *BF* biochemical failure; *ASTRO* initial American Society for Radiation Oncology definition for biochemical recurrence after radiation therapy for prostate cancer (three consecutive rises in serum PSA); Phoenix: definition of biochemical failure according to the RTOG-ASTRO Phoenix Consensus Conference (PSA-rise of $\geq$ 2 ng/ml above the nadir)

such as overall survival and disease-specific survival is still unclear, with different dose relationships detected in different studies. Currently, several phase III randomised trials published in the recent years provided their long-term results with high level of evidence.

2 Randomised Dose Escalation Trials

Five randomised dose-escalated phase-III studies with overall 2,332 patients published between 2005 and 2010 provided the long-term results with high level of evidence (Table 1).

3 Influence of Radiation Therapy Dose on Progression-Free Survival

The long-term data from five randomised trials published between 2005 and 2010 confirmed the advantage of high dose radiation therapy for patients with localised adenocarcinoma of the prostate (Fig. 1).[1]

Dearnaley et al. (2005) published the results of a Royal Marsden NHS Trust and Institute of Cancer Research (RMH) phase III dose escalation pilot study. The total of 126 men with localised (T1–T3b) prostate cancer were randomised after an initial 3–6 month period of androgen suppression to deliver a dose of 64 Gy with or without a 10 Gy boost (64 and 74 Gy arms) between 1995 and 1997. The results showed that freedom from PSA failure was higher in the 74 Gy arm compared to the 64 Gy arm, but this did not reach conventional levels of statistical significance with 5-year actuarial control rates of 71 % in the 74 Gy arm vs. 59 % in the 64 Gy arm ($p = 0.10$). There was no difference in the time to restarting hormone therapy between the randomised groups (5-year actuarial rate 15–16 % in each group).

The following randomised Medical Research Council (MRC) RT01 trial with 843 men with localised prostate cancer (T1–T3a, PSA < 50 nag/mL), which were randomly assigned to escalated dose (74 Gy; $n = 422$) or standard-dose (64 Gy; $n = 421$) conformal radiotherapy was published by Dearnaley et al. (2007). After a median follow-up of 63 months, 5 year biochemical progression-free survival (bPFS) was a 71 % in the escalated and a 60 % in the standard group ($p = 0.0007$). In the subgroup analysis, no heterogeneity of effect on bPFS according to risk groups was found. Neither of these analyses showed that escalated dose treatment is more or less beneficial in either of these risk groups. The bPFS at 5 years for the standard and escalated groups were 79 and 85 % in the low-risk group, 70 and 79 % in the intermediate-risk group and 43 and 57 % in the high-risk group, respectively. No significant benefits were detected for clinical progression-free survival ($p = 0.064$), local control ($p = 0.16$), freedom from salvage androgen suppression ($p = 0.12$), and metastases-free survival ($p = 0.21$).

Al-Mamgani et al. (2008) presented the analysis of the Dutch dose escalation trial of radiotherapy for prostate cancer. A total of 669 patients with localised prostate cancer

[1] Metaanalysis from W. Budach. 95 % confidence intervals were calculated for each trial using "Dose Effect Analysis Module" from XLmTAT®.

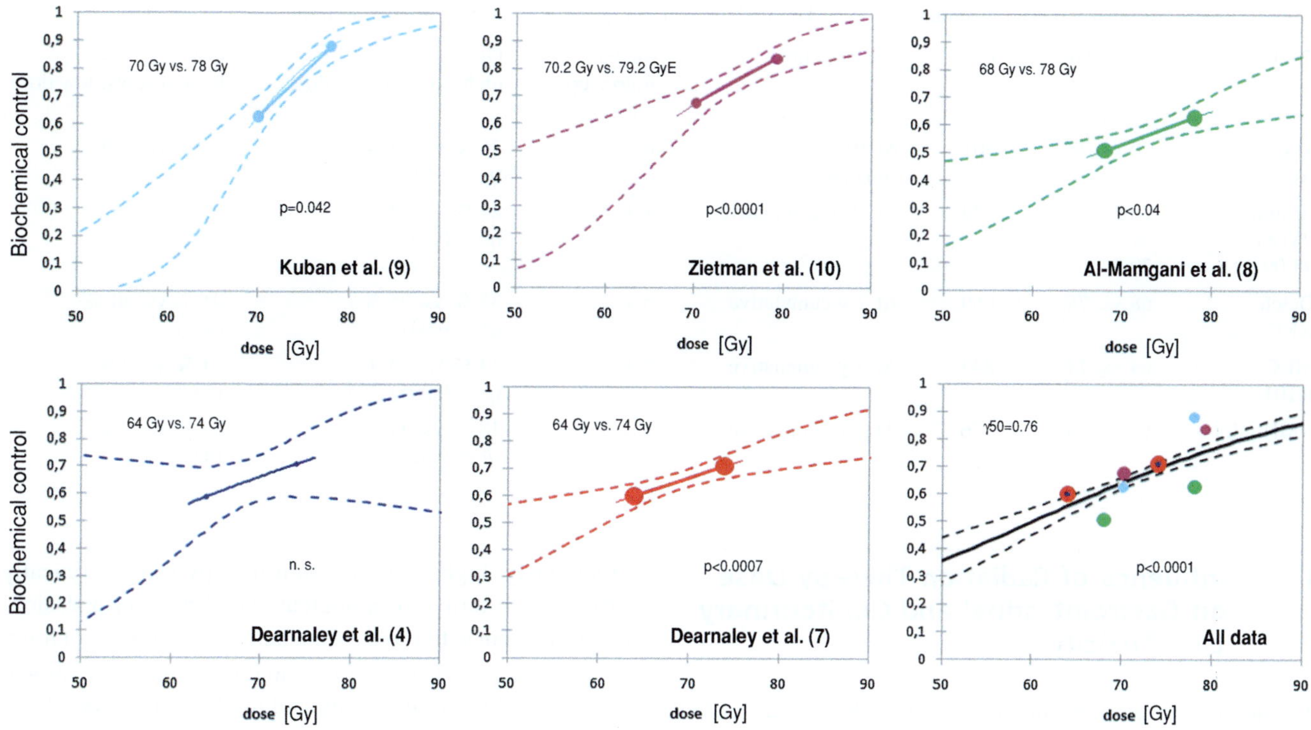

Fig. 1 Dose response curves in randomised trials on prostate cancer; *broken lines* 95 % confidence interval (patient numbers and dose were extracted from the respective publications, a correction for censored cases could not be carried out, thus the confidence intervals might be estimated a bit to narrow)

(T1–T4, PSA $<$ 60 ng/mL) were randomly assigned 1997–2003 to receive either 68 or 78 Gy. After a median follow-up of 70 months, freedom from biochemical or clinical failure (FFF) using the ASTRO definition was significantly better in the 78-Gy arm than in the 68-Gy arm (7-year FFF rate, 54 % vs. 47 %, respectively; $p = 0.04$). The FFF using the Phoenix definition was also significantly better in the 78-Gy arm than in the 68-Gy arm (7-year FFF rate, 56 % vs. 45 %, respectively; $p = 0.03$). However, no difference was found between the high- and low-dose arms in freedom from clinical failure (70 % vs. 68 % at 7 years, respectively, $p = 0.68$).

Between 1993 and 1998, the M. D. Anderson Cancer Centre (MDA) enrolled 301 patients with localised (T1–T3) prostate cancer in phase III dose escalation trial using 70 Gy versus 78 Gy (Pollack et al. 2002, 2004; Kuban et al. 2003). The long-term results with median follow-up 8.7 years reported in 2008 by Kuban et al. (2008) showed superior FFF with the ASTRO definition for the 78 Gy arm (78 %) compared with the 70-Gy arm (59 %) for all patients ($p = 0.004$), increasing with time. In a subgroup analysis an even greater benefit was seen in patients with an initial PSA $>$ 10 ng/mL (78 % vs. 39 % at 8 years, $p = 0.001$). The clinical failure rate was significantly reduced in the dose-escalated arm (7 % vs. 15 %, $p = 0.014$).

Zietman et al. (2010) published an update from the PROG 95-09 randomised trial with 393 men with early stage (T1–T2b, PSA $\leq$ 15 ng/mL) prostate cancer treated between 1996 and 1999 to a total dose of 70.2 or 79.2 Gy using a combination of proton and photon beams (Peeters et al. 2006; Zietman et al. 2005). Median follow-up was 8.9 years. The 10-year ASTRO biochemical failure (BF) rates were 32.4 % for conventional dose and 16.7 % for high dose radiation therapy ($p = 0.0001$). Men receiving high dose radiation therapy were significantly less likely to have local failure ($p < 0.0001$). This difference held when only those with low-risk disease ($n = 227$; 58 % of the total population) were examined for ASTRO BF: 28.2 % for conventional and 7.1 % for high dose ($p = 0.0001$). There was a strong trend in the same direction for the intermediate-risk patients ($n = 144$; 37 % of the total cohort; 42.1 % vs. 30.4 %, $p = 0.06$). Eleven percent of the patients subsequently required androgen deprivation because of recurrence after conventional dose compared with 6 % after high dose ($p = 0.047$).

In summary, dose escalation results in significantly improved biochemical as well as clinical freedom from failure, even in the presence of hormonal treatment. In the subgroup analyses all risk groups seem to have a similar benefit from dose escalation.

Table 2 Gastrointestinal (GI) and genitourinary (GU) late toxicity (RTOG grade ≥ 2) in dose escalation trials

Trial	Dose (Gy)	*n*	Analyses time	Median follow-up (years)	GI high dose vs. low dose	GU high dose vs. low dose
M.D. Anderson	70 vs. 78	301	At 10 y cumulative	8.7	26 % vs. 13 % ($p = 0.013$)	13 % vs. 8 % (n.s.)
Boston PROG 95-09	70.2 vs. 79.2	393	At 10 y cumulative	8.9	24 % vs. 13 % ($p = 0.09$)	29 % vs. 25 % (n.s.)
Dutch NKI	68 vs. 78	669	At 7 y cumulative	5.8	35 % vs. 25 % ($p = 0.04$)	41 % vs. 40 % (n.s.)
MRC RT01	64 vs. 74	843	At 5 y cumulative	5.3	33 % vs. 24 % ($p = 0.005$)	11 % vs. 8 % (n.s.)
RMH pilot	64 vs. 74	126	At 2 y cumulative	6.2	18 % vs. 11 % ($p = 0.02$)	13 % vs. 8 % (n.s.)

4 Influence of Radiation Therapy Dose on Gastrointestinal and Genitourinary Late Toxicity

All the dose escalation randomised trials showed increased risk of Radiation Therapy Oncology Group (RTOG) grade ≥ 2 late bowel toxicity, particularly rectal bleeding, in the higher dose arms at the follow-up time of 5 years. For example, in the MDA trial gastrointestinal (GI) toxicity grade 2 or higher occurred twice as often in patients treated in the dose escalation group, although genitourinary (GU) toxicity grade 2 or higher was less and not statistically significantly different (Kuban et al. 2008).

In the Boston study, there was a small increase in late grade ≥ 2 rectal morbidity in the high dose arm of the trial, but no difference in grade ≥ 3 toxicity. Similar to the MDA trial results there was no statistical significant difference in the late grade ≥ 2 GU toxicity (Zietman et al. 2010).

No difference of late grade 2 or higher genitourinary toxicity was seen in the conventional and dose escalation groups in the Dutch trial (Al-Mamgani et al. 2008, 2011). However, the cumulative incidence of late grade 2 or greater gastrointestinal toxicity was increased in the 78 Gy arm compared to the 68 Gy arm.

The MRC RT01 trial (Dearnaley et al. 2007) showed significantly increased bowel toxicity in the escalated group according to the RTOG grade ≥ 2 scale within 5 years of starting treatment. Late bladder toxicity was slightly increased with an increased incidence of RTOG grade ≥ 2 toxicity in this study.

Late bowel side effects (RTOG ≥ 2) were recorded more commonly in the 74 Gy group in the first 2 years after randomisation in the Royal Marsden pilot study (Dearnaley et al. 2005). No significant differences in late bladder side effects were seen between the randomised groups using the RTOG scoring system.

Obviously, high dose radiation therapy seems clinically worthwhile in terms of biological and clinical progression-free survival but at the costs of an increased incidence of long-term adverse events. The dose escalation using 3D-treatment planning results in a significant, but moderate increase of late gastrointestinal and genitourinary toxicity (Table 2).

5 Influence of Radiation Therapy Dose on Overall Survival

The benefit of higher dose has been shown mainly for biochemical progression rates to date. Because prostate cancer mostly occurs in an elderly population with competing causes of death and the majority of patients do not have the aggressive type of disease, it is very difficult to prove an overall survival advantage, even in randomised trials.

Accordingly, no overall survival benefit was observed for patients treated with dose escalation in all randomised trials yet. The RMH pilot study (Dearnaley et al. 2005) observed seven of nine prostate cancer death in men treated in the 64 Gy group. And the MRC RT01 trial (Dearnaley et al. 2007) reported 7-year overall survival rates of 75 % in both treatment arms ($p = 0.45$), however, both trials were underpowered for this endpoint. Furthermore, a difference in overall survival rates between the treatment arms was neither demonstrated in Dutch (Al-Mamgani et al. 2008) trial (75 % vs. 75 % at 7 years, $p = 0.45$) nor in the Boston (Zietman et al. 2010) trial (78.4 % vs. 83.4 % at 10 years, $p = 0.41$).

No survival advantage for the whole treatment group or for any subgroup of patients was detected in dose-escalated arm of the MDA trial after 8-years of follow-up. The actual survival update recently published in 2011 by Kuban et al. (2011) showed, that 10-years survival for the dose-escalated group was slightly higher in the 78 Gy arm but this did not reach significance. Patients under 70 years of age at treatment died of prostate cancer nearly three times more frequently than of other causes when they were irradiated to 70 Gy, whereas those treated to 78 Gy died of other causes more frequently. Patients aged 70 years or older treated to 70 Gy died of prostate cancer as often as of other causes, and those receiving 78 Gy never died of prostate cancer within 10 years of follow-up. Factors predicting for death from prostate cancer were pre-treatment PSA >10.5 ng/mL, Gleason score 9 and 10, recurrence within 2.6 years of radiation, and doubling time of <3.6 months at the time of recurrence.

Although dose escalation results in fewer deaths from prostate cancer in this trial no overall survival benefit was observed.

More prospective trials with extended follow-up and, furthermore, an endpoint of disease-specific survival are needed to support the influence of radiotherapy dose on prostate cancer-specific mortality.

References

Al-Mamgani A, van Putten WLJ, Heemsbergen WD et al (2008) Update of Dutch multicenter dose-escalation trial of radiotherapy for localized prostata cancer. Int J Radiat Oncol Biol Phys 72:980–988

Al-Mamgani A, van Putten WLJ, van der Wielen GJ et al (2011) Dose escalation and quality of life in patients with localized prostata cancer treated with radiotherapy: long term results of the Dutch dose-escalation trial (CKTO 96-10 trial). Int J Radiat Oncol Biol Phys 79:1004–1012

Dearnaley DP, Hall E, Lowrence D et al (2005) Phase II pilot study of dose escalation using conformal radiotherapy in prostate cancer: PSA control and side effects. Br J Cancer 92:488–498

Dearnaley DP, Sydes MR, Graham JD et al (2007) Escalated-dose versus standard-dose conformal radiotherapy in prostate cancer: First results from the MRC RT01 randomised controlled trial. Lancet Oncol 8:475–487

Kuban DA, Thames HD, Levy LB et al (2003) Long-term multi-institutional analysis of stage T1–T2 prostate cancer treated with radiotherapy in the PSA era. Int J Radiat Oncol Biol Phys 57:915–927

Kuban DA, Tucker SL, Dong L et al (2008) Long-term results of the M.D. Anderson randomized dose-escalation trial for prostate cancer. Int J Radiat Oncol Biol Phys 70:67–75

Kuban DA, Levy LB, Cheung MR et al (2011) Long-term failure patterns and survival in a randomized dose-escalation trial for prostate cancer. Who dies of disease? Int J Radiat Oncol Biol Phys 79:1310–1317

Peeters ST, Heemsbergen WD, Koper PC et al (2006) Dose-response in radiotherapy for localized prostate cancer: results of the Dutch multicenter randomized phase III trial comparing 68 Gy of radiotherapy with 78 Gy. J Clin Oncol 24:1990–1999

Pollack A, Zagars GK, Starkschall G et al (2002) Prostate cancer radiation dose response: results of the M.D. Anderson Phase III randomized trial. Int J Radiat Oncol Biol Phys 53:1097–1116

Pollack A, Hanlon AL, Horwitz EM et al (2004) Prostate cancer radiotherapy dose response: an update of the Fox Chase experience. J Urol 171:1132–1145

Zietman AL, DeSilvio ML, Slater JD et al (2005) Comparison of conventional-dose vs high-dose conformal radiation therapy in clinically localized adenocarcinoma of the prostate: a randomized controlled trial. JAMA 294:1233–1240

Zietman AL, Bae K, Slater JD et al (2010) Randomized trial comparing conventional-dose with high-dose conformal radiation therapy in early stage adenocarcinoma of the prostate: long term results from proton radiation oncology group/American college of radiology 95-09. J Clin Oncol 28:1106–1111

Intensity-Modulated Radiation Therapy for Clinically Localized Prostate Cancer

Marisa A. Kollmeier and Michael J. Zelefsky

Contents

Abstract

The goal of the following chapter is to discuss the role of intensity-modulated radiation therapy (IMRT) for clinically localized prostate cancer. We review the important aspects of patient selection for this therapeutic modality as well as discuss the relevant published literature on dose escalation. Additionally, a comprehensive review of techniques and delivery of treatment are presented. Finally, we discuss both the potential acute and late toxicities associated with IMRT.

1 Introduction

Prostate cancer incidence is increasing in most developed countries worldwide, and currently represents the second most common cause of cancer and the sixth leading cause of cancer deaths worldwide (Center et al. 2012). Fortunately, prostate cancer mortality is decreasing or stable in most of these countries, likely due to the earlier detection of disease through PSA screening. Currently, prostate cancer patients with clinically localized disease are presented with numerous therapeutic options including radical prostatectomy, interstitial brachytherapy, and external beam radiation therapy with increasing choices within these modalities. At present, randomized data do not exist favoring one strategy over another. Hence, patients are often faced with choosing among treatments based on differences in quality-of-life outcomes. External beam radiation therapy (EBRT) can be regarded as the most widely available radiotherapy approach.

Intensity-modulated radiation therapy (IMRT) was introduced into clinical use in the mid-1990s and is currently the most common form of radiotherapy used for the treatment of prostate cancer in the United States (Nguyen et al. 2011). The widespread adoption of IMRT stems from its ability to deliver higher treatment doses to the prostate while sparing normal surrounding tissues as compared to more conventional approaches such as three-dimensional

M. A. Kollmeier (✉) · M. J. Zelefsky
Department of Radiation Oncology,
Memorial Sloan-Kettering Cancer Center,
1275 York Ave, Box 22 New York,
NY 10021, USA
e-mail: kollmeiM@mskcc.org

H. Geinitz et al. (eds.), *Radiotherapy in Prostate Cancer*, Medical Radiology. Radiation Oncology,
DOI: 10.1007/174_2013_930,
Published Online: 21 February 2014

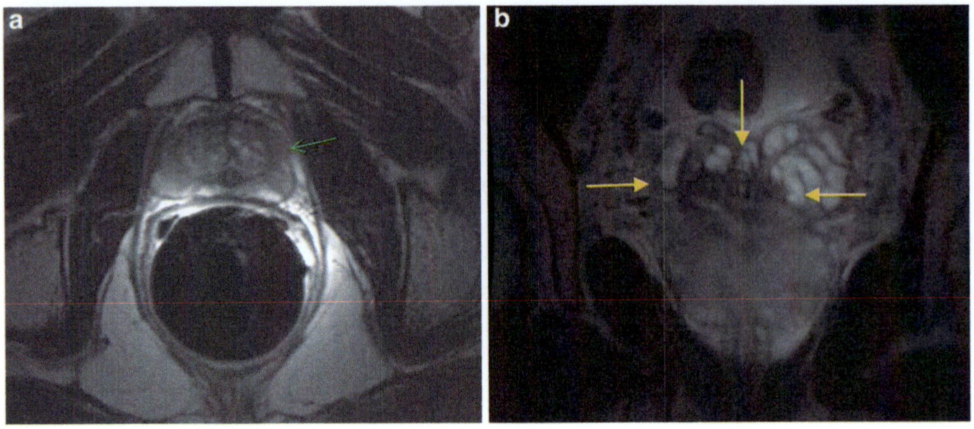

Fig. 1 Magnetic resonance imaging (MRI) demonstrating extracapsular spread on axial image (*green arrow*) (**a**) and seminal vesicle involvement on coronal image (*orange arrows*) (**b**)

conformal radiation therapy (3D-CRT). This is critical as it has been well established that higher radiation doses provide optimal treatment outcomes (Beckendorf et al. 2011; Cesaretti et al. 2007; Kuban et al. 2008; Peeters et al. 2006; Zietman et al. 2010). The use of IMRT is particularly important when doses $\geq$80 Gy are implemented in order to reduce normal tissue doses, particularly to minimize the risk of radiation proctitis (Zelefsky et al. 2000). Image-guided techniques have further contributed to advancing the precision, and ideally, the effectiveness of IMRT and will be discussed in a subsequent chapter.

In this chapter, the methods of IMRT treatment planning and delivery will be reviewed. This chapter will also describe the long-term therapeutic outcomes and the potential acute and long-term toxicities associated with IMRT. Finally, recent innovations will be described.

2 Patient Selection

Selecting the appropriate candidates for external beam radiotherapy using IMRT is important in order to optimize patient outcomes. A pretreatment workup optimally includes a magnetic resonance imaging (MRI) of the prostate preferably with endorectal coil or, if available, a 3 tesla machine, to assess the extent of local disease (extracapsular extension, seminal vesicle invasion, or nodal spread) (Fig. 1). Such information is often helpful when defining target volumes during the treatment planning process. In addition, important information regarding prostate volume can be assessed. For patients with very large prostate volumes, particularly in relation to small bladder volumes, dosimetric constraints for the bladder may be exceeded during treatment planning. In these cases, neoadjuvant cytoreductive hormone therapy may be useful to downsize the prostate gland and optimize dose distribution to the target and normal tissues. In the case of extracapsular extension and/or seminal vesicle involvement, decisions regarding expansion of the planning target volume (PTV) can be made including the decision to encompass pelvic nodal regions if appropriate.

Some patients may not be optimal candidates for EBRT and may be better suited for other modalities. These include patients with bilateral hip replacements in whom accurate CT-based treatment planning is technically challenging due to prosthesis artifact. In such cases, MRI-based simulation or the use of CT-MRI fusion techniques can be used to define the target more accurately with less artifact interference. Alternatively, ultrasound-guided brachytherapy may be selected where the prostate can be visualized more precisely. It is critical when planning EBRT to be able to deliver a therapeutic dose to the prostate while minimizing excess dose to the bowel and bladder. Patients with excessive small bowel adjacent to the prostate target volume or those who have received prior courses of pelvic radiotherapy for non-prostate cancer malignancies such as rectal cancers or testicular seminoma may not be able to receive tumoricidal dose levels of external beam radiotherapy safely and may be better managed with alternative modalities, i.e., brachytherapy.

3 Dose Escalation

EBRT for prostate cancer has evolved dramatically since the mid-1980s. Traditionally, bony landmarks were used to delineate field boundaries designed to encompass the pelvic lymph nodes, prostate and seminal vesicles (also known as a 4-field "box" technique). Using these fields, large volumes of normal tissue were irradiated. This limited the radiation dose that was safely deliverable to the prostate to 64 to 70 Gy and doses above these levels were associated with a significant morbidity risk, particularly with respect to the rectum and bowel (Smit et al. 1990). Newer techniques which use three-dimensional treatment planning and delivery such as 3D CRT and IMRT have refined EBRT markedly allowing more precise treatment delivery leading to more effective treatment with improved tumor control and morbidity outcomes.

Five randomized trials have been reported to date demonstrating a clear advantage to dose-escalated EBRT in terms of biochemical control and are discussed further in another section. Although there remains some controversy over which patients benefit most from dose escalation, it appears that intermediate and higher risk groups may derive a larger benefit (Kim et al. 2012; Pollack et al. 2002).

Despite improvements achieved by dose escalation with 3D CRT, increasing radiation dose came at a cost. Approximately 15–35 % of patients receiving doses ≥70 Gy developed grade ≥2 rectal toxicity (Dearnaley et al. 2007; Kuban et al. 2008; Zietman et al. 2010). In the M.D. Anderson randomized trial comparing 70 and 78 Gy, grade ≥2 gastrointestinal toxicity rates were observed in 13 and 23 % of patients, respectively (Pollack et al. 2002). Peeters et al. reported an increased rate of rectal bleeding requiring laser/transfusion ($p = 0.07$) in patients treated to 78 Gy compared with 68 Gy (Peeters et al. 2006). Urinary morbidity has been less consistently altered by dose escalation with some studies showing similar outcomes (Michalski et al. 2010) and some showing worse toxicity with dose escalation (Dearnaley et al. 2007).

In order to further establish the benefits of dose escalation, the Memorial Sloan-Kettering Cancer Center initiated a phase I/II protocol in 1988, whereby the prescription dose was increased from 64.8 to 86.4 Gy in successive increments of 5.4 Gy (Leibel et al. 1994; Zelefsky et al. 1998). In 1996, IMRT was introduced as a therapeutic tool to overcome the increased rectal toxicity seen with dose escalation using 3D-CRT at doses ≥75.6 Gy. The first report demonstrating the potential benefits of IMRT over 3D conformal approaches was published by Zelefsky et al. in 2000 (Zelefsky et al. 2000). In that study, 61 patients received 81 Gy with 3D-CRT and 171 patients received the same dose with IMRT. Twenty randomly selected patients were planned with both IMRT and 3D-CRT. Toxicity and dosimetric analyses comparing the two techniques demonstrated that IMRT resulted in better coverage of the CTV by the prescription dose than 3D-CRT ($p < 0.01$) and reduced the volumes of rectal and bladder walls receiving 75 Gy ($p < 0.01$). Clinically, this translated into a reduced rate of late grade 2 and 3 rectal bleeding in the IMRT group (2 vs. 10 %, $p < 0.001$). In 2002, Zelefsky et al. reported the safety of delivering doses of 81 Gy to the prostate using IMRT in a larger cohort of 772 patients (Zelefsky et al. 2002). In that series, the 3-year actuarial likelihood of developing grade ≥2 late genitourinary and gastrointestinal toxicity was 15 and 4 %, respectively. Although at the time follow-up was limited, IMRT resulted in at least equivalent biochemical control rates as non-IMRT approaches, quelling concerns that IMRT may result in underdosing of the target due to constricted dose distributions. In a recent update of these data with a median follow-up of 7 years, the 8-year likelihood of developing grade ≥2 late genitourinary and gastrointestinal toxicity was 15 and <2 %, confirming the long-term safety of this treatment (Cahlon et al. 2008). In addition, biochemical control rates remained excellent with 8-year actuarial PSA relapse-free survival rates for patients in favorable, intermediate, and unfavorable risk groups of 89, 78, and 67 %, respectively ($p = 0.0004$).

Others have found similar benefits of dose-escalated IMRT. Vora et al. reported biochemical and toxicity outcomes of dose-escalated IMRT (75.6 Gy) compared with conventional doses (68.4 Gy) in a series of 272 patients and found a 14 % improvement in 5-year biochemical control in the high dose group (Vora et al. 2007). Higher dose IMRT was well tolerated as there were no significant differences in toxicity between the two groups. In a series of 133 patients treated with 74–76 Gy using IMRT reported by De Meerleer et al., toxicity was also noted to be low with 17 and 19 % of patients experiencing late grade 2 GI and GU toxicity, respectively (De Meerleer et al. 2007). Additionally, biochemical outcome was excellent with 3-year biochemical control rates of 100, 94, and 74 % for low-, intermediate-, and high-risk patients, respectively.

The most updated analysis of the MSKCC dose escalation experience has recently been reported including over 1,000 patients treated with IMRT to a dose of 86.4 Gy (Spratt et al. 2013). With a median follow-up of 5.5 years, the 7-year biochemical relapse-free survival rates were 98.8, 85.6, and 67.9 % for low-, intermediate-, and high risk patients, respectively. Late toxicity was minimal with <1 and 2.2 % of patients experiencing late grade 2 or higher GI and GU toxicity, respectively. The rate of acute grade 2 of higher GI and GU toxicity was 4.4 and 21.1 %, respectively.

4 Techniques of IMRT Treatment Planning and Delivery

The development of three-dimensional treatment planning techniques has significantly improved the accuracy of EBRT. Dedicated treatment planning CT and MRI scanners in radiation oncology simulation suites allow the capture of complete volumetric anatomical information which can be directly imported into the treatment planning software. Radiation therapy treatment plans are generated by a careful definition of the target and normal tissues from which customized beams can be individually shaped allowing better shielding of organs at risk. The dose distributions can then be analyzed either graphically in a dose–volume histogram (DVH) or on axial, sagittal, and/or coronal CT images. By using volumetric parameters to evaluate dose, a more careful and complete analysis of target and normal tissue dose distribution is achievable.

4.1 IMRT Treatment Planning

Three-dimensional (3D) conformal radiotherapy uses a forward treatment planning process, whereby the dosimetrist selects beam specifications (e.g., direction, weight, shapes, and modifiers) and calculations are made based on these settings. A trial and error-based approach is used to select the best dose distribution from these specifications. With IMRT, a mathematical approach called inverse planning is used. In this process, the target dose and coverage are chosen, and then normal tissue dose and volume constraints are loaded into the computer program. An optimization algorithm modifies the intensity profile of each radiation beam and the specific shape of each treatment field or aperture in an iterative fashion until the desired dose distribution is achieved. Each beam is nonuniform such that the intensity of the beam varies across the treatment field. By modulating the intensity of each beam, a steep dose gradient is created between the PTV, rectum, and bladder, typically allowing at least 85–90 % of the PTV to receive the prescription dose while maintaining rectal and bladder doses within established tolerances. Doses to organs overlapping the PTV such as the bladder and rectum are often constrained to receive <100 % of the prescription. Given the steep falloff of the dose gradient, accurate targeting becomes increasingly important when implementing an IMRT plan. Treatment planning studies have shown improved conformality of dose distributions around the PTV compared with 3D conformal treatment planning (De Meerleer et al. 2000; Ling et al. 1996).

During the past 10–15 years, many techniques for IMRT treatment have been implemented (e.g., 'step and shoot', sliding window, helical fan beam, volumetric modulated arc therapy (VMAT)), although they all share a goal of creating a concave dose distribution by using multiple coplanar fields arranged at each or nearly equal spacing about the patient. At MSKCC, a 5–7 field beam arrangement is used to encompass the PTV to dose levels of 81 Gy or higher (Fig. 2). Other techniques include arc-based treatments or specialized tomotherapy units which provide similar but slightly different dose distributions (Fig. 3).

4.2 IMRT Treatment Delivery

In order to optimize the use of 3D conformal radiotherapy and/or IMRT, improved methods of recognition and correction of geometric uncertainties such as setup error and organ

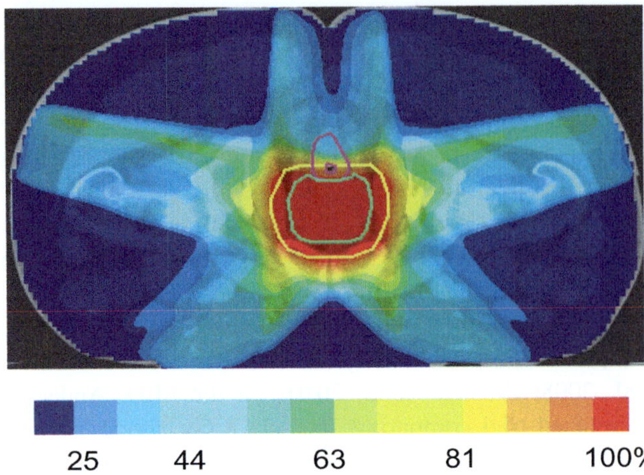

Fig. 2 Dose distribution (% prescription dose) for a 5-field IMRT plan

motion are necessary to integrate into treatment delivery. Organ motion during a course of radiation therapy introduces the potential for day-to-day variations in the position of the prostate (interfraction motion) as well as during a 15–20 min treatment session (intrafraction motion). Image-guided approaches have provided a means to account for target motion during radiation therapy and are discussed further in other chapters. Briefly, several methods of image-guided external beam radiotherapy are available and in the current clinical use. One of the simplest techniques includes the use of implanted gold fiducial markers which can be visualized on two-dimensional X-ray images obtained immediately prior to daily treatment from which positional corrections can be made. Other methods include an ultrasound-based system to detect and correct prostate, bladder, and rectum positioning using B-mode acquisition and targeting (BAT; Nomos Corp., Sewickley, PA). The most recent and the most complex approach includes the use of linear accelerators equipped with CT capability which can be co-registered with treatment planning CT scans.

At the Memorial Sloan-Kettering Cancer Center, we routinely use intraprostatic fiducial marker placements to guide the IMRT treatment. The placement of three radio-opaque (typically gold) markers into the prostate via a transrectal ultrasound-guided approach provides a simple way of tracking motion of the prostate during radiotherapy. The fiducial markers are placed prior to simulation and digitally reconstructed radiographs (DRR images) can be created on which the markers can be clearly seen (Fig. 4). Daily imaging using an electronic portal imaging device allows accurate pretreatment detection, verification, and correction of the prostate position. Several studies have shown this technique to have less user variability than ultrasound-based methods, which require specialized training (Langen et al. 2003). Marker placement is generally

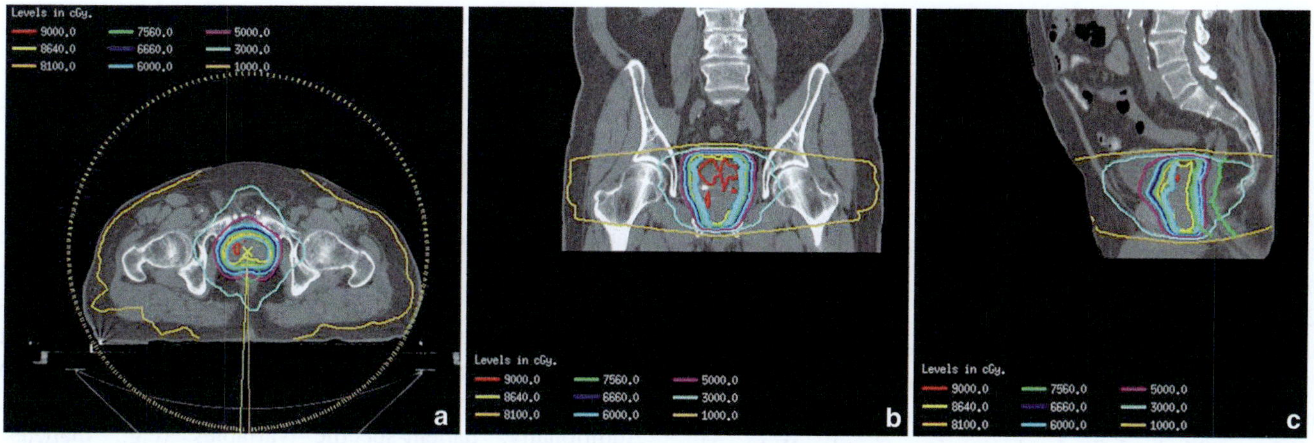

Fig. 3 Isodose distribution of VMAT (volumetric modulated arc therapy) plan **a** axial view, **b** coronal view, **c** sagittal view

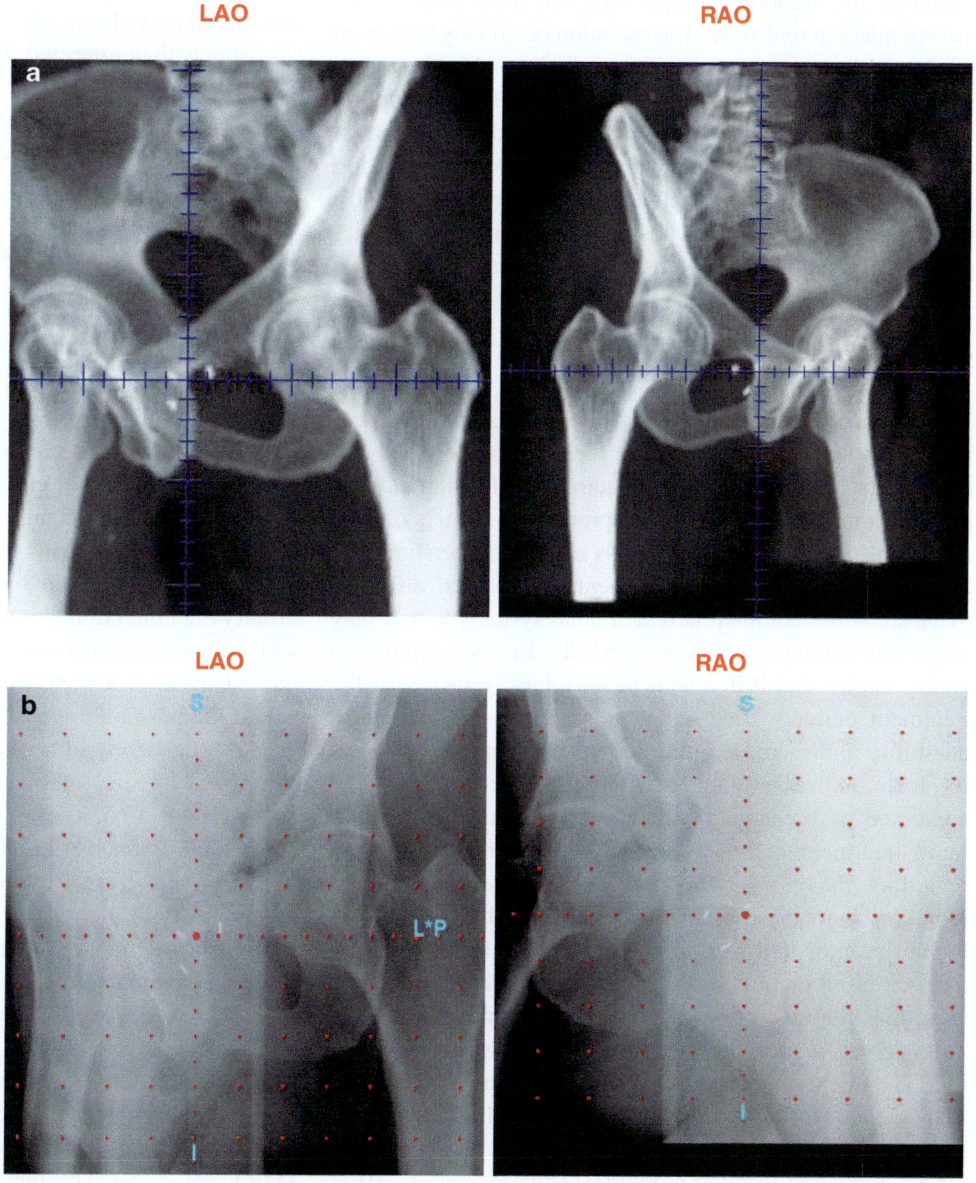

Fig. 4 Fiducial markers placed in prostate visible on left anterior oblique and right anterior oblique digitally reconstructed radiograph (**a**) and portal image (**b**)

well tolerated and marker migration is relatively rare (Trichter and Ennis 2003). We recently reported the toxicity profiles and biochemical outcomes from a cohort of 186 patients undergoing high-dose image-guided radiotherapy (IGRT) for localized prostate cancer which were retrospectively compared with a similar cohort of 190 patients treated with non-image-guided therapy (nIGRT) (Zelefsky et al. 2012). For the IGRT cohort, the rate of grade 2 or higher urinary toxicity was significantly less (10.4 vs. 20.0 %; $p = 0.02$) with no significant differences seen in the rectal toxicity or biochemical outcomes.

A new system has been developed which allows for monitoring of prostate motion during treatment delivery (Calypso Medical Technologies Inc, Seattle, WA). This system uses transponders, also placed transrectally, which emit an electromagnetic signal when excited. Detection of the signal by an alternating current magnetic array localizes the transponders in real-time. The radiation beam may be turned off should the target stray out of the radiation field or beyond a preset motion constraint. Unpredictable intrafraction motion shifts which would otherwise be unaccounted for are detectable and able to be corrected with this system. By increasing the accuracy of treatment delivery in this way, smaller PTV margins may be feasible and possibly further improve toxicity profiles, although this is yet to be clinically established.

4.3 Disadvantages of IMRT

Despite the clear benefits of IMRT in terms of dose escalation and normal-tissue sparing, there are some disadvantages. First, IMRT treatment requires careful and precise planning and quality assurance procedures which can be time-consuming and complex. This can be cumbersome and have an impact on the departmental resources, although there are some commercially available systems which may offset this efficiency concern. Secondly, the use of multiple gantry angles and differential beam intensity increases the treatment delivery time which may impact patient reproducibility and increase intrafraction organ motion variability. Increased uncertainty regarding target accuracy may be addressed by implanted trackable fiducial markers or more rapid treatment delivery (e.g., VMAT). Another concern regarding the use of IMRT is an increase in low dose radiation to non-target tissue (i.e., integral dose) due to higher monitor unit (MU) requirements for IMRT delivery and increased number of beams which raises some concern regarding the risk of secondary radiation-induced cancer. Zelefsky et al. recently reported a comparison of 2,658 IMRT, radical prostatectomy, and brachytherapy patients with median follow-up of >7.5 years and did not identify an increased secondary malignancy risk with the use of IMRT compared to other modalities (Zelefsky et al. 2012). Additional studies and long-term follow-up of IMRT patients will be important to confirm these findings.

5 Sequelae of IMRT: Acute and Late Toxicity

Radiation dose to normal tissues plays a major role in the development of acute and long-term side effects from radiotherapy; yet the relationship between dose and effect is complex. In general, this relationship is sigmoidal such that at low doses there is little observed effect; however with larger doses, increasing and predictable effects are observed. Additionally, patient-specific variables (e.g., diabetes, smoking, collagen vascular disease, previous surgery) can significantly affect this relationship. Known and unknown genetic factors (e.g., ataxia telangiectasia mutated [ATM] mutations) may also predispose some patients to more severe side effects than expected (Cesaretti et al. 2007).

5.1 Urinary Sequelae

Urinary symptoms are the most common acute toxicities associated with external beam radiation therapy for prostate cancer. Typical acute urinary symptoms include both irritative (i.e., frequency, urgency, dysuria) and obstructive-type (i.e., weak stream, incomplete emptying) symptoms. The mechanism of injury is from urethral and bladder neck irritation and inflammation. These symptoms are typically gradual in onset and often respond to alpha blocker or anti-inflammatory medications. Anti-cholinergic medication may help patients with a significant urgency, but should be used with caution in patients with obstruction. Since patients undergoing radiotherapy may be at risk of developing a urinary tract infection, this should be ruled out with urinalysis and culture in patients with significant dysuria. For radiation-related dysuria, a diet excluding bladder irritants such as acidic foods and liquids is often helpful. Urinary analgesics such as phenazopyridine may also be useful. Most patients' symptoms are mild; however, reported rates of grade ≥3 acute urinary toxicity range from 0 to 15 % (Al-Mamgani et al. 2009; Pollack et al. 2006; Zelefsky et al. 2000).

Following treatment, radiation-related acute urinary symptoms typically resolve over 6–12 months. Late toxicity is typically defined as symptoms occurring >90 days following treatment. Late grade 2 urinary toxicity occurs in 10–20 % of patients who undergo conformal radiotherapy and may include similar symptoms as in the acute setting. The mechanism of injury includes bladder neck and urethral microvascular changes leading to fibrosis and stricture formation. The reported rates of urethral stricture with IMRT are <2 %. The incidence of urinary incontinence is rare with reported rates of 0.5 to 2 % in patients with a history of TURP, hence these patients may not be amenable to dose escalation >81 Gy. Hematuria, typically painless, is a common yet rarely serious side effect that may occur related to vascular changes in the urethra or bladder neck and can be confirmed via cystoscopy.

5.2 Gastrointestinal Sequelae

Irradiation of the rectum and/or bowel can cause gastrointestinal sequelae in patients receiving radiation therapy for prostate cancer. Acute gastrointestinal symptoms may include abdominal bloating, gas, rectal urgency, tenesmus, increased bowel frequency, or diarrhea. Often dietary modification, especially fiber supplementation, and/or over the counter medications are effective and all that is necessary to manage these symptoms during treatment. Some patients may require brief courses of prescription anti-diarrheal medication. Patients with a history of active inflammatory bowel disease may be particularly predisposed to more severe gastrointestinal symptoms and should be considered for alternative therapy rather than radiotherapy.

Radiation proctitis is the most common late rectal toxicity and occurs in 10–20 % of patients. Remarkably, with the more modern techniques described above such as IMRT and IGRT, the incidence of grade 2 proctitis is less than 5 %. In approximately 1–2 % of treated patients, severe rectal toxicity such as persistent bleeding or ulcer development (grade 3 toxicity) associated with pain can be observed. Typical endoscopic changes include hyperemia and neovascularization. Symptomatically, patients may experience intermittent rectal bleeding, often with straining or constipation 1–2 years or more following treatment. Conservative measures, including stool softeners and steroid suppositories, are often all that is required. For the rare patient with persistent, severe rectal bleeding, telangiectatic vessels may be treated cautiously with endoscopic argon plasma coagulation. Hyperbaric oxygen (HO) has been shown to induce angiogenesis and may be helpful for refractory symptoms. A randomized trial comparing HO to sham therapy for refractory radiation proctitis demonstrated an improvement in symptoms with HO (Oliai et al. 2012).

5.3 Erectile Sequelae

Erectile dysfunction is a common late effect of conformal radiotherapy and occurs in 30–40 % of previously potent patients (Pinkawa et al. 2009). Younger patients and those who are optimally potent prior to EBRT are more likely to retain potency following radiotherapy. A history of smoking and/or vascular disease may predispose patients to a more significant posttreatment erectile dysfunction. The precise mechanism of radiation damage to erectile tissue is unclear, but likely relates to endothelial damage (Akbal et al. 2008). The damage to vasculature leads to penile arterial and venous insufficiency as well as nerve damage. Phosphodiesterase-5 (PDE-5) inhibitors such as sildenafil citrate are often effective in the treatment of erectile dysfunction following radiotherapy in approximately 60–70 % of affected patients and may play a role in preventing radiation-induced damage (Kedia et al. 1999; Mulhall et al. 2005). Predictors of failure to respond to PDE-5 inhibitors include older age, longer time after RT, duration of androgen deprivation (>4 months), and higher RT dose (Teloken et al. 2009).

6 Conclusion

Several technological advances over the last several decades have paved the way for a more precise and effective radiation therapy for prostate cancer. IMRT has greatly improved the ability for dose escalation while reducing late radiation-induced morbidity and improving local tumor control. Better local tumor control has translated into improved distant metastases-free survival, particularly for patients with intermediate- and high-risk disease and might eventually lead to better survival. Further improvements in these techniques are necessary to further optimize outcome while low-risk patients may benefit from strategies aimed at reducing treatment-related toxicity.

References

Akbal C, Tinay I, Simşek F et al (2008) Erectile dysfunction following radiotherapy and brachytherapy for prostate cancer: pathophysiology, prevention and treatment. Int Urol Nephrol 40:355–363

Al-Mamgani A, Heemsbergen WD, Peeters ST et al (2009) Role of intensity-modulated radiotherapy in reducing toxicity in dose escalation for localized prostate cancer. Int J Radiat Oncol Biol Phys 73:685–691

Beckendorf V, Guerif S, Le Prisé E et al (2011) 70 gy versus 80 gy in localized prostate cancer: 5-year results of getug 06 randomized trial. Int J Radiat Oncol Biol Phys 80:1056–1063

Cahlon O, Zelefsky MJ, Shippy A et al (2008) Ultra-high dose (86.4 gy) IMRT for localized prostate cancer: toxicity and biochemical outcomes. Int J Radiat Oncol Biol Phys 71:330–337

Center MM, Jemal A, Lortet-Tieulent J et al (2012) International variation in prostate cancer incidence and mortality rates. Eur Urol 61:1079–1092

Cesaretti JA, Stock RG, Atencio DP et al (2007) A genetically determined dose-volume histogram predicts for rectal bleeding among patients treated with prostate brachytherapy. Int J Radiat Oncol Biol Phys 68:1410–1416

De Meerleer GO, Fonteyne VH, Vakaet L et al (2007) Intensity-modulated radiation therapy for prostate cancer: late morbidity and results on biochemical control. Radiother Oncol 82:160–166

De Meerleer GO, Vakaet LA, De Gersem WR et al (2000) Radiotherapy of prostate cancer with or without intensity modulated beams: a planning comparison. Int J Radiat Oncol Biol Phys 47:639–648

Dearnaley DP, Sydes MR, Graham JD et al (2007) Escalated-dose versus standard-dose conformal radiotherapy in prostate cancer: first results from the MRC RT01 randomised controlled trial. Lancet Oncol 8:475–487

Kedia S, Zippe CD, Agarwal A et al (1999) Treatment of erectile dysfunction with sildenafil citrate (viagra) after radiation therapy for prostate cancer. Urology 54:308–312

Kim MM, Hoffman KE, Levy LB et al (2012) Prostate cancer-specific mortality after definitive radiation therapy: who dies of disease? Eur J Cancer 48:1664–1671

Kuban DA, Tucker SL, Dong L et al (2008) Long-term results of the M. D. Anderson randomized dose-escalation trial for prostate cancer. Int J Radiat Oncol Biol Phys 70:67–74

Langen KM, Pouliot J, Anezinos C et al (2003) Evaluation of ultrasound-based prostate localization for image-guided radiotherapy. Int J Radiat Oncol Biol Phys 57:635–644

Leibel SA, Zelefsky MJ, Kutcher GJ et al (1994) Three-dimensional conformal radiation therapy in localized carcinoma of the prostate: Interim report of a phase 1 dose-escalation study. J Urol 152: 1792–1798

Ling CC, Burman C, Chui CS et al (1996) Conformal radiation treatment of prostate cancer using inversely-planned intensity-modulated photon beams produced with dynamic multileaf collimation. Int J Radiat Oncol Biol Phys 35:721–730

Michalski JM, Bae K, Roach M et al (2010) Long-term toxicity following 3d conformal radiation therapy for prostate cancer from the RTOG 9406 phase I/II dose escalation study. Int J Radiat Oncol Biol Phys 76:14–22

Mulhall J, Ahmed A, Parker M et al (2005) The hemodynamics of erectile dysfunction following external beam radiation for prostate cancer. J Sex Med 2:432–437

Nguyen PL, Gu X, Lipsitz SR et al (2011) Cost implications of the rapid adoption of newer technologies for treating prostate cancer. J Clin Oncol 29:1517–1524

Oliai C, Fisher B, Jani A et al (2012) Hyperbaric oxygen therapy for radiation-induced cystitis and proctitis. Int J Radiat Oncol Biol Phys 84:733–740

Peeters ST, Heemsbergen WD, Koper PC et al (2006a) Dose-response in radiotherapy for localized prostate cancer: results of the Dutch multicenter randomized phase III trial comparing 68 gy of radiotherapy with 78 gy. J Clin Oncol 24:1990–1996

Peeters STH, Heemsbergen WD, Koper PC et al (2006b) Dose-response in radiotherapy for localized prostate cancer: results of the Dutch multicenter randomized phase III trial comparing 68 gy of radiotherapy with 78 gy. J Clin Oncol 24:1990–1996

Pinkawa M, Gagel B, Piroth MD et al (2009) Erectile dysfunction after external beam radiotherapy for prostate cancer. Eur Urol 55:227–234

Pollack A, Hanlon AL, Horwitz EM et al (2006) Dosimetry and preliminary acute toxicity in the first 100 men treated for prostate cancer on a randomized hypofractionation dose escalation trial. Int J Radiat Oncol Biol Phys 64:518–526

Pollack A, Zagars GK, Starkschall G et al (2002) Prostate cancer radiation dose response: results of the M. D. Anderson phase III randomized trial. Int J Radiat Oncol Biol Phys 53:1097–1105

Smit WG, Helle PA, van Putten WL et al (1990) Late radiation damage in prostate cancer patients treated by high dose external radiotherapy in relation to rectal dose. Int J Radiat Oncol Biol Phys 18:23–29

Spratt DE, Pei X, Yamada J et al (2013) Long-term survival and toxicity in patients treated with high-dose intensity modulated radiation therapy for localized prostate cancer. Int J Radiat Oncol Biol Phys 85:686–692

Teloken PE, Parker M, Mohideen N et al (2009) Predictors of response to sildenafil citrate following radiation therapy for prostate cancer. J Sex Med 6:1135–1140

Trichter F, Ennis RD (2003) Prostate localization using transabdominal ultrasound imaging. Int J Radiat Oncol Biol Phys 56: 1225–1233

Vora SA, Wong WW, Schild SE et al (2007) Analysis of biochemical control and prognostic factors in patients treated with either low-dose three-dimensional conformal radiation therapy or high-dose intensity-modulated radiotherapy for localized prostate cancer. Int J Radiat Oncol Biol Phys 68:1053–1058

Zelefsky MJ, Fuks Z, Happersett L et al (2000) Clinical experience with intensity modulated radiation therapy (IMRT) in prostate cancer. Radiother Oncol 55:241–249

Zelefsky MJ, Fuks Z, Hunt M et al (2002) High-dose intensity modulated radiation therapy for prostate cancer: early toxicity and biochemical outcome in 772 patients. Int J Radiat Oncol Biol Phys 53:1111–1116

Zelefsky MJ, Kollmeier M, Cox B et al (2012a) Improved clinical outcomes with high-dose image-guided radiotherapy compared with non-IGRT for the treatment of clinically localized prostate cancer. Int J Radiat Oncol Biol Phys 84:125–129

Zelefsky MJ, Leibel SA, Gaudin PB et al (1998) Dose escalation with three-dimensional conformal radiation therapy affects the outcome in prostate cancer. Int J Radiat Oncol Biol Phys 41:491–500

Zelefsky MJ, Pei X, Teslova T et al (2012b) Secondary cancers after intensity-modulated radiotherapy, brachytherapy and radical prostatectomy for the treatment of prostate cancer: incidence and cause-specific survival outcomes according to the initial treatment intervention. BJU Int 110:1696–1701

Zietman AL, Bae K, Slater JD et al (2010) Randomized trial comparing conventional-dose with high-dose conformal radiation therapy in early-stage adenocarcinoma of the prostate: long-term results from Proton Radiation Oncology Group/American College of Radiology 95-09. J Clin Oncol 28:1106–1111

IGRT: How and When

Marciana Nona Duma and Patrick Kupelian

Contents

Abstract

This chapter gives an overview of IGRT techniques employed in prostate cancer. The described techniques include portal imaging using Megavoltage sources (porta films and electronic portal imaging devices), Kilovoltage radiographs (room-based or gantry-based systems, transabdominal ultrasound, and in-room CTs. An ideal IGRT system would allow for daily prostate imaging without possible introduction of errors due to image acquisition itself, it would do so within a reasonable time frame, without the necessity for implanted radio-opaque markers and preferentially without exposing the patient to radiation. A solution that combines all these features is inexistent so far. For the existing IGRT techniques, there is a considerable lack of data whether they lead to a reduced acute and chronic toxicity profile in comparison with the non-IGRT approach, or if they are associated with an improved local control. Nevertheless, given the increasingly higher doses and smaller treatment margins utilized, combined with the trend to hypofractionate radiation therapy, daily IGRT for prostate cancer has become a necessity as an accurate and precise way of delivering the intended dose to the PTV and the OARs. The problem of interfractional prostate movement and the possibility of setup errors are optimally accounted for.

Techniques such as IMRT now provide a higher conformality in dose distribution (see chapter on IMRT). With the increased use of dose escalation using tighter margins in the treatment of localized prostate cancer patients, proper localization of target areas and organs at risk has become necessary. Thus, image-guided radiation therapy (IGRT) has become an integral part of prostate cancer radiotherapy. Techniques that are able to depict the location of the tumor as well as surrounding organs, in order to avoid potential losses in local or regional control, are more and more introduced

M. N. Duma (✉)
Klinik und Poliklinik für Strahlentherapie und Radiologische Onkologie, Klinikum rechts der Isar, TU München, Ismaninger Str. 22, 81675 München, Germany
e-mail: Marciana.Duma@mri.tum.de

P. Kupelian
Department of Radiation Oncology, UCLA, 200 UCLA Medical Plaza, Str. B265, Los Angeles, CA 90095-6951, USA

H. Geinitz et al. (eds.), *Radiotherapy in Prostate Cancer*, Medical Radiology. Radiation Oncology,
DOI: 10.1007/174_2014_1009,
Published Online: 6 July 2014

into daily clinical practice (Hammoud et al. 2008). This chapter gives an overview of IGRT techniques employed in prostate cancer.

1 Techniques

Several methods of target localization are available in prostate cancer: portal imaging devices using megavoltage (MV) sources or imaging using kilovoltage (kV) X-rays, transabdominal ultrasound, and in-room CT scanning. Although other methods, such as electromagnetic guidance, are available to perform proper target localization in prostate radiotherapy, this chapter is limited to the actual *image*-based methods mentioned above.

1.1 Portal Imaging Using Megavoltage Sources: Portal Films and Electronic Portal Imaging Devices

This widely used technique is based on X-ray imaging generated by the megavoltage treatment source. The conventional way of X-ray imaging on special films, called portal films, was in the last decade replaced by electronic portal imaging devices (EPID). The development of the semiconductor detector systems (amorphous silicone flat-panel detectors) offered imaging with a quality far better than prior film-based systems.

1.1.1 Bone Matching EPID

Routine evaluation is done by comparing the bony structures of the pelvis in the simulator generated image and the megavoltage treatment source image. The most important flaw of bone matching EPID is evident: there is no direct correlation to the real position of the prostate. To cope with this situation, the visualization of the target volume was provided by implanting imaging radiopaque markers into the prostate.

1.1.2 Implanted Markers EPID

Usually three gold seeds are placed within the prostate using brachytherapy needles: one at each side of the base and one at the apex. They are easily seen on EPID and their variation within the prostate is very small over time. The intermarker distance, a measure of the stability of these implanted fiducials, has been documented to remain within 1 mm over a course of treatment (Kupelian et al. 2005).

When comparing skin alignment or bony alignment to implanted markers EPID, Beltram et al. found out that implanted markers allow a reduction of safety margins (Beltran et al. 2008). The safety margins needed from the clinical target volume (CTV) to the planning target volume (PTV) when daily localization is based on the implanted markers were 4.8 mm left–right (LR), 5.4 mm (inferior–superior) IS, and 5.2 mm anterior–posterior (AP) (Beltran et al. 2008).

1.2 Kilovoltage Radiographs: Room-Based or Gantry-Based Systems

Two different types of kV imaging devices can be used for guidance for prostate cancer: single or dual kV X-ray tubes on the gantry of the linear accelerator (on-board imaging system—OBI) (Jaffray et al. 1995; Takai et al. 2004; Huntzinger et al. 2006) and in-room kV imaging systems (Shirato et al. 1999).

Both approaches are designed to localize the bony structure or fiducial markers as previously described for the EPID. There is a better quality in imaging than the MV portal imaging, but there is still no information available on soft tissue or internal organ changes.

1.3 Transabdominal Ultrasound

The transabdominal ultrasound (US) was the first widely used technique for daily soft tissue/prostate localization in the treatment room. Several devices are available (Serago et al. 2002; Langen et al. 2003). However, the agreement between daily transabdominal US and implanted marker registration is very low. Less than 51 % of the fractions have an agreement within ±3 mm and the mean distance discrepancy is 8.8 mm (Johnston et al. 2008; Scarbrough et al. 2006).

Further, daily transabdominal ultrasound is prone to large interobserver variability. In a study by Langen et al., the average range of couch shifts due to contour alignment variability amongst eight users on the ultrasound were 7, 7, and 5 mm in the anteroposterior (AP), superoinferior, and lateral directions, respectively (Langen et al. 2003).

The effectiveness of daily ultrasound guided alignments to an off-line correction protocol of daily bone alignment plus a correction factor for systematic internal prostate displacement was tested in a study by O'Daniel et al. (O'Daniel et al. 2008). The daily bone alignment plus the factor for systematic internal prostate displacement provided better daily alignment precision and equivalent dose coverage compared with daily US alignment (O'Daniel et al. 2008).

1.4 In-Room CT

1.4.1 Kilovoltage CT

1.4.1.1 *CT-On-Rail*

This relatively uncommon configuration requires a very precise knowledge of the geometric relationship to the linear accelerator's isocenter for placing a conventional CT scanner in the treatment room to allow IGRT. Uematsu et al. have developed this approach for several years using a CT-on-rails (Siemens Primatom; Siemens Medical Solutions, Concord, CA). Patients are set up with opaque BB (branch-and-bound) marks on the triangulated fiducial skin marks on the Linac table. The table is then rotated 180° to allow the CT-on-rails to pass over the treatment table. The exact position of the prostate gland is identified on CT images of the treatment day and is compared to the position seen on the simulation CT scans. The anterior, posterior, superior, inferior, left, and right extreme points of the prostate glands are plotted manually or recorded using an image fusion software. From these points, the day-to-day movements of the prostate glands are derived. The patient is treated with the newly derived isocenter (Wong et al. 2005, 2008; Fung et al. 2005; Cheng et al. 2003).

1.4.1.2 *Cone-Beam CT*

Owing to the recent development of large area flat-panel detector technology, volumetric images can be acquired in a single revolution of the gantry by using a cone of rays emanating from the source. The cone-beam CT (CBCT) device is mounted on the gantry of the linear accelerator. An automatic matching of the CBCT image and the kV CT planning image is performed.

1.4.2 Megavoltage CT

There are different techniques to generate megavoltage CT (MVCT) scans for image-guided radiation therapy, such as single-slice, cone-beam MVCT, and tomotherapy helical MVCT.

1.4.2.1 *Single Slice Technique*

The single slice technique has very little use in radiation therapy. Nakagawa et al. have used MVCT for on-line correction in the clinical setting. The procedure involves positioning the patient according to skin markers, collecting a single MVCT slice, evaluating it, and adjusting the patient's position accordingly (Nakagawa et al. 2000). Obviously, the data provided by the single slice technique are very limited.

1.4.2.2 *Cone Beam MVCT*

The technique of a cone-beam CT (CBCT) has been previously described. The MV CBCT is using as a cone beam source, the megavoltage treatment source.

Table 1 CT dose to normal tissue (fx: fraction)

CT	Rectum (Dose in cGy/fx)	Bladder (Dose in cGy/fx)	Femoral heads (Dose in cGy/fx)
Diagnostic multidetector CT	1.74	1.83	4.05
kV CBCT	1.70	1.73	3.14
MVCT	1.05	1.04	1.02

1.4.2.3 *Tomotherapy Helical MVCT*

The megavoltage image is completed in a manner analogous to a helical CT scanner. After the MVCT image is acquired and reconstructed, it is registered with the kV CT image to determine corrections to the patient's position in the lateral, longitudinal, vertical, and roll directions. For the automatic registration, the algorithm can be chosen by bone anatomy, bone and tissue anatomy, or full image registration. The system allows after automatic registration to apply manual shifts to the setup. An automatic and manual couch shift to the indicated position by the matching of the CTs is done before applying the treatment.

Summary Several papers are available on IGRT by CT in prostate cancer (Zhu et al. 2009; Nairz et al. 2008; Song et al. 2006, 2007; Enmark et al. 2006; Gayou and Miften 2008; Barney et al. 2011). There is significant CT versus implanted markers agreement. More than 70 % of the fractions have an agreement within ±5 mm (LR 97.2 %; SI 72.7 %, and AP 72.4 %, respectively) (Gayou and Miften 2008; Barney et al. 2011). However, an automatic fusion with a gray-value-based algorithm is not sufficient. Shi et al. compared an automatic kV CBCT alignment to a manual alignment to fiducial markers (Shi et al. 2011). The mean 3D distance discrepancy between the two techniques was 7.5 mm (range 0.4–20.6 mm). The fusion of the daily CT to the planning CT should be done manually. Further, performing a daily CT comes at a cost of additional radiation dose to organs at risk/normal tissue (Table 1) (Ding et al. 2010; Shah et al. 2008).

2 Clinical Implications

Because of the relatively new employment of the previously described IGRT techniques in the daily routine, there is a lack of data regarding the clinical implications and reduction of toxicities in comparison with non-IGRT approaches. Thus far, studies have shown that these strategies are feasible in terms of treatment accuracy, with the attendant reduction in margins and radiation exposure to nearby critical organs.

Table 2 Mean CTV to PTV margins for different IGRT techniques (Beltran et al. 2008; Johnston et al. 2008; Gayou and Miften 2008)

Daily IGRT technique	LR (mm)	AP (mm)	SI (mm)
Implanted markers	5	5	5
Transabdominal ultrasound	9	16	12
CT	2	4	3

Table 2 depicts the mean CTV to PTV margins when different daily IGRT techniques are employed (Beltran et al. 2008; Johnston et al. 2008; Gayou and Miften 2008).

However, whether these improvements lead to reduced toxicities, as reported by patients, is uncertain. Song et al. performed an evaluation of image-guided radiation therapy technologies and their impact on the outcomes of hypofractionated prostate cancer treatments by using NTCP and TCP models (Song et al. 2006). The tattoo registered technique had a significant reduction in TCP as the prescription dose decreased. The differences between the techniques other than the tattoo registered (image-guided alignment to bony landmarks, to the daily CTV volume, or alignment to the CTV volume with daily monitor units updates), however, were small (<2.7 %) (Song et al. 2006).

No randomized trials are available. For the existing data, greater patient populations and longer follow-up is needed to determine the importance of IGRT in reducing the acute and chronic toxicities. A study by Jereczek-Fossa et al. (Jereczek-Fossa et al. 2011) assessed in a nonrandomized fashion the acute toxicity of image-guided hypofractionated radiotherapy. 179 patients were treated within the prospective study with 70.2 Gy/26 fractions (equivalent to 84 Gy/42 fractions, α/β 1.5 Gy) using IGRT (transabdominal ultrasound, ExacTrac X-Ray system, or cone-beam computer tomography) techniques. The data of these patients were compared to retrospective data of non-IGRT patients. The acute toxicity rates were low and similar in both study groups (Jereczek-Fossa et al. 2011). Similar results were achieved in Klinkum rechts der Isar, Munich Germany (Geier et al. 2012).

3 Conclusion

An ideal IGRT system would allow for daily prostate imaging without possible introduction of errors due to image acquisition itself, it would do so within a reasonable time frame, without the necessity for implanted radio-opaque markers and preferentially without exposing the patient to radiation (Soete et al. 2008).

A solution that combines all these features is inexistent so far. For the existing IGRT techniques, there is a considerable lack of data whether they lead to a reduced acute and chronic toxicity profile in comparison with the non-IGRT approach, or if they are associated with an improved local control. Nevertheless, given the increasingly higher doses and smaller treatment margins utilized, combined with the trend to hypofractionate radiation therapy, daily IGRT for prostate cancer has become a necessity as an accurate and precise way of delivering the intended dose to the PTV and the OARs. The problem of interfractional prostate movement and the possibility of setup errors are optimally accounted for.

References

Barney BM, Lee RJ, Handrahan D, Welsh KT, Cook JT, Sause WT (2011) Image-guided radiotherapy (IGRT) for prostate cancer comparing kV imaging of fiducial markers with cone beam computed tomography (CBCT). Int J Radiat Oncol Biol Phys 80:301–305

Beltran C, Herman MG, Davis BJ (2008) Planning target margin calculations for prostate radiotherapy based on intrafraction and interfraction motion using four localization methods. Int J Radiat Oncol Biol Phys 70:289–295

Cheng CW, Wong J, Grimm L, Chow M, Uematsu M, Fung A (2003) Commissioning and clinical implementation of a sliding gantry CT scanner installed in an existing treatment room and early clinical experience for precise tumor localization. Am J Clin Oncol 26:e28–e36

Ding A, Gu J, Trofimov AV, Xu XG (2010) Monte Carlo calculation of imaging doses from diagnostic multidetector CT and kilovoltage cone-beam CT as part of prostate cancer treatment plans. Med Phys 37:6199–6204

Enmark M, Korreman S, Nystrom H (2006) IGRT of prostate cancer; is the margin reduction gained from daily IG time-dependent? Acta Oncol 45:907–914

Fung AY, Wong JR, Cheng CW, Lisa Grimm S, Uematsu M (2005) A comparison of two image fusion techniques in ct-on-rails localization of radiation delivery. Phys Med 21:113–119

Gayou O, Miften M (2008) Comparison of mega-voltage cone-beam computed tomography prostate localization with online ultrasound and fiducial markers methods. Med Phys 35:531–538

Geier M, Astner ST, Duma MN et al (2012) Dose-escalated simultaneous integrated-boost treatment of prostate cancer patients via helical tomotherapy. Strahlenther Onkol 188:410–416

Hammoud R, Patel SH, Pradhan D et al (2008) Examining margin reduction and its impact on dose distribution for prostate cancer patients undergoing daily cone-beam computed tomography. Int J Radiat Oncol Biol Phys 71:265–273

Huntzinger C, Munro P, Johnson S et al (2006) Dynamic targeting image-guided radiotherapy. Med Dosim 31:113–125

Jaffray DA, Chawla K, Yu C, Wong JW (1995) Dual-beam imaging for online verification of radiotherapy field placement. Int J Radiat Oncol Biol Phys 33:1273–1280

Jereczek-Fossa BA, Zerini D, Fodor C et al (2011) Acute toxicity of image-guided hypofractionated radiotherapy for prostate cancer: nonrandomized comparison with conventional fractionation. Urol Oncol 29:523–532

Johnston H, Hilts M, Beckham W, Berthelet E (2008) 3D ultrasound for prostate localization in radiation therapy: a comparison with implanted fiducial markers. Med Phys 35:2403–2413

Kupelian PA, Willoughby TR, Meeks SL et al (2005) Intraprostatic fiducials for localization of the prostate gland: monitoring intermarker distances during radiation therapy to test for marker stability. Int J Radiat Oncol Biol Phys 62:1291–1296

Langen KM, Pouliot J, Anezinos C et al (2003) Evaluation of ultrasound-based prostate localization for image-guided radiotherapy. Int J Radiat Oncol Biol Phys 57:635–644

Nairz O, Merz F, Deutschmann H et al (2008) A strategy for the use of image-guided radiotherapy (IGRT) on linear accelerators and its impact on treatment margins for prostate cancer patients. Strahlenther Onkol 184:663–667

Nakagawa K, Aoki Y, Tago M, Terahara A, Ohtomo K (2000) Megavoltage CT-assisted stereotactic radiosurgery for thoracic tumors: original research in the treatment of thoracic neoplasms. Int J Radiat Oncol Biol Phys 48:449–457

O'Daniel JC, Dong L, Zhang L et al (2008) Daily bone alignment with limited repeat CT correction rivals daily ultrasound alignment for prostate radiotherapy. Int J Radiat Oncol Biol Phys 71:274–280

Scarbrough TJ, Golden NM, Ting JY et al (2006) Comparison of ultrasound and implanted seed marker prostate localization methods: Implications for image-guided radiotherapy. Int J Radiat Oncol Biol Phys 65:378–387

Serago CF, Chungbin SJ, Buskirk SJ, Ezzell GA, Collie AC, Vora SA (2002) Initial experience with ultrasound localization for positioning prostate cancer patients for external beam radiotherapy. Int J Radiat Oncol Biol Phys 53:1130–1138

Shah AP, Langen KM, Ruchala KJ, Cox A, Kupelian PA, Meeks SL (2008) Patient dose from megavoltage computed tomography imaging. Int J Radiat Oncol Biol Phys 70:1579–1587

Shi W, Li JG, Zlotecki RA et al (2011) Evaluation of kV cone-beam ct performance for prostate IGRT: a comparison of automatic grey-value alignment to implanted fiducial-marker alignment. Am J Clin Oncol 34:16–21

Shirato H, Shimizu S, Shimizu T, Nishioka T, Miyasaka K (1999) Real-time tumour-tracking radiotherapy. Lancet 353:1331–1332

Soete G, Verellen D, Storme G (2008) Image guided radiotherapy for prostate cancer. Bull Cancer 95:374–380

Song WY, Schaly B, Bauman G, Battista JJ, Van Dyk J (2006) Evaluation of image-guided radiation therapy (IGRT) technologies and their impact on the outcomes of hypofractionated prostate cancer treatments: a radiobiologic analysis. Int J Radiat Oncol Biol Phys 64:289–300

Song WY, Wong E, Bauman GS, Battista JJ, Van Dyk J (2007) Dosimetric evaluation of daily rigid and nonrigid geometric correction strategies during on-line image-guided radiation therapy (IGRT) of prostate cancer. Med Phys 34:352–365

Takai YMM, Yamada S, Mostafavi H, Marc M,Van Antwerp C, Mansfield S (2004) Development of a dual kV X-ray on-board imager for patient setup and dynamic tumor tracking. In: Proceedings 10th varian European users meeting 2004

Wong JR, Grimm L, Uematsu M et al (2005) Image-guided radiotherapy for prostate cancer by CT-linear accelerator combination: prostate movements and dosimetric considerations. Int J Radiat Oncol Biol Phys 61:561–569

Wong JR, Gao Z, Uematsu M et al (2008) Interfractional prostate shifts: review of 1870 computed tomography (CT) scans obtained during image-guided radiotherapy using CT-on-rails for the treatment of prostate cancer. Int J Radiat Oncol Biol Phys 72:1396–1401

Zhu X, Bourland JD, Yuan Y et al (2009) Tradeoffs of integrating real-time tracking into IGRT for prostate cancer treatment. Phys Med Biol 54:N393–N401

Part IV

Locally Advanced Disease

Techniques of Pelvic Irradiation

Ute Ganswindt and Claus Belka

Contents

Abstract

Even if irradiation of pelvic lymph nodes in prostate cancer is still under debate, there is abundant evidence that a well-defined subgroup of prostate cancer patients benefit from such treatment. Thus, the management of high risk and node-positive patients has evolved significantly in the past few years. New imaging tools such as MR, PET, and sentinel procedures now allow surgeons and radiation oncologists to better target lymph nodes or nodal metastasis. Derived from surgical lymphadenectomy series, sentinel lymph node, or PET/MR imaging data, there exist precise guidelines for target volume delineation. In addition, improved radiation technologies such as IMRT and IGRT enable to deliver high-dose conformal radiation to a target volume while minimizing toxicities to normal tissues and allow differentiated dose prescriptions. In this regard, adjuvant regions (suspected microscopic involvement) are most often treated with 45–50 Gy overall dose. In cases of macroscopic lymph node involvement, overall dose on localized lymph node metastasis should be escalated to ≥60 Gy, depending on tumor volume and surrounding normal tissues. Besides conventional fractionation schemes, first series using a moderate hypofractionation to the prostate in combination with pelvic node irradiation was reported. The encouraging results must be validated in prospective clinical trials.

1 Introduction

Even if the irradiation of pelvic lymph nodes in prostate cancer is still a matter of debate, it regained considerable interest after the results of the randomized EORTC (European Organisation for Research and Treatment of Cancer) 22863 (Bolla et al. 2002) and RTOG (Radiation Therapy Oncology Group) 94-13 (Roach et al. 2003) trials were published.

U. Ganswindt (✉) · C. Belka
Department of Radiation Oncology, Ludwig-Maximilians-University (LMU), Marchioninistr. 15, 81377 Munich, Germany
e-mail: ute.ganswindt@med.uni.muenchen.de

H. Geinitz et al. (eds.), *Radiotherapy in Prostate Cancer*, Medical Radiology. Radiation Oncology,
DOI: 10.1007/174_2014_1036, © Springer-Verlag Berlin Heidelberg 2014
Published Online: 7 October 2014

The EORTC 22863 trial randomized patients to receive radiotherapy of the prostate and pelvic lymph nodes with long term (3 years) versus no hormonal ablation. After the 10 years follow-up had revealed a significant benefit in overall survival for the combined treatment arm (58.1 % vs. 39.8 %) without difference to an age-adjusted healthy cohort (Bolla et al. 2010), it is the current standard therapy for high-risk prostate cancer patients besides surgery. However, this trial only randomized long term versus no hormonal ablation therapy, but not the additional irradiation of pelvic nodes. Thus, the benefit of an enlarged treatment volume remained unclear.

The RTOG 94-13 trial randomized patients with an estimated risk for lymph node involvement exceeding 15 % ("Roach formula") in four arms to receive either radiotherapy only to the prostate with additional neoadjuvant or adjuvant hormonal ablation or radiotherapy to the prostate and the pelvic lymph nodes with additional neoadjuvant or adjuvant hormonal ablation. Improved rates of biochemical no evidence of disease (bNED) were observed in patients receiving both neoadjuvant/concomitant hormonal ablation and whole pelvis irradiation (Roach et al. 2003). A follow-up analysis confirmed the initial report (Lawton et al. 2007). Additionally, an analysis of field sizes revealed that larger field sizes correlated significantly with improved outcome (Roach et al. 2006; Roach 2009).

In contrast, the randomized French GETUG (Groupe d'Etude des Tumeurs Uro-Génitales) trial published in 2007 did not corroborate that adjuvant inclusion of the pelvic nodes increased the bNED rates (Pommier et al. 2007). However, the inclusion criteria were different to the RTOG and EORTC trials in regard to patients' lower risk profile and not defined hormonal ablation therapy.

Thus, at present, the role of adjuvant coverage of the lymphatic drainage area is not yet finally clear. Chapters "Treatment of Clinically Involved Lymph Nodes" and "Hypo-fractionation in Prostate Cancer: Biological Aspects" will discuss this topic in detail.

In addition to the results from the randomized trials, data from PET-based studies provide—at least circumstantial—evidence that the inclusion of the local lymphatics in adjuvant radiation portals may be of importance for a subset of patients. In this regard, several authors provide evidence for effective salvage therapies for patients with isolated and choline PET-diagnosed lymph node relapses (Rinnab et al. 2008; Budiharto et al. 2011; Passoni et al. 2014; Wurschmidt et al. 2011).

Thus, at the moment, it can be assumed that a defined subgroup of patients will substantially benefit from an additional radiation treatment of the pelvic lymphatic drainage. However, the result of a surgical or radiotherapeutic adjuvant treatment relies on an adequate definition of potentially involved lymphatic drainage areas.

2 Basic Considerations—Pelvic Target Volume Definition

Before wide implementation of CT-based three-dimensional (3D) radiotherapy planning in the later 1990s, radiotherapy planning was performed on two-dimensional radiographics. Thus, the pelvic target volume was oriented to bony anatomical landmarks derived from historical lymphography series.

Only after implementation of 3D conformal radiotherapy planning in clinical practice CT planning image information was available for each individual patient. However, for a long time, radiotherapy was usually applied using simple box techniques. Conventional four-field-techniques did not allow precise individualizations of target volumes with conformally effective sparing of organs at risk (Fig. 1). The randomized EORTC, RTOG, and GETUG trials started patient recruitment in the 1990s. Thus, necessarily they did not include highly conformal radiotherapy techniques or individualized target volume concepts.

Finally, modern radiotherapy techniques such as IMRT (intensity modulated radiotherapy) required new approaches for pelvic target volume definition as well as conceptions for sparing organs at risk.

Whereas for several other solid pelvic neoplasms (for example rectal cancer), detailed studies regarding the distribution of locoregional failures are available, there are hardly such data for prostate cancer.

This is related to the fact that—for decades—the major endpoint for outcome definition after curative treatment of prostate cancer is biochemical failure rather than patho-anatomically defined failure. Thus, in the past, it was not exactly shown where and how often patients with prostate cancer finally experience local, locoregional, and distant failure. In addition, the rapid initiation of hormonal ablation therapy after biochemical relapse often had blurred the further topographic attribution of the individual relapse.

Therefore, available topographic data about microscopic pelvic or lymph node involvements in prostate cancer had to be considered since IMRT planning allowed and required individualized target volumes.

3 Surgical Lymphadenectomy Data

Prostate cancer patients who are treated by radical prostatovesiculectomy are mostly undergoing simultaneous pelvic lymphadenectomy. Up to now, the therapeutic importance of a lymphadenectomy procedure regarding potential survival benefits is not finally clear. However, there are some lines of evidence, that progression-free survival is improved when lymphadenectomy is performed (Allaf et al. 2004; Bader et al. 2003; Cheng et al. 2001; Hull et al. 2002).

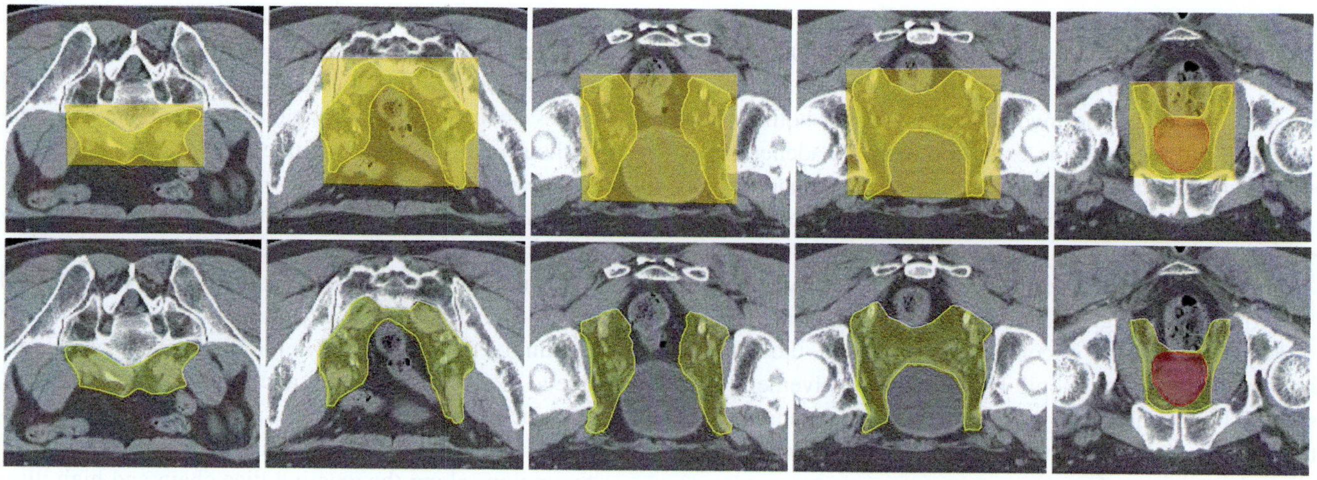

Fig. 1 Target volume definition of whole pelvis irradiation. *Upper row* CTV 3D-four-field planning. *Lower row* CTV IMRT planning

Fig. 2 Lymphadenectomy techniques; 1 + 2 = modified (standard), 2 = minimal, 1 + 2 + 3 = extended lymphadenectomy (Bader et al. 2002)

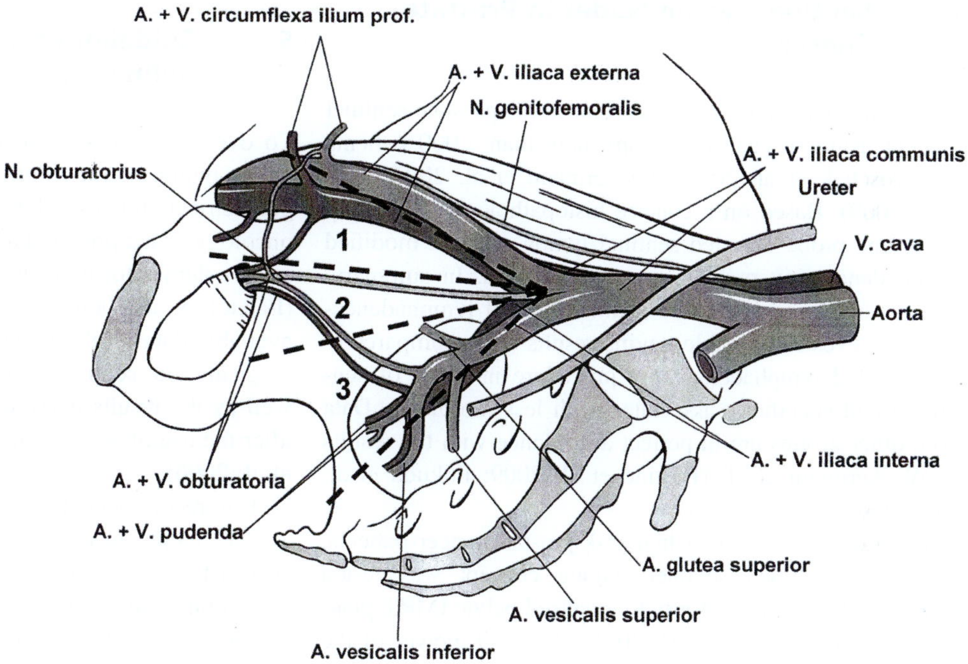

Aside of its questionable therapeutic role, lymphadenectomy has to be understood as a staging procedure followed by potential relevant therapy recommendations.

However, there are relevant differences with regard to detailed lymphadenectomy modalities. In general, the anatomic extension of pelvic lymph node surgery must be distinguished between "minimal/limited," "modified/standard," and "extended" lymphadenectomy. The minimal lymphadenectomy technique only includes the obturator fossa region, and the standard technique furthermore includes the lymphatic area along the external iliac veins, whereas the extended lymphadenectomy area additionally contains all lymph nodes along external, internal, and common iliac vessels (Fig. 2).

Derived from large lymphadenectomy series in the recent years with precise histopathological work-up procedures (Allaf et al. 2004; Bader et al. 2002; Weckermann et al. 2005, 2006; Burkhard et al. 2002, 2005; Heidenreich et al. 2002; Briganti et al. 2006, 2007; Shariat et al. 2003; Pagliarulo et al. 2006; Ferrari et al. 2006; Miyake et al. 2007; Stone et al. 1997; Joslyn and Konety 2006) following key conclusions can be drawn:

- the risk of locoregional seeding is higher than previously assumed
- only for patients at a very low risk for lymph node involvement the procedure of lymphadenectomy seems to be dispensable with regard to morbidity or questionable benefit

- at least 10 lymph nodes should be removed when lymphadenectomy is performed (Briganti et al. 2006; Joslyn and Konety 2006)
- rates of lymph node involvement are rising both by risk profile and by anatomic extension of lymphadenectomy
- the individual lymphatic drainage in prostate cancer patients is more variable than previously suspected
- nomograms based on limited or standard lymphadenectomy data may underestimate rates of pelvic lymph node involvement (Cagiannos et al. 2003; Partin et al. 1997)

From a radiation oncologist's view point the lack of information on microscopic lymph node involvement is of special importance with regard to individual radiotherapy treatment decisions—aiming in at least being comparable to clinical outcomes of surgical strategies.

4 Sentinel Lymph Nodes in Prostate Cancer

Weckermann and co-workers developed the prostate sentinel concept using surgical data from more than 2,000 patients (Wawroschek et al. 2003; Weckermann et al. 2007; Holl et al. 2009). Based on a concise histopathological work-up of gamma probe detected sentinel lymph nodes a modified lymphadenectomy procedure was developed. In summary, their findings suggest that a sentinel-guided lymphadenectomy achieves comparable staging results when compared to an extended lymphadenectomy procedure in terms of sensitivity and specificity associated with less morbidity. Data from other groups are in perfect accordance with the results of Weckermann et al. (Bastide et al. 2009; Fukuda et al. 2007; Jeschke et al. 2008).

In an own series on 61 high-risk prostate cancer patients, a SPECT-CT-based sentinel-imaging concept was tested regarding the feasibility for individualized pelvic IMRT planning (Ganswindt et al. 2007, 2011). Although power of the analysis is somewhat limited by the fact that a histological work-up is inherently impossible, the observations regarding number, location, and anatomical distribution of sentinel lymph nodes were very similar to the available surgical sentinel data.

A key result is the fact that up to 30 % of putatively involved lymph nodes would have been missed when standardized radiation portal or standard lymphadenectomy areas would have been used (Fig. 3a, b). Thus, the following key conclusions of the sentinel node concept in prostate cancer can be drawn:

1. There is a considerable inter-individual pelvic drainage with a highly complex and variable lymph node architecture
2. Contrary to most other solid tumors in most cases more than one sentinel node is detectable
3. The sentinel node concept has a high sensitivity (up to 98 %) and specificity—the rate of false negative but histological positive sentinel nodes is in the range of 6 % (Weckermann et al. 2007; Holl et al. 2009).

- Lymph nodes next to histopathological positive sentinel nodes often show microscopic lymph node involvement without being sentinel positive
- Macroscopic lymph node involvement decreases sensitivity and specificity of the sentinel method—especially with increasing risk profile
- "Sentinel-only" imaging data correlate well with surgical data—partially with the exception of regions with close proximity to bladder and seminal vesicles (potentially due to bladder inside radio-nuclide accumulation)
- Risk of a geographic miss is predominant in the perirectal and sacral lymphatic drainage areas, followed by the regions along the external iliac chain and high iliac/paraortic nodes

5 Guidelines for Pelvic Target Volume Definition

To overcome the significant variations in the definition of pelvic lymph nodes volumes in the past leading to possible geometrical misses, the RTOG genitourinary radiation oncology group prepared a consensus paper on pelvic lymph node volumes for high-risk prostate cancer patients in 2009 (Lawton et al. 2009). It contains a concise summary of all available data on the prostate lymphatic drainage including surgical and sentinel-guided lymphadenectomy series as well as the results derived from patterns of relapse studies after the use of several radiation volume approaches (Roach et al. 2006).

Key recommendations are:

1. The inclusion of following adjuvant areas in high-risk prostate cancer patients: "distal common iliac, presacral lymph nodes (S1–S3), external iliac lymph nodes, internal iliac lymph nodes, and obturator lymph nodes."
2. The lymph node clinical target volume include the vessels (artery and vein) and a 7 mm radial margin being careful to "carve out" bowel, bladder, bone, and muscle.
3. Volumes begin at the L5/S1 interspace and end at the superior aspect of the pubic bone.
4. External iliac contours stop at top of femoral heads (boney landmark for inguinal ligament), obturator contours stop at top of symphysis pubis.

In addition to the RTOG consensus paper, the contouring guidelines are at present available online (http://www.rtog.org/CoreLab/ContouringAtlases/ProstatePelvicLymphNodes.aspx).

Irrespectively of these standardized target volume recommendation, any individual diagnostic finding (including sentinel, MRI- or PET data) on suspicious lymph nodes or anatomic abnormalities in individual patients should possibly

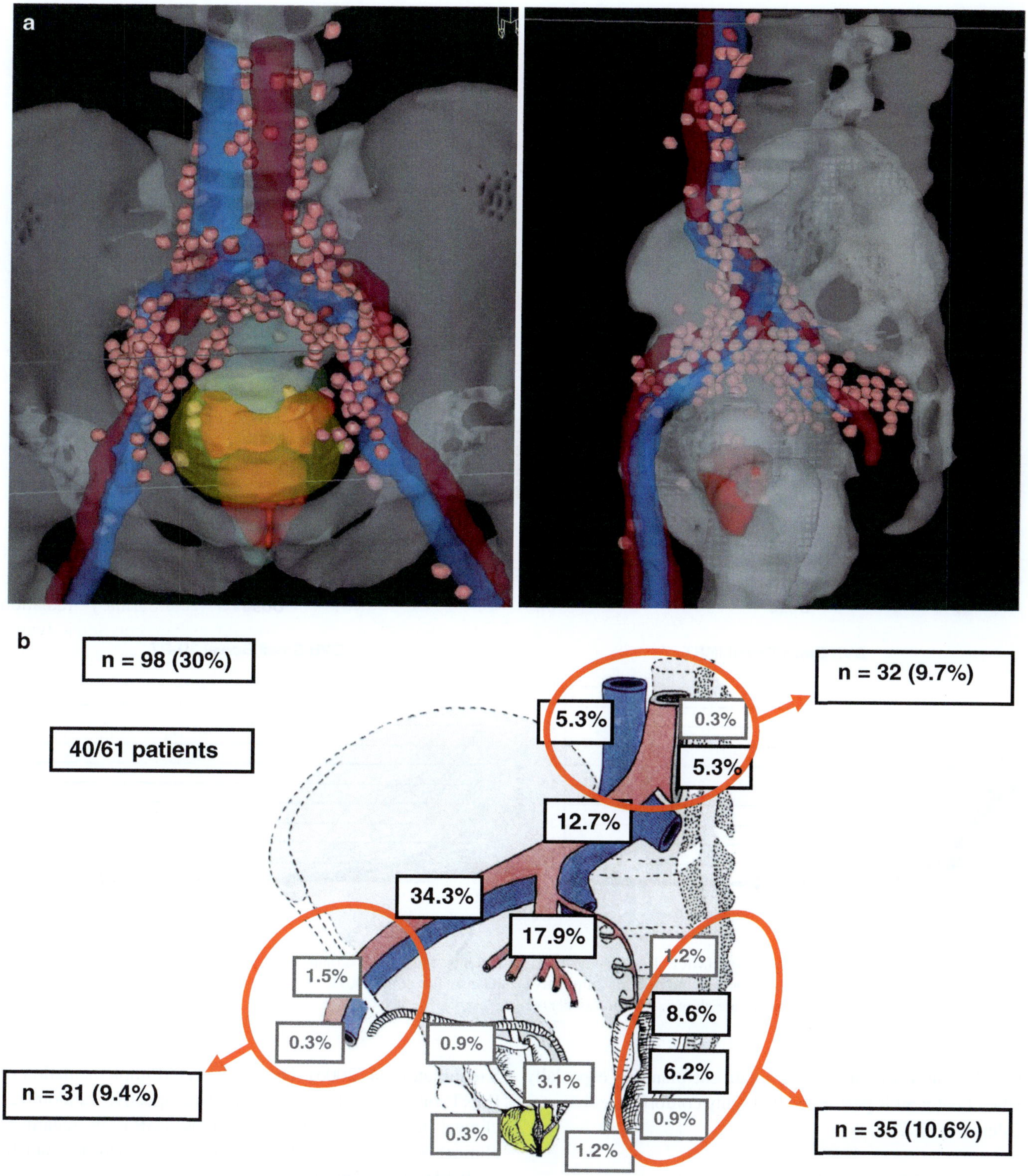

Fig. 3 **a** Cumulative sentinel lymph node distribution (virtual data set) in 61 patients (*left* view from ventral above; *right* view from the *left side*; sentinel nodes = *pink*, prostate = *red*, bladder = *green*, vessels = *blue/red*) (Ganswindt et al. 2011). **b** Areas and anatomical distributions of sentinel nodes with a potential geographic miss. A geographic miss was observed in 98/324 (30 %) sentinel lymph nodes in 40/61 patients (65.6 %) (Ganswindt et al. 2011)

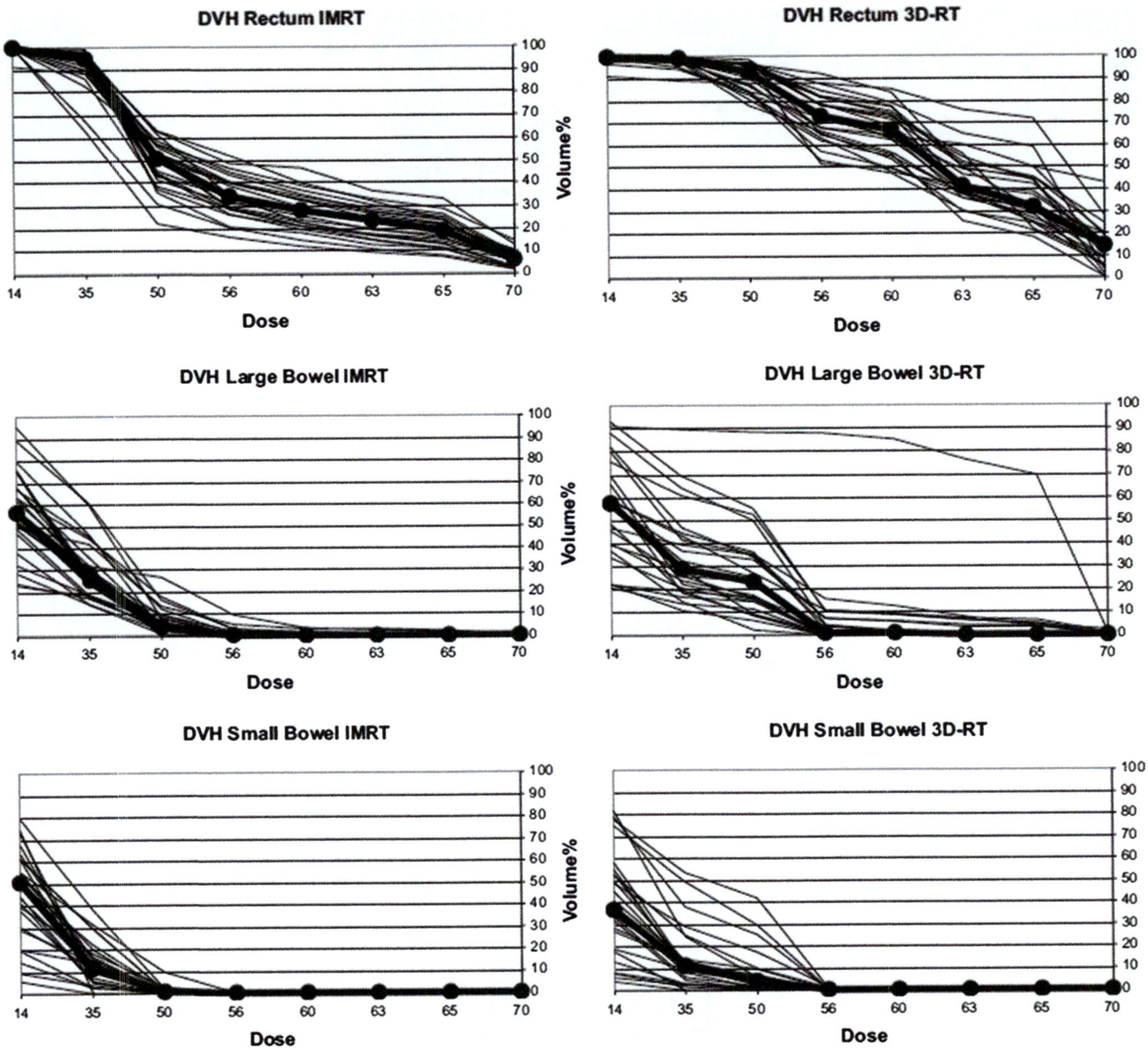

Fig. 4 3D conformal radiotherapy versus IMRT dose-volume histogram comparison of small bowel, large bowel, and rectum. Cumulative dose-volume-histograms of 25 patients are shown. *Solid lines* denote patients 1–25; *lines* connecting *dots* denote median of 25 patients. (Ganswindt et al. 2007)

be taken into account during treatment planning especially when treatment is performed by highly conformal techniques (Meijer et al. 2013).

6 Treatment Planning 3D versus IMRT

Until today, numerous planning studies comparing 3D conformal radiotherapy with IMRT for the treatment of pelvic nodes in prostate cancer patients exist (Ganswindt et al. 2005b, 2007; Nutting et al. 2000; Luxton et al. 2004; Sanguineti et al. 2006). Due to the rapid implementation of IMRT into clinical practice, valid prospective randomized clinical trials comparing 3D versus IMRT in regard to clinical outcome and toxicities are missing and will not be available in the future.

However, approximately all planning studies based on equal target volumes indicate a superiority of IMRT in terms an improved sparing of organs at risk (bladder, small bowel, rectum, bone), especially for high-radiation dose areas (Fig. 4). In selected cases, target volume coverage may be worse—depending on the individual constraints chosen.

In summary, the use of IMRT allows to apply higher doses to the prostate without increasing acute or late toxicities and in parallel allows for an highly conformal dose coverage of pelvic lymph nodes with low acute and late toxicity profiles (Ganswindt et al. 2007; Guckenberger et al. 2008; Sharma et al. 2011; Zelefsky et al. 2012; Vora et al. 2007; Al-Mamgani et al. 2009; Eade et al. 2008).

7 IMRT Planning and Treatment

Pelvic clinical target volume (CTV) delineation should be routinely performed on a CT planning data set in exact treatment position. Usually 3- or 5-mm CT slices are applied, depending on different requirements for dose calculation algorithms being used in a given institution.

In selected cases, a prone position (with belly board) allows improved sparing of small bowel especially when large parts of small bowel are located within the distal pelvic area. However, in general, a supine position results in a more stable patient position, still with adequate sparing of the small bowels. Furthermore, it allows the use of image guidance modalities including ultrasound imaging which is impossible when patients are positioned in a prone position.

Planning and treatment should be performed with nearly empty rectum and comfortably filled bladder. Bladder filling improves sparing of relevant bladder wall and bowel volumes. The irradiation with an empty rectum seems to be associated with better clinical outcomes and less rectal toxicities (Heemsbergen et al. 2007; Engels et al. 2009; Reddy et al. 2009; Jain et al. 2012).

Reasonable safety margins from CTV to PTV are in the range of 5–10 mm; however, the choice of safety margins depends substantially on individual positioning and image guidance strategy being implemented in the given institution. Besides influencing bladder and rectal filling modern image guidance tools as cone beam computed tomography, ultrasound or fiducial markers allow to correct the related position of the prostate during daily radiation treatment. In this regard, it is of special importance not only to focus on the moving prostate position, but also to sufficiently cover the rather immobile pelvic node CTV (Ferjani et al. 2013; Adamczyk et al. 2013; Xia et al. 2010).

8 Dose Prescriptions

Historically, the RTOG used 50.4 Gy to the pelvic nodes followed by a boost to the prostate to cumulative 70.2 Gy (single doses 1.8 Gy, 5/week) and EORTC trial prescribed 50 Gy (pelvic nodes) and 70 Gy (prostate), respectively, but in single doses of 2.0 Gy, 5/week.

Currently, a cumulative dose of 70 Gy to the prostate in a high-risk constellation is considered to be suboptimal (Hanks et al. 2000; Pollack et al. 2002; Peeters et al. 2006; Ganswindt et al. 2005a). Thus, when using pelvic IMRT, a cumulative dose of 74–76 Gy to the prostate region seems advisable. Several trials have shown that this is feasible without increased toxicity profiles (Guckenberger et al. 2008; Zapatero et al. 2005).

One of the key features of IMRT technique is the possibility to employ different dose levels simultaneously (simultaneous integrated boosts [SIB]) within one treated volume. Thus, a dose prescription to the pelvic nodes of 50.4 Gy (single dose 1.8 Gy per fraction) and simultaneously of 2.0 Gy single dose to the prostate is commonly used in clinical practice at present. After these first 28 fractions with SIB, irradiation is continued by a different boost treatment plan of 14 Gy (18 Gy, respectively) without any dose split.

Dose constraints to the given organs at risk (bladder, small bowel, rectum, colon, bone) should aim for a minimum dose adherent to the recent QUANTEC data (Jackson et al. 2010). Thus, each individual IMRT plan needs to be reviewed consequently in order to optimize irradiated normal tissue volumes.

In how far different IMRT techniques [static (step and shoot) techniques and dynamic techniques (sliding windows with or without simultaneous gantry rotation, tomotherapy)] may be advantageous has not been finally determined in clinical trials. Based on theoretical assumptions, fast dynamic techniques (intensity modulated arc therapy, IMAT, "Rapid Arc") may turn out to be advantageous in terms of shortened treatment time and thus reduced intrafractional organ movements. However, on the other hand, the exact dosimetry and quality assurance of highly modulated IMRT may impose new and unexpected problems.

In how far particle therapy may improve the treatment of prostate cancer pelvic nodes has not been determined at present (Sheets et al. 2012). The fact that many pelvic organs are mobile, air filled, and display extreme variations in organ filling, indicate that these targets may not be optimal targets for particle approaches.

In parallel with the implementation of standard IMRT techniques covering prostate and the adjuvant pelvic lymph nodes with normal fractionation schemata, several small series using a moderate hypo-fractionation to the prostate in combination with pelvic node irradiation were reported (Alongi et al. 2012; Norkus et al. 2013; Krause et al. 2012). Guckenberger recently reported on 41 patients treated with 32 × 2.3 Gy SIB to the prostate, according to 80 Gy 2 Gy-equivalent. The 5-year freedom from biochemical failure (FFBF) was 78 % for high-risk disease with low rates of observed toxicity by the use of IMRT and accurate image guided radiotherapy (IGRT) (Guckenberger et al. 2014).

9 IMRT Techniques in Node-positive Patients

Widespread PSA screening has certainly led to increased diagnosis of lower risk prostate cancer and recent studies found a dropping incidence of lymph node metastases (even less than 10 %) (Nguyen et al. 2009; Paul et al. 2010). However, the number of patients with nodal involvement at baseline remains high in subgroups (up to 30–40 % in high-risk patients (Crehange et al. 2012))—particularly when the extension of lymphadenectomy and pathological work-up procedures are taken into account (Briganti et al. 2008). Furthermore, as mentioned above, the real risk of lymphonodular seeding is higher than previously assumed (Weckermann et al. 2006; Heidenreich et al. 2002; Briganti et al. 2006; Shariat et al. 2003; Pagliarulo et al. 2006; Miyake et al. 2007).

At a minimum, there are three different clinical start points regarding node-positive prostate cancer patients and radiation treatment approaches:

Firstly,
: patients with prostate cancer at the time of first diagnosis and synchronously macroscopic lymph node metastasis (cN1) without any surgery.

Secondly,
: patients with newly diagnosed prostate cancer and synchronously clinical or subclinical lymphatic involvement, but after surgery/lymphadenectomy (pN1).

Thirdly,
: patients after primary treatment of prostate cancer and metachronously loco-regional relapse at a site of the pelvic lymphatic region (rN1).

Provided that lymph node involvement is considered as origin, and not merely as surrogate for distant metastatic spread, a loco-regional approach may be appropriate.

Ad 1 (cN1 patients):

Derived from some older retrospective series (Sands et al. 1995; Whittington et al. 1995; Wiegel and Bressel 1995) and a number of subset-analyses of RTOG trials (75-06 (Hanks et al. 1998), 85-31 (Lawton et al. 2005) and 92-02 (Hanks et al. 2003)) there is strong evidence that also lymph node-positive patients could achieve excellent local control rates when pelvic irradiation is combined with hormone therapy. Thereby, the RTOG 85-31 subset analysis in 173 N1 patients revealed biochemical progression-free survival rates at 5/9 years of 33 %/4 % and 54 %/10 %, respectively, in favor of the combined treatment arm. Yet while the previously used "box technique" did not allow higher radiation doses to involved lymph nodes due to bowel toxicity, the dose required to treat with a curative intent positive nodes is higher (i.e. ≥60 Gy).

In this context, new technologies such as IMRT and IGRT make it possible to escalate the dose to positive nodes beyond 50 Gy (Wang-Chesebro et al. 2006; Engels et al. 2009) and, in the meantime, this approach is recommendable in cases of clinically detectable lymph node involvement (Crehange et al. 2012). In an own series of 39 patients, we demonstrated the feasibility of a "SIB technique" in node-positive patients with moderate early and late toxicities after a median follow up of 70 months [Fig. 5 (Muller et al. 2012)].

Ad 2 (pN1 patients):

There is no randomized controlled study that tested the role of adjuvant pelvic radiotherapy in node-positive patients after radical prostatectomy and lymphadenectomy. Da Pozzo et al. (2009) and Briganti et al. (2011) performed a large retrospective matched analysis in >700 consecutive patients treated 1986–2002 with adjuvant hormone therapy compared with conventional radiotherapy combined with hormone therapy. A total of 85 % of the irradiated patients had 4-field box inclusion of the pelvic lymph node areas treated with a median dose of 50.4 Gy, while the prostate bed was treated postoperatively with a median dose of 68.4 Gy. With a mean follow-up of 100.8 months, patients in the combined treatment arm had significantly higher cancer-specific and overall survival rates compared with patient treated with hormone therapy alone at 5, 8, and 10 years after surgery (95, 91, and 86 % vs. 88, 78, and 70 %, and 90, 84, and 74 % vs. 82, 65, and 55 %, respectively; $p = 0.004$ and $p < 0.001$, respectively). A follow-up analysis of 1107 patients confirmed adjuvant radiotherapy as an independent predictor of better cancer control outcomes (10-year cancer-specific mortality-free rate 87 %) in this multimodal setting (Abdollah et al. 2014).

Ad 3 (rN1 patients):

The cases of lymph node recurrent prostate cancer provide an unfavorable situation in medical aftercare practice following primary treatment. In general, the gold standard is systemic hormone therapy (Iversen and Roder 2008). However, there are increasing data on salvage treatment strategies within the meaning of surgical or/and irradiation approaches.

Recently, a retrospective study in 59 patients with lymph node metastases detected by [11C] choline PET/CT analyzed the impact of pelvic/retroperitoneal salvage lymphadenectomy (Suardi et al. 2014). With a median follow-up of 81 months, 35 patients (59.3 %) achieved biochemical response (defined as PSA < 0.2 ng/ml 40 days after surgery). The 8-year biochemical recurrence-free survival rate was 23 %, the 8-year clinical recurrence-free and cancer-specific survival were 38 and 81 %, respectively. The only predictors for clinical recurrence were preoperative PSA level (<4 vs. ≥4 ng/ml) and the presence of retroperitoneal lymph node metastases. In addition, just under two thirds of the patients subsequently received androgen deprivation therapy.

Similarly, Jilg et al. evaluated 47 PET positive patients treated by salvage lymphadenectomy. A total of 27 patients received adjuvant radiotherapy (mean dose 50.8 Gy) limited

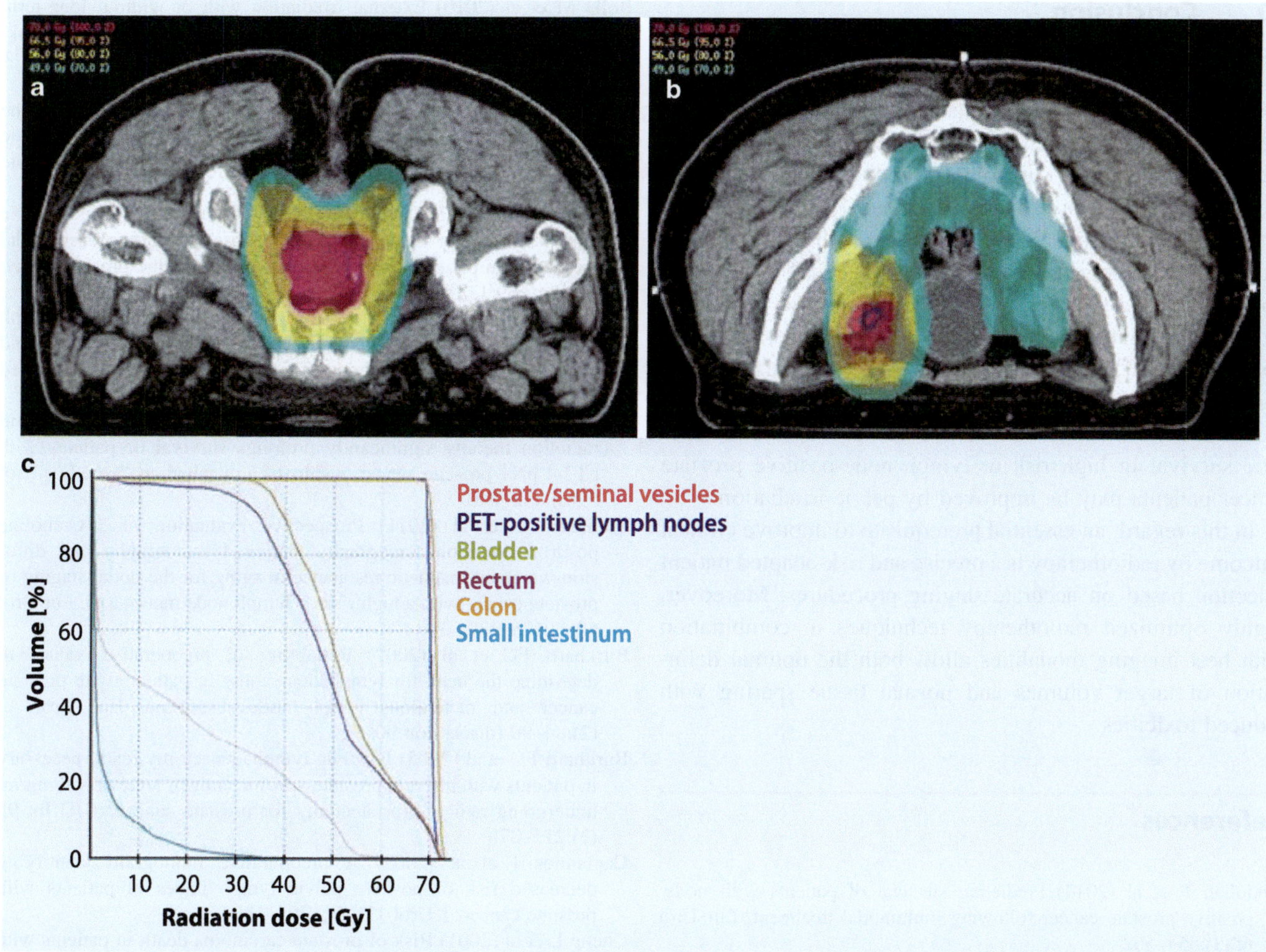

Fig. 5 Example of pelvic IMRT with nodal SIB. Treatment plans with related isodoses (70 %/80 %/95 %/100 %) are shown for primary tumor (**a**) and affected nodes (**b**). Related dose-volume-histograms of target volumes and organs at risk are demonstrated in (**c**) (Muller et al. 2012).

to the affected lymph node regions (Jilg et al. 2012). Even if adjuvant radiotherapy in this small heterogeneous cohort had no significant advantage, the 5-year cancer-specific survival of 77.7 % was comparable to the results mentioned above.

Applying these promising results to a definitive radiotherapy treatment option for (PET positive) rN1 patients, it is highly important to use higher radiation doses to macroscopically involved lymph nodes due to the given dose-effect relationship in prostate cancer. In a recent series, 83 patients were treated with a mean dose of 52 Gy to the complete lymphatic drainage and simultaneously escalated radiation doses to PET positive lymph nodes (mean SIB dose 65 Gy) (Picchio et al. 2014). With a median follow-up of 22 months in 70.2 % of the patients a complete biochemical response could be observed. In 89.4 % of the patients, a PET metabolic response was documented (43 % complete and 47 % partial response, respectively). Only 6 % of patients showed metabolic progression at the treated area, but in 57.4 % new disease at distant sites occurred. Around two third of patients received additive androgen deprivation therapy and observed toxicities were low.

However, up to now there is no clear recommendation regarding the target volume areas in rpN1 patients. Thus, bearing in mind that PET or sentinel positive imaging of lymph nodes may underestimate real microscopic involvement (often located in close proximity to the detected lymph nodes) (Allaf et al. 2004; Bader et al. 2002; Weckermann et al. 2005, 2006; Burkhard et al. 2002, 2005; Heidenreich et al. 2002; Briganti et al. 2006, 2007; Shariat et al. 2003; Pagliarulo et al. 2006; Ferrari et al. 2006; Miyake et al. 2007; Stone et al. 1997; Joslyn and Konety 2006), in the absence of reliable data an inclusion of at least adjuvant areas or even the complete lymphatic drainage may be more plausible from the present point of view.

10 Conclusion

In the past few years, the management of high risk and node-positive prostate cancer patients has evolved significantly. New imaging tools such as MR, PET, and sentinel node procedures now allow surgeons and radiation oncologists to identify and target nodal metastasis and/or lymph nodes with a high risk of subclinical involvement. In addition, improved radiation technologies such as IMRT and IGRT give radiation oncologists the ability to deliver high-dose conformal radiation to a target volume while minimizing toxicities to normal tissues. Despite the lack of large randomized trials, particularly with respect to increasingly complex treatment constellations, there is abundant evidence that cancer-specific survival in high risk or lymph node-positive prostate cancer patients may be improved by pelvic irradiation.

In this regard, an essential prerequisite to improve clinical outcome by radiotherapy is a precise and risk-adapted patient selection based on accurate staging procedures. Moreover, highly optimized radiotherapy techniques in combination with best imaging modalities allow both the optimal delineation of target volumes and normal tissue sparing with reduced toxicities.

References

Abdollah F et al (2014) Predicting survival of patients with node-positive prostate cancer following multimodal treatment. Eur Urol 65(3):554–562

Adamczyk M et al (2013) Dosimetric consequences of prostate-based couch shifts on the precision of dose delivery during simultaneous IMRT irradiation of the prostate, seminal vesicles and pelvic lymph nodes. Phys Med 30(2):228–233

Allaf ME et al (2004) Anatomical extent of lymph node dissection: impact on men with clinically localized prostate cancer. J Urol 172 (5 Pt 1):1840–1844

Al-Mamgani A et al (2009) Role of intensity-modulated radiotherapy in reducing toxicity in dose escalation for localized prostate cancer. Int J Radiat Oncol Biol Phys 73(3):685–691

Alongi F et al (2012) Moderate hypofractionation and simultaneous integrated boost with volumetric modulated arc therapy (RapidArc) for prostate cancer. Report of feasibility and acute toxicity. Strahlenther Onkol 188(11):990–996

Bader P et al (2002) Is a limited lymph node dissection an adequate staging procedure for prostate cancer? J Urol 168(2):514–518 (discussion 518)

Bader P et al (2003) Disease progression and survival of patients with positive lymph nodes after radical prostatectomy. Is there a chance of cure? J Urol 169(3):849–854

Bastide C et al (2009) Radioisotope guided sentinel lymph node dissection in patients with localized prostate cancer: results of the first 100 cases. Eur J Surg Oncol 35(7):751–756

Bolla M et al (2002) Long-term results with immediate androgen suppression and external irradiation in patients with locally advanced prostate cancer (an EORTC study): a phase III randomised trial. Lancet 360(9327):103–106

Bolla M et al (2010) External irradiation with or without long-term androgen suppression for prostate cancer with high metastatic risk: 10-year results of an EORTC randomised study. Lancet Oncol 11 (11):1066–1073

Briganti A et al (2006) Validation of a nomogram predicting the probability of lymph node invasion based on the extent of pelvic lymphadenectomy in patients with clinically localized prostate cancer. BJU Int 98(4):788–793

Briganti A et al (2007) Critical assessment of ideal nodal yield at pelvic lymphadenectomy to accurately diagnose prostate cancer nodal metastasis in patients undergoing radical retropubic prostatectomy. Urology 69(1):147–151

Briganti A et al (2008) Impact of surgical volume on the rate of lymph node metastases in patients undergoing radical prostatectomy and extended pelvic lymph node dissection for clinically localized prostate cancer. Eur Urol 54(4):794–802

Briganti A et al (2011) Combination of adjuvant hormonal and radiation therapy significantly prolongs survival of patients with pT2-4 pN+ prostate cancer: results of a matched analysis. Eur Urol 59(5):832–840

Budiharto T et al (2011) Prospective evaluation of 11C-choline positron emission tomography/computed tomography and diffusion-weighted magnetic resonance imaging for the nodal staging of prostate cancer with a high risk of lymph node metastases. Eur Urol 60(1):125–130

Burkhard FC et al (2002) Reliability of preoperative values to determine the need for lymphadenectomy in patients with prostate cancer and meticulous lymph node dissection. Eur Urol 42 (2):84–90 (discussion 90–92)

Burkhard FC et al (2005) Is pelvic lymphadenectomy really necessary in patients with a serum prostate-specific antigen level of <10 ng/ml undergoing radical prostatectomy for prostate cancer? BJU Int 95 (3):275–278

Cagiannos I et al (2003) A preoperative nomogram identifying decreased risk of positive pelvic lymph nodes in patients with prostate cancer. J Urol 170(5):1798–1803

Cheng L et al (2001) Risk of prostate carcinoma death in patients with lymph node metastasis. Cancer 91(1):66–73

Crehange G et al (2012) Management of prostate cancer patients with lymph node involvement: a rapidly evolving paradigm. Cancer Treat Rev 38(8):956–967

Da Pozzo LF et al (2009) Long-term follow-up of patients with prostate cancer and nodal metastases treated by pelvic lymphadenectomy and radical prostatectomy: the positive impact of adjuvant radiotherapy. Eur Urol 55(5):1003–1011

Eade TN et al (2008) A comparison of acute and chronic toxicity for men with low-risk prostate cancer treated with intensity-modulated radiation therapy or (125)I permanent implant. Int J Radiat Oncol Biol Phys 71(2):338–345

Engels B et al (2009a) Conformal arc radiotherapy for prostate cancer: increased biochemical failure in patients with distended rectum on the planning computed tomogram despite image guidance by implanted markers. Int J Radiat Oncol Biol Phys 74(2):388–391

Engels B et al (2009b) Helical tomotherapy with simultaneous integrated boost for high-risk and lymph node-positive prostate cancer: early report on acute and late toxicity. Technol Cancer Res Treat 8(5):353–359

Ferjani S et al (2013) Alignment focus of daily image guidance for concurrent treatment of prostate and pelvic lymph nodes. Int J Radiat Oncol Biol Phys 87(2):383–389

Ferrari AC et al (2006) Molecular load of pathologically occult metastases in pelvic lymph nodes is an independent prognostic marker of biochemical failure after localized prostate cancer treatment. J Clin Oncol 24(19):3081–3088

Fukuda M et al (2007) Detection of sentinel node micrometastasis by step section and immunohistochemistry in patients with prostate cancer. J Urol 177(4):1313–1317 (discussion 1317)

Ganswindt U et al (2005a) 70 Gy or more: which dose for which prostate cancer? J Cancer Res Clin Oncol 131(7):407–419

Ganswindt U et al (2005b) Intensity modulated radiotherapy for high risk prostate cancer based on sentinel node SPECT imaging for target volume definition. BMC Cancer 5:91

Ganswindt U et al (2007) Optimized coverage of high-risk adjuvant lymph node areas in prostate cancer using a sentinel node-based, intensity-modulated radiation therapy technique. Int J Radiat Oncol Biol Phys 67(2):347–355

Ganswindt U et al (2011) Distribution of prostate sentinel nodes: a SPECT-derived anatomic atlas. Int J Radiat Oncol Biol Phys 79 (5):1364–1372

Guckenberger M et al (2008) Does intensity modulated radiation therapy (IMRT) prevent additional toxicity of treating the pelvic lymph nodes compared to treatment of the prostate only? Radiat Oncol 3:3

Guckenberger M, Lawrenz I, Flentje M (2014) Moderately hypofractionated radiotherapy for localized prostate cancer : Long-term outcome using IMRT and volumetric IGRT. Strahlenther Onkol 190 (1):48–53

Hanks GE et al (1998) Ten-year outcomes for pathologic node-positive patients treated in RTOG 75-06. Int J Radiat Oncol Biol Phys 40 (4):765–768

Hanks GE et al (2000) Dose selection for prostate cancer patients based on dose comparison and dose response studies. Int J Radiat Oncol Biol Phys 46(4):823–832

Hanks GE et al (2003) Phase III trial of long-term adjuvant androgen deprivation after neoadjuvant hormonal cytoreduction and radiotherapy in locally advanced carcinoma of the prostate: the radiation therapy oncology group protocol 92-02. J Clin Oncol 21(21):3972–3978

Heemsbergen WD et al (2007) Increased risk of biochemical and clinical failure for prostate patients with a large rectum at radiotherapy planning: results from the Dutch trial of 68 GY versus 78 Gy. Int J Radiat Oncol Biol Phys 67(5):1418–1424

Heidenreich A, Varga Z, Von Knobloch R (2002) Extended pelvic lymphadenectomy in patients undergoing radical prostatectomy: high incidence of lymph node metastasis. J Urol 167(4):1681–1686

Holl G et al (2009) Validation of sentinel lymph node dissection in prostate cancer: experience in more than 2,000 patients. Eur J Nucl Med Mol Imaging 36(9):1377–1382

Hull GW et al (2002) Cancer control with radical prostatectomy alone in 1,000 consecutive patients. J Urol 167(2 Pt 1):528–534

Iversen P, Roder MA (2008) The early prostate cancer program: bicalutamide in nonmetastatic prostate cancer. Expert Rev Anticancer Ther 8(3):361–369

Jackson A et al (2010) The lessons of QUANTEC: recommendations for reporting and gathering data on dose-volume dependencies of treatment outcome. Int J Radiat Oncol Biol Phys 76(3 Suppl): S155–S160

Jain S et al (2012) The effect of radiation technique and bladder filling on the acute toxicity of pelvic radiotherapy for localized high risk prostate cancer. Radiother Oncol 105(2):193–197

Jeschke S et al (2008) Laparoscopic radioisotope-guided sentinel lymph node dissection in staging of prostate cancer. Eur Urol 53(1):126–132

Jilg CA et al (2012) Salvage lymph node dissection with adjuvant radiotherapy for nodal recurrence of prostate cancer. J Urol 188 (6):2190–2197

Joslyn SA, Konety BR (2006) Impact of extent of lymphadenectomy on survival after radical prostatectomy for prostate cancer. Urology 68 (1):121–125

Krause S et al (2012) Hypofractionated helical intensity-modulated radiotherapy of the prostate bed after prostatectomy with or without the pelvic lymph nodes—the PRIAMOS trial. BMC Cancer 12:504

Lawton CA et al (2005) Androgen suppression plus radiation versus radiation alone for patients with stage D1/pathologic node-positive adenocarcinoma of the prostate: updated results based on national prospective randomized trial Radiation Therapy Oncology Group 85-31. J Clin Oncol 23(4):800–807

Lawton CA et al (2007) An update of the phase III trial comparing whole pelvic to prostate only radiotherapy and neoadjuvant to adjuvant total androgen suppression: updated analysis of RTOG 94-13, with emphasis on unexpected hormone/radiation interactions. Int J Radiat Oncol Biol Phys 69(3):646–655

Lawton CA et al (2009) RTOG GU Radiation oncology specialists reach consensus on pelvic lymph node volumes for high-risk prostate cancer. Int J Radiat Oncol Biol Phys 74(2):383–387

Luxton G, Hancock SL, Boyer AL (2004) Dosimetry and radiobiologic model comparison of IMRT and 3D conformal radiotherapy in treatment of carcinoma of the prostate. Int J Radiat Oncol Biol Phys 59(1):267–284

Meijer HJ et al (2013) Geographical distribution of lymph node metastases on MR lymphography in prostate cancer patients. Radiother Oncol 106(1):59–63

Miyake H et al (2007) Quantitative detection of micrometastases in pelvic lymph nodes in patients with clinically localized prostate cancer by real-time reverse transcriptase-PCR. Clin Cancer Res 13 (4):1192–1197

Muller AC et al (2012) Toxicity and outcome of pelvic IMRT for node-positive prostate cancer. Strahlenther Onkol 188(11):982–989

Nguyen PL et al (2009) Predicting the risk of pelvic node involvement among men with prostate cancer in the contemporary era. Int J Radiat Oncol Biol Phys 74(1):104–109

Norkus D et al (2013) A randomized hypofractionation dose escalation trial for high risk prostate cancer patients: interim analysis of acute toxicity and quality of life in 124 patients. Radiat Oncol 8(1):206

Nutting CM et al (2000) Reduction of small and large bowel irradiation using an optimized intensity-modulated pelvic radiotherapy technique in patients with prostate cancer. Int J Radiat Oncol Biol Phys 48(3):649–656

Pagliarulo V et al (2006) Detection of occult lymph node metastases in locally advanced node-negative prostate cancer. J Clin Oncol 24 (18):2735–2742

Partin AW et al (1997) Combination of prostate-specific antigen, clinical stage, and Gleason score to predict pathological stage of localized prostate cancer. A multi-institutional update. Jama 277 (18):1445–1451

Passoni NM et al (2014) Utility of [(11)C]choline PET/CT in guiding lesion-targeted salvage therapies in patients with prostate cancer recurrence localized to a single lymph node at imaging: Results from a pathologically validated series. Urol Oncol 32(1):38e9–38e16

Paul A et al (2010) Oncologic outcome after extraperitoneal laparoscopic radical prostatectomy: midterm follow-up of 1115 procedures. Eur Urol 57(2):267–272

Peeters ST et al (2006) Dose-response in radiotherapy for localized prostate cancer: results of the Dutch multicenter randomized phase III trial comparing 68 Gy of radiotherapy with 78 Gy. J Clin Oncol 24(13):1990–1996

Picchio M et al (2014) ^{11}C-Choline PET/CT as a guide to radiation treatment planning of lymph-node relapses in prostate cancer patients. Eur J Nucl Med Mol Imaging 41(7):1270–1279

Pollack A et al (2002) Prostate cancer radiation dose response: results of the M. D. Anderson phase III randomized trial. Int J Radiat Oncol Biol Phys 53(5):1097–1105

Pommier P et al (2007) Is there a role for pelvic irradiation in localized prostate adenocarcinoma? Preliminary results of GETUG-01. J Clin Oncol 25(34):5366–5373

Reddy NM et al (2009) Influence of volumes of prostate, rectum, and bladder on treatment planning CT on interfraction prostate shifts during ultrasound image-guided IMRT. Med Phys 36(12):5604–5611

Rinnab L et al (2008) [11C]choline PET/CT for targeted salvage lymph node dissection in patients with biochemical recurrence after primary curative therapy for prostate cancer. Preliminary results of a prospective study. Urol Int 81(2):191–197

Roach M 3rd (2009) Targeted radiotherapy against clinically localized prostate cancer: is pelvic radiotherapy the standard of care for high risk prostate cancer? In: 3rd international symposium on cancer metastasis and the lymphovascular system: basis for rational therapy, San Francisco, Abstract book, pp 56–57

Roach M 3rd et al (2003) Phase III trial comparing whole-pelvic versus prostate-only radiotherapy and neoadjuvant versus adjuvant combined androgen suppression: radiation therapy oncology group 9413. J Clin Oncol 21(10):1904–1911

Roach M 3rd et al (2006) Whole-pelvis, "mini-pelvis," or prostate-only external beam radiotherapy after neoadjuvant and concurrent hormonal therapy in patients treated in the Radiation Therapy Oncology Group 9413 trial. Int J Radiat Oncol Biol Phys 66 (3):647–653

Sands ME, Pollack A, Zagars GK (1995) Influence of radiotherapy on node-positive prostate cancer treated with androgen ablation. Int J Radiat Oncol Biol Phys 31(1):13–19

Sanguineti G et al (2006) Is IMRT needed to spare the rectum when pelvic lymph nodes are part of the initial treatment volume for prostate cancer? Int J Radiat Oncol Biol Phys 64(1):151–160

Shariat SF et al (2003) Detection of clinically significant, occult prostate cancer metastases in lymph nodes using a splice variant-specific rt-PCR assay for human glandular kallikrein. J Clin Oncol 21(7):1223–1231

Sharma NK et al (2011) Intensity-modulated radiotherapy reduces gastrointestinal toxicity in patients treated with androgen deprivation therapy for prostate cancer. Int J Radiat Oncol Biol Phys 80 (2):437–444

Sheets NC et al (2012) Intensity-modulated radiation therapy, proton therapy, or conformal radiation therapy and morbidity and disease control in localized prostate cancer. JAMA 307(15):1611–1620

Stone NN, Stock RG, Unger P (1997) Laparoscopic pelvic lymph node dissection for prostate cancer: comparison of the extended and modified techniques. J Urol 158(5):1891–1894

Suardi N et al (2014) Long-term outcomes of salvage lymph node dissection for clinically recurrent prostate cancer: results of a single-institution series with a minimum follow-up of 5 years. Eur Urol. pii:S0302-2838(14)00130-4

Vora SA et al (2007) Analysis of biochemical control and prognostic factors in patients treated with either low-dose three-dimensional conformal radiation therapy or high-dose intensity-modulated radiotherapy for localized prostate cancer. Int J Radiat Oncol Biol Phys 68(4):1053–1058

Wang-Chesebro A et al (2006) Intensity-modulated radiotherapy improves lymph node coverage and dose to critical structures compared with three-dimensional conformal radiation therapy in clinically localized prostate cancer. Int J Radiat Oncol Biol Phys 66 (3):654–662

Wawroschek F et al (2003) The influence of serial sections, immunohistochemistry, and extension of pelvic lymph node dissection on the lymph node status in clinically localized prostate cancer. Eur Urol 43(2):132–136 (discussion 137)

Weckermann D, Wawroschek F, Harzmann R (2005) Is there a need for pelvic lymph node dissection in low risk prostate cancer patients prior to definitive local therapy? Eur Urol 47(1):45–50 (discussion 50–51)

Weckermann D et al (2006) Incidence of positive pelvic lymph nodes in patients with prostate cancer, a prostate-specific antigen (PSA) level of < or =10 ng/mL and biopsy Gleason score of < or =6, and their influence on PSA progression-free survival after radical prostatectomy. BJU Int 97(6):1173–1178

Weckermann D et al (2007) Sentinel lymph node dissection for prostate cancer: experience with more than 1,000 patients. J Urol 177 (3):916–920

Whittington R et al (1995) Combined hormonal and radiation therapy for lymph node-positive prostate cancer. Urology 46(2):213–219

Wiegel T, Bressel M (1995) Stage D1 prostate cancer–is radiotherapy and early hormonal therapy equivalent to radical prostatectomy, radiotherapy, and early hormonal therapy? (regarding Sands et al (1995) IJROBP 31:13–19). Int J Radiat Oncol Biol Phys 32 (3):896–897

Wurschmidt F et al (2011) [18F]fluoroethylcholine-PET/CT imaging for radiation treatment planning of recurrent and primary prostate cancer with dose escalation to PET/CT-positive lymph nodes. Radiat Oncol 6:44

Xia P et al (2010) Comparison of three strategies in management of independent movement of the prostate and pelvic lymph nodes. Med Phys 37(9):5006–5013

Zapatero A et al (2005) Risk-adapted androgen deprivation and escalated three-dimensional conformal radiotherapy for prostate cancer: does radiation dose influence outcome of patients treated with adjuvant androgen deprivation? A GICOR study. J Clin Oncol 23(27):6561–6568

Zelefsky MJ et al (2012) Improved clinical outcomes with high-dose image guided radiotherapy compared with non-IGRT for the treatment of clinically localized prostate cancer. Int J Radiat Oncol Biol Phys 84(1):125–129

Prophylactic Treatment of the Pelvic Lymphatics in Patients with High-Risk Prostate Cancer: Pro Radiation

Mack Roach III

Contents

Abstract

The role of prophylactic whole pelvic irradiation in men with clinically localized intermediate to high prostate cancer continues to be one of the most hotly debated topics among Radiation Oncologist. This review focuses on the "Pro" side of the argument providing data from prospective randomized trials, retrospective studies, and studies based on patients receiving adjuvant or salvage external beam radiation following a radical prostatectomy. The preponderance of data appears to support pelvic nodal irradiation in appropriately selected patients, however the author acknowledges the need for Phase III Trials to confirm the benefits of this approach.

1 Introduction

Gleason Score (GS), T-Stage, percent positive biopsies, and the level of the prostate specific antigen (PSA) when combined are can be used to predict the probability of lymph node involvement (LNI), which strongly correlates with the risk of death from prostate cancer (Roach et al. 2006c; Eggener et al. 2011). For patients with locally advanced disease the use external beam radiotherapy (EBRT) combined with hormone therapy (HT) is now well established as the standard of care (Roach et al. 2000; Roach 2010). Although, the addition of HT to RT has consistently demonstrated improvements in survival compared to EBRT alone, to-date dose escalated EBRT has not been shown to prolong survival (Roach 2007). This observation implies that control of local disease alone may be inadequate for the cure of patients with the high-risk disease, invoking the notion that regional and/or systemic disease need to addressed as well. Similarly, systemic treatment with HT alone has been shown to be inferior to HT plus EBRT, providing support for the notion that effective local/regional therapy are also critical for cure of

M. Roach III (✉)
Chair Department of Radiation Oncology,
Helen Diller Family Comprehensive Cancer Center,
University of California San Francisco (UCSF),
San Francisco, CA, USA
e-mail: roach@radonc.ucsf.edu

H. Geinitz et al. (eds.), *Radiotherapy in Prostate Cancer*, Medical Radiology. Radiation Oncology,
DOI: 10.1007/174_2013_906,
Published Online: 7 September 2013

high risk patients. Thus, neither local, nor systemic therapy, is enough. Perhaps regional therapy is required as well?

In theory, the effectiveness of high-dose EBRT directed only at the prostate is likely to be limited by the presence of disease outside of the field irradiated, including the pelvic lymph nodes. Whole pelvic radiotherapy (WPRT) could potentially improve the outcomes in patients with pelvic LNI by sterilizing microscopic disease. Although, prophylactic irradiation of lymph nodes is recommended in head and neck, breast, and many others solid tumors, doubts remain about the merits of this approach in prostate cancer patients (Roach 2008).

There is a growing body of literature addressing the role of WPRT versus prostate only radiation therapy (PORT) with supporting the former compared to the latter (Morikawa and Roach 2011). Most of these data come from retrospective studies, and most studies assess the benefits of WPRT based on biochemical outcomes using serum PSA. In this review, I discuss the rationale for treatment of regional disease with WPRT combined with HT in patients with clinically localized prostate who have significant risk of LNI.

2 Pelvic Nodal Metastasis: Who, how often and where?

Partin and associates were among the first to incorporate pretreatment parameters to allow estimates to be made as to the risk of LNI (Partin et al. 1993). Based on this data Roach developed an equation (percent probability of LNI $= 2/3$ PSA $+ [(GS - 6) \times 10]$ (Roach 1993). This equation was subsequently validated and although the accuracy of Partin's Nomogram and the "Roach Equation" has have recently been questioned the preponderance of evidence supports their utility (Roach et al. 1994; Spevack et al. 1996; Roach 2009a, b; Nguyen et al. 2009). The data used to derive the so-called Partin's Tables and the data used to criticism the Tables and the "Roach Equation", were almost entirely derived based on patients undergoing a so-called "standard lymph node dissection" (SLD). Other investigators who have performed extended lymph node dissections (ELD) have reported that ~40 % of involved nodes would have been missed by SLD (Heidenreich et al. 2002, 2007). They concluded that the ELD was associated with high rate of node metastasis outside of SLD field, and recommended ELD in all patients with PSA >10 ng/ml and a biopsy GS ≥7. Briganti et al. have demonstrated that >10 pelvic nodes should be sampled to give a reasonable chance of detecting involved nodes but most of series alluded to above on average include patients with far fewer nodes (Briganti et al. 2007).

Perhaps the most compelling support for the so-called "Roach Equation" comes from an even more recent validation study performed using a cohort of patients undergoing an ELD (Abdollah et al. 2012). These investigators concluded, "The Roach formula is still accurate and does not overestimate the rate of LNI in contemporary prostate cancer patients …". Also of note, given the fact that 40–50 % of metastatic pelvic lymph nodes lay out side of the SLD areas, an additional 5–10 % outside of the typical ELD areas and a false negative rate up to 30 % of pathologic involved nodes, it is plausible that the true estimate of LNI is higher than estimated based on any available nomogram or equation (Pagliarulo et al. 2006; Shariat et al. 2003; Ferrari et al. 2006; Miyake et al. 2007a, b).

3 Pelvic Lymph Node Irradiation: What is the Evidence for Prostate Cancer?

The evidence concerning the potential value of WPRT in conjunction with EBRT can be divided into three general categories: (1) randomized trials; (2) retrospective studies involving definitive radiotherapy and; and (3) retrospective studies involving adjuvant and salvage EBRT post-radical prostatectomy (RP). Data for these categories are summarized in Tables 1, 2 and 3 below. As shown, most studies suggest that the use of WPRT is associated with better outcomes. In general, most of the studies failing to reach this conclusion used a field size that was less than inclusive of the whole pelvis. Several studies suggest that small pelvic fields are unlikely to encompass the majority of the lymph nodes at risk in high-risk patients (Morikawa and Roach 2011).

3.1 Randomized Trials Evaluating Prophylactic Radiotherapy

Table 1 summarizes the major phase III randomized trials addressing WPRT either completed or in progress. Radiation Therapy Oncology Group (RTOG) 7706 was the first prospective trial comparing prostatic versus pelvic irradiation and it failed to demonstrate a benefit to WPRT (Asbell et al. 1988; Hanks et al. 1994). However, this study was conducted in the pre-PSA era was relatively small and was largely composed of patients with low risk disease. Low risk patients (some of whom were surgically staged and proven to be node negative), are the patients least likely to benefit from WPRT, thus this study does not address the role of WPRT in higher risk patients.

GETUG-01 was a small-randomized trial conducted in France (n = 444) including patients clinically staged as T1b-T3, N0 and randomized to WPRT or PORT. The

Table 1 Phase III randomized trials evaluating WPRT versus PORT

First author	Study design	Key findings
Asbell et al. (1988) and Hanks et al. (1991)	Eligible patients (pts) had A2 (occult disease >3 + chips & poorly differentiated) and Stage B without clinical (imaging) or biopsy + LNI, randomized to PORT or WPRT to 45 Gy then a boost to 65 Gy	At a median fu has been 7 yrs, (n = 445), no benefit with WPRT. Path node (-) had a better outcome
Roach et al. (2003, 2006a)	Phase Randomized Trial III testing whether WPRT improves progression-free survival (PFS), with either neoadjuvant (NHT) or adjuvant (AHT) HT	WPRT improves PFS. Larger fields associated with better outcome with NHT
Pommier et al. (2007)	444 pts with T1b-T3N0M0 randomized to 66-70 Gy to prostate ± 46 Gy (top border S1/S2). 4–8 mo NHT allowed for "high-risk" pts. ~55 % of pts had LN risk <15 % (Roach equation)	WPRT did not improve OS or PFS but *none* of the pts received WPRT defined as superior border at L5 S1
Pollack RTOG 0534	Salvage RT & High-risk PORT versus WPRT	Ongoing
Roach RTOG 0924	Trial target 2580 int. & High-risk PORT versus WPRT	Ongoing

Modified from Morikawa and Roach (2011). *HT* hormonal therapy; *int* intermediate; *fu* follow up; *LNI* lymph node involvement; *path* pathological; *WPRT* whole pelvic radiotherapy; *PORT* prostate only radiotherapy; *PFS* progression-free survival; *OS* overall survival

authors concluded that 5-year PFS and overall survival were similar in the two arms with 42 months follow up (Pommier et al. 2007). However, patients in the WPRT arm had the superior limit of the pelvic fields placed at the level of S1/S2, and 55 % of patients in this study had pelvic lymph node risk for metastasis <15 % (Roach equation). In addition, not all patients received HT (critical to the findings of RTOG 9413, discussed below). Furthermore, the ASTRO definition was used to assess biochemical failure, which lacks sensitivity and specificity for clinical failure and death in patients treated with HT compared with Phoenix definition (Roach et al. 2006b). Therefore, the results of GETUG-01 should not be considered definitive proof against WPRT due to the small size of the study, small field sizes used for pelvic EBRT and patient selection.

The RTOG conducted the largest phase III Trial testing the value of WPRT completed to date (Roach et al. 2003). RTOG 9413 included a total of 1,323 patients with intermediate to high-risk PC with risk of LN involvement ≥15 % (Roach's equation). This study compared WPRT versus PORT as well as adjuvant HT (AHT) versus neoadjuvant plus concurrent HT (NHT) with progression-free survival (PFS) as the primary end point. This study demonstrated that there was an improvement in PFS with NHT + WPRT.

The importance of field size on outcome was highlighted in a post hoc analysis looking at field size among patients treated on the NHT arms (chosen to avoid the timing bias favor AHT). In this analysis we compared Arm 1 (NHT + WPRT) (defined as having a superior border placed at the L5 S1 junction, being ~17 cm in length) versus Arm 2 divided into two subgroups based on the median field size used among patients randomized to this arm. The larger of the PORT subgroups was called "mini-pelvis" (MP) and was corresponded approximately to the bottom of the sacroiliac joints (maximum field size ≤11 × 11 cm but >10 × 11 cm) and compared to the subgroup treated with the smaller field, called "prostate only" with a maximum field size being <10 × 11. This analysis showed that the 7-year DFS was 40, 35, and 27 % for patients treated to WPRT, MP and "prostate only", respectively ($p = 0.02$) (Roach et al. 2006a). Thus, there appears to be a clear relationship between PFS and field size in patients with intermediate to high-risk disease. On this basis RTOG 0924 was designed to use even larger fields than 9413. An intermediate update of RTOG 9413 continued to show an improvement in PSA control with NHT + WPRT compared to NHT + PORT but perhaps due to the timing bias (favoring the adjuvant arms), and death from other causes (included in the PFS definition), PFS survival differences were reduced (Lawton et al. 2007).

3.2 Retrospective Studies of Definitive Prophylactic WPRT

Most retrospective studies support the role of WPRT as shown in Table 2. Investigators from UCSF reported better PSA control rates when WPRT was administered with NHT particularly when patients had the risk of LNI between 15 and 35 % (Seaward et al. 1998a, b). Investigators from University of Michigan divided their patients into 3 categories of LNI : low, 0–5 %; intermediate, >5–15 %; and high, >15 % (Partin) and in the multivariate analysis concluded that there was a statistically significant benefit with WPRT (Pan et al. 2002). In a retrospective study from Yale,

Table 2 Definitive retrospective series evaluating WPRT versus PORT

First author	Study design	Key findings
Seaward et al. (1998b)	Retrospective analysis of patients undergoing prostate only or WPRT with and without HT	WPRT improves PFS
Pan et al. (2002)	Retrospective analysis 3D-CRT (n = 1832), 3 categories of LNI: low, 0–5 %; int., >5–15 %; and high, >15 % (Partin Tables)	Benefit for int-risk pts with WPRT 2-year PSA control, 90 % versus 81 % (p = 0.02)
Jacob et al. (2005)	Retrospective, pts with risk +LN >15 % pelvic RT versus, partial pelvic, or prostate only (n = 420). Concluded RT dose the major determinant of PSA control	No benefit to WPRT. Criticism none of the pts received WPRT as defined by RTOG 9413
Aizer et al. (2009)	Retrospective, 277 pts with ≥15 % risk of LNI treated with prostate only (75.5 %) or WPRT (24.5 %)	WPRT improved 4 yr control (69.4 % versus 86.3 %)
Milecki et al. (2009)	Retrospective analysis including men with High-Risk Disease (n = 162) with and without WPRT	5-yr CSS were 90 % versus 79 % (p = 0.01) & PSA control 52 % versus 40 % (p = 0.07)

Modified from Morikawa and Roach (Morikawa and Roach 2011). *HT* hormonal therapy; *LNI* lymph node involvement; *WPRT* whole pelvic radiotherapy; *PORT* prostate only radiotherapy; *WPRT* whole pelvic radiotherapy; *PORT* prostate only radiotherapy; *PFS* progression-free survival; *CSS* Cause specific survival

Table 3 Post Op and/or pathologic node positive series evaluating WPRT versus PORT

First author	Study design	Key findings
Spiotto et al. (2007)	160 patients underwent adjuvant or salvage RT after RP. WPRT resulted in PSA control in high-risk patients at 5-years 47 % versus. 21 % (p = 0.008)	Better PSA control for high-risk pts receiving WPRT after RP
Da Pozzo et al. (2009) and Briganti et al. (2011)	Retrospective, 250 pts with LNI. 129 pts (51.6 %) with WPRT & HT & 121 pts (48.4 %) HT alone	RT improved PSA control & CSS (p = 0.002 & 0.009)
	Matched comparison 117 pts AHT + RT with 247 pts with RT alone	RT improved CSS & OS (p = 0.004 & < 0.0012)
Moghanaki et al. (2013)	Study compared outcomes for pts who received SRT with WPRT (n = 112) versus (PORT) (n = 135). 247 pts were analyzed with a median fu of 4 yrs	Pts with PSA ≥ 0.4 ng/mL, WPRT improve PSA control (P = 0.03)
Johnstone et al. (2007)	Surveillance Epidemiology End Results (SEER) registry used to evaluate the efficacy of post-op RT in 1921 node + pts who underwent RP alone, or RP & RT	No significant survival benefit for +LN pts receiving post-op RT
Tward (2013)	Retrospective analysis using SEER data including men with High-Risk Disease (cT1-T4, cN1) with and without WPRT	5-yr CSS: 90 versus 79 % (p = 0.01) & PSA control 52 versus 40 % (p = 0.07), respectively

Modified from Morikawa and Roach (Morikawa and Roach 2011). *HT* hormonal therapy; *AHT* adjuvant hormonal therapy; *RP* radical prostatectomy; *LNI* lymph node involvement; *SRT* Salvage Radiotherapy; *WPRT* whole pelvic radiotherapy; *PORT* prostate only radiotherapy; *CSS* Cause specific survival; *OS* overall survival

Aizer et al. reported on 277 patients with at least a 15 % likelihood of LNI, that the 4-year PSA control rate was 69.4 % in the PORT and 86.3 % in the WPRT group (Aizer et al. 2009). In contrast, investigators from Fox Chase concluded there was no benefit to the addition of WPRT in patients with a risk of LNI >15 % (Roach Equation) (Jacob et al. 2005). However, none of the patients included in their study were treated with WPRT as defined on RTOG 9413, most were treated with a MP field, and very few received NHT and most were much more favorable than those treated on RTOG 9413. Milecki et al. retrospectively studied 162 high-risk patients and concluded that WPRT combined with NHT improved cause specific survival (CSS) and PSA control compared to PORT and HT.

3.3 Prophylactic WPRT Post Prostatectomy and/or Nodal Sampling

Table 3 summarizes the outcomes of patients undergoing post-operative radiotherapy. The patients included in these series included those at high risk for LNI as well as those known to have positive nodes pathologically as well as those at risk for additional nodal involvement but without gross nodal involvement by imaging. Spiotto et al. compared PSA control among patients receiving WPRT to prostate bed RT (PBRT) after RP (Spiotto et al. 2007). PSA control was improved with WPRT compared to PBRT in patients with a risk of LNI >15 %. Moghanaki et al. reported similar findings among patients treated with salvage radiotherapy (SRT) (Moghanaki et al. 2013). This inter-institutional retrospective study compared outcomes for patients who received SRT at 2 separate academic institutions with one favoring WPRT and the other favoring PBRT. They concluded that "WPRT was not independently associated with biochemical PFS in the multivariate model (adjusted HR, 0.79; P = 0.20)". However, they also concluded that "... restricting the analysis to patients with pre-SRT PSA levels >/=0.4 ng/mL ... WPRT was independently associated with a 53 % reduction in the risk of biochemical progression (adjusted HR, 0.47; P = 0.03)."

Da Pozzo, Briganti, and Tward focused their post-operative series on patients with proven LNI (Da Pozzo et al. 2009; Briganti et al. 2011; Johnstone et al. 2007; Tward 2013). In their retrospective series from Italy Da Pozza and Briganti showed that patients appeared to have improved outcomes with the addition of EBRT although the technical details (e.g., field sizes and doses) were not uniformly applied, however roughly 85 % were believed to have had WPRT.

Johnstone et al. used the Surveillance Epidemiology End Results (SEER) registry database to assess the efficacy of post-operative RT for patients + for LNI after RP, while Tward studied patients spared the RP (Johnstone et al. 2007; Tward 2013). Johnstone analyzed 1921 patients with clinically localized prostate cancer who underwent RP alone, or RP followed by RT and documented LNI. They concluded that there was no significant relative survival benefit for +LN patients receiving post-operative RT and discouraged the routine use of post-operative RT in patients with LNI (p = 0.270). However, Tward et al. used SEER data to evaluate the role of EBRT in patients with lymph node positive disease *without* a prostatectomy. They concluded that the addition of EBRT (presumably including pelvic nodes) was associated with an improvement in cause specific and all cause survival.

4 Conclusions

Improvement technology should allow us to more effectively cover pelvic lymph nodes, while escalating doses and lowering morbidity associated with WPRT (Chan et al. 2008). Additional Trials are needed to confirm the role of WPRT in patients with an intermediate to high risk of LNI and to this end, in 2011 the RTOG launched RTOG 0924. Despite a negative staging workup, occult LNI is a well-known problem in high-risk and some intermediate risk prostate cancer patients. It is not logical to ignore the body of literature presented and only irradiate the prostate. To date, essentially all major randomized trials including high-risk patients demonstrating a survival benefit (RTOG 8610 thru 9202 and EORTC studies) incorporated WPRT. Essentially, all of the studies that have failed to show the benefit with "pelvic radiotherapy" did not in fact use true WPRT (per RTOG 9413). The author argues that the results of RTOG 9413 and the body of literature summarized above establish WPRT in conjunction with HT as the standard of care in patients with intermediate and high-risk disease.

References

Abdollah F, Cozzarini C, Suardi N, Gallina A, Capitanio U, Bianchi M, Tutolo M, Salonia A, la Macchia M, di Muzio N, Rigatti P, Montorsi F, Briganti A (2012) Indications for pelvic nodal treatment in prostate cancer should change. Validation of the Roach formula in a large extended nodal dissection series. Int J Radiat Oncol Biol Phys 83:624–629

Aizer AA, Yu JB, McKeon AM, Decker RH, Colberg JW, Peschel RE (2009) Whole pelvic radiotherapy versus prostate only radiotherapy in the management of locally advanced or aggressive prostate adenocarcinoma. Int J Radiat Oncol Biol Phys 75:1344–1349

Asbell SO, Krall JM, Pilepich MV, Baerwald H, Sause WT, Hanks GE, Perez CA (1988) Elective pelvic irradiation in stage A2, B carcinoma of the prostate: analysis of RTOG 77-06. Int J Radiat Oncol Biol Phys 15:1307–1316

Briganti A, Chun FK, Salonia A, Gallina A, Zanni G, Scattoni V, Valiquette L, Rigatti P, Montorsi F, Karakiewicz PI (2007) Critical assessment of ideal nodal yield at pelvic lymphadenectomy to accurately diagnose prostate cancer nodal metastasis in patients undergoing radical retropubic prostatectomy. Urology 69:147–151

Briganti A, Karnes RJ, da Pozzo LF, Cozzarini C, Capitanio U, Gallina A, Suardi N, Bianchi M, Tutolo M, Salonia A, di Muzio N, Rigatti P, Montorsi F, Blute M (2011) Combination of adjuvant hormonal and radiation therapy significantly prolongs survival of patients with pT2-4 pN + prostate cancer: results of a matched analysis. Eur Urol 59:832–840

Chan LW, Xia P, Gottschalk AR, Akazawa M, Scala M, Pickett B, Hsu IC, Speight J, Roach M III (2008) Proposed rectal dose constraints for patients undergoing definitive whole pelvic radiotherapy for clinically localized prostate cancer. Int J Radiat Oncol Biol Phys 72:69–77

da Pozzo LF, Cozzarini C, Briganti A, Suardi N, Salonia A, Bertini R, Gallina A, Bianchi M, Fantini GV, Bolognesi A, Fazio F, Montorsi F, Rigatti P (2009) Long-Term Follow-up of Patients with Prostate Cancer and Nodal Metastases Treated by Pelvic Lymphadenectomy and Radical Prostatectomy The Positive Impact of Adjuvant Radiotherapy. Eur Urol 55:1003–1011

Eggener SE, Scardino PT, Walsh PC, Han M, Partin AW, Trock BJ, Feng Z, Wood DP, Eastham JA, Yossepowitch O, Rabah DM, Kattan MW, Yu C, Klein EA, Stephenson AJ (2011) Predicting 15-year prostate cancer specific mortality after radical prostatectomy. J Urol 185:869–875

Ferrari AC, Stone NN, Kurek R, Mulligan E, McGregor R, Stock R, Unger P, Tunn U, Kaisary A, Droller M, Hall S, Renneberg H, Livak KJ, Gallagher RE, Mandeli J (2006) Molecular load of pathologically occult metastases in pelvic lymph nodes is an independent prognostic marker of biochemical failure after localized prostate cancer treatment. J Clin Oncol 24:3081–3088

Hanks GE, Asbell S, Krall JM, Perez CA, Doggett S, Rubin P, Sause W, Pilepich MV (1991) Outcome for lymph node dissection negative T-1b, T-2 (A-2, B) prostate cancer treated with external beam radiation therapy in RTOG 77–06. Int J Radiat Oncol Biol Phys 21:1099–1103

Hanks GE, Perez CA, Kozar M, Asbell SO, Pilepich MV, Pajak TF (1994) PSA confirmation of cure at 10 years of T1b, T2, N0, M0 prostate cancer patients treated in RTOG protocol 7706 with external beam irradiation. Int J Radiat Oncol Biol Phys 30:289–292

Heidenreich A, Ohlmann CH, Polyakov S (2007) Anatomical extent of pelvic lymphadenectomy in patients undergoing radical prostatectomy. Eur Urol 52:29–37

Heidenreich A, Varga Z, von Knobloch R (2002) Extended pelvic lymphadenectomy in patients undergoing radical prostatectomy: high incidence of lymph node metastasis. J Urol 167:1681–1686

Jacob R, Hanlon AL, Horwitz EM, Movsas B, Uzzo RG, Pollack A (2005) Role of prostate dose escalation in patients with greater than 15% risk of pelvic lymph node involvement. Int J Radiat Oncol Biol Phys 61:695–701

Johnstone PA, Assikis V, Goodman M, Ward KC, Riffenburgh RH, Master V (2007) Lack of survival benefit of post-operative radiation therapy in prostate cancer patients with positive lymph nodes. Prostate Cancer Prostatic Dis 10:185–188

Lawton CA, Desilvio M, Roach M III, Uhl V, Kirsch R, Seider M, Rotman M, Jones C, Asbell S, Valicenti R, Hahn S, Thomas CR Jr (2007) An update of the phase III trial comparing whole pelvic to prostate only radiotherapy and neoadjuvant to adjuvant total androgen suppression: updated analysis of RTOG 94-13, with emphasis on unexpected hormone/radiation interactions. Int J Radiat Oncol Biol Phys, 69:646–55

Milecki P, Baczyk M, Skowronek J, Antczak A, Kwias Z, Martenka P (2009) Benefit of whole pelvic radiotherapy combined with neoadjuvant androgen deprivation for the high-risk prostate cancer. J Biomed Biotechnol 2009:625394

Miyake H, Hara I, Kurahashi T, Inoue TA, Eto H, Fujisawa M (2007a) Quantitative detection of micrometastases in pelvic lymph nodes in patients with clinically localized prostate cancer by real-time reverse transcriptase-PCR. Clin Cancer Res 13:1192–1197

Miyake H, Kurahashi T, Hara I, Takenaka A, Fujisawa M (2007b) Significance of micrometastases in pelvic lymph nodes detected by real-time reverse transcriptase polymerase chain reaction in patients with clinically localized prostate cancer undergoing radical prostatectomy after neoadjuvant hormonal therapy. BJU Int 99:315–320

Moghanaki D, Koontz BF, Karlin JD, Wan W, Mukhopadhay N, Hagan MP, Anscher MS (2013) Elective irradiation of pelvic lymph nodes during postprostatectomy salvage radiotherapy. Cancer 119:52–60

Morikawa LK, Roach M III (2011) Pelvic nodal radiotherapy in patients with unfavorable intermediate and high-risk prostate cancer: evidence, rationale, and future directions. Int j radiat oncol biol phys 80:6–16

Nguyen PL, Chen MH, Hoffman KE, Katz MS, D'Amico AV (2009) Predicting the risk of pelvic node involvement among men with prostate cancer in the contemporary era. Int J Radiat Oncol Biol Phys 74:104–109

Pagliarulo V, Hawes D, Brands FH, Groshen S, Cai J, Stein JP, Lieskovsky G, Skinner DG, Cote RJ (2006) Detection of occult lymph node metastases in locally advanced node-negative prostate cancer. J Clin Oncol 24:2735–2742

Pan CC, Kim KY, Taylor JM, McLaughlin PW, Sandler HM (2002) Influence of 3D-CRT pelvic irradiation on outcome in prostate cancer treated with external beam radiotherapy. Int J Radiat Oncol Biol Phys 53:1139–1145

Partin AW, Yoo J, Carter HB, Pearson JD, Chan DW, Epstein JI, Walsh PC (1993) The use of prostate specific antifen, clinical stage and Gleason score to predict pathological stage in men with localized prostate cancer. J Urol 150:110–114

Pommier P, Chabaud S, Lagrange JL, Richaud P, Lesaunier F, le Prise E, Wagner JP, Hay MH, Beckendorf V, Suchaud JP, Pabot Du Chatelard PM, Bernier V, Voirin N, Perol D, Carrie C (2007) Is there a role for pelvic irradiation in localized prostate adenocarcinoma? Preliminary results of GETUG-01. J Clin Oncol 25:5366–5373

Roach M (1993) Re: The use of prostate specific antigen, clinical stage and Gleason score to predict pathological stage in men with localized prostate cancer. J Urol 150:1923–1924

Roach M III (2007) Dose escalated external beam radiotherapy versus neoadjuvant androgen deprivation therapy and conventional dose external beam radiotherapy for clinically localized prostate cancer: do we need both? Strahlenther Onkol 183 Spec No 2:26–28

Roach M III (2008) Targeting pelvic lymph nodes in men with intermediate- and high-risk prostate cancer, and confusion about the results of the randomized trials. J Clin Oncol, 26:3816–3817; author reply 3817–8

Roach M III (2009a) Predicting pathologic stage, nomograms, and clinical judgment: don't miss the forest for the trees! Int J Radiat Oncol Biol Phys 73:325–326

Roach M III (2009b) Predicting the risk of pelvic node involvement among men with prostate cancer in the contemporary era: change you can believe in, or back to the future? (In regard to Nguyen PL, et al. (Int J Radiat Oncol Biol Phys 2009). Int J Radiat Oncol Biol Phys 75:316; author reply 316

Roach M III, Desilvio M, Lawton C, Uhl V, Machtay M, Seider MJ, Rotman M, Jones C, Asbell SO, Valicenti RK, Han S, Thomas CR Jr, Shipley WS (2003) Phase III trial comparing whole-pelvic versus prostate-only radiotherapy and neoadjuvant versus adjuvant combined androgen suppression: Radiation Therapy Oncology Group 9413. J Clin Oncol 21:1904–1911

Roach M III, Desilvio M, Valicenti R, Grignon D, Asbell SO, Lawton C, Thomas CR Jr, Shipley WU (2006a) Whole-pelvis, "mini-pelvis," or prostate-only external beam radiotherapy after neoadjuvant and concurrent hormonal therapy in patients treated in the Radiation Therapy Oncology Group 9413 trial. Int J Radiat Oncol Biol Phys 66:647–653

Roach M III, Hanks G, Thames H Jr, Schellhammer P, Shipley WU, Sokol GH, Sandler H (2006b) Defining biochemical failure following radiotherapy with or without hormonal therapy in men with clinically localized prostate cancer: recommendations of the RTOG-ASTRO Phoenix Consensus Conference. Int j radiat oncol biol phys 65:965–974

Roach M III, Lu J, Pilepich MV, Asbell SO, Mohiuddin M, Terry R, Grignon D, Lawton C, Shipley W, Cox J (2000) Predicting long-term survival, and the need for hormonal therapy: a meta-analysis of RTOG prostate cancer trials. Int J Radiat Oncol Biol Phys 47:617–627

Roach M III, Marquez C, Yuo HS, Narayan P, Coleman L, Nseyo UO, Navvab Z, Carroll PR (1994) Predicting the risk of lymph node involvement using the pre-treatment prostate specific antigen and Gleason score in men with clinically localized prostate cancer. Int J Radiat Oncol Biol Phys 28:33–37

Roach M III, Weinberg V, Nash M, Sandler HM, Mclaughlin PW, Kattan MW (2006c) Defining high risk prostate cancer with risk groups and nomograms: implications for designing clinical trials. J Urol 176:S16–S20

Roach M, Hsu I-C WK, Carroll P (2010) Prostate cancer. In: HOPPE P, Roach (eds.) Leibel and Phillips textbook of radiation oncology, 3rd ed. Elsevier, Philadelphia

Seaward SA, Weinberg V, Lewis P, Leigh B, Phillips TL, Roach M III (1998a) Identification of a high-risk clinically localized prostate cancer subgroup receiving maximum benefit from whole-pelvic irradiation. Cancer J Sci Am, 4:370–377

Seaward SA, Weinberg V, Lewis P, Leigh B, Phillips TL, Roach M III (1998b) Improved freedom from PSA failure with whole pelvic irradiation for high-risk prostate cancer. Int J Radiat Oncol Biol Phys 42:1055–1062

Shariat SF, Kattan MW, Erdamar S, Nguyen C, Scardino PT, Spencer DM, Wheeler TM, Slawin KM (2003) Detection of clinically significant, occult prostate cancer metastases in lymph nodes using a splice variant-specific rt-PCR assay for human glandular kallikrein. J Clin Oncol 21:1223–1231

Spevack L, Killion LT, West JCJR, Rooker GM, Brewer EA, Cuddy PG (1996) Predicting the patient at low risk for lymph node metastasis with localized prostate cancer: an analysis of four statistical models. Int J Radiat Oncol Biol Phys 34:543–547

Spiotto MT, Hancock SL, King CR (2007) Radiotherapy after prostatectomy: improved biochemical relapse-free survival with whole pelvic compared with prostate bed only for high-risk patients. Int J Radiat Oncol Biol Phys 69:54–61

Tward JD, Kokeny, Kristine E, Shrieve, Dennis C (2013) Radiation therapy for clinically node-postive adenocarcinoma is correlated with improved overall and prostate cancer-specific survival. Practical Radiation Oncology 3:234–240

Prophylactic Treatment of the Pelvic Lymphatics: Contra

Pascal Pommier

Contents

P. Pommier (✉)
Radiotherapy Department, Centre Léon Bérard,
28 Rue Laënnec, 69373 Lyon CEDEX 08, France
e-mail: pascal.pommier@lyon.unicancer.fr

Abstract

According to the opinion of the author, to date—applying evidence-based medicine—physicians should not perform prophylactic pelvic lymph node irradiation in routine practice for locally advanced prostate cancer because of the lack of any demonstrated benefit. In addition, this treatment has a higher risk of acute and late toxicities. Standard prognostic factors and nomograms, failed to identify a subgroup of patients who may benefit from pelvic lymph nodes irradiation. Several biases including technical radiotherapy features (target volume, dose) are discussed. Radiation oncologists should be encouraged to participate in the ongoing RTOG 094 international randomized study.

1 Pelvic Radiotherapy in Locally Advanced Prostate Cancer: What are the Evidences?

To date, three published prospective randomized trials (RTOG 77-06, RTOG 94-13, and GETUG-01) have been conducted to answer that question. None of them have demonstrated any benefit (nor even of a trend for a benefit) for overall survival, metastases free survival nor biological free survival. In addition, a higher risk for acute and late toxicity has been observed with a significant higher incidence of late grade 3 or more gastrointestinal toxicity in the whole pelvic arm (5 vs. 1 % in the RTOG study) (Asbell et al. 1988, 1998; Roach et al. 2003; Lawton et al. 2007; Pommier et al. 2007).

The conclusion appears to be obvious: referring to an evidenced-based medicine approach, standard of care for radiotherapy modality in patients with locally advanced prostate cancer staged as cN0 or pN0 is not to irradiate the pelvic nodes as long as a new phase III trial demonstrates its benefit.

H. Geinitz et al. (eds.), *Radiotherapy in Prostate Cancer*, Medical Radiology. Radiation Oncology,
DOI: 10.1007/174_2013_949, © Springer-Verlag Berlin Heidelberg 2014
Published Online: 11 January 2014

2 Are there Some Subgroups of Patients who may Benefit from Pelvic Node Radiotherapy?

In general, pelvic radiotherapy may be beneficial only to patients with lymph node involvement (LNI), no distant metastases and a cancer locally controlled within the prostate.

2.1 "Is Node-Positive Prostate Cancer Always a Systemic Disease?"

Indeed a potential benefit of pelvic radiotherapy may have been masked especially with the outcome of bone metastases as patients with high risk for LNI also have a high risk of infra-clinic bone metastases (Briganti et al. 2008).

This has been indirectly shown by the long-term results of the RTOG77-06 revealing that patients with a pN0 status after laparotomy compared to patients staged only by lymphangiogram had a higher 12-year overall survival (48 vs. 38 %, p: 0.02) and disease-free survival (38 vs. 26 %, *p*: 0.003) and developed less frequently bone metastases (14 vs. 27 %, p: 0.003) (Asbell et al. 1998). The absence of any therapeutic gain with pelvic irradiation in any of these two subgroups may signified that there is no need for pelvic irradiation in pN0 patients (subject to the accuracy of the staging!), and that patients with LNI do not benefit from from pelvic radiotherapy as most of them will develop bone metastases.

Indeed, the answer to the above-quoted question raised by Briganti in his 2008 editorial (Briganti et al. 2008) is fortunately "no," as long-term overall survival and disease-free survival has been reported for patients with pathologically proven positive nodes. Therefore some patients may benefit from pelvic radiotherapy provided that there are accurate tools to appropriately select those with pN1 M0 disease, with a limited number of pelvic lymph nodes involved (Briganti et al. 2008a, b, 2009; Swanson et al. 2006).

Unfortunately, the nomograms developed to predict lymph node involvement have not only a low positive and negative predictive value they also do not permit to identify patients with a limited node involvement who may benefit from pelvic radiotherapy.

2.2 May Patients with Low-Risk Features for Node Metastasis Benefit from Pelvic Radiotherapy?

The risk of pelvic LNI is possibly not negligible in patients classified as low risks. Indeed, in a selected population with a PSA value $\leq$10 ng/ml and a Gleason score $\leq$6, the prevalence of LNI detected by scintigraphically guided surgery was 5.4 and 11.3 %, respectively, for unilateral and bilateral positive core biopsies in the Weckermann experience (Weckermann et al. 2006).

The GETUG-01 study allowed assessing the role of pelvic radiotherapy in a subgroup of patients with a low risk for LNI thanks to the stratification between "low risk patients" (corresponding to the low-risk group according to the D'Amico classification) versus a "high risk group" including patients that may have been classified as intermediate and high-risk groups by the D'Amico classification (D'Amico et al. 1998). In this low-risk group (92 patients,) with a median follow-up of 3.5 years, the 5 years progression free survival was 83.9 versus 75.1 %, respectively, in favor of whole pelvis irradiation, however this difference was not significant ($p = 0.21$) (Pommier et al. 2007). Moreover, in the multivariate analysis that considered three level of node involvement risk stratified with the Roach formula (Roach et al. 1994) (>15 vs. 15–35 vs. > 35 %) as well as concomitant hormonal therapy, pelvic radiotherapy was not significant for progression free survival ($p = 0.82$).

2.3 May Patients with Intermediate and/or High-Risk Features for Node Metastasis Benefit from Pelvic Radiotherapy?

The literature data is quite confusing regarding analysis of more homogeneous subgroup with either intermediate or high-risk features for LNI, first because of the nomogram used to define the subgroups that do not lead to the same outcome (i.e., Roach formula vs. Partin tables) and second because of opposite conclusions.

In a subgroup analysis of the RTOG 94-13 patients with "intermediate risk" for LNI (defined as GS of 2 to 6 and PSA >30 ng/ml or GS of 7 to 10 and PSA <30 ng/ml) a significant difference was observed between the 4 arms in favor of the whole pelvic RT associated with a neoadjuvant and concomitant hormonotherapy (Roach et al. 2003).

Similar results have been published by Pan et al. (2002) in a retrospective matched paired analysis. Patients were retrospectively stratified in three groups using the updated Partin tables (709 low-risk, 263 intermediate risk, and 309 high-risk patients). Multivariate analysis demonstrated a statistically significant relative risk reduction for biological progression for the entire population treated with pelvic RT, but the beneficial effect appeared to be limited to the intermediate risk group (>5–15 % according to Partin tables).

However, two other large retrospective studies using the Roach formula to individualize patients in three LNI prognostic groups failed to find any benefit for pelvic irradiation in multivariate analysis (Vargas et al. 2005; Jacob et al. 2005).

2.4 Does a Competitive Negative Effect of a Lack of Prostate Local Control may have Masked a Pelvic Radiotherapy Benefit?

A dose effect has been demonstrated in terms of DFS linked to a higher local control rate in case of exclusive RT in intermediate risk patients (Pollack et al. 2002). However, the role of dose escalation in case of combined EBRT and HT is still under evaluation (i.e., the GETUG18 trial for high-risk patients).

In that setting, the GETUG-01 methodology may be criticized as many patients with high-risk features received quite a low dose to the prostate bed (66–70 Gy) and no hormonal therapy. There was a higher but nonsignificant percentage of patients receiving exclusive low dose RT (<70 Gy) in the pelvic arm. The RTOG-94-13 also used doses that are at present considered as low (70 Gy), but all the patients received an androgen blockage either adjuvant or neoadjuvant and concomitant.

However, the rate of documented local relapse is quite low in both randomized series and was similar in both arms. Documented local progressions at 4 years for prostate + pelvis versus prostate only arms were, respectively, 8.9 versus 9.9 % in the GETUG-01 (*personal updated data*), and 9.1 versus 8 % in the RTOG-94-13 trial (Roach et al. 2003) with no statistically significant difference among the four arms ($p = 0.67$) (Lawton et al. 2007). Therefore, the lack of local control in these randomized studies is not likely to have hidden a potential benefit of pelvic radiotherapy.

Vargas et al. (Vargas et al. 2005) assessed the role of pelvic RT in 596 patients with high risk of LNI (between 15 and 30 in 422 and above 30 % in 174 applying the Roach formula) treated in three institutions with a high dose RT with a combination of external beam RT and high dose rate BT (average biologic effective dose $\geq$100 Gy). The policy of two of the three institutions was to treat the pelvis nodes (46–50 Gy) (312 pts), whereas the treated volume was limited to the prostate and seminal vesicles in the third one (284 pts). Short-term neoadjuvant/adjuvant HT was given in 42 % of patients. With a 4.3 years median follow-up, local recurrence was low (3.1 and 5.2 % respectively for LNI risk >15–30 and $\geq$30 %) and no benefit was seen in the 5-year rates of clinical failure, cause-specific survival, or overall survival with pelvic radiation.

In Jacob et al. (Jacob et al. 2005) series including 420 patients with a >15 % risk of LNI, radiation dose to the prostate was the most significant independent prognostic factor of 5 years of freedom from biochemical failure in the multivariate analysis, Gleason score, and initial prostate-specific antigen level were also significant but the radiation field size (e.g., "whole pelvis" vs. partial pelvis" vs. prostate only) and androgen deprivation were not.

3 Is Radiotherapy Ineffective for Pelvic Nodes, or is it Just a Matter of "Technique, Pelvic Dose and Hormonal Manipulation"?

3.1 Is There an Interaction Between Pelvic Irradiation and Hormonal Therapy?

The observed trend toward a statistical significance for progression free survival and overall survival in favor of a neoadjuvant and concomitant hormonal therapy compared to an adjuvant only HT in the "whole pelvic arm" of the RTOG 94-13 protocol may be due to the supra-additive role of concomitant hormonal therapy and radiotherapy.

On the other hand, in Vargas et al. large series of patients treated with high dose to the prostate (combining EBRT and HDR-BT) with or without pelvic RT, not only pelvic nodal irradiation did not demonstrate any benefit, but a detrimental role of short course of neoadjuvant HT has been observed (Vargas et al. 2005, 2006).

3.2 Treated Volume: "Too Large" for Prostate only Radiotherapy?

A potential bias in disfavor of the "pelvic arm radiotherapy" in the RTOG94-13 trial is that first pelvic nodes relay may have been irradiated in the "prostate only" (PO) arm due to the use of standard techniques.

To assess that question Roach et al. performed a subgroup analysis excluding patients randomized in the post-radiotherapy adjuvant HT. Patients randomized in the "PO" arm were dichotomized by median field size (10 × 11 cm) ("MP field" vs. "PO field"). A slight (not significant?) difference was observed for 7-year PFS in favor of "MP Field" compared to "PO field" (respectively 31 and 21 %) but there was no difference between these two groups regarding the 5 years biochemical failure (respectively 45 and 44 % in pairwise comparisons with whole pelvic RT) (Roach et al. 2006).

In the GETUG-01 study, three-dimensional treatment plan were mandatory for prostate bed irradiation and that should limit the bias of an undesirable pelvic node irradiation in the PO arm.

Therefore, it is unlikely that the true treated volume in these two major randomized study may have mask a potential benefit of pelvic node irradiation.

3.3 Treated Volume: "Not Enough" for Pelvic Radiotherapy?

According to the RTOG 75-06 randomized trial, irradiation of periaortic nodes in addition to pelvic nodes in patients with stage C or with stage A-2 or B with evidence of pelvic nodes involvement does not improve distant metastases occurrence, disease-free and overall survival (Pilepich et al. 1986).

Extended pelvic lymphadenectomy have permitted to assess precisely the sites at risk for LNI and to demonstrate that some of them (especially presacral and deep inguinal nodes) are not encompassed by standard four-fields irradiation technique applied in the randomized studies (Heidenreich et al. 2007). Based on these observations, several recommendations has been proposed to delineate more accurately the pelvic nodes clinical target volume (CTVN) (Taylor et al. 2005; Shih et al. 2005; Lawton et al. 2009) and to promote the use of IMRT to ensure a better coverage of this CTV with a lower toxicity than standard fields RT (Wang-Chesebro et al. 2006; Ganswindt et al. 2007).

3.4 Pelvic Dose

In the three randomized trials, dose delivered to the pelvic nodes was equivalent (50.4 Gy with fractions of 1.8 or 46 Gy with fractions of 2 Gy) and are still considered to be a standard. This low dose may be insufficient to control metastatic lymph nodes and explain the lack of benefit for pelvic radiotherapy in these trials.

Thanks to the development of IMRT, there are some attempts to escalate the dose to the pelvic nodes but to date no data are available on a potential dose effect on cancer control outcomes (Muren et al. 2008; Hwang et al. 2012; Guerrero Urbano et al. 2010).

4 Conclusion and Perspectives

To date, applying evidence-based medicine should lead physicians not to perform prophylactic pelvic nodes irradiation in routine practice for locally advanced prostate cancer because of the lack of any demonstrated benefit and because of the higher risk of acute and late toxicities.

Indeed, the most important challenge for patients staged as N0M0 would be to individualize the subgroup of patients with a high probability of pN1 and at the same time a low probability of having infra-clinic metastases. Partin tables and Roach formula are very likely to under-estimate the real percentage of patients with LNI as demonstrated by the data from extended pelvic lymph node dissections (EPLND) (Heidenreich et al. 2007) and new nomograms have been recently developed and validated (Briganti et al. 2012; Walz et al. 2012).

Modern imaging and less invasive surgical procedure may also permit to prospectively assess in selected patients the frequency and the characteristics of pelvic recurrence (isolated or associated with concomitant local recurrence or distant metastases) after prostate radiotherapy (with or without pelvic irradiation), that means to perform a complete restaging (i.e., using multi-parametric MRI and new imaging modalities as Choline PET-CT) in case of biological recurrence before starting palliative hormonal therapy. Some of these patients may possibly beneficiate from a salvage upfront or postoperative radiotherapy (Jilg et al. 2012; Jereczek-Fossa et al. 2012).

4.1 Is a Fourth Prospective Randomized Trial (RTOG 0924) Necessary?

Non-accurate patient selection and several confounding factors including inadequate irradiation technique and dose may explain the negative results of the already published three phase III studies. Every radiation oncologist should therefore be encouraged to include patients in the international recently launched RTOG 0924.

The high number of patients to be included (2580) may at least permit to identify the characteristics of a subgroup that potentially benefits from pelvic radiotherapy based on already known prognostic factors but also based on "biomarkers" to be extracted from the prospective collection of biological material for *"planned and future translational research."*

References

Asbell SO, Krall JM, Pilepich MV et al (1988) Elective pelvic irradiation in stage A2, B carcinoma of the prostate: analysis of RTOG 77-06. Int J Radiat Oncol Biol Phys 15(6):1307–1316

Asbell SO, Martz KL, Shin KH et al (1998) Impact of surgical staging in evaluating the radiotherapeutic outcome in RTOG #77-06, a phase III study for T1BN0M0 (A2) and T2N0M0 (B) prostate carcinoma. Int J Radiat Oncol Biol Phys 40(4):769–782

Briganti A, Chun FK, Karakiewicz P et al (2008) Is node-positive prostate cancer always a systemic disease? Eur Urol 54(2):243–246

Briganti A, Karnes J, Da Pozzo L et al (2008b) Two positive nodes represent a significant cut-off value for cancer specific survival in patients with node positive prostate cancer. A new proposal based on a two-institution experience on 784 consecutive N+ patients. Eur Urol 7:303

Briganti A, Karnes JR, Da Pozzo LF et al (2009) Two positive nodes represent a significant cut-off value for cancer specific survival in patients with node positive prostate cancer. a new proposal based on a two-institution experience on 703 consecutive N+ patients treated with radical prostatectomy, extended pelvic lymph node dissection and adjuvant therapy. Eur Urol 55(2):261–270

Briganti A, Larcher A, Abdollah F et al (2012) Updated nomogram predicting lymph node invasion in patients with prostate cancer undergoing extended pelvic lymph node dissection: the essential importance of percentage of positive cores. Eur Urol 61(3):480–487

D'Amico AV, Whittington R, Malkowicz SB et al (1998) Biochemical outcome after radical prostatectomy, external beam radiation therapy, or interstitial radiation therapy for clinically localized prostate cancer. JAMA 280:969–974

Ganswindt U, Paulsen F, Corvin S et al (2007) Optimized coverage of high-risk adjuvant lymph node areas in prostate cancer using a sentinel node-based, intensity-modulated radiation therapy technique. Int J Radiat Oncol Biol Phys 67(2):347–355

Guerrero Urbano T, Khoo V, Staffurth J et al (2010) Intensity-modulated radiotherapy allows escalation of the radiation dose to the pelvic lymph nodes in patients with locally advanced prostate cancer: preliminary results of a phase I dose escalation study. Clin Oncol (R Coll Radiol) 22(3):236–244

Heidenreich A, Ohlmann CH, Polyakov S (2007) Anatomical extent of pelvic lymphadenectomy in patients undergoing radical prostatectomy. Eur Urol 52:29–37

Hwang AB, Chen J, Nguyen TB et al (2012) Irradiation of the prostate and pelvic lymph nodes with an adaptive algorithm. Med Phys 39(2):1119–1124

Jacob R, Hanlon AL, Horwitz EM et al (2005) Role of prostate dose escalation in patients with greater than 15 % risk of pelvic lymph node involvement. Int J Radiat Oncol Biol Phys 61:695–701

Jereczek-Fossa BA, Beltramo G, Fariselli L et al (2012) Robotic image-guided stereotactic radiotherapy, for isolated recurrent primary, lymph node or metastatic prostate cancer. Int J Radiat Oncol Biol Phys 82(2):889–897

Jilg CA, Rischke HC, Reske SN et al (2012) Salvage lymph node dissection with adjuvant radiotherapy for nodal recurrence of prostate cancer. J Urol 188(6):2190–2197

Lawton CA, DeSilvio M, Roach M et al (2007) An update of the phase III trial comparing whole pelvic to prostate only radiotherapy and neoadjuvant to adjuvant total androgen suppression: updated analysis of RTOG 94-13, with emphasis on unexpected hormone/radiation interactions. Int J Radiat Oncol Biol Phys 69:646–655

Lawton CA, Michalski J, El-Naqa I et al (2009) RTOG GU Radiation oncology specialists reach consensus on pelvic lymph node volumes for high-risk prostate cancer. Int J Radiat Oncol Biol Phys 74(2):383–387

Muren LP, Wasbø E, Helle SI et al (2008) Intensity-modulated radiotherapy of pelvic lymph nodes in locally advanced prostate cancer: planning procedures and early experiences. Int J Radiat Oncol Biol Phys 71(4):1034–1041

Pan CC, Kim KY, Taylor JM (2002) Influence of 3D-CRT pelvic irradiation on outcome in prostate cancer treated with external beam radiotherapy. Int J Radiat Oncol Biol Phys 53:1139–1145

Pilepich MV, Krall JM, Johnson RJ et al (1986) Extended field (periaortic) irradiation in carcinoma of the prostate–analysis of RTOG 75-06. Int J Radiat Oncol Biol Phys 12(3):345–351

Pollack A, Zagars GK, Starkschall G et al (2002) Prostate cancer radiation dose response: results of the MD Anderson phase III randomized trial. Int J Radiat Oncol Biol Phys 53:1097–1105

Pommier P, Chabaud S, Lagrange JL et al (2007) Is there a role for pelvic irradiation in localized prostate adenocarcinoma? Preliminary results of GETUG-01. J Clin Oncol 25:5366–5373

Roach M, Marquez C, Yuo HS et al (1994) Predicting the risk of lymph node involvement using the pre-treatment prostate specific antigen and Gleason score in men with clinically localized prostate cancer. Int J Radiat Oncol Biol Phys 28:33–37

Roach M III, DeSilvio M, Lawton C et al (2003) Phase III trial comparing whole-pelvic versus prostate-only radiotherapy and neoadjuvant versus adjuvant combined androgen suppression: radiation Therapy Oncology Group 9413. J Clin Oncol 21: 1904–1911

Roach M 3rd, DeSilvio M, Valicenti R et al (2006) Whole-pelvis, "mini-pelvis," or prostate-only external beam radiotherapy after neoadjuvant and concurrent hormonal therapy in patients treated in the radiation therapy oncology group 9413 trial. Int J Radiat Oncol Biol Phys 66(3):647–653

Shih H, Harisinghani M, Zietman A et al (2005) Mapping of nodal disease in locally advanced prostate cancer: rethinking the clinical target volume for pelvic nodal irradiation based on vascular rather than bony anatomy. Int J Radiat Oncol Biol Phys 63:1262–1269

Swanson GP, Thompson IM, Basler J (2006) Treatment options in lymph node-positive prostate cancer. Cancer 106(12):2531–2539

Taylor A, Rockall A, Reznek R et al (2005) Mapping pelvic lymph nodes: guidelines for delineation in intensity-modulated radiotherapy. Int J Radiat Oncol Biol Phys 63:1604–1612

Vargas CE, Galalae R, Demanes J et al (2005) Lack of benefit of pelvic radiation in prostate cancer patients with a high risk of positive pelvic lymph nodes treated with high-dose radiation. Int J Radiat Oncol Biol Phys 63:1474–1482

Vargas C, Martínez A, Galalae R et al (2006) High-dose radiation employing external beam radiotherapy and high-dose rate brachytherapy with and without neoadjuvant androgen deprivation for prostate cancer patients with intermediate- and high-risk features. Prostate Cancer Prostatic Dis 9(3):245–253

Walz J, Bladou F, Rousseau B et al (2012) Head to head comparison of nomograms predicting probability of lymph node invasion of prostate cancer in patients undergoing extended pelvic lymph node dissection. Urology 79(3):546–551

Wang-Chesebro A, Xia P, Coleman J, Akazawa C, Roach M 3rd (2006) Intensity-modulated radiotherapy improves lymph node coverage and dose to critical structures compared with three-dimensional conformal radiation therapy in clinically localized prostate cancer. Int J Radiat Oncol Biol Phys 66(3):654–662

Weckermann D, Goppelt M, Dorn R et al (2006) Incidence of positive pelvic lymph nodes in patients with prostate cancer, a prostate-specific antigen (PSA) level of < or = 10 ng/mL and biopsy Gleason score of < or = 6, and their influence on PSA progression-free survival after radical prostatectomy. BJU Int 97(6): 1173–1178

Hormonal Therapy and Radiation Therapy: Randomized and Prospective Trials

Michel Bolla, Camille Verry, Violaine Brun Baronnat, and Alexandre Tessier

Contents

Abstract

In high risk prostate cancer (PCa), the aim of androgen deprivation therapy (ADT) is to improve the therapeutic ratio of radiotherapy (RT) by potentiating irradiation whatever its technique and destroying the infraclinical disease located outside the irradiated volume. Many phase III randomized trials have paved the way for establishing the indications of the combination of ADT with external irradiation. For locally advanced PCa, long-term ADT ($\geq$2 years) with LHRH agonists combined with external irradiation is a gold standard (level 1a of evidence); should there be a significant comorbidity, a reticence of the patients who want to remain potent or a poor tolerance, a 6-month duration may be proposed unless to choose an anti-androgen monotherapy. For high risk localized PCa 4–6-months complete ADT is recommended (level 2a evidence). For intermediate risk localized PCa, patients may benefit from a combined approach with a short-term ADT. IMRT has replaced conventional irradiation and allows a dose escalation recommended for high risk PCa, offering also the opportunity to treat intermediate risk localized PCa without ADT. Patients have to be informed of the potential morbidity of ADT and a close cooperation is needed with general practitioners and specialists to prevent or minimize harmful side effects as much as possible and to maintain quality of life.

1 Introduction

To better control the growth of high risk prostate cancer (PCa) the combination of a local treatment with a systemic treatment has become mandatory, due to the limited curative potential of definitive conventional irradiation (Bagshaw et al. 1988; Hanks et al. 1995). High risk PCa include men with locally advanced PCa (T3-4 N0-X M0) or localized PCa (T1-2 N0-X M0) with either a Gleason score 8–10 and/or a

M. Bolla (✉) · C. Verry · V. Brun Baronnat · A. Tessier
Clinique Universitaire de Cancérologie-Radiothérapie, Centre Hospitalier Universitaire Albert Michallon, BP 217 38043 cedex 9, Grenoble, France
e-mail: MBolla@chu-grenoble.fr

H. Geinitz et al. (eds.), *Radiotherapy in Prostate Cancer*, Medical Radiology. Radiation Oncology, DOI: 10.1007/174_2014_999, © Springer-Verlag Berlin Heidelberg 2014
Published Online: 17 May 2014

baseline PSA >20 ng/ml (Scardino et al. 2003). Huggins and Hodges introduced androgen deprivation therapy (ADT) in the 1940s (Huggins et al. 1941), with surgical castration or oestrogens, based on the dependence of prostatic epithelial and adenocarcinoma cells on androgenic hormones, which explains that more than 80 % of the patients respond to orchidectomy or oestrogens (Schröder 1990). Their side effects obliged clinicians to replace them by agonists of the luteinising hormone-releasing hormone (LHRH) which had the same efficacy (Parmar et al. 1985) with reversibility. As a result of screening (Schroder et al. 2009), the incidence of locally advanced PCa is decreasing while the incidence of localized PCa is increasing, but ADT remains an important part of the therapeutic panoply.

The positive results of phase III randomized trials have promoted long-term adjuvant ADT (≥2 years) as a standard of care for locally advanced PCa, while short-term ADT (4–6 months) is proposed to patients with intermediate or poor risk localized PCa. Far from compensating a non optimal RT, ADT has to be combined with optimal modalities of RT because local control remains of paramount importance, all the more as intensified modulated RT has replaced conventional irradiation and enables radiation oncologists to increase the dose without increasing morbidity (Zelefsky et al. 2008). We would like to consider here: (i) the rationale of this combined approach, (ii) the results of phase III randomised controlled trials focusing on the duration and the chronology of HT with respect to RT, (iii) the new options linked to the breakthrough of radiation techniques and/or drugs, (iv) the morbidity and quality of life referring to ADT, (v) the on-going phase III trials.

2 Rationale

The objectives of combining androgen deprivation with external beam RT are: (i) to decrease both prostate gland volume and prostate cancerous tissue, thereby decreasing the clinical target volume (CTV) and improving bladder and/or rectum dose volume histograms. (ii) to reduce the risk of local relapse within the planning target volume by inhibiting repopulation during irradiation. (iii) to decrease—thanks to a spatial cooperation—the occurrence of distant metastases due to the presence of an infraclinical disease at the time of diagnosis, analog to breast cancer (EBCTCG 2005). (iv) to improve the effectiveness of radiation by an additive or supra-additive effect. To assess the effect of sequencing of ADT by the means of castration and RT on PCa growth, animal studies have been carried out on transplantable androgen-dependant tumor, treated by radiation alone, radiation preceded by orchiectomy, radiation followed by orchiectomy ± androgen restauration. Zietman et al. (1997) at the Massachusetts General Hospital have used a transplantable murine mammary androgen-dependant tumor (Shionogi tumour model) as allografts in the hind limbs of athymic nude mice and have shown that neoadjuvant ADT (given 12 days before RT) provides the greatest effect according to TCD 50. Joon et al. (1997) used Dunning R3327-G rat prostate tumors transplanted in the flanks of Copenhagen rats, and a supra-additive apoptotic response was obtained when castration was initiated 3 days prior to radiation. Kaminski et al. (2003) have used R3327-G rat prostate tumors implanted in the flanks of Copenhagen rats and have calculated the tumor volume doubling time: the results suggest that neoadjuvant ADT may result in prolonged suppression of tumor growth, even after testosterone replacement. All these results were obtained from animal models under experimental conditions that do not allow hormonal treatment during and after irradiation to be delivered in a more protracted way.

3 Combined Androgen Deprivation Therapy and Radiation Therapy: Results of Randomized Controlled Trials (Table 1)

3.1 Locally Advanced Prostate Cancer

The main trials showing a benefit on overall survival were launched by the Radiation Therapy Oncology Group (RTOG) and the RTOG of the European Organization on Treatment and Research on Cancer (EORTC). Devoted to T3-4 N0-X M0 patients and sometimes bulky T2 patients, these trials deal with an agonist analog of LHRH. Two trials were carried out before the introduction of LHRH agonists using conventional modalities of castration. One of these trials, conducted at the MD Anderson Cancer Centre on a cohort of T3 NX M0 patients ($n = 78$) treated with pelvic RT ± diethylstilbestrol (DES, 5 mg), has shown a striking difference in 15-year disease-free survival in favor of the combined treatment, that did not translate into an improvement of overall survival (Zagars et al. 1988). The other trial, launched by the Medical Research Council (Fellows et al. 1992), focused on 277 T2-4 NX M0 cases treated by castration ($n = 90$), RT ($n = 88$) or combined treatment ($n = 99$): irradiation was left to the discretion of each center. Results of that trial showed that orchiectomy delayed the onset of distant metastases, and RT or orchiectomy proved equally effective in controlling local disease.

3.1.1 Concomitant and Long-Term LHRH Adjuvant Androgen Deprivation Therapy

The EORTC trial 22863 was the first to show a gain in overall survival (Bolla et al. 1997). It recruited 415 patients classified as T1-2 NO histological grade 3 WHO or T3-4 N0

Table 1 Phase III studies addressing the use of androgen deprivation in combination with radiation therapy as an adjuvant treatment for prostate cancer

Study	Year of publication	TNM 2002	Number of patients	Androgen suppression therapy	External irradiation	Effect of overall survival
Androgen suppression + radiotherapy versus radiotherapy alone						
(a) *Adjuuvant (+/– concomittant) androgen suppression*						
EORTC 22863 Bolla et al. (2010)	2002	T1–2 poorly differentiated M0 or T3–4N0-1 M0	415	LHRHa for 3 years	70 Gy RT	Significant benefit for combined treatment (HR = 0.51, 95 % CI: 0.36–0.73, $p = 0.0002$)
RTOG 85-31 Pilepich et al. (2005)	2005	T3 or N1M0	977	Orchiecotomy or LHRHa	65–70 Gy RT	Significant benefit for combined treatment ($p = 0.002$) seems mostly caused by patients with Gleason score 7–10
Granfors et al. (2006)	2006	T3N0–1M0	91	Orchiectomy	65 Gy RT	Significant benefit ($p = 0.02$), mainly caused by lymph node positive tumors
D'Amico et al. (2008a)	2008	T2N0M0 (localized unfavorable risk)	206	LHRHa + flut. 6 months	70 Gy 3D-CRT	Significant benefit (HR = 0.55, 95 % CI: 0.34–0.90, $p = 0.01$) that may pertain only to men with no or minimal comorbidity
(b) *Neiadjuvant and concomittant androgen suppression*						
TROG 96-01 Denham et al. (2005)	2005	T2b–T4 N0M0	802	Goserelin + flutamide 3 or 6 months before + concomitant	66 Gy	No significant difference in overall survival reported. Benefit in prostate-cancer-specific survival (HR = 0.56 [0.32–0.98], $p = 0.04$)
RTOG 94-13 Lawton et al. (2007)	2007	T1c–T4N0-1M0	1,292	2 months neoadjuvant + concomitant versus 4 months adjuvant	Whole pelvic RT versus prostate only 70.2 Gy	No significant difference in neoadjuvant + concomitant versus adjuvant ADT groups (interaction suspected)
RTOG 86-10 Roach et. al. (2008)	2008	T2–4N0-2	456	Goserelin + flutamide 2 months before + concomitant	65–70 Gy	No significant difference at 10 years
Short-versus long-term androgen suppression adjuvant (± concomittant) to radiotherapy						
RTOG 92-02 Horwitz et al. (2010)	2008	T2c–4N0-1M0	1,554	LHRHa 2 years adjuvant after 4 months neoadjuvant	65–70 Gy RT	$p = 0.73$ overall. Significant benefit ($p = 0.044$) in subset with Gleason 8–10
EORTC 22961 Bolla et al. (2009)	2009	T1c–T2abN1M0 T2c–4N0-1M0	970	LHRHa 6 months versus 3 years	70 Gy 3D-CRT	Better result with 3-year treatment than with 6 months (+3.8 % survival at 5 year)
Androgen suppression therapy + radiotherapy versus androgen suppression alone						
SPCGF-7/SFUO-3 Widmark et al. (2009)	2009	T1b-T2 Grade 2–3 T3N0M0	880	LHRHa 3 months + continuous flutamide	70 Gy RT versus no RT	Significantly better survival with combined treatment (HR = 0.68.95 % CI: 0.52–0.89, $p = 0.004$)
NCIC CTG PR.3 MRC PRO7/SWOG Warde et al. (2010)	2010 ASCO	T3-4 N0M0	1,205	Continuous LHRHa	60–65 Gy RT versus no RT	Significant benefit in favor of combined treatment (HR = 0.77.95 % CI 0.61–0.98, $p = 0.033$)
French study Mottet et al. (2010)	2010 ASCO	T3–4 N0M0	273	LHRHa for 3 years	70 Gy 3D-RT versus no RT	Significant reduction of clinical progression. Effect on overall survival not reported

Table 3 from Bolla et al. (2010a), Lancet Oncology, page 1071, authorization given

M0 to compare RT with concomitant and adjuvant ADT to RT alone, and a deferred ADT in case of relapse; 82 % of the patients were T3, 10 % T4, and 89 % N0. The hormone treatment was oral cyproterone acetate, 50 mg 3 times daily for 1 month, beginning 1 week before the start of RT and subcutaneous injection of Zoladex® 3.6 mg every 4 weeks for 3 years starting on the first day of RT. The pelvic target volume received 50 Gy and the prostatic target volume 20 Gy. With a median follow-up of 66 months, there was a significant difference in overall survival, 78 % in favor of the combination versus 62 % for RT alone ($p = 0.001$) (Bolla et al. 2002). The 10-year results (median follow-up of 9.1 years), confirm that the addition of HT increased the clinical disease-free survival from 22.7 to 47.7 % ($P < 0.0001$), distant progression free survival (PFS) from 30.2 to 51.0 % ($P < 0.0001$), and overall survival from 39.8 to 58.1 % ($P = 0.0004$). The 10-year PCa mortality was 30.4 % with RT alone and 10.3 % with long-term ADT combined with RT ($P < 0.001$) (Bolla et al. 2010a) and no significant difference in cardiovascular mortality was noted between treatment groups.

3.1.2 Long-Term LHRH Adjuvant Androgen Deprivation Therapy

The RTOG Trial 85-31 was designed to evaluate the effectiveness of indefinite Zoladex® alone after RT; 977 patients with stages T3–T4 M0 with or without lymph node involvement, or pT3 after radical prostatectomy in the event of capsule invasion, positive margins, or seminal vesicle involvement were included. Monthly administration of Zoladex® was started during the last week of RT and was continued indefinitely or until relapse (arm 1) or started at relapse (arm 2); no antiandrogen was given at the very start of Zoladex® to inhibit the initial rise of LH and then of testosterone. Fifteen percent of patients had undergone radical prostatectomy in arm 1 and 14 % in arm 2, and 29 and 26 % had lymph node involvement, respectively. The pelvic target volume received 45 Gy and the prostate target volume 65–70 Gy. Patients with a pT3 tumor received 60–65 Gy to the postoperative target volume. The combined approach has been associated with all 8-year efficacy endpoints except overall survival (49 % vs. 47 % ($p = 0.36$)); subset analysis by Gleason score, revealed a significant overall survival ($p = 0.036$) in favor of the adjuvant HT arm for centrally reviewed Gleason 8–10 patients who had not previously undergone prostatectomy (Lawton et al. 2001). In the updated results of the trial after a median follow-up time of 7.6 years, statistical significances were reached in favor of the adjuvant HT arm for 10-year overall survival (49 % vs 39 %, $p < 0.002$), 10-year incidence of distant metastases (24 % vs 39 %, $p < 0.001$), and disease specific mortality (16 % vs 22 %, $p = 0.005$) (Pilepich et al. 2005).

A subset analysis of the RTOG 85-13 trial evaluated 173 patients with biopsy proven pN1 lymph nodes of whom 98 received RT plus adjuvant HT; with a median follow-up of 6.5 years multivariate analysis revealed that the combined approach had a statistical impact on all endpoints: overall survival ($p = 0.03$), disease-specific failure ($p = 0.014$), metastatic failure ($p < 0.0005$), and biochemical control ($p < 0.0001$) (Lawton et al. 1997). These data are in keeping with those of Gransfors et al. (1998) who compared for T1-4 pN0-3 M0 patients, the combination of orchiectomy and RT ($n = 45$) to RT alone and androgen ablation deferred at clinical disease progression ($n = 46$). The study was prematurely closed due to an insufficient accrual, and after a median follow-up of 9.3 years there was a significant difference in overall survival ($p = 0.02$) and progression free survival ($p = 0.005$) in favor of the combined arm; this difference was mainly caused by lymph node positive tumors. In conclusion, patients with pathologically or clinically involved pelvic lymph nodes should be considered for RT plus immediate long-term HT (level of evidence 2b).

3.1.3 Long-Term Anti-Androgen Adjuvant Monotherapy

The Early PCa Program consisting of 3 randomized, double-blind placebo-controlled trials included 1370 patients with T1-4, any N M0 PCa. A nonsteroidal antiandrogen—bicalutamide (Casodex®) 150 mg/day orally was given as immediate adjuvant to RT during 2 years (trial 23), 5 years (trial 24), or until progression (trial 25), as an alternative to castration due to the potential benefits in term of sexual interest, physical capacity, and maintenance of bone mineral density. At a median follow-up of 5.3 years (Tyrell et al. 2005) bicalutamide 150 mg significantly reduced the risk of disease progression ($p = 0.003$) in patients with locally advanced PCa ($n = 305$).

3.1.4 Neoadjuvant and Concomitant Short-Term Androgen Deprivation Therapy

The RTOG trial 86-10 was designed to test the potential value of a combined ADT prior (2 months) and during RT (2 months) with respect to RT alone, or at relapse: 471 patients with bulky (5 × 5 cm) tumors (T2-4) with or without regional lymph node involvement were included: 7 % had a positive nodal status in the combined treatment arm versus 9 % in the RT alone arm. Thirty percent of patients had a T2 tumor, and 70 % were classified as T3-4. Hormonal treatment consisted of oral flutamide (250 mg 3 × day) and a subcutaneous injection of Zoladex® 3.6 mg every 4 weeks (Pilepich et al. 2001). The pelvis received 45 Gy and the prostate target volume 65–70 Gy. At 8 years, ADT has been associated with all efficacy endpoints except overall survival, but subset analysis demonstrated that a significant enhancement in overall survival was seen in patients with Gleason score 2–6: 70 % versus 52 %; $p = 0.015$. These results were maintained at 10-year with a significant difference in disease specific mortality (23 % vs. 36 %; $p = 0.01$), distant metastases (35 % vs. 47 %; $p = 0.006$), disease-free survival (11 % vs. 3 %; $p < 0.0001$), but no difference in 10-year overall survival (43 % vs. 34 %; $p = 0.12$) (Roach et al. 2008).

The Trans-Tasman Radiation Oncology Group 96.01 trial has included 818 men randomly assigned to RT alone (66 Gy/ 33 fractions) (Scardino et al. 2003; Denham et al. 2005) 3 months' androgen deprivation with goserelin and flutamide starting 2 months before RT; or 6 months' ADT with the same regimen starting 5 months before RT. After a median follow-up of 10.6 years, compared with patients assigned RT alone, those assigned to 3 months' ADT had a decrease cumulative incidence of PSA progression ($p = 0.003$), and local progression ($p = 0.0005$), and event-free survival ($p = 0.0001$). Six months' ADT-reduced PSA progression ($p < 0.0001$) and local progression ($p = 0.0001$) and led to a greater improvement in event-free survival ($p < 0.0001$); moreover 6 months' ADT decreased distant progression ($p = 0.001$), cancer-specific mortality ($p = 0.0008$), and all-cause mortality ($p = 0.0008$) compared with RT alone (Denham et al. 2011).

These two trials suggest that the significant impact of HT on disease-specific survival is certainly due to the concomitant component of HT during RT. In the trial reported by Crook's et al. (2004), 378 patients were randomized between 3 months or 8 months neoadjuvant combined ADT with flutamide and gosereline before RT (66 Gy): with a median follow-up of 44 months there was no impact on biochemical control or survival.

Nevertheless, starting ADT 2 or 3 months before RT (and continuing it during RT) may be useful to decrease the tumor volume of high risk PCa and to improve the dose to organs at risk.

3.1.5 Short-Term Neoadjuvant Versus Short-Term Adjuvant Combined Androgen Deprivation Therapy with Whole Pelvis or Prostate Only Radiotherapy

RTOG 94-13 study is a four arm trial devoted to 1323 patients T1c-4 N0 M0 PSA <100 ng with an estimated risk of lymph node involvement >15 % based on the equation: risk of positive nodes = (2/3) PSA + ((GS)-6) × 10). The first randomization is done between neoadjuvant concurrent ADT (NCADT)—2 months before and 2 months during RT—and 4-month adjuvant hormone therapy (AADT) after RT; the second randomization took place between whole pelvis radiotherapy (WPRT) followed by a boost to the prostate or prostate only radiotherapy (PORT). WPRT plus NCADT improved the 4-year progression free survival (61 %) compared with PORT + NCADT (45 %), PORT + AADT (49 %) and WPRT + AADT (47 %) ($p = 0.008$) and there was no advantage to WPRT over PORT without neoadjuvant ADT (Roach et al. 2003). With longer follow-up progression free survival and biochemical failure (Phoenix definition) continue to favor the WPRT arm ($p = 0.034$ and 0.0098, respectively) but we await the major secondary endpoints, cause-specific and overall survival, since not enough events had occurred (Lawton et al. 2007).

3.1.6 Long-Term Androgen Deprivation Therapy Alone is Inferior to Long-Term Androgen Deprivation Therapy Plus Radiation Therapy

The above-mentioned studies have shown the efficacy of hormonal treatment combined with RT, but the impact of LTADT alone was not assessed so far. The SPCG-7/SFUO-3 trial has included 875 patients T1b–T2, G2–G3, or T3 any WHO histological grade (1–3) (78 % of T3) with baseline PSA < 70 ng/ml; patients were randomly allocated to endocrine treatment alone with 3 months of total androgen blockade followed by continuous flutamide ($n = 439$ patients), or to the same endocrine treatment combined with RT ($n = 436$ patients). After a median follow-up of 7.6 years, the cumulative incidence at 10 years for PCa specific mortality was 23.9 % in the endocrine alone group and 11.9 % in the endocrine plus RT group for a relative risk of 0.44 (0.30–0.66); the cumulative incidence for overall mortality was 39.4 % and 29.6 % with a relative risk of 0.68 (0.52–0.89) (Widmark et al. 2009). In conclusion, in patients with locally advanced or high risk localized PCa, the combination of RT to HT halved the 10-year PCa specific mortality and decreased overall mortality with fully acceptable risk of side-effects, compared to HT alone.

Protocol NCIC CTG PR-3/MRC PR07/SWOG included 1205 patients with T3-4 ($n = 1057$) or T2, PSA > 40 ng/ml ($n = 119$), or T2, PSA > 20 ng and Gleason > 8 ($n = 25$) and N0-X M0 PCa who were randomized to lifelong ADT (bilateral orchidectomy or LHRH agonist) with or without RT (65–70 Gy to prostate ± 45 Gy to pelvic lymph nodes). With a median follow-up of 6 years, the addition of RT to ADT significantly reduced the risk of death ($p = 0.033$) and the risk of specific death ($p = 0.001$) (Warde et al. 2010).

The Mottet trial included 273 patients with locally advanced PCa T3-4 or pT3 N0 M0 randomly assigned to lifelong ADT by LHRH agonist (leuproreline) with or without RT (70 Gy to prostate plus 48 ± 2 Gy to pelvic lymph nodes). With a median follow-up of 67 months, there was a significant improvement of the 5-year disease-free survival ($p < 0.001$), metastatic disease-free survival ($p < 0.018$) loco-regional progression free survival ($p < 0.0002$), but the effect on overall survival was not reported (Mottet et al. 2010).

3.1.7 Short-Term Androgen Deprivation Therapy is Inferior to Long-Term Androgen Deprivation

The aim of RTOG protocol 92-02 devoted to 1554 patients classified T2c-4N0, was to investigate the value of a long-term adjuvant ADT (LTADT) after a short-term ADT (STADT). All patients received 2 months of CADT with Zoladex® and flutamide before RT, followed during RT; a radiation dose of 65–70 Gy was given to the prostate. Patients were randomly assigned to receive no additional therapy or 24 months of Zoladex®. Compared with the STADT, the LTADT arm showed significant improvement in all efficacy endpoints except 5-year overall survival; in a subset of patients Gleason scores 8–10, the LTADT arm had significantly better overall survival: 81 % versus 70.7 % ($p = 0.04$) (Hanks et al. 2003). The 10-year results confirmed significant benefits in all 10-year efficacy endpoints terms except overall survival ($p = 0.35$); in a subset analysis the overall survival benefit was limited to patients with Gleason score 8–10 ($p = 0.006$) (Horwitz et al. 2008).

EORTC (22863) and RTOG (85–31) trials have demonstrated that LTADT (>2 years) is recommended for high risk PCa (level I evidence) but they do not determine the optimal duration of hormonal treatment combined with external beam RT. That is why the EORTC equivalence trial 22961 randomly assigned patients who had received 3D-CRT plus 6 months of ADT in two groups: one to receive no further treatment (STADT) and the other to receive 2.5 years of further treatment (LTADT) with a LHRH agonist, triptoreline, Decapeptyl 11.25 mg®. An outcome of noninferiority of STADT as compared to LTADT required a hazard ratio of more than 1.35 for overall survival, with a one-sided alpha level of 0.05. An interim analysis showed futility, and the results are presented with an adjusted one-sided alpha level of 0.0429. 970 patients were randomized: 483 STADT and 487 LTADT. At a median follow-up of 6.4 years, the 5-year overall survival shows 84.8 % for the LTADT arm and 81 % for the STADT arm with an estimated hazard ratio of 1.42 ($P = 0.008$). The 5-year clinical progression free survival was 80.5 % for the LTADT arm and 68.7 % for STADT arm ($P < 0.0001$). The 5-year biochemical progression free survival was 77.7 % on the LTADT arm versus. 56.8 %on the STAD arm P < 0.0001. In conclusion, the combination of RT plus 6 months of ADT provides inferior survival as compared with RT plus 3 years of ADT (Bolla et al. 2009).

Additional support can be found in a retrospective analysis assessing combined HT with RT (median follow-up >45 months) which showed that long-term ADT (median duration 25.6 months) improves 5-year overall survival (87.5 %) with respect to short-term ADT (75 %) ($p = 0.009$) in patients with a PSA level >20 ng/ml, irrespective of Gleason score and T stage (Berthelet et al. 2005).

3.2 Intermediate and High Risk Localized Prostate Cancer

3.2.1 6-Month Neoadjuvant and Concomitant Short-Term Androgen Deprivation Therapy

The Boston group published a small trial concerning 206 men with localized (T1b-T2b N0-X M0) but unfavorable-risk PCa (baseline PSA $\geq$ 10 ng/ml and $\leq$40 ng or a Gleason score of at least 7); patients were randomized to receive RT alone (70 Gy 3D-CRT) or RT plus 6 months of ADT; low risk patients were ineligible unless they had radiologic evidence of extracapsular extension or seminal vesicle invasion. After a median follow-up of 4.5 years, patients who received 3D-CRT plus ADT had a higher survival ($p = 0.04$) and a lower cancer-specific mortality ($p = 0.02$) (D'Amico et al. 2004). With a median follow-up of 7.6 years, overall survival was higher for men who were randomized RT and ADT compared with RT: 74 % versus 61 % ($p = 0.01$), but the survival benefit varies according comorbidity: among the 49 patients with moderate or severe comorbidity, the 8-year overall survival was 25 % for those randomized to RT and ADT as compared to 54 % for those with RT ($p = 0.08$) (D'Amico et al. 2008a).

3.2.2 4-Month Neoadjuvant and Concomitant Short-Term Androgen Deprivation Therapy

In RTOG trial 94-08 (Jones et al. 2011) which has accrued 1979 patients with T1b–T2b localized PCa, a stratification was done with PSA ($\leq$ 20 ng/ml), histological grade and nodal status. Patients were randomized between neodjuvant CADT, 2 months before conventional RT (66.6 Gy) and 2 months during RT versus RT alone. The 10-year overall survival was 62 % for the combined approach as compared with 57 % ($p = 0.03$) among patients receiving RT alone. Biochemical failure, distant metastases, and the rate of positive findings on repeat prostate biopsy at 2 years were significantly improved with RT plus STADT, but the gains in overall survival and reductions in disease specific mortality were mainly limited to men in the intermediate risk subgroup.

In conclusion, 6-month of neoadjuvant and concomitant CADT combined with 3D-CRT (70 Gy) improved overall survival in men with intermediate or poor-risk localized PCa without moderate or severe comorbidity, meanwhile a conventional RT (66.6 Gy) plus 4-month of CADT improves overall survival only in men with intermediate localized PCa.

4 New Trends

4.1 4–6 Month Combined Androgen Deprivation Therapy Versus 6-Month LHRH Analog

The rationale of using an anti-androgen in association with an LHRH agonist is: (1) to block the androgens of adrenal origin, which are left free to continue to stimulate PCa (Labrie et al. 1993); (2) to block the androgen receptors (AR) to prevent the so-called "flare" that can result due to the surge in testosterone resulting from the use of LHRH agonist; and (3) to contribute independent anti-tumor activity. To know the optimal duration of combined androgen blockade in high risk patients would require a large phase III randomized trial. Since a meta-analysis of 27 randomized trials devoted to advanced PCa has shown that the addition of an anti-androgen to androgen deprivation, improved the 5-year survival by about 2 or 3 %, with a range of uncertainty between 0 and 5 %, it is unlikely that the effect would be very large (PCTCG 2000); but a small effect in patients with metastatic disease might be larger in men with high risk localized PCa analogous to the benefits of adjuvant 5-Fu chemotherapy for regional as compared to metastatic disease (Bauer and Spitz 1998; Colucci et al. 1999; Focan et al. 2000). Considering the positive impact of 4-month (Jones et al. 2011) or 6-month (D'Amico et al. 2008a) CADT on the overall survival of intermediate and high risk localized PCa and the positive impact of 6-month CADT on locally advanced PCa (Denham et al. 2011), CADT has to be preferred to LHRH agonists alone. Moreover, it has been shown that men with localized but unfavorable-risk PCa who were treated with RT and 6-month of planned combined ADT appear to have an increased risk of recurrence when treated with less than as compared with 6 months of the antiandrogen; recurrence risk was significantly decreased ($p = 0.001$) with each additional month of antiandrogen use after analysis adjustment for prognostic factors (D'Amico et al. 2008b).

4.2 Androgen Deprivation Therapy Plus Dose Escalation

IMRT and image-guided RT allow dose escalation without increasing acute or late toxicity; a meta-analysis of 7 randomized controlled trials accruing 2812 patients showed a significant reduction in the incidence of biochemical failure in those patients treated with high dose RT ($p < 0.0001$) (Viani et al. 2009). The MD Anderson Cancer Center phase III trial (Kuban et al. 2008), which accrued 301 patients with stage T1b to T3, was the first to show an improvement in freedom from biochemical failure or clinical failure in favor of the 78 Gy arm: 78 % as compared with 59 % for the 70 Gy arm ($p = 0.004$) with an even greater benefit in patients with initial PSA >10 ng/ml: 78 % versus 39 % ($p = 0.0014$). Dose escalation will be more developed in a further chapter devoted to that topic.

4.2.1 Intermediate Risk Localized Prostate Cancer

Two phase III trials have shown the gain in overall survival linked to the combination of conventional RT with ADT (D'Amico et al. 2008a; Jones et al. 2011). A retrospective analysis on a cohort of 1044 patients with intermediate ($n = 782$) or high risk ($n = 262$) PCa treated with dose escalated external beam RT alone, brachytherapy or high dose rate brachytherapy plus pelvic external beam RT, has shown—with a 5-year median follow-up- that no advantages in any clinical endpoints at 8 years were associated with ADT administration: the loco-regional failure rate was 5 % with or without ADT and the 8-year cause-specific survival was 97 % with ADT versus 99 % without ($p = 0.20$) (Krauss et al. 2011). Another retrospective study concerning 919 stage T1–T3 N0M0 patients—with a median follow-up of 97 months—treated with RT alone supports such an approach: the 7-year local failure rate stratified by dose group (<72 Gy, >72 but <82 Gy, and >82 Gy was 6, 2 and 2 %, respectively ($p = 0.012$) and the 7-year distant metastases rate 9, 6 and 1 %, respectively ($p = 0.008$) (Kupelian et al. 2008). The GETUG 14 randomized trial has addressed this question in 377 patients with localized intermediate risk PCa; lymphadenectomy was mandatory when the risk of node involvement was >10 %. Patients were randomly assigned to high dose RT (prostate 80 Gy; seminal vesicles 46 Gy) either alone or in combination with 4-month CADT (flutamide + Decapeptyl® starting 2 months before RT). With 37 months median follow-up, the 3-year biochemical or clinical control probabilities were 86 % and 92 % in RT and CADT-RT groups, respectively ($p = 0.09$) and the 3-year biochemical control probabilities 91 % and 97 % ($p = 0.04$) (Dubray et al. 2011).

Dose escalation alone may be proposed to patients who are reticent to short-term ADT due to comorbidities or because they want to preserve their sexual health, provided the prostate dose delivered by image-guided IMRT is around 80 Gy.

4.2.2 High risk Localized Prostate Cancer

We do not have data comparing high dose RT alone (78/80 Gy) vs 70 Gy plus ADT; the combined approach has to remain with a dose escalation. Dearnaley et al. reported the findings of the MRC Trial RT01 with 843 men with localized PCa randomly assigned to standard dose (64 Gy) or escalated dose (74 Gy), both delivered with conformal RT with neoadjuvant CADT. The freedom from PSA failure was better ($p = 0.0007$) for the dose escalated arm and the

5 year control rate was 71 % for the dose escalated arm compared to 60 % for conventional dose arm ($p = 0.16$). Of note, there was also a trend for improved freedom from salvage ADT ($p = 0.12$) and metastases-free survival ($p = 0.21$) (Dearnaley et al. 2007).

4.2.3 Locally Advanced Prostate Cancer

Dose escalation will certainly have an impact on survival outcomes, as suggested by the Zapatero trial (2005) based on a cohort of 416 patients: low risk treated by 3D-CRT alone ($n = 181$), intermediate risk allocated to receive neoadjuvant 4–6 months before and during 3D-CRT ($n = 160$) and high risk receiving neoadjuvant and adjuvant 3D-CRT 2 years after RT ($n = 75$). With a stratification for treatment groups the 5-year biochemical disease-free survival for high risk patients with ADT was 63 % for dose <72 Gy and, 84 % for dose $\geq$72 Gy ($p = 0.003$). In a MSKCC retrospective analysis (Zelefsky et al. 2008), 296 T3 patients were treated with dose escalation and 189 patients (43 %) were treated with STAS prior to RT. They noted that 3D-CRT ± IMRT was associated with excellent tumor control and survival outcomes with a 10-year local control rates of 88 % and a 10-year cause-specific survival of 83 %, respectively 88 % for T3a and 79 % for T3b. The incidence of late grade 3 urinary and rectal toxicities was remarkable at only 4 and 1 %.

In conclusion, in the management of locally advanced PCa treated by a combined approach-despite the absence of level I evidence for a significant impact on overall survival—dose escalation with IMRT is recommended up to 76–78 Gy.

4.3 Pelvic Lymph Node Irradiation

This topic remains controversial. The RTOG 94-13 trial (Crook et al. 2004; Roach et al. 2003; Lawton et al. 2007) has shown a positive impact of neoadjuvant ADT on progression free survival with whole pelvic RT, not confirmed by the GETUG-01 trial (Pommier et al. 2007): (i) the GETUG trial included 444 T1b-T3 N0-pNX M0 patients while more than 1200 were recruited in RTOG 94-13. (ii) the GETUG trial allowed a STADT, but not required it for patients in the high risk group; also 56.8 % of the patients in that trial had a lymph node risk lower than 15 % according to the Roach formula (thus the number of patients at risk for positive nodes was much smaller than in RTOG 94-13) (Roach et al. 2006). (iii) in GETUG no patients received whole pelvic RT using the RTOG cut-off at the L5 S1 interspace, which is considered by RTOG investigators to be a critical determinant of outcome (Pommier et al. 2007). (iv) no difference in 5-year PFS between the pelvic (46 Gy) and prostate RT (66–70 Gy) arm was noted in the GETUG trial, with a 42-month median follow-up. The definition of the limit of the pelvic fields is of paramount importance and Shih et al. (Shih et al. 2005) have shown that by using lymphotropic nanoparticules-enhanced magnetic resonance imaging, 80 % of the metastatic nodes were located only in the pelvis with a superior border of 2 cm above the common iliac bifurcation; moreover lateral rectal shielding to reduce the rectal dose contribution resulted in an underdosage of the presacral lymph nodes (Sanguineti et al. 2006).

In daily practice, pelvic irradiation is not considered for localized or intermediate risk localized PCa; conversely high risk and locally advanced PCa required pelvic irradiation all the more as an RTOG consensus on pelvic lymph node CTVs was reached available as web-based computed tomography images allowing to choose an optimal IMRT technique to cover the correct lymph node volume and to prescribe an appropriate dose Lawton et al. (2009a, b).

4.4 Adjuvant Chemotherapy

Taxanes are radiosensitizing agents, which block the cell cycle during the G2/M-phase, inhibit the antiapoptotic effect of *bcl-2*, and induce apoptosis (Milas et al. 1999; Schiff et al. 1979). Moreover, docetaxel has been shown to produce a cytotoxic effect during the S-phase, known to be radioresistant (Hennequin et al. 1995). In androgen-dependent and independent human PCa xenografts, docetaxel showed a significant antitumoral effect in hormone-sensitive tumors compared with mitoxantrone and estramustine (Oudard et al. 2003). In patients with castration-resistant prostate cancer, the results of randomized trials showed a significant improvement in biological response and survival in favor of docetaxel-containing regimens compared with the reference treatment (Petrylak et al. 2004; Tannock et al. 2004). These results have prompted testing the drug in locally advanced PCa within the frame of phase II trials assessing the feasibility of concomitant (Kumar et al. 2004) or concomitant and adjuvant docetaxel (Bolla et al. 2010b) with RT and phase III randomized trials assessing the role of adjuvant docetaxel with ADT and RT (RTOG 2009). The GETUG 12 trial has addressed the role of neoadjuvant chemotherapy with docetaxel on PFS in a cohort of 413 high risk patients defined as $\geq$1 of the following criteria: T3-4, Gleason score $\geq$8, PSA $\geq$20 ng/ml, pN + ; patients were randomly assigned to either goserelin 10.8 mg every 3 months for 3 years and 4 cycles of docetaxel 70 mg/m^2 q3w plus estramustine 10 mg/kg/d d1-5 (arm 1) or goserelin alone (arm 2). Local the RT rapy was administered at 3 months which consisted of RT in 358 patients (87 %). Toxicity included grade 3–4 neutropenia (27 %) with neutropenic fever in 2 % but no toxicity-related death and no secondary leukemia. With a median follow-up of 4.6 years, the 4-year PFS was 85 % in arm 1 versus 81 % in arm 2 ($p = 0.26$) (Fizazi et al. 2011), but data need to mature.

5 Health-Related Quality of Life-Related to Androgen Deprivation Therapy

ADT with LHRH agonists is known to adversely affect quality of life, leading to hot flushes, fatigue, impact on cognitive function, depression, sexual side effects, anemia, weight gain, insulin-resistance, bone mineral density loss (Israeli et al. 2008; Shahinian et al. 2005), increased diagnoses of cardiac disease (D'Amico et al. 2007), and metabolic side effects Smith et al. (2008a). These side effects assessed by a self-administered questionnaire (Potosky et al. 2001) are in relation with the prevalent comorbidities of the patients and the duration of the treatment. With regard to cardiovascular mortality the retrospective analysis made on the data of the EORTC and RTOG trials by taking into account all deaths linked to cardiovascular disease have shown that LTADT did not increase the cumulative incidence estimates of cardiovascular mortality as compared with short term or no ADT Bolla et al. (2009, 2010a; Efstathiou et al. 2008, 2009). Using data of the 92-02 RTOG trial, Smith et al. (2008b) have found that weight, but not prevalent diabetes is associated with PCa mortality in men undergoing combined treatment, but prevalent diabetes was associated with greater all-cause and non PCa mortality. Many studies have demonstrated that chronic ADT was associated with an increased risk of fractures: Shahinian et al. (2005) studying records from the Surveillance, Epidemiology, and end results database and Medicare, mention that of men surviving at least 5 years, 19.4 % of those who received ADT had a fracture versus 12.6 % of those not receiving this treatment ($p < 0.001$). After RT and 6 months of androgen blockade, fatigue, hot flushes, and sexual problems increased significantly both statistically ($p < 0.001$) and clinically (Bolla et al. 2009); for patients continuing ADT after 6 months for 2.5 years more, there were statistically significant differences between the groups in term of insomnia ($p = 0.006$), hot flushes ($p < 0.001$), and sexual interest and activity ($p < 0.001$), but overall quality of life did not differ significantly between the two groups ($p = 0.37$) (Bolla et al. 2009) . In the phase III bicalutamide trial, the adverse events among patients receiving 150 mg plus RT ($n = 694$) were breast pain (74.8 %), gynaecomastia (66.6 %), diarrhoea (15.4 %), asthenia (13.4 %), impotence (12.7 %), hot flushes (9.8 %) which were mild to moderate >90 % of cases.

All these potential side effects have to be discussed in depth with the patients, taking into account age, WHO performance status, comorbidities, blood count, and the recommendations of a multidisciplinary approach. They must not dissuade radiation oncologists from prescribing LHRH agonists after obtaining an informed consent, however the treating radiation oncologists must advise patients to observe regular physical exercise and modification of diet to prevent or minimize these side effects, and to pay attention to a careful monitoring of blood pressure, lipid, and glucose levels according to the status of the patient with the help of the general practitioner. In case of long-term ADT, an adequate timing for the measurement of bone mineral density by dual-energy X-ray absorptiometry is also recommended to enable a pharmacological treatment by biphosphonate in case of osteoporosis when the T-score is <2.5 (Diamond et al. 2004).

6 Ongoing Prospective Trials

The RTOG-0815 trial is devoted to intermediate risk localized PCa. The aim is to demonstrate an overall survival advantage in favor of dose escalation with respect to a combination of a conventional dose EBRT plus a short-term ADT started 2 months before RT. RT is carried out at the discretion of treating physician with 3D-conformal RT or IMRT, meanwhile dose escalation is achieved with EBRT alone or brachytherapy (LDR or HDR); the target sample size is 1520 patients.

The GETUG 18 phase III trial is assessing the value of a dose escalation (80 Gy/40 fractions versus70 Gy/35 fractions) in patients with a high risk localized PCa submitted to a long-term androgen deprivation. The major end-point is the 5-year biochemical and clinical disease-free survival; the target sample size is 500 patients.

The RTOG 1115 phase III trial is aiming at evaluating the difference in overall survival of patients with high risk PCa treated by EBRT plus 24 months of CAB beginning 2 months before EBRT with respect to the same treatment plus 24 months of steroid 17 alpha-monooxygenase TAK-700. In both arms, patients undergo IMRT or 3D-conformal RT to the whole pelvis, followed by a prostatic boost by EBRT or brachytherapy; the target sample size is 900 patients.

7 Conclusions

In high risk PCa, the aim of ADT is to potentiate irradiation whatever its technique and to destroy the infraclinical disease outside the irradiated volume. Many phase III randomized trials have paved the way for establishing the indications of the combination of ADT with external irradiation. For locally advanced PCa, long-term ADT ($\geq$2 years) with LHRH agonists combined with external irradiation is a gold standard (level 1a of evidence); should there be a significant comorbidity, a reticence of the patient and/or a poor tolerance, a 6-month duration may be proposed. For high risk localized PCa a 4–6-month complete ADT is recommended (level 2a evidence). For intermediate risk localized PCa, patients may benefit from a combined approach with a short-term ADT. Image-guided IMRT allows a dose escalation for high risk PCa and may offer the opportunity to treat intermediate risk localized PCa without ADT. Nobody has the monopoly of the knowledge and the right way to find an adequate compromise is the multidisciplinary approach based on guidelines (Heidenreich et al. 2011). Patients have to be fully informed of the potential morbidity of ADT and a close cooperation is needed with general practitioners and specialists to prevent as much as possible harmful side effects.

References

Bagshaw MA, Cox RS, Ray GR (1988) Status of radiation treatment of prostate cancer at Stanford University. NCI Monogr 7:47–60

Bauer TW, Spitz FR (1998) Adjuvant and neoadjuvant chemoradiation therapy for primary colorectal cancer. Surg Oncol 7:175–181

Berthelet E, Pickles T, Lee KW, Liu M, Truong PT (2005) Long-term androgen deprivation therapy improves survival in prostate cancer patients presenting with prostate-specific antigen levels >20 ng/mL. Int J Radiat Oncol Biol Phys 63:781–787

Bolla M, Gonzalez D, Warde P et al (1997) Improved survival in patients with locally advanced prostate cancer treated with radiotherapy and goserilin. N Engl J Med 337:295–300

Bolla M, Collette L, Blank L et al (2002) Long-term results with immediate androgen suppression and external irradiation in patients with locally advanced prostate cancer (an EORTC study): a phase III randomised trial. Lancet 360:103–106

Bolla M, de Reijke TM, Van Tienhoven G et al (2009) Duration of androgen suppression in the treatment of prostate cancer. N Engl J Med 360:2516–2527

Bolla M, van Tienhoven G, Warde P et al (2010a) External irradiation with or without long-term androgen suppression for prostate cancer with high metastatic risk: 10-year results of an EORTC randmized study. Lancet Oncol 11:1066–1073

Bolla M, Hannoun-Levi JM, Ferrero JM et al (2010b) Concurrent and adjuvant docetaxel with three-dimensional conformal radiation therapy plus androgen deprivation for high-risk prostate cancer: preliminary results of a multicentre phase II trial. Radiother Oncol 197: 312–317

Colucci G, Maiello E, Gebbia V et al (1999) 5-fluorouracil and levofolinic acid with or without recombinant interferon-2b in patients with advanced colorectal carcinoma: a randomized multicenter study with stratification for tumor burden and liver involvement by the Southern Italy Oncology Group. Cancer 85:535–545

Crook J, Ludgate C, Malone S et al (2004) Report of a multicenter Canadian phase III randomized trial of 3 months versus 8 months neoadjuvant androgen deprivation before standard-dose radiotherapy for clinically localized prostate cancer. Int J Radiat Oncol Biol Phys 60:15–23

D'Amico AV, Manola J, Loffredo M, Renshaw AA, DellaCroce A, Kantoff PW (2004) 6-month androgen suppression plus radiation therapy vs radiation therapy alone for patients with clinically localized prostate cancer: a randomized controlled trial. JAMA 292:821–827

D'Amico AV, Denham JW, Crook J et al (2007) Influence of androgen suppression therapy for prostate cancer on the frequency and timing of fatal myocardial infarctions. J Clin Oncol 25:2420–2425

D'Amico AV, Chen MH, Renshaw AA, Loffredo M, Kantoff PW (2008a) Androgen suppression and radiation versus radiation alone for prostate cancer: a randomized trial. JAMA 299:289–295

D'Amico AV, Chen MH, Renshaw AA, Loffredo B, Kantoff PW (2008b) Risk of prostate cancer reccurence in men treated with radiation alone or in conjunction with combined or less than combined androgen suppression therapy. J Clin Oncol 26:2979–2983

Dearnaley DP, Sydes MR, Graham JD et al (2007) Escalated-dose versus standard-dose conformal radiotherapy in prostate cancer: first results from the MRC RT01 randomised controlled trial. Lancet Oncol 8:475–487

Denham JW, Steigler A, Lamb DS et al (2005) Short-term androgen deprivation and radiotherapy for locally advanced prostate cancer: results from the Trans-Tasman Radiation Oncology Group 96.01 randomised controlled trial. Lancet Oncol 6:841–850

Denham JW, Steigler A, Lamb DS, et al. (2011) Short term neoadjuvant androgen deprivation and radiotherapy for locally advanced prostate cancer: 10-year data from the TROG 96.01 randomised trial. Lancet Oncol 12(5): 145–149 (Epub ahead of print)

Diamond TH, Higano CS, Smith MR, Guise TA, Singer FR (2004) Osteoporosis in men with prostate carcinoma receiving androgen-deprivation therapy: recommendations for diagnosis and therapies. Cancer 100:892–899

Dubray BM, Beckendorf V, Guerif S et al (2011) Does short-term androgen depletion add to high-dose radiotherapy (80 Gy) in localized intermediate-risk prostate cancer? Intermediate analysis of GETUG 14 randomized trial (EU-20503/NCT00104741) J Clin Oncol 29(6):726–732:(suppl; abstr 4521)

Early Breast Cancer Trialists Collaboration Group (EBCTCG) (2005) Effects of chemotherapy and hormonal therapy for early breast cancer on recurrence and 15-year survival: an overview of the randomized trials. Lancet 365:1687–1717

Efstathiou JA, Bae K, Shipley WU et al (2008) Cardiovascular mortality and duration of androgen deprivation for locally advanced prostate cancer: analysis of RTOG 92-02. Eur Urol 54:816–823

Efstathiou JA, Bae K, Shipley WU et al (2009) Cardiovascular mortality after androgen deprivation therapy for locally advanced prostate cancer: RTOG 85-31. J Clin Oncol 27:92–99

Fellows GJ, Clark PB, Beynon LL et al (1992) Treatment of advanced localised prostatic cancer by orchiectomy, radiotherapy, or combined treatment. A medical research council study. Urological cancer working party-subgroup on prostatic cancer. Br J Urol 70:304–309

Fizazi K, Lesaunier F, Delva R et al (2011) Docetaxel-estramustine in high-risk localized prostate cancer: first results of the French Genitourinary Tumor Group phase III trial (GETUG12) J Cli Oncol 29 (suppl; abstr 4513)

Focan C, Bury J, Beauduin M et al (2000) Importance of 5-fluorouracil dose-intensity in a double randomised trial on adjuvant portal and systemic chemotherapy for Dukes B2 and C colorectal cancer. Anticancer Res 20:4665–4672

Granfors T, Modig H, Damber JE, Tomic R (1998) Combined orchiectomy and external radiotherapy versus radiotherapy alone for nonmetastatic prostate cancer with or without pelvic lymph node involvement: a prospective randomized study. J Urol 159:2030–2034

Granfors T, Modig H, Damber JE, Tomic R (2006) Long-term followup of a randomized study of locally advanced prostate cancer treated with combined orchiectomy and external radiotherapy versus radiotherapy alone. J Urol 176:544–547

Hanks GE, Corn BW, Lee WR, Hunt M, Hanlon A, Schultheiss TE (1995) External beam irradiation of prostate cancer. Conformal treatment techniques and outcomes for the 1990. Cancer 75:1972–1977

Hanks GE, Pajak TF, Porter A et al (2003) Phase III trial of long-term adjuvant androgen deprivation after neoadjuvant hormonal cytoreduction and radiotherapy in locally advanced carcinoma of the prostate: the Radiation Therapy Oncology Group Protocol 92-02. J Clin Oncol 21:3972–3978

Heidenreich A, Bellmunt J, Bolla M et al (2011) EAU Guidelines on Prostate Cancer. Part 1: Screening, Diagnosis, and Treatment of Clinically Localized Disease. Eur Urol 59(6):1–71

Hennequin C, Giocanti N, Favaudon V (1995) S-phase specificity of cell killing by docetaxel (Taxotere) in synchronised HeLa cells. Br J Cancer 71:1194–1198

Horwitz EM, Bae K, Hanks GE et al (2008) Ten-year follow-up of radiation therapy oncology group protocol 92-02: a phase III trial of the duration of elective androgen deprivation in locally advanced prostate cancer. J Clin Oncol 26:2497–2504

Huggins C, Stevens RE, Hodges CV (1941) Studies on prostatic cancer. The effects of castration on advanced carcinoma of the prostate gland. Arch Surg 43:209–243

Israeli RS, Ryan CW, Jung LL (2008) Managing bone loss in men with locally advanced prostate cancer receiving androgen deprivation therapy. J Urol 179:414–423

Jones CU, Hunt D, McGowan DG et al (2011) Radiotherapy and short-term androgen deprivation for localized prostate cancer. N Engl J Med 365:107–118

Joon DL, Hasegawa M, Sikes C et al (1997) Supraadditive apoptotic response of R3327-G rat prostate tumors to androgen ablation and radiation. Int J Radiat Oncol Biol Phys 38:1071–1077

Kaminski JM, Hanlon AL, Joon DL, Meistrich M, Hachem P, Pollack A (2003) Effect of sequencing of androgen deprivation and radiotherapy on prostate cancer growth. Int J Radiat Oncol Biol Phys 57:24–28

Krauss D, Kestin L, Ye H et al (2011) Lack of benefit for the addition of androgen deprivation therapy to dose-escalated radiotherapy in the treatment of intermediate and high risk prostate cancer. Int J Radiat Oncol Biol Phys 80:1064–1071

Kuban DA, Tucker SL, Dong L et al (2008) Long-term results of the M. D. Anderson randomized dose-escalation trial for prostate cancer. Int J Radiat Oncol Biol Phys 70:67–74

Kumar P, Perrotti M, Weiss R et al (2004) Phase I trial of weekly docetaxel with concurrent three-dimensional conformal radiation therapy in the treatment of unfavorable localized adenocarcinoma of the prostate. J Clin Oncol 22:1909–1915

Kupelian PA, Ciezki J, Chandana AR et al (2008) Effect of increasing radiation doses on local and distant failures in patients with localized prostate cancer. Int J Radiat Oncol Biol Phys 71:16–22

Labrie F, Belanger A, Simard J, Labrie C, Dupont A (1993) Combination therapy for prostate cancer. Endocrine and biologic basis of its choice as new standard first-line therapy. Cancer 71:1059–1067

Lawton CA, Winter K, Byhardt R et al (1997) Androgen suppression plus radiation versus radiation alone for patients with D1 (pN+) adenocarcinoma of the prostate (results based on a national prospective randomized trial, RTOG 85-31). Radiation Therapy Oncology Group. Int J Radiat Oncol Biol Phys 38:931–939

Lawton CA, Winter K, Murray K et al (2001) Updated results of the phase III Radiation Therapy Oncology Group (RTOG) trial 85-31 evaluating the potential benefit of androgen suppression following standard radiation therapy for unfavorable prognosis carcinoma of the prostate. Int J Radiat Oncol Biol Phys 49:937–946

Lawton CA, DeSilvio M, Roach M 3rd et al (2007) An update of the phase III trial comparing whole pelvic to prostate only radiotherapy and neoadjuvant to adjuvant total androgen suppression: updated analysis of RTOG 94-13, with emphasis on unexpected hormone/radiation interactions. Int J Radiat Oncol Biol Phys 69:646–655

Lawton CA, Michalski J, El-Naqa I et al (2009a) Variation in the definition of clinical target volumes for pelvic nodal conformal radiation therapy for prostate cancer. Int J Radiat Oncol Biol Phys 74:377–382

Lawton CA, Michalski J, El-Naqa I et al (2009b) RTOG GU Radiation Oncology specialists reach consensus on pelvic lymph node volumes for high-risk prostate cancer. Int J Radiat Oncol Biol Phys 74:383–387

Maximum androgen blockade in advanced prostate cancer: an overview of the randomised trials. Prostate Cancer Trialists' Collaborative Group (2000) Lancet 355:1491–1498

Milas L, Milas MM, Mason KA (1999) Combination of taxanes with radiation: preclinical studies. Semin Radiat Oncol 9:12–26

Mottet N, Peneau M, Mazeron J et al (2010) Impact of radiotherapy (RT) combined with androgen deprivation (ADT) versus ADT alone for local control in clinically locally advanced prostate cancer. Proc Am Soc Clin Oncol 28(19):3107–3114 abstr CRA4505

Oudard S, Legrier ME, Boye K et al (2003) Activity of docetaxel with or without estramustinephosphate versus mitoxantrone in androgen dependent and independent human prostate cancer xenografts. J Urol 169:1729–1734

Parmar H, Philipps RH, Lightman SL, Edwards L, Allen L, Schally AV (1985) Randomised controlled study of orchidectomy versus long-acting D-Trp-6-LHRH microcapsules in advanced prostatic carcinoma. Lancet 2:1201–1205

Petrylak DP, Tangen CM, Hussain MH et al (2004) Docetaxel and estramustine compared with mitoxantrone and prednisone for advanced refractory prostate cancer. N Engl J Med 351:1513–1520

Pilepich MV, Winter K, John MJ et al (2001) Phase III radiation therapy oncology group (RTOG) trial 86-10 of androgen deprivation adjuvant to definitive radiotherapy in locally advanced carcinoma of the prostate. Int J Radiat Oncol Biol Phys 50:1243–1252

Pilepich MV, Winter K, Lawton CA et al (2005) Androgen suppression adjuvant to definitive radiotherapy in prostate carcinoma–long-term results of phase III RTOG 85-31. Int J Radiat Oncol Biol Phys 61:1285–1290

Pommier P, Chabaud S, Lagrange JL et al (2007) Is there a role for pelvic irradiation in localized prostate adenocarcinoma? Preliminary results of GETUG-01. J Clin Oncol 25:5366–5373

Potosky AL, Knopf K, Clegg LX et al (2001) Quality-of-life outcomes after primary androgen deprivation therapy: results from the Prostate Cancer Outcomes Study. J Clin Oncol 19:3750–3757

Roach M 3rd, DeSilvio M, Lawton C et al (2003) Phase III trial comparing whole-pelvic versus prostate-only radiotherapy and neoadjuvant versus adjuvant combined androgen suppression: Radiation Therapy Oncology Group 94-13. J Clin Oncol 21:1904–1911

Roach M 3rd, DeSilvio M, Valicenti R et al (2006) Whole-pelvis, "mini-pelvis," or prostate only external beam radiotherapy after neoadjuvant, concurrent hormonal therapy in patients treated in the Radiation Therapy Oncology Group 9413 trial. Int J Radiat Oncol Biol Phys 66:647–653

Roach M 3rd, Bae K, Speight J et al (2008) Short-term neoadjuvant androgen deprivation therapy and external-beam radiotherapy for locally advanced prostate cancer: long-term results of RTOG 86-10. J Clin Oncol 26:585–591

RTOG 05-21:A phase III protocol of androgen suppression (AS) and 3D CRT/IMRT vs AS and 3D CRT/IMRT followed by chemotherapy with docetaxel and prednisone for localized high risk prostate cancer. [PDF]. 2009; http://rtog.org/members/protocols/0521/0521.pdf. Accessed 8 April, 2010

Sanguineti G, Cavey ML, Endres EJ, Brandon GG, Bayouth JE (2006) Is IMRT needed to spare the rectum when pelvic lymph nodes are part of the initial treatment volume for prostate cancer? Int J Radiat Oncol Biol Phys 64:151–160

Scardino PT, Abbas F, Adolfson J (2003) Management of localized and regional diseases. In: Denis K, Bartsch G, Khoury S, Murai M, Partin A (eds) Prostate cancer: the 3rd international consultation on prostate cancer. Health Publications, Paris, pp 219–247

Schiff PB, Fant J, Horwitz SB (1979) Promotion of microtubule assembly in vitro by taxol. Nature 277:665–667

Schröder FH (1990) What is new in endocrine therapy of prostatic cancer? EORTC Genitourinary Group Monograph 7. In: Newling DWW, Jones WG (eds) Prostate cancer and testicular cancer. Wiley-Liss, New York, pp 45–52

Schroder FH, Hugosson J, Roobol MJ et al (2009) Screening and prostate-cancer mortality in a randomized European study. N Engl J Med 360:1320–1328

Shahinian VB, Kuo YF, Freeman JL (2005) Goodwin JS (2007) Risk of fracture after androgen deprivation for prostate cancer. N Engl J Med 352:154–164

Shih HA, Harisinghani M, Zietman AL, Wolfgang JA, Saksena M, Weissleder R (2005) Mapping of nodal disease in locally advanced prostate cancer: rethinking the clinical target volume for pelvic nodal irradiation based on vascular rather than bony anatomy. Int J Radiat Oncol Biol Phys 63:1262–1269

Smith MR, Lee H, McGovern F et al (2008a) Metabolic changes during gonadotrophin-releasing hormone agonist therapy for prostate cancer. Differences from the classic metabolic syndrome. Cancer 112:2188–2194

Smith MR, Bae K, Efstathiou JA et al (2008b) Diabetes and mortality in men with locally advanced prostate cancer. J Clin Oncol 26:4333–4339

Tannock IF, de Wit R, Berry WR et al (2004) Docetaxel plus prednisone or mitoxantrone plus prednisone for advanced prostate cancer. N Engl J Med 351:1502–1512

Tyrell CJ, Payne H, Wa See et al (2005) Bicalutamide ('Casodex') 150 mg as adjuvant to radiotherapy in patients with localised or locally advanced prostate cancer:results from the randomised early prostate cancer programme. Radiat Oncol 76:4–10

Viani GA, Stefano EJ, Afonso SL (2009) Higher-than-conventional radiation doses in localized prostate cancer treatment: a meta-analysis of randomized, controlled trials. Int J Radiat Oncol Biol Phys 74:1405–1418

Warde PR, Mason MD, Sydes MR et al (2010) Intergroup randomized phase III study of androgen deprivation therapy (ADT) pus radiation therapy (RT) in locally advanced prostate cancer (CaP)(NCIC-CTG, SWOG, MRC-UK,INT:T94-0110;NCT00002633). Proc Am Soc Clin Oncol. 28 abstr CRA4504

Widmark A, Klepp O, Solberg A et al (2009) Endocrine treatment, with or without radiotherapy, in locally advanced prostate cancer (SPCG-7/SFUO-3): an open randomised phase III trial. Lancet 373:301–308

Zagars GK, Johnson DE, von Eschenbach AC, Hussey DH (1988) Adjuvant estrogen following radiation therapy for stage C adenocarcinoma of the prostate: long-term results of a prospective randomized study. Int J Radiat Oncol Biol Phys 6:1085–1091

Zapatero A, Valcarcel F, Calvo FA et al (2005) Risk-adapted androgen deprivation and escalated three-dimensional conformal radiotherapy for prostate cancer: Does radiation dose influence outcome of patients treated with adjuvant androgen deprivation? A GICOR study. J Clin Oncol 23:6561–6568

Zelefsky MJ, Yamada Y, Kollmeier MA, Shippy AM, Nedelka MA (2008) Long-term outcome following three-dimensional conformal/intensity-modulated external-beam radiotherapy for clinical stage T3 prostate cancer. Eur Urol 53:1172–1179

Zietman AL, Prince EA, Nakfoor BM, Park JJ (1997) Androgen deprivation and radiation therapy: sequencing studies using the Shionogi in vivo tumor system. Int J Radiat Oncol Biol Phys 38:1067–1070

Treatment of Clinically Involved Lymph Nodes

Arne Grün

Contents

Abstract

Today long-term survival in patients present with lymphatic disease is not uncommon although treatment approaches for prostate cancer patients with pelvic nodal disease without further metastatic spread is highly individual as no clear evidence on the superiority of any approach exists. Practical aproaches can be extrapolated from studies on high-risk patients.

Abbreviations

ADT	Androgen deprivation therapy
CSS	Cancer-specific survival
DFS	Disease free survival
DSS	Disease-specific survival
EBRT	External beam radiotherapy
ePLND	Extensive pelvic lymph node dissection
FU	Follow-up
LAPC	Locally advanced prostate cancer
LN	Lymph node
PFS	Progression-free survival
OS	Overall survival

1 Treatment of Clinically Involved Lymph Nodes

Lymph node metastases are a major prognostic factor in prostate cancer (Gervasi et al. 1989). Studies correlating the number of positive lymph nodes with cancer outcome show a negative trend for progression-free survival (PFS) and overall survival (OS) with increasing nodal tumor burden (Boorjan et al. 2007; Briganti et al. 2009).

A. Grün (✉)
Department for Radiation Oncology and Cyberknife Cente, Charité - University Medicine Berlin Campus Virchow-Clinic, Augustenburger Platz 1, 13353 Berlin, Germany
e-mail: arne.gruen@charite.de

H. Geinitz et al. (eds.), *Radiotherapy in Prostate Cancer*, Medical Radiology. Radiation Oncology,
DOI: 10.1007/174_2014_1025, © Springer-Verlag Berlin Heidelberg 2014
Published Online: 4 October 2014

Since the dawn of the PSA-era a shift toward early localized disease has occurred and the relative number of lymph node-positive prostate cancer patients has decreased (Palapattu et al. 2004). Nowadays the prevalence of pN+ disease in RRP-series is 2.5–5 % (Nguyen et al. 2009; Paul et al. 2009), a cN+ situation is even more rare. Data solely concerning the subgroup of cN+ patients is sparse and hence the optimal treatment approach for clinically LN-positive prostate cancer patients is unclear. Evidence can only be extrapolated from large studies either pooling stage III-IV patients (thus also including locally advanced T3-4 patients or pN+ patients with histologically proven nodal metastases) or studies on "high-risk" patients (which might also include patients with a statistically high risk for lymphatic disease predicted by nomograms without overt metastatic disease).

Although the 7th edition of the AJCC cancer staging manual groups N+ and M+ patients together as stage IV, today long-term survival in patients with lymphatic disease is not uncommon. According to the current NCCN treatment guideline on prostate cancer (version 2.2014) cN+ patients should either receive ADT alone or RT in conjunction with 2–3 years of neoadjuvant/concomitant or adjuvant ADT.

Patients unable or unwilling to undergo any treatment can also be offered observation. Due to the fact that even in patients with node-positive prostate cancer the onset of symptomatic disease progression might take months to years, observation might prove a reasonable approach in elderly patients or patients unable or unwilling to go through local or systemic treatment. EORTC 30891 looked at histologically confirmed prostate cancer patients (T0-4) with or without nodal involvement (cN0-2) without metastatic disease (M0) ineligible for local treatment and randomized between immediate and deferred ADT. In the delayed treatment arm ADT was initiated when symptomatic disease progression occurred. At a median FU of 7.8 years there was a small but statistically significant difference concerning OS favoring immediate ADT of 42 versus 48 %. An advantage in DSS or symptom free survival could not be shown. Median time to initiation of ADT in the deferred arm was 7 years (Studer et al. 2006).

In a recent SEER-data analysis Tward and co-workers identified 1,100 patients diagnosed between 1988 and 2006 with histologically confirmed prostate cancer with nodal involvement receiving either radiotherapy or no definitive treatment (Tward et al. 2013). With a median FU of 90 months the 10-year CSS was 50.3 % for patients without definitive treatment and 62.5 % for patients receiving radiotherapy (HR 0.66, 95 % CI 0.93–0.99, p 0.01). On multivariate analyses radiotherapy, year of diagnosis, and low and intermediate grade were correlated with improved CSS.

Hormonal treatment alone might offer effective disease control in patients with limited life expectancy or who are unable or unwilling to undergo definitive treatment. From trials including pN+ patients we know that ADT alone may achieve similar OS and DFS rates at 5 years compared to definitive local treatment approaches. In a series published by Zagars et al. on pN+ patients treated with ADT alone a poignant drop-off in survival was seen at 8 years to 57 % where it had been as good as 80 % at 5 years. No clear predictive factors on outcome could be identified. Tumor grade affected the risk for progression but not OS (Zagars et al. 1994). This accords with the results presented by Aus et al. on ADT alone in pN+ patients who could only show a trend toward worse CSS in dependence of tumor grade (Aus et al. 2003).

Combination procedures offer a greater chance of long-term cure and hence higher probability of prevention of symptoms caused by recurrent or progressive disease. From the large RCTs (RTOG trials 85-31, 86-10, 92-02, and EORTC trial 22961) we know that the combination of EBRT with hormonal therapy can produce excellent long-term disease control even in locally advanced prostate cancer patients. All of those trials included pN+ and cN+ patients. Doses to the prostate ranged from 65 to 70 Gy with 44–50 Gy to the pelvic lymphatics.

The pivotal EORTC trial published by Bolla et al. compared EBRT and no further treatment vs. EBRT plus 3 years of an LHRH agonist in LAPC patients (T3-4, N0-1). With a median FU of 66 months OS and DSS at 5 years could be increased from 62 to 78 % and from 79 to 94 % respectively (Bolla et al. 2002). These results could be confirmed in the 10 year update published in 2010 (Bolla et al. 2010).

There were large differences in the duration of hormonal therapy in the aforementioned studies. The EORTC 22961 study corroborated the superiority of long-term ADT (3 years) over short-term ADT (6 months) with a statistical benefit in 5 year prostate-specific mortality (Bolla et al. 2009). Hence, current guidelines recommend the use of long-term (2–3 years) over short-term (6 months) ADT in LAPC patients receiving EBRT.

2 Practical Guideline

If standard noninvasive staging procedures remain inconclusive and surgical staging-approaches cannot be performed a PET-scan might help identifying nodal disease. To avoid unnecessary extension of radiation portals due to suspicious nodes in atypical localizations, it might be warranted to obtain a lymph-node biopsy.

Treatment approaches for prostate cancer patients with pelvic nodal disease without further metastatic spread is highly individual since no clear evidence on the superiority of any approach exists. An EBRT-only approach including 45–50 Gy to the pelvic lymphatics will not be able to eradicate bulky nodal disease. Curative doses of ~70 Gy to bulky nodal sites will seldom be possible without exceeding constraints to organs at risk.

Hence, we would start a cN+ patient in whom no surgical intervention is planned on 3 month neoadjuvant ADT to down-size nodal disease. In a CR situation 45–50 Gy to the pelvic lymphatics should suffice to eradicate microscopic residual disease. A PR situation can either call for a prolongation of neoadjuvant ADT by another 3 months or a boost of ~60 Gy can be delivered simultaneously or sequentially to remaining nodal disease. In a situation with persisting bulky nodal disease high precision techniques such as SBRT or Cyberknife^{TM} might enable one to apply curative doses to remaining sites without exceeding constraints to organs at risk (Jereczek-Fossa et al. 2012).

References

Aus G, Nordenskjöld K, Robinson D (2003) Prognostic factors and survival in node-positive (N1) prostate cancer—a prospective study based on data from a swedish population-based cohort. Eur Urol 43:627–631

Bolla M, Collette L, Blank L et al (2002) Long-term results with immediate androgen suppression and external irradiation in patients with locally advanced prostate cancer (an EORTC study): a phase III randomised trial. Lancet 360:103–108

Bolla M, de Reijke TM, van Tienhoven G (2009) Duration of androgen suppression in the treatment of prostate cancer. N Engl J Med 360:2516–2527

Bolla M, van Tienhoven G, Warde P et al (2010) External irradiation with or without long-term androgen suppression for prostate cancer with high metastatic risk: 10-year results of an EORTC randomised study. Lancet Oncol 11:1066–1073

Boorjian SA, Thompson RH, Siddiqui S (2007) Long-term outcome after radical prostatectomy for patients with lymph node positive prostate cancer in the prostate specific antigen era. Urol 178:864–870

Briganti A, Karnes JR, Da Pozzo LF et al (2009) Two positive nodes represent a significant cut-off value for cancer specific survival in patients with node positive prostate cancer. a new proposal based on a two-institution experience on 703 consecutive N+ patients treated with radical prostatectomy, extended pelvic lymph node dissection and adjuvant therapy. Eur Urol 55:261–270

Gervasi LA, Mata J, Easley JD et al (1989) Prognostic significance of lymph node metastases in prostate cancer. J Urol 142:332–336

Jereczek-Fossa BA, Beltramo G, Fariselli L et al (2012) Robotic image-guided stereotactic radiotherapy, for isolated recurrent primary, lymph node or metastatic prostate cancer. Int J Radiat Oncol Biol Phys 82:889–897

Nguyen PL, Chen MH, Hoffman KE et al (2009) Predicting the risk of pelvic node involvement among men with prostate cancer in the contemporary era. Int J Radiat Biol Phys 74:104–109

Palapattu GS, Allaf ME, Trock BJ et al (2004) Prostate specific antigen progression in men with lymph node metastases following radical prostatectomy: results of long-term follow-up. J Urol 172: 1860–1864

Paul A, Ploussard G, Nicolaiew N et al (2009) Oncologic outcome after extraperitoneal laparoscopic radical prostataectomy: midterm follow-up of 1115 procedures. Eur Urol 57:267–272

Studer UE, Whelan P, Albrecht W et al (2006) Immediate or deferred androgen deprivation for patients with prostate cancer not suitable for local treatment with curative intent: European organisation for research and treatment of cancer (EORTC) trial 30891. J Clin Oncol 24:1868–1876

Tward JD, Kokeny KE, Shrieve DC (2013) Radiation therapy for clinically node-positive prostate adenocarcinoma is correlated with improved overall and prostate cancer-specific survival. Pract Radiat Oncol 3:234–240

Zagars G, Sands ME, Pollack A (1994) Early androgen ablation for stage D1 (N1 to N3, M0) prostate cancer: prognostic variables and outcome. J Urol 151:1330–1333

Part V

Hypofractionation

Hypo-fractionation in Prostate Cancer: Biological Aspects

Nicolaus Andratschke and Klaus-Rüdiger Trott

Contents

N. Andratschke (✉)
Department of Radiation Oncology,
University Hospital Zurich, Raemistrasse 100,
Zürich 8091, CH, Switzerland
e-mail: n_andratschke@yahoo.com

K.-R. Trott
Department of Oncology, University College London,
London, UK

Abstract

Recent radiobiological modeling of experimental and clinical data suggests a low α/ß ratio for prostate cancer. If this assumption holds true, it represents a unique opportunity for exploiting a therapeutic window with hypo-fractionated radiotherapy schedules, especially in case α/ß for prostate cancer is lower than that for rectal complications. This chapter will—after general considerations on fractionation and the α/ß ratio—summarize the current scientific status on the assumed α/ß for prostate cancer and relevant normal tissue complications and discuss the potential and the caveats of hypo-fractionation for prostate cancer.

1 History and Radiobiological Basis of Dose Fractionation in Radiotherapy

Dose fractionation in radiotherapy was originally based on systematic clinical studies by French radiotherapists, in particular by Regaud in the 1920s, performed mainly in head and neck cancer. The criterion was a treatment schedule, which provided the best balance between local tumor control and unacceptable normal tissue complications. Since the 1930s, daily fractionation for 4–6 weeks became generally accepted as providing the best treatment outcome. Minor modifications were made depending on tumor histology and normal tissue sensitivity. Biological mechanisms did not play any role in the general concept of fractionation schedules in radiation oncology.

This approach changed radically with the publications by Withers (1975, 1985). He identified four different biological processes which take place during the intervals between dose fractions thus determining the overall treatment response of tumor and normal tissues. They are generally known as the four R's of fractionated radiotherapy:

R1 Recovery from sublethal radiation damage
R2 Reoxygenation

H. Geinitz et al. (eds.), *Radiotherapy in Prostate Cancer*, Medical Radiology. Radiation Oncology,
DOI: 10.1007/174_2014_1019, © Springer-Verlag Berlin Heidelberg 2014
Published Online: 15 July 2014

R3 Redistribution
R4 Repopulation

Whereas R1, recovery from sublethal radiation damage depends mostly on the dose per fraction, R2–4 depend on time, i.e., the duration of the interval between fractions and overall treatment time. It was generally accepted that the most important factor was recovery from sublethal radiation damage, which had been demonstrated first by Elkind and Sutton in 1960 in vitro (Elkind and Sutton 1960). This new paradigm also lead to a thorough re-evaluation of the formalisms of how to describe the shape of cell survival curves. The old formulas which were based on target theory were replaced by the linear quadratic formula which originated from the dual radiation action model of Rossi (1979).

Notwithstanding this theoretical background of either formalism, neither is really supported by radiobiological mechanisms involved in tumor cure or early and late normal tissue damage. Nevertheless, the linear quadratic formula is widely accepted due to the fact that it "works": it is easy to use and, as long as it is not overstressed, it is safe.

2 The Dependence of the Tumor Cure Dose on the Dose Per Fraction: The Alpha/Beta Ratio of Tumors

In vitro experiments by Elkind and Sutton in 1960 demonstrated that with each successive radiation dose in multiple fraction experiments, the surviving fractions of clonogenic cells decreased by a constant factor (Elkind and Sutton 1960). Therefore, with increasing radiation dose, the number of clonogenic cells in a cell population decreases exponentially. The same effect has been demonstrated to happen in murine tumors in vivo. Considering a course of 30 fractions of 2 Gy and a surviving fraction after 2 Gy of 50 %, the total effect of this treatment would result in a surviving fraction of 10^{-9}. This means that if the tumor contained 1 billion tumor stem cells, only one cell on average would survive, and according to the rules of Poisson statistics, there would be a probability of local tumor control of 37 %. Therefore and most importantly, minor differences in surviving fractions at 2 Gy would result in major differences in cure probability. These considerations are the reason for using as one simple criterion of tumor radiosensitivity the SF2 value, i.e., the surviving fraction after 2 Gy. Whereas in fractionated irradiation, cell survival decreases strictly according to an exponential survival curve with the slope defined by the surviving fraction of the first dose, the exact shape of the survival curve for a single dose and its deviation from an exponential is defined by the "shoulder," which is usually determined by a parameter derived from the linear quadratic formula, the α/ß ratio. The lower the alpha beta ratio, the more does the effect of fractionation depend on the dose per fraction. Therefore, the α/ß ratio is generally used as the most important criterion of fractionation sensitivity of a normal tissue or of a tumor. The only safe way to determine the alpha beta ratio in vivo (and in vitro) is by comparing isoeffective doses given in fractionated irradiation with different doses per fraction, following the equation proposed by Withers et al. (1983):

$$D1 * \left(1 + \frac{d1}{\alpha/\beta}\right) = D2 * \left(1 + \frac{d2}{\alpha/\beta}\right) = D3 * \left(1 + \frac{d3}{\alpha/\beta}\right) \tag{1}$$

D1, D2, and D3 are isoeffective total doses, e.g., doses which cause 50 % of local tumor control (TCD-50); d1, d2, and d3 are the respective doses per fraction; α/ß is a tissue, effect, or tumor-specific constant.

The validity of the α/ß value derived this way depends crucially on the condition that except for the different dose fractionations under study all other conditions in both arms of the fractionation study are equal, in particular tumor size and stage, follow-up and treatment outcome criterion, dose specification, other treatments and, above all, overall treatment time. This is difficult to achieve in human tumors if retrospective studies are analyzed but can be precisely achieved in experiments using transplanted mouse tumors.

Using this method, α/ß ratios have been determined for a large number of experimental tumors, in particular isogenic mouse tumors. These values have been collated by Williams et al. (1985). Values of α/ß ratios from 48 different experimental tumors ranged from 1 to 35 Gy with a mean value of approximately 10 Gy. Based on this review, it is generally recommended that in case no specific data are available for the particular tumor under consideration, a default α/ß value of 10 Gy should be used for tumors.

3 The Dependence of Human Tumor Cure Doses on the Dose Per Fraction: The Alpha/Beta Ratio of Human Cancers, in Particular of Prostate Cancer

The number of clinical studies which permit the reliable analysis of α/ß values is limited. In skin cancers, Trott and colleagues calculated a value of about 10 Gy (Trott et al. 1981). Several studies in squamous cell carcinomas of the head and neck found similar results (Stuschke and Thames 1999). However, there was considerable variation due to the fact that the different tumor groups differed with regard to size, dose distribution, or overall treatment time.

The first cancer in which clinical radio resistance was attributed to a high fractionation sensitivity/low α/ß value was malignant melanoma. In vitro, large variation between different cell lines isolated from human malignant melanomas with α/ß values ranging from 1 to 50 Gy and SF2 values ranging from 0.15 to 0.75 have been observed (Rofstad 1986). Studies of transplantable mouse melanomas yielded α/ß values between 6 and 14 Gy. Early retrospective evaluation of clinical fractionation schedules yielded conflicting results by either showing a higher (Habermalz 1981) or lower (Trott et al. 1981) rate of complete response rate with higher doses per fraction. In the largest retrospective study on fractionation sensitivity an α/ß ratio of 2.5 Gy was estimated (Overgaard et al. 1986), which was later recalculated to be equal to 0.6 Gy (Bentzen et al. 1989). Finally, a randomized clinical study performed on 126 patients with metastatic melanomas comparing the results of four fractions of 8 Gy with 20 fractions of 2.5 Gy did not record any difference in outcome (Sause et al. 1991). In conclusion, the retrospective analyses of response rates of melanomas to different fractionation protocols have produced conflicting results rendering reliable α/ß estimation impossible.

More recently, a low α/ß ratio for breast cancer has been postulated by Whelan et al. (2002). This lead to a large randomized clinical study called START, which is still in progress but various interim reports have been published (Haviland et al. 2013).

To date, the most important retrospective clinical analyses on fractionation sensitivity of human cancers are those on prostate cancer and a wealth of α/ß estimates have been published since then.

In vitro experiments and calculation of PSA doubling times after external beam radiotherapy from clinical data yielded a slow cell cycle time for prostate cancer compared to other tumor types (Pollack et al. 1994; Haustermans et al. 1997). Based on the assumption that the potential cell doubling time of a particular tumor is associated with the fractionation sensitivity, the experimental findings were considered not compatible with a presumed α/ß ratio >8 Gy. This notion formed the initial basis to reconsider the presumed α/ß ratio of prostate cancer and resulted in the seminal work by Brenner and Hall (1999) as well as Fowler et al. (2001) to estimate and derive a α/ß ratio from retrospective clinical data. As detailed above, in order to calculate a α/ß value, isoeffective fractionation schedules have to be employed. Brenner and Hall used two datasets on isoeffective treatments from external beam radiotherapy and low dose rate iodine seed brachytherapy to arrive at an estimated α/ß value of 1.5 Gy (95 % CI 0.8–2.2 Gy). Extending this approach to include isoeffective LDR implant strategies with 103-Paladium (Fowler et al. 2001) and to then available hypo-fractionated data (Chappell et al. 2004), a similar α/ß ratio around 1.5 Gy was established again.

Still, one has to bear in mind that in order to derive a α/ß value with this approach simplified assumption were made the most relevant will be discussed briefly.

To eliminate the ß component in their calculation and for the lack of available hypo-fractionation datasets, Brenner and Hall (1999) used data from LDR brachytherapy where complete sublethal damage repair could be assumed. Though elegant in principle, a completely different dose distribution with inherent dose heterogeneity and dose rate in LDR brachytherapy was compared to homogenous EBRT, all factors differently affecting biologically effective dose. It was even reported that implantation edema may negatively affect dose rate and hence BED (Van Gellekom et al. 2002).

Looking at the derived parameters for α and ß, the assumed number of clonogenic cells was claimed to be considerably underestimated and not congruent between LDR and EBRT.

However, each of these retrospective analyses were based on the assumption that repopulation during a course of radiotherapy of prostate cancer can be neglected and that there was no "time factor." As repopulation in prostate cancer with an assumed T_{pot} of 42 days was not considered relevant during a course of normo-fractionated radiotherapy, it had not been taken into account. Still, at least with protracted treatments such as LDR brachytherapy it should have been considered.

Though criticized for uncertainties to the assumption inherent to this approach, these initial analyses stirred a wealth of research interest, especially as data of hypo-fractionated regimens became available and were incorporated to overcome the limitations in comparing EBRT and BT datasets.

To overcome some of the limitations when using brachytherapy datasets, several groups compared large EBRT only patients cohorts and calculated α/ß values between 1.4 and 3.7 (Williams et al. 2007; Proust-Lima et al. 2011; Leborgne et al. 2012).

Interestingly, no difference of α/ß ratios between the different prostate cancer risk groups were found so far (Nickers et al. 2010; Miralbell et al. 2012).

The analysis of a nine-institution database of nearly 5,000 patients treated for prostate cancer with different radiotherapy schedules by Thames et al. (2010) proved that overall treatment times is a significant determinant of outcome of radiotherapy in low and intermediate-risk patients treated to 70 Gy or higher. A time factor equivalent to 0.24 Gy/d was estimated. This lead Baumann et al. (2010) to suggest that the apparent low α/ß ratio was artificially caused by the different overall treatment times of hypo-fractionated and

Table 1 Published α/ß estimates based on clinical data comparing different fractionation schedules either as external beam radiotherapy (EBTRT) or high-/low-dose brachytherapy (HDR-BT or LDR-BT)

Author	Radiation treatment	Estimated α/ß value (95 % CI)
Brenner and Hall (1999)	EBRT, LDR-BT	1.5 Gy (0.8–2.2 Gy)
King et al. (2000)	EBRT, LDR-BT	4.96 Gy (4.1–5.6 Gy)
Fowler et al. (2001)	EBRT, LDR-BT	1.49 Gy (1.25–1.76 Gy)
Brenner et al. (2002)	EBRT + HDR-BT	1.2 Gy (0.03–4.1 Gy)
Wang et al. (2003)[a]	EBRT + HDR-BT	3.41 Gy (2.56–4.26 Gy)
Chappell et al. (2004)	EBRT, LDR-BT	1.44 Gy (1.22–1.76 Gy)
Bentzen et al. (2005)	EBRT	1.12 Gy (3.3–5.6 Gy)
	EBRT (Hyperfractionation)	8.3 Gy (0.7–16)
Wiliams et al. (2007)	all pts.	2.6 Gy (0.9–4.8 Gy)
	EBRT pts. only	3.6 Gy (0.9–∞)
Nickers et al. (2010)	EBRT	3.41 Gy (2.56–4.26 Gy)
Shaffer et al. (2011)	EBRT, LDR	>30 Gy (5.5–∞)
Proust-Lima et al. (2011)	EBRT only	1.55 Gy (0.46–4.52 Gy)
Nickers et al. (2010)	EBRT	3.41 Gy (2.56–4.26 Gy)
Leborgne et al. (2012)	EBRT	1.86 Gy (0.7–5.1)
Miralbel et al. (2012)	EBRT	1.4 (0.9–2.2 Gy)
Vogelius and Bentzen (2012)[a]	EBRT	1.93 Gy (0.27–4.14)

[a] The only studies taking a time factor into consideration

the conventional treatment schedules. Vogelius and Bentzen (2012) estimated a mean time factor from several studies of 0.3 Gy/day. Incorporating this time factor into the analysis of the α/ß value also correcting for the lack of isoeffectiveness of the different schedules using a logistic dose response with a gamma-50 of one increased the α/ß value from close to zero to 4 Gy (Table 1).

Recalculations taking the different confounding factors into consideration still mostly arrived at α/ß ratios below 5 Gy.

In conclusion, with regard to the available data the α/ß value of prostate cancer indeed seems considerably lower compared to other common tumor entities and may be assumed to be at around 3–4 Gy. Therefore, we regard the α/ß value derived by Vogelius and Bentzen (2012) as the most reliable figure, which we will use in the discussion of the radiobiological justification of hypo-fractionated radiotherapy of prostate cancer.

Due to the inherent uncertainties in the derivation of the α/ß ratio in all theoretical analyses of retrospective data, a reliable α/ß estimate with narrower confidence intervals is only to be expected from large prospective randomized trials comparing different EBRT fractionation schedules with sufficient long-term follow-up but this is unlikely to be available in the near future.

4 The Fractionation Sensitivity of Critical Normal Tissues in Radiotherapy

The radiobiological justification of hypo-fractionated radiotherapy rests on the assumption that the fractionation sensitivity or α/ß ratio of the cancer tissue is significantly lower than that of the critical complications in the normal tissues inevitable exposed to high radiation doses. In their seminal work, Brenner and Hall (1999) estimated an α/ß value of prostate cancer tissue of 1.5 Gy and an α/ß value for rectal complications of 5 Gy. If these values would be correct, there would not be any further discussion on the radiobiological basis of hypo-fractionation in radiotherapy of prostate cancer. But there are serious doubts on the validity, not only of the fractionation sensitivity of the cancer tissue but even more so on the validity of the value for rectal complications.

One of the most critical normal tissues to be considered in the optimization of prostate cancer radiotherapy is the recto-sigmoid, the rectum, and anal canal. In clinical practice, severity scores are used to report treatment outcome but these scores are a mixture of different manifestations of late radiation damage. These scores have been developed, e.g., by the RTOG to compare severity and rates of complications from different treatment protocols, however, they are of very limited value for clinical radiobiology research such as estimating α/ß ratios (Trott et al. 2012). Four different types of symptoms following the development of late normal tissue damage in the rectum of patients after treatment for prostate cancers have been identified, namely rectal bleeding, urgency/frequency, tenesmus, and fecal incontinence (Trott et al. 2012). Each of these symptoms is likely to be caused by a different pathogenic mechanism; each of them is also related to a different distribution of the radiation dose in the rectum. This means that volume-based or surface-based NTCP models which have been used to normalize dose distributions are of very limited value for clinical research. The severity of bleeding is related to the area of the rectal wall which exceeds a threshold dose. Urgency and frequency are also related to the area of rectal mucosa which develops severe early reactions. However, a different geometric dose distribution is likely to influence severity. Fecal incontinence is an effect, which depends on the radiation dose in the anal sphincter. Experimental data suggest that not only does the critical target area/volume differ between the different complication types, but also the effects of dose per fraction are likely to be different (Trott et al. 1981). Whereas for telangiectasia, the α/ß ratio is low and may be <3 Gy, it is higher for the chronic inflammation causing fibrosis. No data are available for sphincter damage. To use a single value for the four different radiobiological mechanisms of potential ano-rectal complications of radiotherapy for prostate cancer as it has been done in the justification of hypo-fractionation in radiotherapy for prostate cancer is certainly inadequate.

Several studies used results from randomized and non-randomized clinical studies comparing hypo-fractionation and conventional fractionation in radiotherapy of prostate cancer to estimate α/ß values (Marzi et al. 2009; Tucker et al. 2011; Leborgne et al. 2012) and all arrived at values only little smaller than the original estimate of Brenner and Hall (1999). This is probably due to the fact that all used essentially the same approach, comparing incidence of RTOG scores of grade 2 or more. The confidence limits of these estimates were high, including the accepted value of the α/ß ratio for the prostate cancer tissue. The main aim is to prevent quality of life impairing late complications (e.g., greater or equal than grade 3). However, complications of this severity are rare (<1 % of all patients, whereas the rate of grade 2 complications is >10 %). It is for this reason that the moderate severity complications are used for analysis hoping that the fractionation sensitivity of severe complications is the same as that for moderate severity complications but there is no scientific evidence supporting this assumption. It is obvious that a direct estimate of the fractionation sensitivity of severe rectal complications cannot be derived from clinical trials data alone, for the various reasons listed above.

There are only few experimental data available which could be used to assist in this task. Dubray and Thames (1994) analyzed the existing data from animal experiments on the response of the rodent rectum to fractionated or low dose rate exposure, in particular the experiments performed by the Munich group and summarized by (Trott et al. 1981). They concluded that the α/ß value was about 4–5 Gy, similar to the values used in the justification of hypo-fractionated treatment schedules. However, Kummermehr and Trott (1994) pointed out that these values are the result of pooling data, which are related to very different radiobiological mechanisms. A large proportion of "late" normal tissue damage in patients as well as in rats, such as ulceration, severe telangiectasia, severe fibrosis is a typical consequential late normal tissue damage which is associated with a very different fractionation sensitivity, i.e., much less than "genuine" late normal tissue damage. Pooling fractionation data from both clinical endpoints into one endpoint is likely to yield an alpha beta value half-way between that for early damage and late damage. Kummermehr and Trott (1994) warned that pooling late normal tissue effects which may not represent the response of the same tissue component in the various treatment protocols may produce unsafe results. A major factor in this interaction of early and late normal tissue damage is related to regenerative processes such as repopulation which crucially depends on overall treatment time. Also Dubray and Thames (1994) warned to combine early and late injury of the rectum in order to produce the clinical endpoint (which may be telangiectasia, fibrosis, chronic inflammation) and that therefore an increase of "late" rectal radiation damage might be expected to occur with decrease in overall treatment time.

However, besides dose per fraction and overall treatment time, the anatomical dose distribution in the rectal wall is another, probably even more important determinant of the type and severity of rectal complications. Yet, no established consensus on how to delineate the rectum/rectal wall and which criteria/constraints to use for a "safe" dose-volume histogram has been developed to date.

5 Therapeutic Ratio of Hypo-fractionation: Clinical Evidence and Their Limitations

Most of the aforementioned studies arrived at the conclusion that prostate cancers are particularly sensitive to changes in dose per fraction and that this would be compatible with a very low α/ß ratio of <2 Gy. Since this value would be lower than that for late complications of critical normal tissues for which a value of 3 Gy has been generally recommended, an improved therapeutic ratio could be expected from hypo-fractionation. This intriguing situation would allow for two approaches to significantly improve the therapeutic window for the cure of prostate cancer.

Isotoxic dose escalation: While the current standard treatment with conventionally fractionated radiotherapy >70 Gy employing modern image-guided and intensity-modulated radiotherapy already yields low toxicity rates, further radiation dose intensification seems possible maintaining the same theoretical toxicity profile without unnecessary prolongation of treatment duration.

Isoeffective dose reduction: As not all risk groups may benefit from dose intensification, another approach could be to reduce biologically effective dose to normal tissues while maintaining an isoeffective tumor dose. While reducing again overall treatment time, patients could benefit from negligible risk of serious side effects.

Several randomized clinical studies have been initiated following this argument, although due to considerable uncertainties to estimate the α/ß value with tight confidence

Table 2 Selected isoeffective schedules for fractionation schemes used in clinical studies recalculated for different α/ß ratios for prostate cancer and rectal toxicity

Fx schedule (dose per fraction/total dose)	NTD_{2Gy}		NTD_{2Gy}		Reference
	Prostate cancer		Rectal toxicity		
	α/ß = 1.5 Gy	α/ß = 3.0 Gy	α/ß = 2.0 Gy	α/ß = 8.0 Gy	
2.625 Gy/52.5	61, 9 Gy	59, 1 Gy	60, 7 Gy	55, 8 Gy	Lukka et al. (2005)
3.13 Gy/50 Gy	66, 2 Gy	61, 4 Gy	64, 2 Gy	55, 7 Gy	Livsey et al. (2003)
3.0 Gy/57.0 Gy	73, 3 Gy	68, 4 Gy	71, 3 Gy	62, 7 Gy	Khoo and Dearnaley (2008)
2.5 Gy/70.0 Gy	80, 0 Gy	77, 0 Gy	78, 8 Gy	73, 5 Gy	www.rtog.org/members/protocols/0415/0415.odf
2.7 Gy/70.2 Gy	84, 2 Gy	80, 0 Gy	82, 5 Gy	75, 1 Gy	Pollack et al. (2006)
3.63 Gy/58.1 Gy	85, 1 Gy	77, 0 Gy	81, 7 Gy	67, 5 Gy	Ritter et al. (2007)
7.25 Gy/36.25 Gy	90, 6 Gy	74, 3 Gy	83, 8 Gy	55, 3 Gy	Pawlicki et al. (2007)

Only hypo-fractionated schedules were selected in case of randomized phase III trials. NTD_{2Gy}: normalized total dose 2 Gy

intervals, the assumption of a tumor α/ß value of 1.5 Gy as a basis to derive isoeffective/isotoxic schedules has to be viewed with caution. Some of these studies now start to yield mature data to derive tentative α/ß estimates. Yet, clinical results are very encouraging even though they indicate a low a/b value of 3–4 Gy rather than the presumed 1.5 Gy (Arcangeli et al. 2012; Lukka et al. 2005; Pollack et al. 2006; McBride et al. 2011).

Contrary to the wide-spread trend toward hypo-fractionation in radiotherapy for prostate cancer, Valdagni et al. (2005) initiated a prospective clinical trial, which compared a dose of 74 Gy in 2 Gy fractions with hyper fractionation of 79 Gy in two daily doses of 1.2 Gy, completing treatment in about the same overall treatment time. The results published so far are in favor of a hyper fractionated approach.

Table 2 shows the theoretical divergence for presumed isoeffective treatment schedules if the initial assumptions on prostate cancer (1.5 Gy) or rectal toxicity (3 Gy) prove to be inaccurate as outlined in Chaps. 17.3 and 17.4. The α/ß values chosen for recalculation represent the more realistic α/ß ratio of four for prostate cancer and theoretical α/ß values for different toxicity endpoints of rectal toxicity.

As seen in Table 2, a clinically relevant large therapeutic window can be achieved sparing normal tissue while at the same time significantly escalating the dose to the tumor. Especially, extreme hypo-fractionation seems an appealing approach in this scenario. If the assumptions on α/ß for prostate cancer and normal tissue hold true, this would represent a unique opportunity for radiotherapy of malignant tumors. Even if α/ß for prostate cancer approximates 3–4 Gy rather than the presumed 1.5 Gy in most clinical trials, a benefit in terms of significantly reducing overall treatment time while maintaining isoeffectivity and isotoxicity can still be derived.

On the other hand, there is the theoretical risk that all assumption prove wrong and the gain from hypo-fractionation solely relies on reducing overall treatment time overcoming repopulation. In this case some of the proposed schedules should prove inferior. Especially, extreme hypo-fractionated schedules would be prone to such deviations in estimated α/ß ratios, since in addition the validity of the LQ model has been questioned for single fraction doses greater than 8 Gy.

Long-term follow-up with late toxicity data need to be awaited to truly judge whether a therapeutic gain can be reached with an intermediate α/ß value for prostate cancer (approx. 3–4 Gy) which is similar or little higher than the α/ß value for rectal toxicity.

6 Conclusion

Though most studies point to a low alpha-beta ratio of prostate cancer, a reliable value with tight confidence values has not yet been established. Since a time factor has been neglected so far, clinical results for hypo-fractionation still could partly reflect isoeffectiveness due to reduction in overall treatment time (as compensation for repopulation) and not solely a low alpha-beta ratio. In addition, the assumption of a single alpha-beta ratio for rectal toxicity has to be reconsidered. Different effects may be observed for different treatment schedules depending upon fractionation, clinical and planning target volumes as well as how normal tissues are being delineated and late normal tissue damage is being quantified and scored.

Therefore, some uncertainty remains as to whether α/ß of prostate cancer is really lower than that for rectal toxicity and whether biological optimization of treatment schedules should only rely on one parameters of dose fractionation.

Nevertheless, if the assumptions on α/ß for prostate cancer and normal tissue hold true, this would represent a unique opportunity for radiotherapy of prostate cancer with regard to either dose escalation or normal tissue sparing or shortening overall treatment time for those patients many of whom are of very advanced age.

The euphoric assumptions have already triggered different clinical studies ranging from moderate to ultra fractionated schedules. So far, clinical results are encouraging and indicative of low a/b value though it rather approximates to 3–4 Gy than the presumed 1.5 Gy. Long-term evaluation with regard to biochemical failure rates and late toxicity and prudent evaluation und interpretation of the results is necessary before implementing these schedules in routine clinical practice.

Despite all these cautious caveats, (moderate) hypo-fractionation combined with modern IGRT and IMRT techniques is an intriguing model of optimally pairing radiobiology with radiation physics and has the potential to significantly improve outcomes in prostate cancer.

References

Arcangeli S, Strigari L, Gomellini S, et al (2012) Updated results and patterns of failure in a randomized hypofractionation trial for high-risk prostate cancer. Int J Radiat Oncol Biol Phys 84:1172–1178

Baumann M, Holscher T, Denham J (2010) Fractionation in prostate cancer is it time after all? Radiother Oncol 96:1–5

Bentzen SM, Overgaard J, Thames HD et al (1989) Clinical radiobiology of malignant melanoma. Radiother Oncol 16:169–182

Bentzen SM, Ritter MA (2005) The alpha/beta ratio for prostate cancer: what is it, really? Radiother Oncol 76:1–3

Brenner DJ, Hall EJ (1999) Fractionation and protraction for radiotherapy of prostate carcinoma. Int J Radiat Oncol Biol Phys 43:1095–1101

Brenner DJ, Martinez AA, Edmundson GK et al (2002) Direct evidence that prostate tumors show high sensitivity to fractionation (low alpha/beta ratio), similar to late-responding normal tissue. Int J Radiat Oncol Biol Phys 52:6–13

Chappell R, Fowler J, Ritter M (2004) New data on the value of alpha/beta-evidence mounts that it is low. Int J Radiat Oncol Biol Phys 60:1002–1003

Dubray BM, Thames HD (1994) Chronic radiation damage in the rat rectum: an analysis of the influences of fractionation, time and volume. Radiother Oncol 33:41–47

Elkind MM, Sutton H (1960) Radiation response of mammalian cells grown in culture. 1. Repair of X-ray damage in surviving Chinese hamster cells. Radiat Res 13:556–593

Fowler J, Chappell R, Ritter M (2001) Is alpha/beta for prostate tumors really low? Int J Radiat Oncol Biol Phys 50:1021–1031

Habermalz HJ (1981) Irradiation of malignant melanoma: experience in the past and present. Int J Radiat Oncol Biol Phys 7:131–133

Haustermans KM, Hofland I, Van Poppel H et al (1997) Cell kinetic measurements in prostate cancer. Int J Radiat Oncol Biol Phys 37: 1067–1070

Haviland JS, Owen JR, Dewar JA et al (2013) The UK standardisation of breast radiotherapy (START) trials of radiotherapy hypofractionation for treatment of early breast cancer: 10-year follow-up results of two randomised controlled trials. Lancet Oncol 14:1086–1094

Khoo VS, Dearnaley DP (2008) Question of dose, fractionation and technique: ingredients for testing hypofractionation in prostate cancer—the CHHiP trial. Clin Oncol (R Coll Radiol) 20:12–14

Kummermehr J, Trott KR (1994) Chronic radiation damage in the rat rectum: an analysis of the influences of fractionation, time and volume. Radiother Oncol 33:91–92

King CR (2000) What is the T(pot) for prostate cancer? Radiobiological implications of the equivalent outcome with(125)I or (103)Pd. Int J Radiat Oncol Biol Phys 47:1165–1167

Leborgne F, Fowler J, Leborgne JH et al (2012) Later outcomes and alpha/beta estimate from hypofractionated conformal three-dimensional radiotherapy versus standard fractionation for localized prostate cancer. Int J Radiat Oncol Biol Phys 82:1200–1207

Livsey JE, Cowan RA, Wylie JP et al (2003) Hypofractionated conformal radiotherapy in carcinoma of the prostate: five-year outcome analysis. Int J Radiat Oncol Biol Phys 57:1254–1259

Lukka H, Hayter C, Julian JA et al (2005) Randomized trial comparing two fractionation schedules for patients with localized prostate cancer. J Clin Oncol 23:6132–6138

Marzi S, Saracino B, Petrongari MG et al (2009) Modeling of alpha/beta for late rectal toxicity from a randomized phase II study: conventional versus hypofractionated scheme for localized prostate cancer. J Exp Clin Cancer Res 28:117

McBride SM, Wong DS, Dombrowski JJ et al (2011) Hypofractionated stereotactic body radiotherapy in low-risk prostate adenocarcinoma: preliminary results of a multi-institutional phase 1 feasibility trial. Cancer 118:3681–3690

Miralbell R, Roberts SA, Zubizarreta E, et al (2012) Dose-Fractionation sensitivity of prostate cancer deduced from radiotherapy outcomes of 5,969 patients in seven international institutional datasets: alpha/beta = 1.4 (0.9–2.2) Gy. Int J Radiat Oncol Biol Phys 82(1):e17–e24

Nickers P, Hermesse J, Deneufbourg JM et al (2010) Which alpha/beta ratio and half-time of repair are useful for predicting outcomes in prostate cancer? Radiother Oncol 97:462–466

Overgaard J, Overgaard M, Hansen PV et al (1986) Some factors of importance in the radiation treatment of malignant melanoma. Radiother Oncol 5:183–192

Pawlicki T, Cotrutz C, King C (2007) Prostate cancer therapy with stereotactic body radiation therapy. Front Radiat Ther Oncol 40:395–406

Pollack A, Hanlon AL, Horwitz EM et al (2006) Dosimetry and preliminary acute toxicity in the first 100 men treated for prostate cancer on a randomized hypofractionation dose escalation trial. Int J Radiat Oncol Biol Phys 64:518–526

Pollack A, Zagars GK, Kavadi VS (1994) Prostate specific antigen doubling time and disease relapse after radiotherapy for prostate cancer. Cancer 74:670–678

Proust-Lima C, Taylor JM, Secher S et al (2011) Confirmation of a low alpha/beta ratio for prostate cancer treated by external beam radiation therapy alone using a post-treatment repeated-measures model for PSA dynamics. Int J Radiat Oncol Biol Phys 79:195–201

Ritter MA, Forman JD, Kupelian PA et al (2007) A phase I/II trial of dose-per-fraction escalation for prostate adenocarcinoma. Int J Radiat Oncol Biol Phys 69:S174

Rofstad EK (1986) Radiation biology of malignant melanoma. Acta Radiol Oncol 25:1–10

Rossi HH (1979) The role of microdosimetry in radiobiology. Radiat Environ Biophys 17:29–40

Sause WT, Cooper JS, Rush S et al (1991) Fraction size in external beam radiation therapy in the treatment of melanoma. Int J Radiat Oncol Biol Phys 20:429–432

Shaffer R, Pickles T, Lee R et al (2011) Deriving prostate alpha-beta ratio using carefully matched groups, long followup and the phoenix definition of biochemical failure. Int J Radiat Oncol Biol Phys 79:1029–1036

Stuschke M, Thames HD (1999) Fractionation sensitivities and dose-control relations of head and neck carcinomas: analysis of the randomized hyperfractionation trials. Radiother Oncol 51: 113–121

Thames HD, Kuban D, Levy LB, et al (2010) The role of overall treatment time in the outcome of radiotherapy of prostate cancer: an analysis of biochemical failure in 4,839 men treated between 1987 and 1995. Radiother Oncol 96:6–12

Trott KR, Doerr W, Facoetti A et al (2012) Biological mechanisms of normal tissue damage: importance for the design of NTCP models. Radiother Oncol 105:79–85

Trott KR, von Lieven H, Kummermehr J et al (1981) The radiosensitivity of malignant melanomas part I: experimental studies. Int J Radiat Oncol Biol Phys 7:9–13

Tucker SL, Dong L, Bosch WR et al (2011) Late rectal toxicity on RTOG 94-06: analysis using a mixture Lyman model. Int J Radiat Oncol Biol Phys 78:1253–1260

Valdagni R, Italia C, Montanaro P et al (2005) Is the alpha-beta ratio of prostate cancer really low? A prospective, non-randomized trial comparing standard and hyperfractionated conformal radiation therapy. Radiother Oncol 75:74–82

Van Gellekom MP, Moerland MA, Kal HB et al (2002) Biologically effective dose for permanent prostate brachytherapy taking into account postimplant edema. Int J Radiat Oncol Biol Phys 53:422–433

Vogelius IR, Bentzen SM (2012) Meta-analysis of the alpha/beta ratio for prostate cancer in the presence of an overall time factor: bad news, good news, or no news? Int J Radiat Oncol Biol Phys 118(21):5432–5440

Wang JZ, Li XA, Yu CX et al (2003) The low alpha/beta ratio for prostate cancer: what does the clinical outcome of HDR brachytherapy tell us? Int J Radiat Oncol Biol Phys 57:1101–1108

Whelan T, MacKenzie R, Julian J et al (2002) Randomized trial of breast irradiation schedules after lumpectomy for women with lymph node-negative breast cancer. J Natl Cancer Inst 94: 1143–1150

Williams MV, Denekamp J, Fowler JF (1985) A review of alpha/beta ratios for experimental tumors: implications for clinical studies of altered fractionation. Int J Radiat Oncol Biol Phys 11:87–96

Williams SG, Taylor JM, Liu N et al (2007) Use of individual fraction size data from 3,756 patients to directly determine the alpha/beta ratio of prostate cancer. Int J Radiat Oncol Biol Phys 68:24–33

Withers HR (1975) The four R's of radiotherapy. Adv Radiat Biol 5:241–247

Withers HR (1985) Biologic basis for altered fractionation schemes. Cancer 55:2086–2095

Withers HR, Thames HD Jr, Peters LJ (1983) A new isoeffect curve for change in dose per fraction. Radiother Oncol 1:187–191

Hypofractionation and Stereotactic Treatment: Clinical Data

Giorgio Arcangeli, Stefano Arcangeli, and Lidia Strigari

Contents

G. Arcangeli (✉) · S. Arcangeli · L. Strigari
Regina Elena National Cancer Institute, Rome, Italy
e-mail: arcangeli.gio@tiscali.it

Abstract

During the last decade, improved physical sparing of normal tissues with the most recent technologies and a better understanding of prostate cancer radiobiology has prompted a number of moderate as well as extreme hypofractionation trials using different treatment schedules with the aim of exploring the outcome and toxicity of shorter regimens. The hypofractionated regimes appear to be associated with excellent results and toxicity similar to that observed after conventional fractionation courses, in spite of the numerous variables relative to different distributions in the risk categories or androgen deprivation delivery in the trials. However, the relatively short follow-up and the single-arm nature of these reports do not permit any meaningful comparisons with the conventional regimes. Until now, six controlled randomized trials of moderate hypofractionation have been published. Notwithstanding the similar outcome and toxicity results between hypo and conventional fractionation, two of these studies used a 2D technique delivering total doses that are now considered insufficient and inconclusive for treating prostate cancer. In the most recent trial, reporting equivalent 2 year toxicity rates, the follow-up is still too short to evaluate the clinical outcome of the two schedules. The three remaining trials report similar biochemical outcomes between the short and standard regimes. Only one trial has a sufficiently long follow-up to confirm the equivalence of the two regimes in terms of biochemical, clinical local and distant failure, and overall and disease-specific survival. This trial also shows that in some subgroups of patients, i.e., those with a pretreatment PSA $\leq$ 20 ng/mL or with a T-stage $\geq$ 2c, hypofractionation may be better than conventional fractionation in terms of both local failure and disease-specific survival. These results suggest that moderate hypofractionation for prostate cancer does not increase treatment-related toxic effects or decrease efficacy, although they still need

H. Geinitz et al. (eds.), *Radiotherapy in Prostate Cancer*, Medical Radiology. Radiation Oncology,
DOI: 10.1007/174_2013_871,
Published Online: 18 July 2013

to be confirmed by trials with more patients. The premature results of extreme hypofractionation (or SBRT) studies, although associated with good treatment tolerance, excellent early biochemical outcomes and low late toxicity rates, do not lead to any firm conclusions on the clinical benefits of these regimes in comparison to escalated conventional dose fractionation. Given that a certain number of uncertainties exist in extrapolating biological effects to very large fraction size, the results of extreme hypofractionation need to be confirmed by appropriate randomized trials with a sufficiently long follow-up and accurate evaluation of long-term tolerance and toxicity.

1 Introduction

The better physical sparing of normal tissues using three-dimensional (3D) or intensity modulated radiation (IMRT) techniques has resulted in a re-evaluation of the use of a few large dose fractions with shorter treatment duration. The delivery of a reduced number of higher dose fractions (hypofractionation) is based on the assumption that prostate cancer has a low α/β ratio. In radiobiology, the α/β ratio, defined as the dose at which killing of cells by linear (α) and quadratic (β) components is equal, is used to quantify the fractionation sensitivity of tissues and tumours. Recent analyses and reviews of tumour control in prostate cancer (Fowler et al. 2001; Brenner et al. 2002; Williams et al. 2007) have suggested an α/β value to the order of 1–3 Gy, which is somewhat lower than the value typically ascribed to the adjacent late-responding normal tissues (Steel 2003). If this is indeed the case, hypofractionation would offer a unique opportunity to optimize the therapeutic ratio taking advantage of the potential heightened sensitivity of prostate cancer to radiation dose fractions in comparison to the surrounding organs at risk (i.e., rectum, bladder, and urethra). Fewer but larger-than-conventional fractions for a lower total dose should achieve efficacy equivalent to higher doses delivered with conventional fraction sizes. On the other hand, a radiotherapy course given in a reduced number of sessions should be less distressing for elderly patients with prostate cancer, especially when they live some distance from the radiotherapy center, and for those who might be more attracted by quicker treatments, such as radical prostatectomy, or even non-definitive approaches such as androgen deprivation therapy (ADT). A decrease in overall treatment time of 3–4 weeks by hypofractionation with respect to conventional fractionation would have a substantial effect on the quality of life and health costs.

A further reduction in the number of fractions and overall treatment time can be delivered by the technique known as "extreme hypofractionation" which is synonymous with stereotactic body radiotherapy (SBRT) and consists of the delivery of few fractions (usually 4–5) of very large doses (usually 7–8 Gy per fraction). The safe delivery of such treatment regimes, however, other than the favorable therapeutic ratio offered by the low α/β ratio of prostate cancer, also requires the employment of highly focused radiation beams delivering full doses to the target volume with a rapid fall-off to minimize the dose absorbed by the surrounding critical normal tissues. Because of the delivery of very large doses per fraction, extreme hypofractionation also requires the use of techniques employing daily image guidance, which allow the use of a minimal CTV to PTV margin, and maximizes the treatment accuracy by daily patient repositioning and correction for the inter- and—in case of continuous or multiple imaging or tracking during treatment—intra-fraction organ movements.

2 Moderate Hypofractionation

The possibility of reducing the number of fractions has prompted several hypofractionation trials using different treatment schedules with the aim of exploring the outcomes and toxicity of hypofractionation regimens. The trials with longer follow-ups are listed in Table 1 together with the available published randomized phase III studies. The hypofractionated regimes appear to be associated with excellent results and toxicity similar to that observed after conventional fractionation, in spite of numerous uncontrolled variables like different distributions in risk categories or differences in the frequency of ADT in these trials. However, the relatively short follow-up and the single-arm nature of most of these reports do not permit any meaningful comparisons with conventional regimes (Fonteyne et al. 2012; Kupelian et al. 2007; Leborgne and Fowler 2009; Miralbel et al. 2012; Cowan et al. 2007; Faria et al. 2011; Higgins et al. 2006; Livsay et al. 2003; Rene et al. 2010; Thomson et al. 2012; Ritter et al. 2001; Martin et al. 2007).

3 Results from Randomized Studies

3.1 Tumour Control

All published randomized phase III hypofractionation trials are also summarized in Table 1. In the Canadian study (Lukka et al. 2005), a total of 936 patients were randomized to receive 66 Gy in 33 fractions in 6.5 weeks or 52.4 in 20 fractions in 4 weeks, which corresponds to an equivalent dose given at 2.0 Gy per fraction (EQD2) of 61.9 Gy for an α/β of 1.5 Gy. None of the patients received ADT. There was a trend toward a better 5-year Freedom From

Table 1 Nonrandomized and randomized* hypofractionation trials: Schedules, equivalent doses in 2 Gy fractions and biochemical outcome

Reference	No. Pts	Dose/fx size/# fxs	EQD2 $\alpha/\beta = 1.5$ Gy (tumor) (Gy)	EQD2 $\alpha/\beta = 3$ Gy (late effects) (Gy)	Med F/U (mos)	Risk class	% 5-year FFBF
Fonteyne et al. (2012)	113	55 Gy/3.4 Gy/16 fx	77.0	70.4	47	L-I-H	94
Kupelian et al. (2007)	770	70 Gy/2.5 Gy/28 fx	80	77	45	L-I-H	82
Leborgne and Fowler (2009)	130	78 Gy/2 Gy/39fx	78	78	49	L-I-H	90
	89	61.5 Gy/3.1 Gy/20fx	80.8	75.0		L-I-H	88
Miralbel et al. (2012)	403	74.2 Gy/1.86 Gy/38.5fx	71.2	72.1	52	L-I-H	70
	71	56 Gy/4 Gy/14 fx	88.0	78.4	41	L-I-H	78
Cowan et al. (2007)	325	50 Gy/3.1 Gy/16fx	65.7	61.0	84	L	77
Faria et al. (2011)	89	66 Gy/3 Gy/22fx	84.9	79.2	51	I	95
Livsay et al. (2003)	705	66 Gy/3 Gy/22fx	84.9	79.2	60	L-I-H	56
Higgins et al. (2006)	300	52.5 Gy/2.625 Gy/20 fx	61.9	59.1	58	L-I-H	45
Rene et al. (2010)	129	66 Gy/3 Gy/22fx	84.9	79.2	51	L-I	98
Thomson et al. (2012)	30	60 Gy/3 Gy/20fx	77.1	72.0	84	H	50
	30	57 Gy/2.85 Gy/20fx	70.8	66.7			58
Ritter et al. (2001)		64.7 Gy/2.9 Gy/22fx	81.3	76.3	56	I	91.5
	317	58.1 Gy/3.63 Gy/16fx	85.2	77.0	37	I	96.1 (3y)
		51.6 Gy/4.3 Gy/12fx	85.5	75.3	28	I	98.7 (3y)
Martin et al. (2007)	92	60 Gy/3 Gy/20 fx	77.2	72	38	L-I-H	85
Lukka et al. (2005)*	466	52.5/2.625 Gy/20 fx	61.9	59.1	68	L-I-H	57.7
	470	66 Gy/2 Gy/33 fx	66	66		L-I-H	62.3
Yeoh et al. (2011)*	108	55 Gy/2.75 Gy/20 fx	66.8	63.2	48	L-I-H	57.4
	109	64 Gy/2 Gy/32 fx	64	64		L-I-H	55.5
Pollack et al. (2011)*	150	70.2 Gy/2.7 Gy/26 fx	84.2	80	>60	L-I-H	86.1
	150	76 Gy/2 Gy/38 fx	76	76	>60	L-I-H	85.6
Kuban et al. (2010)*	101	75.6 Gy/1.8 Gy/42 fx	71.3	72.6	56	L-I	92
	101	70.2 Gy/2.7 Gy/26 fx	84.2	80.0		L-I	96
Arcangeli et al. (2012)*	85	80 Gy/2 Gy/40 fx	80.0	80.0	70	H	79
	83	62 Gy/3.1 Gy/20 fx	81.5	75.6		H	85

EQD2 Equivalent Dose in 2 Gy fractions, *L* low risk, *I* intermediate risk, *H* high risk, *FFBF* freedom from biochemical failure

Biochemical Failure (FFBF) rate in the conventional fractionation versus hypofractionation group (59.95 % vs. 52.95 %) with a hazard ratio of 1.18 (95 % CI of 0.99–1.41) with no difference to the overall survival (87.6 % vs. 85.2 %). In the Australian trial (Yeoh et al. 2011), 217 patients were randomized to receive 64 Gy in 32 fractions in 6.5 weeks or 55 Gy in 20 fractions in 5 weeks (EQD2 of 66.8 Gy for an α/β of 1.5 Gy), and none of the patients received ADT. There were no differences between the hypofractionated and conventional schedules with the estimated 5-year FFBF ± Freedom From Clinical Failure (FFCF) of 57.4 % versus 55 %, and overall survival of 86.4 % versus 84.1 %. The total dose delivered by both trials was less than 76–80 Gy, now considered a standard-of-care. Both were designed and performed before the studies suggesting a low α/β for prostate cancer (with no attempt to make the arms isoeffective), and did not provide any conclusive evidence with regard to outcomes (Lukka et al. 2005; Yeoh et al. 2011).

Another two randomized trials have been undertaken in the U.S. (Pollack et al. 2011; Kuban et al. 2010) and their results have only been reported in an abstract form. The randomized trial by Pollack et al. (2011), compared 76 Gy delivered in conventional 2.0 Gy fractions (CIMRT) to 70.2 Gy delivered in 2.7 Gy fractions (HIMRT) in 303 intermediate- and high-risk patients. At 5 years, no statistically significant difference in outcome was observed, with 5-year BF rates of 14.4 and 13.9 %, respectively, between

Table 2 5-year freedom from failure rates according to prognostic factors in a randomized trial of conventional versus hypofractionated radiotherapy (Arcangeli et al. 2012)

FFF rates	Prognostic factors						Total
	iPSA ≤ 20	iPSA > 20	GS ≤ (3 + 4)	GS ≥ (4 + 3)	T < 2c	T ≥ 2c	
Biochemical							
Convent	83	72	94	66	85	74	79
Hypo	95	73	88	83	89	83	85
p-value	*0.02*	*0.4*	*0.5*	*0.01*	*0.3*	*0.08*	*0.06*
Local							
Convent	92	91	97	87	93	90	91
Hypo	100	85	95	91	100	89	93
p-value	*0.01*	*0.5*	*0.5*	*0.15*	*0.05*	*0.9*	*0.35*
Distant							
Convent	87	84	98	76	91	82	86
Hypo	98	81	91	89	89	91	90
p-value	*0.04*	*0.95*	*0.25*	*0.08*	*0.85*	*0.2*	*0.3*

Convent Conventional Fractionation, *Hypo* Hypofractionation, *FFF* freedom from failure, *iPSA* pretreatment PSA, *T* T-stage, *GS* Gleason Score

the two fractionation schedules. Kuban et al. (2010), reported on a randomized trial comparing a conventional CIMRT of 75.6 delivered in 42 fractions to a hypofractionated HIMRT of 72 Gy delivered in 30 fractions for 204 patients, some of whom also received a contemporary ADT. No statistically significant difference in FFBF was observed between the former and latter fractionation groups, with 5-year rates of 92 and 96 %, respectively.

The randomized phase III trial by our group (Arcangeli et al. 2010) was designed to compare the effects of a conventional fractionation of 80 Gy at 2 Gy per fraction in 8 weeks versus a hypofractionation schedule of 62 Gy at 3.1 Gy per fraction in 5 weeks (4 fractions per week) to the prostate and seminal vesicles, using 3D-CRT, in patients with high-risk prostate cancer who were also receiving a 9-month ADT. The two arms were hypothesized to be isoeffective with regard to tumour control, assuming a fairly low α/β ratio of 1.5–1.8 Gy. The results of this trial have recently been updated (Arcangeli et al. 2012). At a median follow-up of 70 months, hypofractionation was only slightly better, with a nonsignificant improvement in actuarial FFBF compared to conventional fractionation, with 5-year rates of 85 % and 79 %, respectively ($p = 0.065$). No difference between the two fractionation schedules was detected in the 5-year rates of Freedom From Local (FFLF: 93 % vs. 91 %, respectively, $p = 0.33$) or Distant Failure (FFDF: 90 % vs. 85 %, respectively, $p = 0.29$). However, the analysis of a subgroup of patients stratified according to the prognostic factors showed that in the subgroup with a pretreatment PSA level of 20 ng/mL or less, hypofractionation was significantly better than conventional fractionation in all three endpoints, with 5-year rates of 95 % versus 83 % ($p = 0.02$), 100 % versus 92 % ($p = 00.01$), and 98 % versus 87 % ($p = 0.04$), for FFBF, FFLF, and FFDF, respectively (Table 2). Also in the subgroup with a Gleason Score ≥(4 + 3), hypofractionation was significantly better than conventional fractionation, but only for FFBF, with 5-year rates of 83 % versus 66 % ($p = 0.01$). For the entire population the actuarial analysis of survival showed no significant difference in either the overall or cancer specific survival between the short and long radiation schedules, with 5-year OS rates of 92 % versus 82 % ($p = 0.16$), respectively, and Cause Specific Survival (CSS) rates of 98 % versus 92 % ($p = 0.13$), respectively. In the subgroup with a pretreatment PSA of 20 ng/mL or less and in that with a T-stage ≥2c, however, the actuarial analysis of CSS, showed a significantly better outcome in the hypo than the conventional fractionation group, with 5-year rates of 100 % versus 89 % ($p = 0.03$), and 100 % versus 87 % ($p = 0.01$), respectively (Table 3). We also looked at mortality, by calculating the Hazard Risk of the Overall (OM) and Cancer Specific Mortality (CSM) as a function of time for both fractionation arms (Fig. 1). While CSM was found to be only a small fraction of OM in the hypofractionation arm, in the conventional fractionation arm most of the deaths resulted from prostate cancer. Hypofractionation was confirmed as a significant predictor of CSS by multivariate analysis (HR = 0.15, CL = 0.019–1.27).

To obtain a rough estimation of efficacy of some fractionation schedules, we plotted the biochemical results of all hypofractionation trials (Table 1) together with those of the most representative dose escalation studies of conventional fractionation, reported in Table 4.

Figure 2 shows a dose response curve of the 5-year biochemical tumour control probability (TCP) versus EQD2. The FFBF points from each trial are plotted relative to their

Table 3 5-year cancer-specific survival rates according to prognostic factors in a randomized trial of conventional versus hypofractionated radiotherapy (Arcangeli et al. 2012)

Prognostic factors	5-year cancer-specific survival rate		*p*-value
	Conventional fraction	Hypofraction	
iPSA ≤ 20	89	100	0.03
iPSA > 20	96	97	0.85
GS ≤ 3 + 4	97	100	0.90
GS ≥ 4 + 3	87	97	0.10
T-stage < 2c	97	96	0.90
T-stage ≥ 2c	87	100	0.01
All patients	*92*	*98*	*0.15*

iPSA pretreatment PSA, *GS* Gleason Score, *T* T-stage

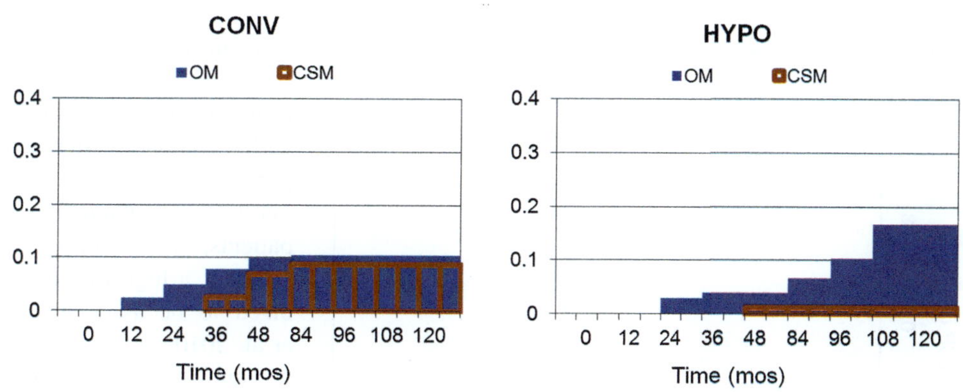

Fig. 1 The Hazard Risk of the Overall (OM) and Cancer Specific Mortality (CSM) as a function of time for both conventional and hypofractionation arms in the randomized trial of conventional versus hypofractionation (Arcangeli et al. 2012)

equivalent EQD2 for an assumed α/β ratio of 1.5. Notwithstanding the numerous unaccounted variables in these trials (patient risk class, use of ADT, etc.), all data from conventional dose escalation and hypofractionation trials are reasonably well fitted by the solid line dose response curve, confirming the low value of α/β for prostate cancer.

3.2 Late Toxicity

All the trials confirmed that moderate hypofractionation for prostate cancer does not increase treatment-related toxic effects or decrease efficacy. Of the five randomized trials reporting the toxicity results at more than 3 years, the Australian and Canadian trials (Lukka et al. 2005; Yeoh et al. 2011) delivered lower EQD2 doses and could not be compared with the more contemporary trials. However, neither trial showed any significant difference in late toxicity between long and short schedules. In the two U.S. trials, the EQD2 doses to normal critical organs, assuming an α/β value of 3 Gy, were higher in the hypofractionated than in the conventional arm. However, Pollack et al. (2011) reported 5-year ≥ G2 late toxicity rates of 8.9 and 13.8 % ($p = 0.2$) for GU, and 4.1 and 5.9 % ($p = 0.5$) for GI toxicity, for the conventional or hypofractionated arm, respectively. The corresponding 5-year ≥ G2 late toxicity rates reported in the Kuban et al. (2010) trial were 19 and 19 % for GU, and 6 and 14 % (p = NS) for GI toxicity.

A recent U.K. trial (Dearnaley et al. 2012) compared 74 Gy delivered in 37 fractions in 153 patients to 57 Gy in 19 fractions and 60 Gy in 20 fractions delivered to 151 and 153 patients, respectively, for stage I–II prostate cancer. In patients with a median follow-up of about 50 months, a comparable toxicity between the three treatment schedules was reached at 2 years. The incidence of side effects subsequently stayed at about the same level, with G2 or worse late GI toxicity in 4.3, 3.6, and 1.4 % of patients receiving 74, 60, and 57 Gy, respectively. Grade 2 or worse late GU toxicity was 2.2, 2.2, and 0 %, respectively. However, long-term follow-up results, especially for late genitourinary toxic effects, are needed, notably because the prostatic urethra and bladder neck still receive high fraction sizes. In the randomized study done by our group, the conventional total dose of 80 Gy was compared with the EQD2 dose of approximately 75 Gy delivered to normal tissues. In the hypofractionation and conventional fractionation schedules, the 3-year late ≥ G2 complication rates were 17 and 14 %, for GI toxicity, and 16 and 11 % for GU toxicity, respectively, with no significant difference between the two arms. The incidence of complications increased with time.

Table 4 Biochemical outcome from the most relevant dose escalation trials

Reference	No. Pts	Dose/fx size/# fxs	Med F/U (mos)	Risk class	% 5-year FFBF (*)
Kuban et al. (2008)	150	70 Gy/2 Gy/35 fx	116	L-I-H	87
	151	78 Gy/2 Gy/39 fx	116	L-I-H	88
Dearnaley et al. (2007)	421	64 Gy/2 Gy/32 fx	64	L-I-H	60
	422	74 Gy/2 Gy/37 fx	63	L-I-H	71
Al-Magmani et al. (2010)	331	68 Gy/2 Gy/34 fx	70	L-I-H	51
	333	78 Gy/2 Gy/39 fx	70	L-I-H	63
Kuban et al. (2003)	1087	67 Gy/2 Gy/33.5 fx	65	L-I-H	36
		78 Gy/2 Gy/39 fx	65	L-I-H	45
Zelefsky et al. (2008)	358	70.2 Gy/1.8 Gy/39 fx	79	L-I-H	61
	471	75.6 Gy/1.8 Gy/42 fx	79	L-I-H	74
	741	81 Gy/1.8 Gy/45 fx	79	L-I-H	85
	477	86.4 Gy/1.8 Gy/48 fx	79	L-I-H	82

L low risk, *I* intermediate risk, *H* high risk, *FFBF* freedom from biochemical failure. (*) Average of FFBF patients with/without ADT

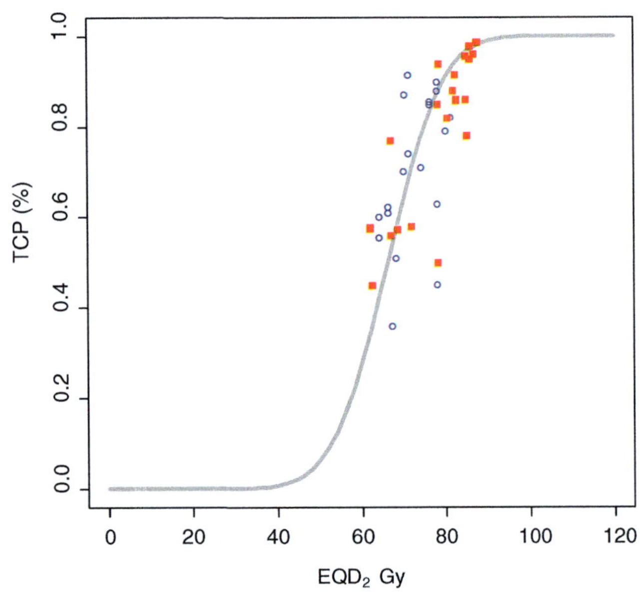

Fig. 2 The dose response curve (*solid line*) of the 5-year FFBF versus equivalent dose at 2 Gy/fraction (EQD2) assuming an α/β ratio of 1.5 Gy for prostate cancer. *Squares* and *circles* represent the 5-year FFBF data for patients treated with hypofractionation or conventional schedules, respectively, as reported in Tables 1 and 4

However, rectal toxicity seemed to reach a plateau in both treatment groups at 20–26 months after treatment, while urinary toxicity continued to increase after 4 years (Arcangeli et al. 2011).

3.3 Acute Toxicity

RTOG scoring criteria are commonly used to report acute toxicity. Most trials report rectal bleeding as the objective end-point, which impacts the quality of life. Differently from late toxicity, acute rectal toxicity occurs during or within 3 months after completion of treatment and is temporary. However, the acute effects may be severe enough to interrupt the planned course of treatment in 10 % of the patients. In addition, with conventional fractionation regimes, a high rate of acute rectal toxicity is now recognized to be associated with late proctopathy (Michalski et al. 2010).

Out of all six randomized trials, a detailed description of acute toxicity was only reported in the U.K. and our study (Dearnaley et al. 2012; Arcangeli et al. 2011). Both studies reported a slightly higher but not statistically significant rate of grade 2 or more GI and GU acute toxicity in the short over the long treatment arms, with an earlier peak for both rectal and urinary toxicity in the former arm. In our study, the median interval to toxicity detection was 22 and 36 days ($p = 0.001$) for GI and 15 and 23 days ($p = 0.002$) for GU in the hypofractionation and conventional fractionation, respectively. However, there was no difference in the duration of either GI or GU toxicities between the two treatment schedules ($p = 0.31$ and 0.34, respectively) (Arcangeli et al. 2011).

We also tested the correlation between acute and late $\geq$ G2 toxicity and found that it was statistically significant for GI and marginally significant for GU in the group of patients treated with conventional fractionation, while no correlation was found for either GI or GU in the hypofractionation arm (Arcangeli et al. 2011), likely because of the higher sensitivity of late damage to high dose/fraction.

Acute effects, on the contrary, are more dependent on overall treatment time and, therefore, to avoid excessive toxicity with hypofractionation schedules, the duration of treatment should be long enough to allow mucosal repopulation. This relationship has been well described by the

Table 5 Summary of outcomes from SBRT trials with a follow-up of more than 30 months and at least 40 enrolled patients

Study	Schedule	Number of patients	Risk class	Medi F/U (mos)	Late grade 3 GU toxicity (%)	Late grade 3 GI toxicity (%)	FFBF (%)
CyberKnife							
Katz et al. (2011)	35–36.25 Gy in 5 fx	304	L-I-H	48	2	–	97, 93, 75 at 4 years
Freeman and King (2011)	35 Gy in 5 fx	41	L	60	<1	–	93 at 5 years
McBride et al. (2011)	36.25–37.5 Gy in 5 fx	45	L	44.5	<1	–	97.7 at 3 years
Fuller et al. (2011)	38 Gy in 4 fx †	49	L-I	36	4	–	96 at 3 years
Kang et al. (2011)	32–36 Gy in 4 fx	44	L-I-H	40	–	–	100, 100, 90.9 at 5 years
King et al. (2012)	36.25 Gy in 5 fx	67	L	32.4	3.5	–	94 at 4 years
Gantry-based systems							
Madsen et al. (2007)	33.5 Gy in 5 fx	40	L	41	–	–	90 at 4 years
Boike et al. (2011)	45–47.50 Gy in 5 fx	45	L-I	30, 18, 12	4	2 plus 1 grade 4	100 at 1–2.5 years

L low, *I* intermediate, *H* high

Fowler formula (Fowler 2005), and by a model developed according to data of our group (Strigari et al. 2009).

4 Extreme Hypofractionation (Stereotactic Body Radiotherapy)

In recent years, several clinical studies have employed only a few very large dose fractions, mainly in low risk, localized prostate cancer, with the aim of exploring the feasibility of such extreme hypofractionation schedules. The attempt to further reduce the treatment duration in prostate cancer is based on the emulation of the HDR- brachytherapy hypofractionated approach in an alternative, more suitable way, allowing for steep dose gradients that resemble brachytherapy dose distributions, without the need for hospitalization, catheterization, and the discomfort of keeping the delivery needles inserted for an extended time period. The rational of extreme hypofractionation in prostate cancer mainly depends upon the extrapolation from results obtained by the moderate hypofractionation which, in turn, have not yet been fully established. Furthermore, there are still significant uncertainties on the validity of the linear quadratic model for predicting the tumour response to such large dose fractions.

Several prospective trials of extreme hypofractionation have already been published and several others are currently underway. The results of the more relevant SBRT trials are summarized in Table 5. Many of these trials were carried out by the Cyberknife® and were planned to explore the feasibility of applying the shorter schedules to treat low/intermediate risk, localized prostate cancer. It is estimated that approximately 10,000 prostate patients have been treated with the CyberKnife® since 2003 (Katz et al. 2010). Katz et al. (2011) published the largest CyberKnife® SBRT series to date with the treatment of 304 prostate cancer patients. The first 50 were treated with 35 Gy in 5 fractions; the remaining 254 patients were escalated to 36.25 Gy in 5 fractions. With a median follow-up of 48 months, no grade 3 late GI toxicity was documented and only one grade 3 late urinary toxicity (2 %) was reported in the escalated group. The actuarial 4 year biochemical control rates were 97, 93, and 75 % in low-, intermediate-, and high-risk patients, respectively. Overall potency preservation was 87 %. Freeman and King (2011) reported on the outcomes for low-risk prostate cancer patients with a median follow-up of 5 years after SBRT administered to a total dose of 35 Gy in 5 fractions: Only one late grade 3 genitourinary toxicity occurred and the actuarial 5-year FFBF rate was 93 %. McBride et al. (2011) reported on 45 patients with low-risk prostate adenocarcinoma treated to a total dose of 36.25–37.5 Gy delivered in five consecutive fractions. After a median follow-up of 44.5 months there was one episode of late grade 3 urinary obstruction, and there were two episodes of late grade 3 proctitis. The FFBF rate at 3 years was 97.7 %. Fuller et al. (2011) reported on 49 low-and intermediate-risk patients treated with 38 Gy delivered in 4 fractions using an HDR-like dose distribution. After a median follow-up of 36 months, no late grade 3 GI toxicity but only 4 % late grade 3 GU toxicity were detected.

The median PSA was 0.4, 0.2 and 0.1 ng/mL at 24, 36 and 48 months, respectively. The 3-year actuarial FFBF was 96 %. Kang et al. (2011) reported the results of a retrospective study on 44 patients with prostate cancer using a schedule of 4 fractions to a total dose of 32–36 Gy. After a median follow-up of 40 months there were no grade 3 or higher treatment-related toxicities and the 5-year FFBF rate of low-, intermediate-, and high-risk patients was 100, 100, and 90.8 %, respectively.

The first long-term outcomes from a prospective trial of SBRT for low-risk prostate cancer were published by King et al. (2012) who pooled 67 low-risk patients who received 35–36.25 Gy delivered in 5 fractions. After a median follow-up of 2.7 years, there were no grade 3 or higher rectal toxicity, no grade 4 urinary toxicity, and 3.5 % grade 3 urinary toxicity. The authors also found that low-grade toxicities were substantially less frequent in the alternate-day (QOD) versus daily dose (QD) regime for both gastrointestinal and genitourinary toxicity. The 4-year actuarial FFBF was 94 %. Madsen et al. (2007) reported a pioneering experience using a linac-based SBRT on 40 patients with localized prostate cancer delivering 33.5 Gy in 5 fractions. After a median follow-up of 41 months, only one acute grade 3 GU toxicity was detected and no instances of late grade 3 or higher toxicity was encountered. The actuarial 4-year FFBF was 90 %. Recently, Boike et al. (2011) evaluated the tolerability of escalating doses of linac-based SBRT in patients with intermediate-risk prostate cancer, by using fiducial markers and either megavoltage or kilovoltage CT for daily set-up verification. Three groups of 15 patients each received 45, 47.5, and 50 Gy (the highest SBRT dose reported to date), respectively, in 5 fractions every other day. After a median follow-up of 30, 18, and 12 months, respectively, grade ≥ 2 and ≥ 3 GI toxicity occurred in 18 and 2 %, respectively, and grade ≥ 2 and ≥ 3 GU toxicity in 31 and 4 %, respectively, of all patients, with a biochemical control rate of 100 %.

The premature results of these studies, although associated with good treatment tolerance, excellent early biochemical outcomes and low, late toxicity rates, did not lead to any firm conclusions on the clinical benefits of these regimens in comparison to escalated conventional dose fractionation. Nevertheless, a strong interest amongst the radiation oncologist community in the adoption of SBRT for localized prostate cancer has recently prompted the Radiation Therapy Oncology Group (RTOG) to open a randomized non-inferiority phase II trial, RTOG 0938 , comparing delivery of 36.25 Gy in 5 fractions over 2 weeks to 51.6 Gy in 12 fractions over 2.5 weeks (Lukka 2012).

The current 3- to 4-year FFBF rates of >90 %, reported in all SBRT published trials with a sufficient follow-up, seem to be consistent with the 5-year rates of ~90–95 % reported in trials of conventional escalated doses of 78–80 Gy. However, given the uncertainties, which exist in extrapolating biological effects to very large fraction size, these results need to be confirmed by appropriate randomized trials with a sufficiently long follow-up and accurate evaluation of long-term tolerance and toxicity, particularly of the urethra which is an unavoidable organ at risk in the irradiation of prostate cancer.

5 Conclusion

Prostate cancer is the leading cancer in men, with more than 382,000 new cases (22 % of all cancer in men) and 89,300 deaths estimated during 2008 in 40 European countries (Ferlay et al. 2012). The current standard options for local treatment include radical prostatectomy, brachytherapy (seed implantation or interstitial HDR), and dose-escalated external beam irradiation given at conventional dose fractions in an exhaustive overall treatment time. Current conventionally fractionated radiotherapy courses for prostate cancer at escalated doses are the longest treatment courses among those used for any tumours. Shorter effective regimes may provide an alternative to the more invasive treatment options with a significant impact on the patient's ability to contine working without the need for numerous daily visits to radiotherapy departments and extended toxicity and recovery time. Although, currently, there is no established evidence that the hypofractionated regimes are at least equivalent to conventional fractionation radiotherapy, several preliminary results from randomized and nonrandomized trials suggest that moderate hypofractionation could be considered as a standard treatment of prostate cancer, once established results with a longer follow-up confirm the early good clinical outcomes and quality of life measures achieved with shorter observation periods.

In spite of the promising results from several, small, and preliminary single-institutional studies, extreme hypofractionation regimes are largely unverified and need to be better evaluated by more adequate randomized studies. The technologic advances required by the SBRT technique, together with precise daily target localization, hold sufficient promise to warrant broader investigation.

References

Al-Magmani AA, Heemsbergen WD, Levendag PC, and Lebesque JV (2010) Subgroup analysis of patients with localized prostate cancer treated within the Dutch-randomized dose-escalation trial. Radiother Oncol 96:13–18

Arcangeli G, Saracino B, Gomellini S et al (2010) A prospective phase III randomized trial of hypofractionation versus conventional

fractionation in patients with high-risk prostate cancer. Int J Radiat Oncol Biol Phys 78:11–18
Arcangeli G, Fowler J, Gomellini S et al (2011) Acute and late toxicity in a randomized trial of conventional versus hypofractionated three-dimensional conformal radiotherapy for prostate cancer. Int J Radiat Oncol Biol Phys 79:1013–1021
Arcangeli S, Strigari L, Gomellini S et al (2012) Updated results and pattern of failures in a randomized hypofractionation trial for high-risk prostate cancer. Int J Radiat Oncol Biol Phys 84:1172–1178
Boike TP, Lotan Y, Cho LC et al (2011) Phase I dose-escalation study of stereotactic body radiation therapy for low- and intermediate-risk prostate cancer. J Clin Oncol 29:2020–2026
Brenner DJ, Martinez AA, Edmundson GK et al (2002) Direct evidence that prostate tumors shows high sensitivity to fractionation (low alpha/beta ratio), similar to late-responding normal tissue. Int J Radiat Oncol Biol Phys 52:6–13
Cowan RA, Mitchel DM, Bottomley IC et al (2007) Hypofractionated conformal radiotherapy for good prognosis carcinoma of the prostate: seven year outcome analysis. J Radiat Oncol Biol Phys 69:S339
Dearnaley DP, Sydes MR, Graham JD et al (2007) Escalated-dose versus standard-dose conformal radiotherapy in prostate cancer: first results from MRC RT01 randomised controlled trial. Lancet Oncol 8:475–487
Dearnaley D, Syndicus I, Sumo G et al (2012) Conventional versus hypofractionated high dose intensity-modulated radiotherapy for prostate cancer: preliminary safety results from CHHiP randomized controlled trial. Lancet Oncol 13:4354
Faria S, Dal Pra A, Cury F et al (2011) Treating intermediate-risk prostate cancer with hypofractionated external beam radiotherapy alone. Radiother Oncol 101:486–489
Ferlay J, Parkin DM, Steliarova-Foucher E (2012) Estimates of cancer incidence and mortality in Europe in 2008. Radiother Oncol 46:765–781
Fonteyne V, Soete G, Arcangeli S et al (2012) Hypofractionated high-dose radiation therapy for prostate cancer: long term results of a multi-institutional phase II trial. Int J Radiat Oncol Biol Phys 84:e483–e490
Fowler JF (2005) The radiobiology of prostate cancer including new aspects of fractionated radiotherapy. Acta Oncol 44(3): 265–276
Fowler J, Chappel R, Ritter M (2001) Is alpha/beta for prostate tumors really low? Int J Radiat Oncol Biol Phys 50:1021–1031
Freeman DE, King CR (2011) Stereotactic body radiotherapy for low-risk prostate cancer: five-year outcomes. Radiat Oncol 6:3
Fuller DB, Shirazi R, Naitoh J et al (2011) Virtual HDR SBRT for localized prostatic carcinoma: efficacy and quality of life assessment. Int J Radiat Oncol Biol Phys 81:S423–S424
Higgins GS, McLaren DB, Kerr GR et al (2006) Outcome analysis of 300 prostate cancer patients treated with neoadjuvant androgen deprivation and hypofractionated radiotherapy. Int J Radiat Oncol Biol Phys 65:982–989
Kang JK, Cho CK, Choi CW et al (2011) Image-guided stereotactic body radiation therapy for localized prostate cancer. Tumori 97:43–48
Katz AJ, Santoro M, Ashley R et al (2010) Stereotactic body radiotherapy for organ-confined prostate cancer. BMC Urol 10:1
Katz AJ, Santoro M, Di Blasio F et al (2011) Stereotactic body radiation therapy for low, intermediate and high-risk prostate cancer: disease control and quality of life. Int J Radiat Oncol Biol Phys 81:S100 (abstract)
King CR, Brooks JD, Gill H et al (2012) Long-term outcomes from a prospective trial of stereotactic body radiotherapy for low-risk prostate cancer. Int J Radiat Oncol Biol Phys 82(2):877–882
Kuban D, Pollack A, Huang E et al (2003) Hazard of dose escalation in prostate cancer radiotherapy. Int J Radiat Oncol Biol Phys 57:1260–1268
Kuban D, Tucker S, Dong L et al (2008) Long-term results of the M.D. Anderson randomized dose-escalation trial for prostate cancer. Int J Radiat Oncol. Biol Phys 70:67–74
Kuban DA, Nogueras-Gonzalez NG, Hamblin L et al (2010) Preliminary report of a randomized dose escalation trial for prostate cancer using hypofractionation. Int J Radiat Oncol Biol Phys 78(suppl):S58
Kupelian P, Willoughby TR, Reddy CA et al (2007) Hypofractionated intensity-modulated radiotherapy (70 Gy at 2.5 Gy per fraction) for localized prostate cancer: Cleveland clinic experience. Int J Radiat Oncol Bio Phys 68:1424–1430
Leborgne F, Fowler J (2009) Late outcomes following hypofractionated conformal radiotherapy vs. standard fractionation for localized prostate cancer: a non randomized contemporary comparison. Int J Radiat Oncol Biol Phys 74(1441):1446
Livsay JE, Cowan RA, Wylie J et al (2003) Hypofractionated conformal radiotherapy in carcinoma of the prostate: five-year outcome analysis. Int J Radiat Oncol Biol Phys 1254–1259
Lukka HR (2012) A randomized phase II trial of hypofractionated radiotherapy for favorable risk prostate cancer-RTOG CCOP study, 201125, Katz AJ Personal communication ASTRO 2012
Lukka H, Hayter C, Julian JA et al (2005) A randomized trial comparing two fractionation schedules for patients with localized prostate cancer. J Clin Oncol 23:6132–6138
Madsen BL, Hsi RA, Pham HT et al (2007) Stereotactic hypofractionated accurate radiotherapy of the prostate (SHARP), 33.5 Gy in five fractions for localized disease: first clinical trial results. Int J Radiat Oncol Biol Phys 67:1099–1105
Martin JM, Rosewall T, Bayley A et al (2007) Phase II trial of hypofractionated image-guided intensity-modulated radiotherapy for localized prostate adenocarcinoma. Int J Radiat Oncol Biol Phys 69:1084–1089
McBride SM, Wong DS, Dombrowski JJ et al (2011) Hypofractionated stereotactic body radiotherapy in low-risk prostate adenocarcinoma: Preliminary results of a multi-institutional phase 1 feasibility trial. Cancer 118:3681–3690
Michalski JM, Gay H, Jackson A, Tucker SL, Deasy JO (2010) Radiation dose-volume effects in radiation-induced rectal injury. Int J Radiat Oncol Biol Phys 76:S20–S27
Miralbel R, Roberts SA, Zubizarreta E et al (2012) Dose-fractionation sensitivity of prostate cancer deduced from radiotherapy outcomes of 5,969 patients in seven international institutional datasets: $\alpha/\beta = 1.4$ (0.9–2.2) Gy. Int J Radiat Oncol Biol Phys 82:e17–e24
Pollack AW, Buyounouski M, Horwitz E et al (2011) Five year results of a randomized external beam radiotherapy hypofractionation trial for prostate cancer. Int J Radiat Oncol Biol Phys 81(suppl):S1
Rene N, Faria S, Cury F et al (2010) Hypofractionated radiotherapy for favorable risk prostate cancer. Int J Radiat Oncol Biol Phys 77:805–810
Ritter MA, Forman JD, Kupelian P et al (2001) Five-year efficacy and toxicity outcomes from phase I/II trial of increasingly hypofractionated radiation therapy for prostate cancer. Int J Radiat Oncol Biol Phys 81(S2):S99
Steel GG (2003) Basic clinical radiobiology. Arnold, London
Strigari L, Arcangeli G, Arcangeli S, Benassi M (2009) Mathematical model for evaluating incidence of acute rectal toxicity during conventional or hypofractionated radiotherapy courses for prostate cancer. Int J Radiat Oncol Biol Phys 73(5):1454–1460
Thomson D, Merrick S, Swindell R et al (2012) Dose-escalated hypofractionated intensity-modulated radiotherapy in high-risk carcinoma of the prostate: outcome and late toxicity. Prostate Cancer. doi:10.1155/2012/450246

Williams SG, Taylor JM, Liu N et al (2007) Use of individual fraction size data from 3756 patients to directly determine the alpha/beta ratio of prostate cancer. Int J Radiat Oncol Biol Phys 68:24–33

Yeoh EE, Botten RJ, Butters J et al (2011) Hypofractionated versus conventionally fractionated radiotherapy for prostate carcinoma: final results of phase III randomized trial. Int J Radiat Oncol Biol Phys 81:1271–1278

Zelefsky MJ, Yamada Y, Fuks Z et al (2008) Long-term results of conformal radiotherapy for prostate cancer: impact of dose escalation on biochemical tumor control and distant metastasis-free survival. Int J Radiat Oncol Biol Phys 71:1028–1033

Focal Therapy and the Index Lesion Hypothesis in Prostate Cancer

Mitchell Kamrava and Patrick Kupelian

Contents

M. Kamrava (✉) · P. Kupelian
Department of Radiation Oncology, University of California Los Angeles, 200 UCLA Medical Plaza, Suite B265, Los Angeles, CA 90095, US
e-mail: mkamrava@mednet.ucla.edu

Abstract

Standard whole gland radiation therapy for prostate cancer results in high cure rates but impacts quality of life. Active surveillance is an alternative but has not been widely embraced. Focal therapy represents a middle ground between these two treatment options. In this paper we will review the rationale, patient selection considerations, technical planning issues, and recent clinical data for prostate focal therapy.

1 Introduction

The majority of newly diagnosed men with prostate cancer will have low risk disease. They will be faced with the decision to pursue definitive treatment or active surveillance. Definitive treatment results in significant changes in long-term quality of life and recent data questions whether treatment in low risk men impacts overall survival compared with observation (Sanda et al. 2008; Wilt et al. 2012). Active surveillance is an alternative to definitive treatment but ideal patient selection and monitoring is challenging and has limited its adoption (Klotz et al. 2010). Focal therapy presents a middle ground between definitive whole gland therapy and active surveillance. The goal of a "male lumpectomy" is to achieve equal cancer control to whole gland therapy but to reduce the risk of short and long term changes in quality of life. The stakes are high as long-term PSA control rates are already in the 90 % range (Grimm et al. 2012) for low risk patients and late toxicities for brachytherapy are about 5–10 % for genitourinary side effects, 1–5 % for gastrointestinal side effects, and 30–40 % for developing erectile dysfunction (Yamada et al. 2012). Ultimately there is still room to improve the therapeutic ratio for prostate cancer treatment and focal therapy may help achieve this. In this paper we will review the rationale,

H. Geinitz et al. (eds.), *Radiotherapy in Prostate Cancer*, Medical Radiology. Radiation Oncology,
DOI: 10.1007/174_2013_913,
Published Online: 7 September 2013

patient selection considerations, technical planning issues, and recent clinical data for prostate focal therapy.

2 Understanding the Rationale for Focal Therapy

One of the strongest arguments against focal therapy is the multifocal nature of prostate cancer is incompatible with partial gland treatment (Mouraviev et al. 2007; Tareen et al. 2009). The index lesion hypothesis is a controversial rebuttal to multifocality being a limitation for focal treatment. It suggests that regardless of whether prostate cancer is multifocal or not disease progression is typically driven by the largest tumor focus, or index lesion (Ahmed 2009). The argument then follows that by treating the index lesion with "active surveillance" of small satellite lesions that focal treatment may be a reasonable alternative to whole gland therapy. To explore the evidence for and against the index lesion hypothesis there are three questions that need to be discussed: (1) Does maximum tumor size correlate with prostate cancer treatment outcomes? (2) Does the index lesion harbor the most aggressive prostate cancer tumor cells? (3) Is there such a thing as insignificant prostate cancer?

2.1 Does Maximum Tumor Size Correlate with Treatment Outcomes?

The staging system for most cancers includes tumor size, however, prostate cancer does not. One of the issues is that prostate cancer growth is irregular and not spherical as in other disease sites. This results in a weaker correlation between maximum tumor diameter and tumor volume. There are also multiple other well-established prognostic factors such as Gleason score which correlate with tumor volume making the independent value of tumor volume on outcomes more difficult to discern. Challenges do exist in correlating tumor volume and treatment outcomes but there is solid data to support a correlation. In an analysis of 379 prostatectomy specimens percent Gleason 4/5, cancer volume, lymph node status, and vascular invasion independently predicted biochemical progression (Stamey Ta 1999). Rates of PSA control were 86 % in men with a cancer volume of 0.5–2.0 cm^3, 61 % with 2.0–6.0 cm^3, 33 % with 6.0–12.0 cm^3, and 3 % for > 12.0 cm^3 of cancer. This data is compelling but can be criticized for representing cases predating the PSA era and therefore not necessarily holding true in a PSA screened population. When reviewing the literature for correlations between maximum tumor volume and outcomes in more contemporary series the literature is mixed in its conclusions. In nine papers tumor volume was an independent predictor of biochemical recurrence while it was not in eight others (Epstein 2011). This discordance is multifactorial and includes variable patient populations, different tumor quantification methods, and interrelated prognostic variables. There is also indirect evidence for maximum tumor volume correlating with outcomes. At least two series show the PSA progression probability for multifocal tumors is better than for unifocal tumors. This suggests that smaller incidental tumors may have little prognostic significance (Wise et al. 2002; Noguchi et al. 2001). Outside the prostatectomy literature there is also data to support an index lesion hypothesis in radiation oncology. Cellini et al. performed a semiquantitative evaluation of the site of prostate cancer recurrence based on clinical examination and imaging prior to and after therapy (Cellini et al. 2002). In 12/118 patients with an intraprostatic recurrence all 12 had recurrence within their initial tumor volume. These findings have subsequently been confirmed in a study of 9 patients showing radiation failures were located at the same location on pretreatment and postradiation MRI. These imaging findings were verified on salvage prostatectomy pathology (Pucar et al. 2007). In another study MR imaging and MR spectroscopy was used in nine patients to show that the site of failure after radiation was at the same location as the dominant baseline tumor in 8/9 cases (Arrayeh et al. 2012). Additional data from salvage prostatectomy series following radiation failure suggests that "recurrent" cancer after radiation does not represent a new tumor but is usually the regrowth or persistence of the original cancer (Arakawa et al. 1995; Cheng et al. 1999). There is certainly data to support a correlation between maximum tumor size with clinical outcomes, however, the evidence is mixed regarding its independent prognostic value. Further evidence based on contemporary series is needed to definitively answer this question.

2.2 Does the Index Lesion Harbor the Most Aggressive Prostate Cancer Tumor Cells?

Studies show that most, if not all, metastatic prostate cancers have a monoclonal origin suggesting that despite prostate cancer being a multifocal and heterogenous disease that a single precursor cancer cell leads to metastatic disease (Mehra et al. 2008; Liu et al. 2009). This data argues that not all cancer foci within the prostate gland are important for predicting clinical outcomes. What remains controversial though is whether this single precursor cancer cell resides within the index lesion. Data supporting that the most aggressive cells are located within the index lesion include the fact that histological features of poor prognosis including Gleason score, extracapsular extension, and seminal vesicle invasion are almost always associated with the index lesion (Karavitakis et al. 2011). In one recent series of 100 radical prostatectomy specimens there was no case where a satellite focus had a higher Gleason score than the index lesion. There were only 2 cases where the satellite foci had extracapsular extension. In one case both the satellite lesion and the index lesion extended beyond the capsule and in the second only the satellite lesion extended outside. In both of these cases the satellite focus actually measured >0.5 cm^3 (a marker of significant disease). No satellite lesion was found to invade the seminal vesicles. The results from this study are compelling but would be strengthened with clinical follow-up data. There are older series showing a correlation between the index lesion and biochemical outcomes. Wise et al. reviewed prostatectomy specimens from 486 patients and correlated the volume of the index tumor versus the index tumor plus satellite lesions with biochemical disease free survival. With a median follow-up of 3.2 years biochemical outcomes were similar when just considering the index tumor volume versus the index tumor plus satellite lesions (Wise et al. 2002). In a much larger series of 1,159 men treated with radical prostatectomy pathologic and biochemical outcomes were compared between patients with unifocal versus multifocal disease (Rice et al. 2009). There were significantly higher rates of positive surgical margins, Gleason score 8–10 disease, and biochemical recurrence in the single focus group. Noguchi et al. also looked at the prognostic value of secondary cancers in 222 patients treated with surgery (Noguchi et al. 2001). 24 % had a single tumor, 39 % had an index tumor with secondary cancers <0.5 mL, and 37 % had an index tumor with secondary cancers >0.5 mL. There were no differences in baseline features between the groups on multivariate analysis. The group with multifocal smaller secondary cancers had better outcomes than those with a single index lesion. These data suggest that multifocal disease in and by itself does not portend a poorer prognosis but that the index lesion is the main driver of outcomes. This data needs, however, to be tempered by other studies showing non-index lesions can determine not only the pathological stage but also be important determinants of blood-borne and lymphatic metastasis (Ruijter et al. 1996; Djavan et al. 1999; Schmidt et al. 2006; Gburek et al. 1997; Miller and Cygan 1994).

2.3 Is There Such a Thing as Insignificant Prostate Cancer?

It is estimated that 20 % of prostate cancer patients have unifocal disease . If only these patients are appropriate candidates for focal therapy then only a small proportion of men will be eligible for this treatment. Alternatively, if we accept that only the index lesion needs to be treated and active surveillance of insignificant disease is appropriate then the pool of candidates for focal therapy dramatically increases. The term insignificant prostate cancer is used somewhat interchangeably in the literature with indolent, minimal, minute, low volume, and microfocal (Trpkov et al. 2010). The most commonly used terms are indolent and insignificant but there are slight differences in their definitions. An indolent cancer is one that, regardless of the lifespan of the patient, would never become clinically manifest (Ploussard et al. 2011). Insignificant cancer is a subset of indolent cancers that factors in patient age and comorbidities (Ploussard et al. 2011). The concept of insignificant disease was based on work by McNeal and presented by Stamey et al. when he reported on the tumor volume of incidental prostate cancer found in 139 cystoprostatectomy specimens (Stamey Ta et al. 1993). They concluded that tumors <0.5 cm^3 are unlikely to become clinically significant during the lifespan of a patient and need not be treated. Epstein et al. subsequently validated this threshold and the "Epstein" criteria are the most commonly used criteria to define insignificant disease (Epstein 1994). Insignificant disease is defined as prostate cancers with Gleason score ≤6, organ confined disease, <3 positive biopsy cores, ≤50 % involvement of any one core, and PSA density <0.15 ng/mL (Epstein 1994; Bastian et al. 2004; Epstein et al. 1998). Clinically, the concept of insignificant disease serves as the cornerstone of active surveillance. The 10 year prostate cancer specific survival for low risk patients on active surveillance is 97 % (Klotz et al. 2010). This suggests that there really is a group of prostate cancer patients with disease that is unlikely to be significant and therefore should just be monitored. The challenge is actually being able to identify this group of patients. The Epstein criteria, for example, are only able to correctly predict a prostate tumor volume <0.5 cm^3 on final pathology 75–80 % of the time (Ploussard et al. 2011). Many other authors have attempted to develop predictive models/nomograms for predicting insignificant disease at the time of surgery yet all of them misclassify patients in 10–20 % of cases (Makarov et al. 2007; Nakanishi et al. 2007; Chun et al. 2008). These data demonstrate that preoperative variables are insufficient to define insignificant disease. When considering the totality of evidence for and against the index lesion hypothesis one is left in limbo regarding which patients to select for focal therapy. Depending on how one interprets the existing literature appropriate focal therapy candidates could run the spectrum from including only those with truly unifocal disease to those with an index lesion and insignificant prostate cancer satellites.

3 Identifying Candidates for Focal Therapy

Regardless of whether one agrees with the index lesion hypothesis or only believes in treating unifocal disease there are limitations in characterizing the location, size, extent, multifocality, and biological potential of prostate cancer. The fact that 80 % of secondary non-index foci within the prostate gland are less than 0.5 mL (Villers et al. 1992) makes it unlikely that existing imaging technologies can characterize all prostate cancer foci. This makes it more realistic to focus patient selection on defining an index lesion and the absence of significant disease elsewhere. This concept of a biologically unifocal tumor was coined by Bostwick et al. and is an important concept in focal therapy patient selection (Bostwick et al. 2006). Estimates for how many men may have biologically unifocal disease ranges in the literature from about 50–65 % (Karavitakis et al. 2012; Bott et al. 2010).

The ideal way to identify patients with biologically unifocal lesions is an area of intense investigation. The greatest controversy centers on the ideal biopsy method to ensure accurate and detailed mapping of the true extent of disease. One thing we know is that a systematic sextant biopsy is a poor sampling tool to accurately predict the extent and significance of disease (Noguchi et al. 2001). Others have examined sextant versus 12 core extended biopsy strategies to predict unilateral prostate cancer. Taking more cores does improve the diagnostic accuracy of predicting unilateral disease (49 vs. 59 %, $p < 0.05$) but this technique is also not ideal (Tsivian et al. 2010). Onik et al. took things a step further and compared 180 patients with biopsy proven unilateral prostate cancer on transrectal ultrasound (TRUS)-guided biopsies with biopsy outcomes using a transperineal mapping (TPM) approach (Onik et al. 2009). Mapping was done using a brachytherapy grid under TRUS guidance and biopsies were taken every 5 mm throughout the prostate. For the 84 patients who had ≥10 cores taken on their initial TRUS (mean 13.9) and were thought to have unilateral disease 60 % actually had bilaterally disease. Of the 100 patients who were thought to have low risk disease 26 % had an increase to Gleason score ≥7 and 50 % thought to have unilateral disease actually had bilateral disease. These results demonstrate that TPM biopsies have a high accuracy in defining the extent of disease.

Although TPM biopsies are currently the most accurate method of finding all disease there are not many studies comparing the chances of finding significant cancer for different biopsy techniques. Computer simulation modeling can provide some insight to determine the ideal biopsy method to find clinically significant disease with one such study doing modeling on 96 prostates acquired at radical cystoprostatectomy. They simulated how well 12 core transrectal, 14 core transrectal, and TPM biopsies are in finding clinically significant disease (Gleason score ≥7 and/or lesion volume 0.5 mL or greater) (Lecornet et al. 2012). Receiver operating curve analysis to detect and rule out clinically significant disease was 0.69, 0.75, 0.82, and 0.91 for 12 core transrectal biopsies with random localization errors of 15 and 10 mm, 14 core transrectal biopsies, and TPM biopsies using a 5 mm sampling frame. All biopsy approaches missed patients with clinically significant prostate cancer, however, only 1 % were missed on TPM biopsies versus about 5–15 % with other transrectal approaches. This suggests that TPM biopsies are the ideal method to identify clinically significant disease. A similar type of simulation was done on radical prostatectomy specimens that compared five different TRUS biopsy techniques to transperineal biopsy. TRUS biopsy missed 30–40 % of lesions ≥0.2 mL and ≥0.5 mL while TPM biopsy missed only 5 % of such lesions (Hu et al. 2012).

While TPM biopsy is the most accurate way to identify clinically significant disease it is expensive, cumbersome, invasive (the above Onik study took a median of 50 cores), and can have complications. Improvements in MRI imaging and in particular multiparametric MRI (mp-MRI) imaging have led some to advocate that mp-MRI with targeted biopsies may rival the accuracy of TPM biopsy.

In one study that used 3T MRI that included diffusion weighted imaging, MR spectroscopy, and dynamic contrast-enhanced MR and did a one-to-one histopathological correlation the positive predictive value of mp-MRI to detect prostate cancer was 98, 98, and 100 % in the overall prostate, peripheral zone, and central gland (Turkbey et al. 2011). There was a significantly higher sensitivity for tumors larger than 5 mm in diameter and for tumors with a Gleason score greater than 7. The positive predictive value for detecting prostate cancer in the peripheral zone using all 4 sequences was 98 % which was significantly higher than using T2 W MRI alone (positive predictive value 69 %). The negative predictive value (83–90 %) was, however, similar for the different sequences and did not improve by using all 4 sequences. These results demonstrate that mp-MRI has a high sensitivity for identifying prostate cancer lesions but is best for finding lesions greater than 5 mm in diameter.

For the lesions that are too small for mp-MRI to reliably characterize it appears that these cancers are of little significance. In one study standard 12 core TRUS followed by TRUS/MRI-fused biopsy of specific target lesions was performed on a group of 125 patients with low suspicion prostate lesions on mp-MRI (Yerram et al. 2012). 77 patients (62 %) on TRUS/MR fusion biopsy had no cancer detected, 38 had Gleason 6, and 10 had Gleason 7 (3 + 4). There were no cases of Gleason 4 + 3 or greater. 15 patients had a prostatectomy and none were upgrade to high risk prostate cancer. In total 88 % either had no cancer or clinically insignificant disease. This data shows that mp-MRI can identify a population of low risk patients that are unlikely to harbor high risk disease.

Given TPM biopsy is the most accurate method for mapping out the extent of disease a comparison between this technique and transperineal mp-MRI-targeted biopsies was carried out in 182 men. The goal was to see whether there were differences in finding clinically significant prostate cancer (maximum cancer core length of $\geq$4 mm and/or Gleason score $\geq$3 + 4). A median of 30 cores was obtained for the TPM biopsies versus 5 for the MRI-targeted approach. The rate of finding clinically significant cancer between the two biopsy methods was similar. The rate of finding insignificant cancer was, however, higher with TPM biopsies versus MRI targeted ones (17 vs. 9.3 %). These results show that a targeted approach has encouraging rates of detecting clinically significant prostate cancer but further study is needed as 16 % of cases in this series defined as having insignificant cancer on targeted biopsy had clinically significant cancer on transperineal biopsies (Kasivisvanathan et al. 2013).

In a different approach a prebiopsy mp-MRI that included diffusion weighted imaging was performed and followed by a 14 core biopsy (8 transperineal and 6 transrectal) (Matsuoka et al. 2012). 135 patients then went on to have radical prostatectomy. They divided patients into those with lobes with no cancer, lobes with indolent cancer, and lobes with significant cancer. Indolent was defined as <0.5 cm^3 and GS $\leq$3 + 4. The negative predictive value of diffusion weighted imaging and the prostate biopsy was 96 % for predicting lobes with significant cancer.

mp-MRI-targeted imaging is improving and further evolution of this technique may soon rival TPM. Until that time TPM biopsies still represent the gold standard for characterizing the full extent of disease.

4 Technical Issues Related to Focal Therapy with Radiation Therapy

There are multiple treatment platforms for delivering focal treatment including high intensity frequency ultrasound (HIFU), cryoablation, laser therapy, photodynamic therapy, and radiation. There is growing literature with non-radiation techniques but relatively little on radiation-based ones. Proposed definitions for different types of focal therapy were presented in a recent consensus statement on focal low dose rate brachytherapy (Langley et al. 2012). Three types of focal brachytherapy were proposed: (1) ultra-focal (treatment of an index lesion plus margin), (2) hemi-focal (treatment to half a gland), and (3) focused therapy (full dose to the involved hemi-gland but a reduced dose to the contralateral gland) (Fig. 1). Definitions for contouring targets were also introduced including F-GTV for the gross visible or clinically demonstrable cancer, F-CTV for the F-GTV plus a margin for clinically insignificant disease, and F-PTV for the F-CTV plus a margin to compensate for uncertainties in image registration and treatment delivery. No recommendations for actual margin sizes were suggested. There is some data from Turkbey et al. that correlated the size of index lesions on mp-MRI with their actual size on prostatectomy specimens for 135 patients (Turkbey et al. 2012). MRI tumor volume tended to overestimate the size of the lesion on final pathology by a mean of 7 % and size correlation was best for lesions >0.5 cm^3. A significant limitation of this study is that a universal shrinkage factor was used. Data on image registration errors between preprocedural MRI and MRI-guided procedures are reported around 1.3 mm while those for TRUS to MRI a bit larger at 2.4 mm (Hu et al. 2012; Fedorov et al. 2012).

Irrespective of the approach (ultra-focal, hemi-focal, focused) there are technical considerations to consider as well. A hemi-focal approach does not require either TRUS/MRI fusion or MRI-based brachytherapy seed/catheter insertion. The target can be adequately encompassed as the urethra serves as the midline and is clearly defined with a foley catheter and aerated jelly. On the other hand if one considers implanting just the peripheral zone as a hemi-focal technique then using ultrasound alone is likely not sufficient. Other more ultra-focal approaches are even riskier in terms of inadequately encompassing the target and should be done using TRUS/MRI fusion or MRI-based approaches. In fact, some have argued that a disadvantage of radiation therapy for focal therapy is the fact that there is no real time feedback of tissue destruction.

There are additional considerations with defining targets based on mp-MRI for focal therapy. mp-MRI shows a lesion in about 84 % of cases (68, 89, and 100 % of patients with NCCN low, intermediate, and high risk disease) (Kamrava et al. 2013). This means approximately 30 % of low risk patients will not have an identifiable target for an ultra-focal approach. When patients do have a lesion it still needs to be biopsied and cannot be assumed to be cancer. A modified version of the European Society of Uroradiology guidelines has been used to stratify the suspicion of cancer for target lesions. Based on TRUS/MRI fusion biopsies, patients with a cancer suspicion score of 5 have a 94 % chance of having prostate cancer but only 29 % of low risk patients have a score of 4–5 (Kamrava et al. 2013; Sonn et al. 2013). So there will be many low risk patients with

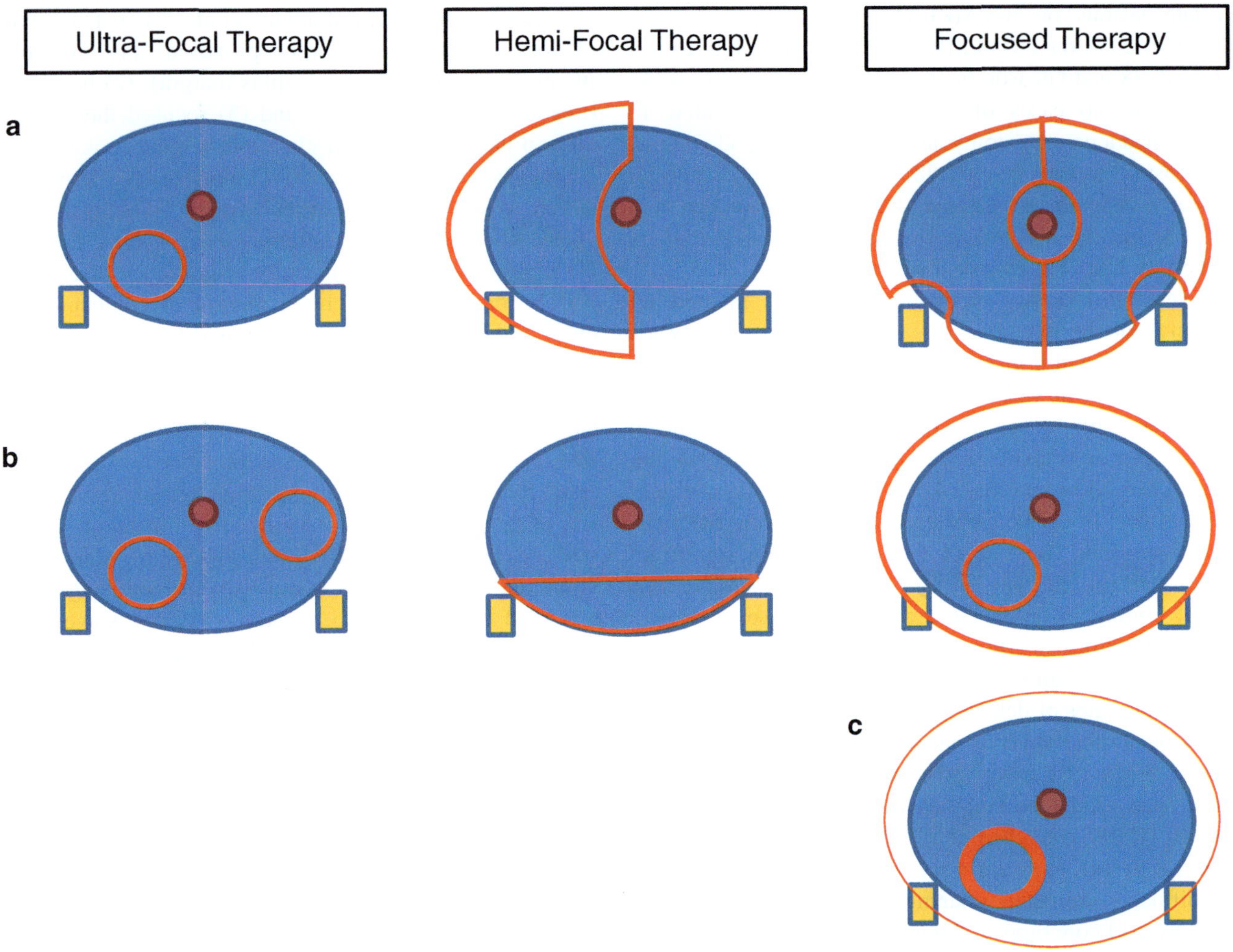

Fig. 1 Examples of different types of focal therapy. Ultra-focal therapy refers to treating **a** a specific target lesion or **b** multiple target lesions with a margin. Hemi-focal therapy refers to treating **a** half the gland with the urethra serving as midline or **b** treating the peripheral zone only. Focused therapy refers to differentially treating parts of the prostate gland. Examples of this include **a** full dose to the prostate gland but with sparing of the urethra and neurovascular bundles, **b** full dose to the prostate gland and a boost to a target lesion, and **c** full dose to a target lesion but less than full dose to the whole prostate gland. *Blue circle* = prostate gland, *red filled circle* = urethra, *red open circles* = treatment target, *orange rectangle* = neurovascular bundle

either no target lesion or a lesion with a low suspicion score. The effect of hormone therapy on the conspicuity of MRI target lesions also needs to be considered as hormones can change the appearance of targets (Groenendaal et al. 2012).

The best radiation technique (low dose rate seeds, high dose rate brachytherapy, stereotactic body radiation therapy, intensity-modulated proton therapy) for focal therapy is also unknown. When using a low dose rate approach the above consensus statement suggests a preplanned approach that ideally includes mp-MRI fusion with TRUS. Real time intraoperative dose planning is also ideal. In deciding between ^{125}I, ^{103}Pd, and ^{131}Cs it was felt ^{125}I has the most favorable characteristics. Stranded or linked seeds were recommended in the periphery with loose seeds centrally to provide more flexibility. Lower seed activity ($\sim$0.5 U) was also felt to be advantageous as it allows for seeds to be spaced closer together.

There are no consensus guidelines for other radiation techniques but there is one dosimetry paper that has examined the magnitude of dose reduction with standard high dose rate brachytherapy whole gland versus hemi-gland treatment (Kamrava et al. 2013) (Fig. 2). 10 whole-gland high dose rate prostate implants were used to generate 10 whole-gland and 20 hemi-gland (consisting of left and right) treatment plans using Inverse Planning Simulation Annealing using Oncentra Masterplan (Nucletron). The hemi-gland contour was a modification of the whole gland contour whereby the urethra was used to divide the volume into a left and right hemi-gland. Hemi-gland treatment decreased the D_{avg} to the rectum, bladder, and urethra by a

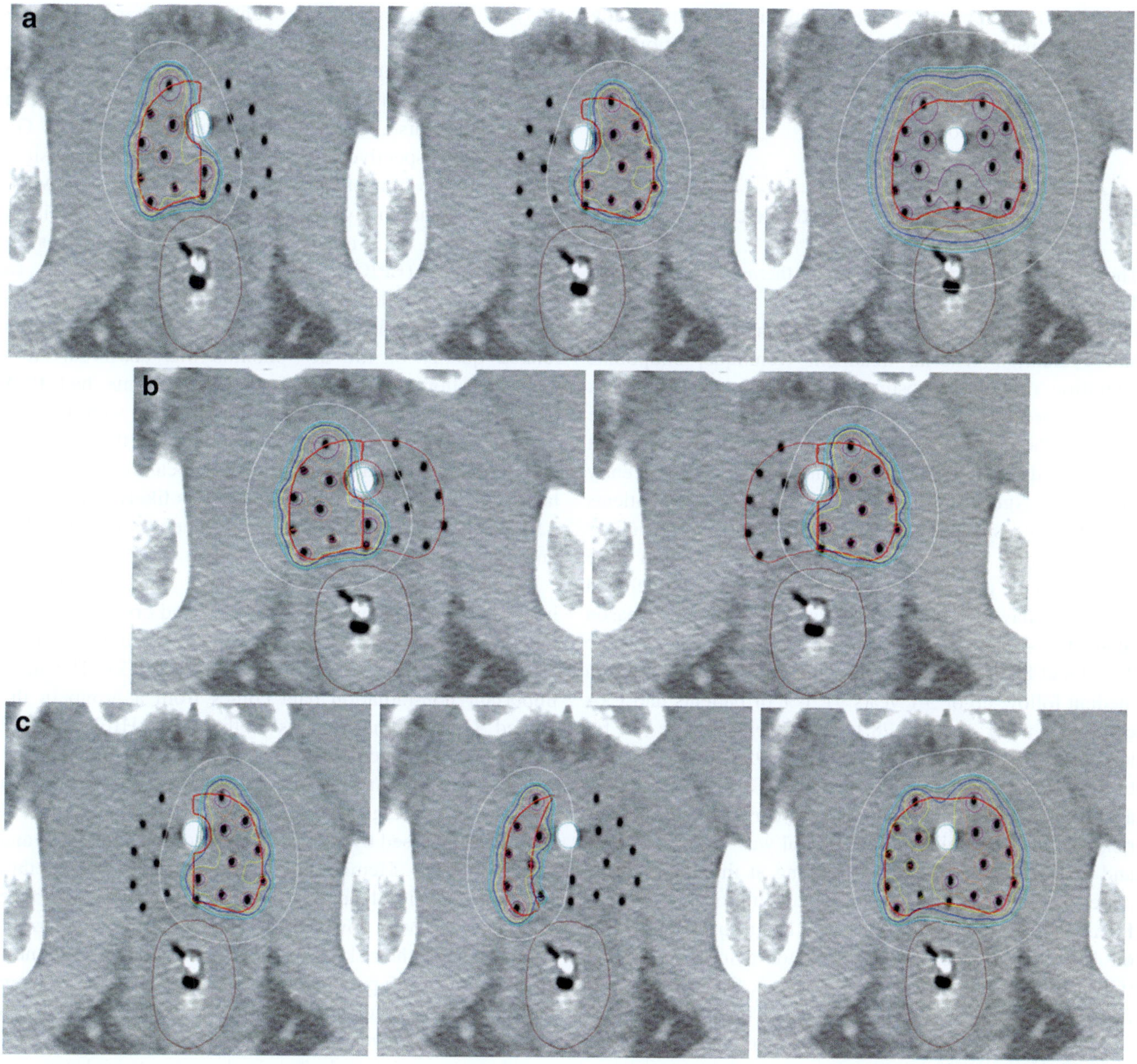

Fig. 2 Examples of the isodose distribution (*blue* = 100 %, *yellow* = 110 %, *white* = 50 %) with high dose rate brachytherapy hemi-gland treatment. These images are axial slices of a high dose rate brachytherapy implant where the whole prostate gland contour was split into right and left hemi-gland contours with the urethra serving as the midline. Figure 2a demonstrates the isodose distribution of a right hemi-gland treatment, a left hemi-gland treatment, and a summation of the right and left hemi-gland plans demonstrating that simply adding the two hemi-gland plans overdoses normal tissues. Figure 2b shows the extent of "spill" from a right and left hemi-gland treatment into the contralateral hemi-gland. Figure 2c demonstrates an example of a left hemi-gland treatment, a matching field in the event of a contralateral failure, and a summation of the two plans showing acceptable doses to organs at risk

difference of 7.0, 5.9, and 16.3 %. Another dosimetric consideration with radiation therapy which is not true with other ablative technologies is the fact that the dose of radiation therapy does not fall off immediately outside of the target. This "spill dose" may be advantageous if this dose is adequate to treat insignificant disease that falls within this "spill dose" region but may be a disadvantage when considering retreatment options. In the above-mentioned HDR dosimetry study the "spill dose" was determined for one case and it was determined that the V_{50} to the contralateral gland was 40 % (Kamrava et al. 2013). This means that if one were to retreat the contralateral hemi-gland and sum the dose from the original plan and the retreatment plan then one would overdose the organs at risk (Kamravaet al. 2013). A modified contour is necessary with a modified dose to meet current dose constraints (Kamrava et al. 2013). The example presented in this dosimetric study did not consider issues such as prostate deformation and size changes following treatment and so the reality of combining dose from an initial implant and retreatment will certainly be more complicated.

5 Clinical Outcomes with Focal Therapy

There is a growing body of focal therapy clinical data. Trying to draw definitive conclusions from the existing literature is challenging. Studies vary greatly in inclusion and evaluation criteria, treatment technique, endpoints, definition of failure, posttreatment assessment protocols, and measures of toxicity. A great deal of insight can still be gleaned, though, from the existing literature. The largest study to date investigating focal therapy was recently updated by Nguyen et al. (Nguyen et al. 2012). 318 patients were treated using intraoperative MRI guidance to deliver low dose rate brachytherapy using ^{125}I (minimum dose 137 Gy) to the peripheral zone only. Entry criteria included being T1c, having a PSA < 15 ng/mL and a biopsy Gleason score 3 + 4 or less. 88 % of patients had Gleason score 3 + 3 and 83 % of the patient cohort was low risk. With a median follow-up of 5.1 years 91.5 % of patients had PSA control by nadir + 2 and 78.1 % at 8 years. Nadir + 2 for low risk patients at 5 and 8 years was 95.1 % and 80.4 % but this improved to 95.6 % and 90.0 % using nadir + 2 and PSA velocity >0.75 ng/mL per year. For intermediate risk patients PSA failure-free survival was 73 % at 5 years and 66.4 % at 8 years. When looking at the cohort of 36 patients who failed by the nadir + 2 definition 16/22 with a PSA velocity >0.75 ng/mL per year had a suspicious lesion on MRI that was biopsy positive for a local recurrence (Gleason 3 + 3 in 5, Gleason 3 + 4 in 2, Gleason 4 + 3 in 2, Gleason 4 + 4 in 1, Gleason 3 + 5 in 1, and Gleason 4 + 5 in 2). For the 10 patients with nadir + 2 failure but PSA velocity <0.75 ng/mL per year only 2 had suspicious lesions on MRI. Both underwent 12 core biopsy and one Gleason score 3 + 3 = 6 disease was found. Based on this data PSA velocity greater than 0.75 ng/mL per year in addition to nadir + 2 better predicts failure in this less than whole gland treatment setting. While this provides some evidence-based guidance, PSA kinetics post partial gland therapy are ultimately not well understood. Our limited understanding of PSA changes post partial gland treatment serves as an impediment to defining ideal follow-up and definitions of failure.

Other focal therapy radiation approaches have used intensity modulated radiation therapy to spare the urethra in a more focused therapy approach. A randomized phase II study of urethra sparing treatment versus standard whole gland therapy for NCCN low risk patients was recently published (Vainshtein et al. 2012). The prescription dose was 75.6 Gy and for the urethral sparing plans the mean proximal and distal urethral doses were limited to 65 Gy and 74 Gy, respectively. Patients had to have no visible lesion within 5 mm of the prostatic urethra seen on MRI. The primary endpoint was a change in urinary health related quality of life at 3 months using the Expanded Prostate Cancer Index (EPIC) quality of life questionnaire. 16 patients were randomized and the trial was subsequently halted as no significant differences in EPIC urinary health related quality of life at 3 months was observed. At a median follow-up of 4.7 years three patients had PSA failure in the urethral sparing group but there were none in the standard treatment group. Two out of the three patients with PSA failure had biopsy proven local failure contralateral to the original site of disease. It is likely that using a 1.5T MRI with no multiparametric sequences that the MRI understaged some of these patients.

Outside of radiation therapy there are a number of important focal therapy studies. HIFU and cryoablation are the most developed techniques, however, multiple other techniques are emerging (Bozzini et al. 2013). The most important non-radiation data comes from a group in the United Kingdom that focuses on the use of HIFU (Ahmed et al. 2011). They conducted a Phase I/II trial in men with either low or intermediate risk disease (PSA ≤ 15, Gleason score ≤4 + 3, stage ≤T2b). They had to have unilateral disease as assessed by TRUS guided biopsies, mp-MRI, and TPM biopsies. Hemi-gland treatment with the urethra defining the mid-gland was delivered using the Sonablate 500. The trial was powered to see if focal therapy significantly reduces the risk of erectile dysfunction at 12 months post-treatment. 20 patients were enrolled and 75 % of them had D'Amico based intermediate risk disease. mp-MRI at 6 months showed residual cancer in the treated lobe in 2 men but no suspicious lesions in the untreated lobe in any. There was an 80 % decrease in PSA seen at 3 months that persisted at 12 months (7.3 vs. 1.5 ng/mL). 2 patients with positive mp-MRI at 6 months had biopsies. Both had low volume disease with 1 mm Gleason 3 + 3 in 1 of 4 and 1 of 5 biopsies. One patient elected to undergo active surveillance and the other was retreated with HIFU. 89 % of patients achieved the trifecta status of pad-free, leak-free continence, and erections sufficient for intercourse. This same group subsequently published the first study using an ultra-focal HIFU approach (Ahmed et al. 2012). Low risk patients (PSA ≤ 15, Gleason score ≤4 + 3, stage ≤T2a) were included and evaluated using 1.5T mp-MRI and transperineal template mapping biopsies. The edges of the ablative zone needed to be at least 10 mm from a neurovascular bundle or at least 5 mm from both neurovascular bundles if disease was bilateral. Untreated areas could not have any histological evidence of prostate cancer. A maximum of two areas could be treated and were treated with at least 3–5 mm margins. Primary outcomes were feasibility, patient acceptability, and side-effect profile. Secondary outcomes were histological and imaging measures of cancer control. 41 men were treated with 49 % receiving unilateral one area ablation, 37 % receiving bilateral two area ablation, and 15 % receiving a midline one area ablation. Median PSA level at baseline was 6.6 ng/mL and at 12 months follow-up was 1.9 ng/mL. 39 patients had a biopsy at 6 months with a mean of 6 cores taken. mp-MRI at 6 months showed signs of residual cancer in the treated areas in nine men and was confirmed on biopsy in seven of them. Two men had negative mp-MRIs but positive biopsies. Both demonstrated clinically insignificant disease. Of the men with positive biopsies five chose active surveillance and four chose retreatment with HIFU. Of the 31 men with good baseline function 84 % achieved the trifecta status of being leak-free, pad-free, erections sufficient for intercourse, and with no evidence of clinically significant disease on mp-MRI at 12 months. Cryotherapy is another very common focal therapy technique and the largest cohort of patients treated with this modality was reported from the Cryo On-Line Database (COLD) registry (Ward and Jones 2012). Focal therapy to a portion of the gland was performed in 1,160 patients (47 % low risk and 41 % intermediate risk) with biochemical control (old ASTRO definition) at 36 months of 75.7 %. This is similar to the biochemical recurrence-free survival of patients treated with whole gland cryotherapy treatment at 75.1 %. Toxicity rates were either similar or better in the focal versus whole gland cryotherapy group: urinary incontinence 1.6 versus 3.1 %, new-onset erectile dysfunction 41.9 versus 67.6 %, rectourethral fistula 0.1 versus 0.4 %, urinary retention 1.2 versus 1.6 %. Definitive conclusions from this data are limited because of the lack of defined criteria for treating patients.

Radiation, HIFU, and cryotherapy are all viable treatment modalities for focal therapy. Whether one modality is superior to another is not known and further studies are needed to determine the ideal use of each modality.

6 Conclusions

Focal therapy for prostate cancer is an emerging treatment option for the overtreatment of prostate cancer. Its goal is to provide equivalent tumor control while reducing acute and late term morbidities. Initial data appears promising, however, much more work is needed to consider this standard of care. Patients interested in focal therapy should be enrolled on well-designed clinical trials so definitive conclusions regarding this treatment approach can be made.

References

Ahmed HU (2009) The index lesion and the origin of prostate cancer. N Engl J Med 361(17):1704–1706

Ahmed HU et al (2011) Focal therapy for localized prostate cancer: a phase I/II trial. J Urol 185(4):1246–1255

Ahmed HU et al (2012) Focal therapy for localised unifocal and multifocal prostate cancer: a prospective development study. Lancet Oncol 13(6):622–632

Arakawa A et al (1995) High grade prostatic intraepithelial neoplasia in prostates removed following irradiation failure in the treatment of prostatic adenocarcinoma. Pathol Res Pract 191(9):868–872

Arrayeh E et al (2012) Does local recurrence of prostate cancer after radiation therapy occur at the site of primary tumor? Results of a longitudinal MRI and MRSI study. Int J Radiat Oncol Biol Physics 82(5):787–e793

Bastian PJ et al (2004) Characteristics of insignificant clinical T1c prostate tumors. Cancer 101(9):2001–2005

Bostwick DG et al (2007) Group consensus reports from the consensus conference on focal treatment of prostatic carcinoma, celebration, florida, February 24, 2006. Urology 70(6, Supplement 1):S42–S44

Bozzini G et al (2013) Focal therapy of prostate cancer: energies and procedures. Urol Oncol Semin Original Invest 31:155–167

Bott SRJ et al (2010) The index lesion and focal therapy: an analysis of the pathological characteristics of prostate cancer. BJU International 106(11):1607–1611

Cellini N et al (2002) Analysis of intraprostatic failures in patients treated with hormonal therapy and radiotherapy: implications for conformal therapy planning. Int J Radiat Oncol Biol Physics 53(3): 595–599

Cheng L et al (1999) Prevalence and distribution of prostatic Intraepithelial neoplasia in Salvage radical prostatectomy specimens after radiation therapy. Am Jo Surg Pathol 23(7):803

Chun FKH et al (2008) Critical assessment of tools to predict clinically insignificant prostate cancer at radical prostatectomy in contemporary men. Cancer 113(4):701–709

Djavan BSM, Bursa B, Basharkhah A, Simak R, Marberger M (1999) Predictability and significance of multifocal prostate cancer in the radical prostatectomy specimen. Tech Urol 5(3):139–142

EpsteinJI CD, Sokoll LJ, Wlash PC, Cox JL, Rittenhouse H, Wolfert R, Carter HB (1998) Nonpalpable stage T1c prostate cancer: prediction of insignificant disease using free/total prostate specific antigen levels and needle biopsy findings. J Urol 160(6 Pt 2): 2407–2411

Epstein JI (2011) Prognostic significance of tumor volume in radical prostatectomy and needle biopsy specimens. J Urol 186(3): 790–797

Epstein Ji WPCCMBCB (1994) PAthologic and clinical findings to predict tumor extent of nonpalpable (stage t1 c) prostate cancer. J Am Med Assoc 271(5):368–374

Fedorov A et al (2012) Image registration for targeted MRI-guided transperineal prostate biopsy. J Magn Reson Imaging 36(4): 987–992

Gburek BM et al (1997) Chromosomal anomalies in stage D1 prostate adenocarcinoma primary tumors and lymph node metastases detected by Fluorescence in situ hybridization. J Urol 157(1): 223–227

Groenendaal G et al (2012) The effect of hormonal treatment on conspicuity of prostate cancer: implications for focal boosting radiotherapy. Radiother Oncol 103(2):233–238

Grimm P et al (2012) Comparative analysis of prostate-specific antigen free survival outcomes for patients with low, intermediate and high risk prostate cancer treatment by radical therapy. Results from the prostate cancer results study group. BJU International 109:22–29

Hu Y et al (2012a) A biopsy simulation study to assess the accuracy of several transrectal ultrasonography (TRUS)-biopsy strategies compared with template prostate mapping biopsies in patients who have undergone radical prostatectomy. BJU Int 110(6):812–820

Hu Y et al (2012b) MR to ultrasound registration for image-guided prostate interventions. Med Image Anal 16(3):687–703

Kamrava M C.M, Kayode O, Wang J, Marks L, Kupelian P, Steinberg M, Park S, Demanes D (2013) Focal high-dose-rate brachytherapy: a dosimetric comparison of hemi-gland versus conventional whole-gland treatment brachytherapy. Brachytherapy 86(5):819–821

Kamrava M, M.S, Banergee R, Raman S, Marks L, Demanes D, Margolis D (2013) Evaluating the utility of a multi-parametric MRI based cancer suspicion score in defining brachytherapy focal therapy targets for prostate cancer. In: Proceedings of the American Brachytherapy society 2013 Annual Meeting

Karavitakis M et al (2011) Histological characteristics of the index lesion in whole-mount radical prostatectomy specimens: implications for focal therapy. Prostate Cancer Prostatic Dis 14(1):46–52

Karavitakis M, Ahmed HU, Abel PD, Hazell S, Winkler MH (2012) Anatomically versus biologically unifocal prostate cancer: a pathological evaluation in the context of focal therapy. Ther Adv Urol 4(4):155–160

Kasivisvanathan V et al (2013) Transperineal magnetic resonance image targeted prostate biopsy versus transperineal template prostate biopsy in the detection of clinically significant prostate cancer. J Urology 189(3):860–866

Klotz L et al (2010) Clinical results of long-term follow-up of a large, active surveillance cohort with localized prostate cancer. J Clin Oncol 28(1):126–131

Langley S et al (2012) Report of a consensus meeting on focal low dose rate brachytherapy for prostate cancer. BJU Int 109:7–16

Lecornet E et al (2012) The accuracy of different biopsy strategies for the detection of clinically important prostate cancer: a computer simulation. J Urol 188(3):974–980

Liu W et al (2009) Copy number analysis indicates monoclonal origin of lethal metastatic prostate cancer. Nat Med 15(5):559–565

Makarov DV et al (2007) Updated nomogram to predict pathologic stage of prostate cancer given prostate-specific antigen level, clinical stage, and biopsy gleason score (partin tables) based on cases from 2000 to 2005. Urology 69(6):1095–1101

Matsuoka Y et al (2012) Combination of diffusion-weighted magnetic resonance imaging and extended prostate biopsy predicts lobes without significant cancer: application in patient selection for hemiablative focal therapy. Eur Urol Oct 16. pii: S0302-2838(12)01229-8

Mehra R et al (2008) Characterization of TMPRSS2-ETS gene aberrations in androgen-independent metastatic prostate cancer. Cancer Res 68(10):3584–3590

Miller GJ, Cygan JM (1994) Morphology of prostate cancer: the effects of multifocality on histological grade, tumor volume and cpsule penetration. J Urol 152(5 Pt 2):1709–1713

Mouraviev V et al (2007) Prostate cancer laterality as a rationale of focal ablative therapy for the treatment of clinically localized prostate cancer. Cancer 110(4):906–910

Nakanishi H et al (2007) A nomogram for predicting low-volume/low-grade prostate cancer. Cancer 110(11):2441–2447

Nguyen PL et al (2012) Updated results of magnetic resonance imaging guided partial prostate brachytherapy for favorable risk prostate cancer: implications for focal therapy. J Urol 188(4): 1151–1156

Noguchi M et al (2001) Relationship between systematic biopsies and histological features of 222 radical prostatectomy specimens: lack of prediction of tumor significance for men with nonpalpable prostate cancer. J Urol 166(1):104–110

Onik G, Miessau M, Bostwick DG (2009) Three-dimensional prostate mapping biopsy has a potentially significant impact on prostate cancer management. J Clin Oncol 27(26):4321–4326

Ploussard G et al (2011) The contemporary concept of significant versus insignificant prostate cancer. Eur Urol 60(2):291–303

Pucar D (2007) et al., Clinically significant prostate cancer local recurrence after radiation therapy occurs at the site of primary tumor: magnetic resonance imaging and step-section pathology evidence. Int J Radiat Oncol Biol Physics 69(1):62–69

Rice KR et al (2009) Clinicopathological behavior of single focus prostate adenocarcinoma. J Urol 182(6):2689–2694

Ruijter ET et al (1996) Histological grade heterogeneity in multifocal prostate cancer. Biological and clinical implications. J Pathol 180(3):295–299

Sanda MG et al (2008) Quality of life and satisfaction with outcome among prostate-cancer survivors. N Engl J Med 358(12): 1250–1261

Schmidt H et al (2006) Asynchronous growth of prostate cancer is reflected by circulating tumor cells delivered from distinct, even SMALL foci, harboring loss of heterozygosity of the PTEN gene. Cancer Res 66(18):8959–8965

Sonn GA et al (2013) Targeted biopsy in the detection of prostate cancer using an office based magnetic resonance ultrasound fusion device. J Urol 189(1):86–92

Stamey Ta FF McNeal JE, Redwine EA, Whittermore AS, Schmid H (1993) Localized prostate cancer. Relationship of tumor volume to clinical significance for treatment of prostate cancer. Cancer 71(S3):993–938

Stamey Ta MJEYCMSBMJIM (1999) BIological determinants of cancer progression in men with prostate cancer.J Am Med Assoc 281(15):1395–1400

Tareen B et al (2009) Appropriate candidates for hemiablative focal therapy are infrequently encountered among men selected for radical prostatectomy in contemporary cohort. Urology 73(2): 351–354

Trpkov K et al (2010) 'Insignificant' prostate cancer on prostatectomy and cystoprostatectomy: variation on a theme 'low-volume/low-grade' prostate cancer? BJU Int 106(3):304–315

Tsivian M et al (2010) Predicting unilateral prostate cancer on routine diagnostic biopsy: sextant versus extended. BJU International 105(8):1089–1092

Turkbey B et al (2011) Multiparametric 3T prostate magnetic resonance imaging to detect cancer: histopathological correlation using prostatectomy specimens processed in customized magnetic resonance imaging based molds. J Urol 186(5):1818–1824

Turkbey B et al (2012) Correlation of magnetic resonance imaging tumor volume with histopathology. J Urol 188(4):1157–1163

Vainshtein J, A.-I.E., Olson KB, Ray ME, Sandler HM, Normolle D, Litzenberg DW, Masi K, Pan C, Hamstra DA (2012) Randomized phase II trial of urethral sparing intensity modulated radiation therapy in low-risk prostate cancer: implications for focal therapy. Radiat Oncol 7(82)

Villers AMJ, Freiha FS, Stamey TA (1992) Multiple cancers in the prostate. Morphologic features of clinically recognized versus incidental tumors. Cancer 70(9):2313–2318

Ward JF, Jones JS (2012) Focal cryotherapy for localized prostate cancer: a report from the national Cryo On-Line Database (COLD) registry. BJU International 109(11):1648–1654

Wilt TJ et al (2012) Radical prostatectomy versus observation for localized prostate cancer. N Engl J Med 367(3): 203–213

Wise AM et al (2002) Morphologic and clinical significance of multifocal prostate cancers in radical prostatectomy specimens. Urology 60(2):264–269

Yamada Y et al (2012) American Brachytherapy Society consensus guidelines for high-dose-rate prostate brachytherapy. Brachytherapy 11(1):20–32

Yerram NK et al (2012) Low suspicion lesions on multiparametric magnetic resonance imaging predict for the absence of high-risk prostate cancer. BJU Int 110(11 Pt B):E783–E788

Part VI

Brachytherapy

Permanent Seed Implantation

Reinhard Thamm

Contents

R. Thamm (✉)
Department of Radiation Oncology,
University of Ulm, Ulm, Germany
e-mail: Reinhard.Thamm@uniklinik-ulm.de

Abstract

Within recent years permanent interstitial brachytherapy of the prostate has become an widely accepted, attractive treatment approach typically for the low-risk prostate cancer. In the hands of an experienced brachytherapist, it is a safe and feasible therapy with acceptable toxicity. Its application might further be extended to intermediate to high risk cancers, possibly in combination with androgen deprivation therapy or external beam radiotherapy. In this chapter, state of the art approaches as well as controversies are discussed, and recent literature is reviewed. While the technical details of this demanding procedure itself are presented elsewhere, the following focuses on selected topics like patient selection, indications and contraindications, dosimetry and definitions of recurrence.

Abbreviations and Acronyms

ABS	American Brachytherapy Society
ADT	Androgen deprivation therapy
BED	Biologically effective dose
BFFF	Biochemical freedom of failure
bNED	Biochemical no evidence of disease
bPFS	Biochemical progression-free survival
CSS	Cause-specific survival
CTV	Clinical target volume
D90	Dose in Gray, which is delivered to 90 % of the contoured volume
DRE	Digital rectal examination
DSS	Disease-specific survival
EBRT	External beam radiotherapy
FFBF	Freedom from biochemical failure
FFP	Freedom from progression
GI	Gastrointestinal
GU	Genitourinary
IIEF	International index or erectile function
IPSS	International prostate symptom score

H. Geinitz et al. (eds.), *Radiotherapy in Prostate Cancer*, Medical Radiology. Radiation Oncology,
DOI: 10.1007/174_2014_1033, © Springer-Verlag Berlin Heidelberg 2014
Published Online: 26 September 2014

LDR	Low dose rate
LUTS	Lower urinary tract symptoms
OS	Overall survival
p/r/u	Prefixes for dosimetric values D90, V100 ("p"—prostate, "u"—urethra, and "r"—rectal contour)
PBC	Positive biopsy cores
PCSM	Prostate cancer specific mortality
PD	Prescribed dose
PDE-5	Phosphodiesterase type 5
PPC	Percentage of positive biopsy cores
PSA	Prostate specific antigen
PSI	Permanent seed implantation
PTV	Planning target volume
SVB	Seminal vesicle biopsy
TRUS	Transrectal ultrasound
TUR-P	Transurethral resection of prostate
V100	Volume in cm^3, which gets 100 % of PD

1 Why Seeds?

The permanent implantation of radioactive seeds (PSI) has become a commonly accepted and effective treatment option mainly for low-risk prostate cancer. Obviously, the one day minimal-invasive treatment procedure provides several advantages for patients. In practice, this technique has to compete with surgical and conservative treatment modalities, thus brachytherapists often need to argue in terms of disease control, toxicity, quality of life and economical burden to support its use.

Excellent long-term outcomes can be achieved with PSI (Taira et al. 2011; Sylvester et al. 2011; Stone and Stock 2014a). It is mainly recommended for low-risk patients, but it also has proven, often in combination with other treatment modalities, its successful use in intermediate- and high-risk tumors.

A recent study emphasized the superior outcome for all risk groups in comparison to other current primary treatment options, when PSI was used alone or in conjunction with external beam radiotherapy (EBRT) or androgen deprivation therapy (ADT) (Grimm et al. 2012).

During EBRT, the prostate and the seminal vesicles show an intrafractional motion of a few millimeters. The longer a single treatment fraction lasts, the higher is the probability of a significant displacement of the target organ. Several approaches like endorectal balloon application, fiducial markers and intrafractional image guidance are undertaken to minimize the problem of inappropriate prostate dose coverage. However, field margins of 0.5–1.5 cm are recommended for EBRT, which can be reduced to 0.5–1 cm with daily portal imaging (Hansen and Roach III 2010). During brachytherapy however, the dose coverage depends on the seed arrangement within the prostate and follows the natural movement of the organ. Hence, a reduction of safety margins to 2–3 mm is possible mainly to cover potential extracapsular extension. Due to the reduced margins, the organs at risk like bladder and rectum can largely be saved from the high dose region, which might ultimatively translate into reduced toxicity. On the other hand, misplacement of seeds can lead to severe injury of adjacent normal tissues.

Some studies regarding patients with low-risk prostate cancer, suggest that PSI results in a more complete ablation of the prostate gland's metabolism than EBRT (Pickett et al. 2004, 2006). This might be an indicator for a superior radiobiological effect of LDR brachytherapy in the treatment of prostate cancer.

2 Guidelines and Recommendations

Brachytherapy of the prostate follows a curative intention, wherefore careful attention should be paid to current treatment recommendations and an appropriate patient selection. These may be the main influencing factor for the effectiveness and (long term) toxicity of this treatment approach. Every treatment outside of guidelines concerning selection of tumor stage and functional characteristics may lead to a reduced tumor control probability or a higher risk for adverse effects.

The American Brachytherapy Society has published a detailed consensus guideline for permanent prostate brachytherapy (Davis et al. 2012). It focuses on patient selection, contraindications, and the pre-, intra- and postoperative procedures.

A shorter overview provides the current guideline of the American Society for Radiation Oncology (Rosenthal et al. 2011) and the National Comprehensive Cancer Network (NCCN) (Mohler et al. 2012; NCCN 2012).

European Guidelines from the European Society for Therapeutic Radiology and Oncology were published by Ash et al. (2000).

In Germany, a collaborative group released an evidence based guideline for the early diagnosis, diagnostic practice and treatment of prostate cancer (Deutsche Gesellschaft für Urologie 2011).

Moreover, summarized results from the Prostate Cancer Results Study Group were published in 2012. This international group conducted a comprehensive literature review and provides detailed informations to assist treatment decisions (Grimm et al. 2012).

Table 1 Risk group criteria for clinically localized prostate cancer T1-T2c N0 M0

	Low risk	Intermediate risk	High risk
Seattle Zelefsky et al. (1998)	(all factors) T1-2 + GS ≤6 + PSA ≤10	(one factor) >T2 / GS ≥7 / PSA >10	2 or 3 factors >T2 / GS ≥7 / PSA >10
Mount Sinai Sylvester et al. (2003)	(all factors) <T2c + GS< 7 + PSA ≤10	(one factor) ≥T2c / GS ≥7 / PSA >10	2 or 3 factors ≥ T2c / GS ≥7 / PSA >10
Boston D'Amico et al. (1998)	T1c-T2a + GS ≤6 + PSA ≤10	T2b / GS = 7 / PSA >10 and ≤20	T2c / GS 8–10 / PSA >20
AUA Thompson et al. (2007)	T1c-T2a + GS ≤6 + PSA ≤10	T2b not qualifying for high risk / GS = 7 / PSA 10–20	T2c / GS 8–10 / PSA >20

+ and; / or; ± and/or; T-Stage AJCC 1992

3 Patient Selection

Usually, treatment decisions are made on clinical risk categories, which predict the future probability of an outcome. According to T-Stage, Gleason pattern and PSA-Value patients can be primarily categorized in three risk groups (low-, intermediate- and high risk) (Tables 1 and 2). Furthermore, functional characteristics affecting functional outcome are taken into account (IPSS, urodynamic parameters, TURP in medical history).

The pre-treatment risk stratification is an area of current debate. Critical prognostic parameters such as tumor extension, invasion of the prostate capsule or the seminal vesicles and Gleason score are ultimately available only after surgery. At primary diagnosis, a clinical T stage is stated by the urologist due to pathological findings in digital rectal examination or transrectal ultrasound, which is prone to significant interobserver variability and staging errors.

Reese et al. found errors in assigning the correct clinical stage in 35.4 % of patients. Most of them resulted in patient downstaging, and TRUS findings are frequently disregarded (Reese et al. 2011). 25 % of patients with Gleason 6 in one or two biopsy cores might reveal a higher Gleason score or extraprostatic extension at prostatectomy (Katz et al. 2011).

In comparison to urologists using pathological findings to predict the outcome after prostatectomy, radiation oncologists have to accept obvious uncertainties in clinical staging categories before therapy. This might strongly affect clinical outcomes.

Concerning this matter, nomograms have been developed to give a more precise prediction of treatment success, complications and acute and long-term morbidity (Stephenson and Kattan 2006; Zelefsky et al. 2012; Kaplan et al. 2012; Roeloffzen et al. 2011). Another nomogram is applied to patients with favorable-risk prostate cancer considered for brachytherapy to estimate the risk for Gleason score upgrading (Bowes et al. 2012b). While these nomograms can help selecting a treatment for prostate cancer, they should not be used as a surrogate for physician's treatment recommendations.

Additional radiological examinations (high-quality magnetic resonance imaging, spectroscopy) could improve evaluation of tumor location and support accuracy in therapy decision and planning. Imaging fusion techniques with ultrasonography have been established for image-guided prostate biopsy (Hoeks et al. 2011) or post-implant dosimetry (Bowes et al. 2013a). In future, image-guided prostate brachytherapy may open up new therapy approaches (e.g. dose escalation in sub-volumes of the prostate, salvage brachytherapy following EBRT). However, in low risk cancer, usually additional examinations including MRT are currently not recommended.

The difficulty in assigning biochemical failure to risk groups in patients following brachytherapy still remains challenging. Some authors discuss the weakness of the existing three-group stratification system in detail (Rodrigues et al. 2012). They mention novel prognostic factors and the introduction of further risk categories, such as very-low-risk and very high-risk strata. Others refer to the inhomogeneity of intermediate-risk group and suggest a division into a low-intermediate risk group and a high-intermediate risk group (Beasley et al. 2008; Williams et al. 2006). However, the author's stratification system did not integrate essential risk factors such as amount of high-grade cancer, Gleason pattern 4+3 versus 3+4.

Table 2 Risk group criteria for prostate cancer

<table>
<tr><th></th><th colspan="2">Low risk</th><th colspan="2">Intermediate risk</th><th colspan="2">High risk</th></tr>
<tr><td>Merrick et al. (2008)</td><td colspan="2">≤T2a
+ GS ≤6
+ PSA ≤10</td><td colspan="2">(one factor)
T2b
/ GS = 7
/ PSA 10–20</td><td colspan="2">2 or 3 factors of intermediate
/ (≥T2c
/ GS 8–10
/ PSA ≥20)</td></tr>
<tr><td>NICE
Great Britain
Graham et al. (2008)</td><td colspan="2">(all factors)
T1-T2a
+ GS ≤6
+ PSA <10</td><td colspan="2">T2b-T2c
/ GS = 7
/ PSA 10–20</td><td colspan="2">T3–T4
/ GS 8–10
/ PSA >20</td></tr>
<tr><td>CaPSURE
USA
Cooperberg et al. (2003)</td><td colspan="2">T1-T2a (1997 TNM system)
+ GS ≤6
+ PSA ≤10</td><td colspan="2">T2b
/ GS = 7
/ PSA 10–20</td><td colspan="2">T3-T4
/ GS 8–10
/ PSA >20</td></tr>
<tr><td>PPC classification
Australia (T1c-T3)
Huang et al. (2012)</td><td colspan="2">+ GS 2–6
+ PSA ≤10
Or
(GS = 7
± PSA 10–20)
+ PPC ≤50 %</td><td colspan="2">not low/high risk</td><td colspan="2">(GS 8–10
± PSA >20)
+ PPC >50%</td></tr>
<tr><td>ESMO
Horwich et al. (2010)</td><td colspan="2">T1-2a
+ GS ≤7
+ PSA <10</td><td colspan="2">not low/high risk</td><td colspan="2">T3–T4
/ GS 8–10
/ PSA >20</td></tr>
<tr><td>Five Level Risk Stratification
(any T)
Australia
Beasley et al. (2008)</td><td colspan="2">PSA <7.5
+ GS ≤6</td><td>Low int.
PSA
7.5–15
+ GS ≤6</td><td>High int.
(PSA 15–20
+ GS ≤6)
/ (PSA ≤10
+ GS ≥7)</td><td>High
(PSA 20–30
+ GS ≤6)
/ (PSA
10–20
+ GS ≥7)</td><td>Extreme
(PSA >20
+ GS ≥7)
/ (PSA >30
+ GS ≤6)</td></tr>
<tr><td>NCCN
USA
NCCN (2012)</td><td>Very low
T1c
+ GS ≤6
+ PSA ≤10
+ PBC <3
+ PPC <50 %
PSA-density <0.15 ng/ml/g</td><td>Low
T1-T2a
+ GS ≤6
+ PSA ≤10</td><td colspan="2">T2b-T2c
/ GS = 7
/ PSA 10–20</td><td>High
T3a
/ GS = 8–10
/ PSA >20</td><td>Very high
T3b–T4:
(locally advanced)</td></tr>
<tr><td>EAU
Heidenreich et al. (2011)</td><td colspan="2">cT1-T2a
+ GS 2–6
+ PSA <10</td><td colspan="2">cT2b-T2c
/ GS = 7
/ PSA 10–20</td><td>cT3a
/ GS 8–10
/ PSA >20</td><td>cT3b-T4 N0
any T, N1</td></tr>
</table>

+ and; / or; ± and/or; T-Stage AJCC 1992

3.1 Patient's Selection

The patient's decision, which therapy fits their needs best, is often influenced by the personal attitude of their physician as well as their own attitude. In one study by Anandanas et al., 60 % of the patients with early prostate cancer, who chose radical prostatectomy (40 %), did so because they wanted physical removal of their tumor. Twenty-seven percent of men with EBRT (31 %) had fear of other treatment options, and the main reason (39 %) for choosing brachytherapy (21 %) was lifestyle consideration. There was no predominant reason for choosing Active Surveillance (8 %). After 2 years, all patient groups (Surgery, EBRT, PSI, and Active Surveillance) showed comparable satisfaction with their treatment decision (Anandadas et al. 2011). Other studies showed a significant better patient satisfaction following PSI compared to Surgery or EBRT (Crook et al. 2011; Wagner et al. 2011).

Remarkably, choosing radiation is generally a more difficult decision than choosing surgery (Sidana et al. 2012). Because "Doctor's recommendation" is the main reason for selecting a treatment, there might be a difference between surgeons and radiation oncologists in terms of persuasive power or argumentation (Patient is "too young for less aggressive treatment", "Avoid RT: difficult to treat recurrence").

Holmes et al. presented a patterns of care study of the relationship between age, the likelihood of extraprostatic cancer and primary therapy. Patients younger than 50 years receive more often primary surgery. In older patients, there may be a higher use of conservative treatment, even with >50 % likelihood of extraprostatic cancer (Holmes et al. 2012). Thus, multidisciplinary consultation should be established as a standard, to result in individualized treatment recommendations based on age, risk strata and comorbidities.

4 Risk Groups

4.1 Low-Risk

Traditionally, PSI is a domain of low-risk cancer, mostly defined as cT1c-2a, Gleason Score 2–6, and PSA ≤10 ng/ml. This stage describes a localized growing tumor with estimation of low malignancy. Therefore, every local treatment approaches should result in comparable high cure rates.

Despite plenty of single institutional studies with presentation of long-term results, randomized studies are rare. In the low-risk group, excellent biochemical relapse-free survival up to 95.6 % (12 year) and 85.9 % (15 year) are reported (Taira et al. 2011; Sylvester et al. 2007). Studies with the largest patient numbers report biochemical freedom of failure (BFFF) in about 88 % of the patients (Stone et al. 2011), with clinical stage, Gleason Score, PSA level and biological effective dose as significant predictors.

A matched-pair analysis proved a superior biochemical control of PSI after 5 years in comparison to EBRT (94 vs. 88 %) (Pickles et al. 2010). For low-risk patients with assumed organ-confined disease, there may be no advantage of additional EBRT.

In studies regarding surgery, it is often unclear if the risk stratification is based on the pre-therapy assumed T-stage, or on the histopathological report. With more accurate knowledge on the exact tumor burden, the risk classification is more reliable, and statistics may show better outcomes for "real" early tumor stages. Therefore, comparison of outcomes after prostatectomy with those following PSI is complex.

Older series should not further be used for argumentation, because of lower radiation doses, higher PSA median in EBRT group and ancient techniques used for PSI (D'Amico et al. 1998).

In a comprehensive review of papers published during 2000–2010, PSI provides superior outcome regarding PSA-free progression in patients with low-risk disease in comparison to surgery, EBRT and other treatment approaches. (Grimm et al. 2012).

A cohort analysis of outcomes after radical prostatectomy or brachytherapy in 371 men with low- or intermediate risk prostate cancer recently was published by Fisher et al. Five years after surgery, bRFS rates for low—and intermediate-risk disease were 96.1 and 90.6 %, and 92.5 and 95.8 % after brachytherapy, respectively (Fisher et al. 2012).

Due to the lack of randomized trials, the Deutsche Krebsgesellschaft (German Cancer Society) has started a preference based study to evaluate surgery, EBRT, PSI and active surveillance in low risk and low-intermediate risk patient groups. Patients participating in this study will be randomized in nine substudies according to their preferred treatment options (PREFEREnce based randomized evaluation of treatment modalities in low or early intermediate risk prostate cancer) (Schmedders et al. 2011).

4.2 Intermediate-Risk

Definitions for intermediate-risk criteria may be different from series to series, therefore outcome results may vary slightly. An intermediate-risk tumor is more aggressive than low risk tumors, but still organconfined. The risk for local infiltration of the prostate's capsula or the base of the seminal vesicles is strikingly increased, thus the extent of periprostatic treatment margins of PSI plays an important role if it is used as a single therapy approach for these patients. Regarding biochemical free progression in the intermediate risk group, PSI alone seems to be equivalent to PSI + EBRT. (Grimm et al. 2012; Merrick et al. 2005).

The direct comparison of surgery with radiotherapy-based approaches like EBRT, PSI or the combination of both to prove the superiorness of any therapy approach is still a reason for intensive disputes between urologists and radiooncologists (Eastham 2004; Petros 2004). In the lack of prospective, randomized trials, this question still remains open.

While some retrospective surveys reported almost comparable results for BRFS in patients with low- and intermediate risk (Fisher et al. 2012; Merrick et al. 2001), other groups seem to clearly recommend radiotherapy-based options in the treatment of all risk strata of prostate cancer (Grimm et al. 2012).

Survival is still high. In a retrospective single institution analysis, Merrick et al. report that at 8 years, 95.7 % of patients (n = 251) were free of biochemical failure after PSI alone for intermediate risk cancer (Merrick et al. 2005).

Survival results may vary, when different risk group scoring schemes are used. Sylvester et al. presented biochemical relapse-free survival results in patients with intermediate risk prostate cancer, treated with PSI plus neoadjuvant EBRT. After 10 years, biochemical relapse-free survival were 77, 93, 90 % for Seattle risk group, Mt. Sinai risk group and D'Amico risk group, respectively (Sylvester et al. 2003). Disease-specific survival rates range between 87 % (10-year) (Hinnen et al. 2010), 95 % (10-year) (Henry et al. 2010) and 99.3 % (12-year) (Taira et al. 2011).

In the intermediate risk group, PSI is often combined with EBRT.

Long-term (8-years) results of RTOG 0019 (Phase II EBRT+PSI, primary endpoint: grade 3–5 genitourinary and gastrointestinal toxicity, closed in 2001) revealed 15 % grade >3 toxicity (urinary frequency, dysuria, proctitis). Forty-two % complained of grade 3 impotence. Unfortunately, EBRT (45 Gy) consisted of a outdated four-field technique (Lawton et al. 2012). Current techniques for PSI and EBRT are able to reduce side-effects when used in combination. Zelefsky reported 4 years after real-time intraoperative planning for PSI combined with intensity-modulated radiotherapy with no gastrointestinal Grade 3–4 complications and only one of 127 patients developed a Grade 3 urethral stricture (Zelefsky et al. 2008). Therefore, modern techniques should claimed as the standard approach when PSI is combined with EBRT.

Data of the randomised RTOG 0232 study, (accrural closed in 2012) are awaited and will report on differences between freedom from progression (FFP) 5 years after EBRT + PSI vs. PSI alone in intermediate risk patients. Remarkably, intermediate risk in that study is defined as Gleason Score = 7 with PSA <10 ng/ml or GS <7 and PSA 10–20 ng/ml, which is a subgroup of D'Amicos intermediate-risk definition (RTOG 2011).

In a retrospective series, Tanaka et al. reported a significantly higher late gastrointestinal (GI) and genitourinary (GU) toxicity in patients with EBRT+PSI. As expected, pre-implantation-IPSS was a significant predictor for acute GU toxicity and the combination of EBRT+PSI was predictive for late GU toxicity. The rectal volume receiving at least 100 % of the prescribed dose (rV100) was associated with late GI toxicity (Tanaka et al. 2013).

As the combination of EBRT and PSI carries the potential risk of increased side effects and complications, this treatment option should only be performed in experienced centers.

The most common indication for the combination of PSI with androgen deprivation (ADT) is prostate size reduction to avoid pubic arch interference during needle insertion. There are no randomized studies proving a benefit for survival. In the retrospective study by Lee et al., the 5-year actuarial freedom from biochemical failure rate increased significantly, when ADT was given 3 months before and after PSI. The best outcome (94 %, n = 40) had patients with a higher implant dose (D90 >140 Gy) and ADT (Lee et al. 2002).

New data suggest a need for additive ADT only in lower dose PSI with BED <150 Gy (Stock et al. 2012b).

When a five-level risk stratification system is used, the cut-off for advantageous use of ADT is the high-intermediate risk group, defined as an initial PSA of 15–20 ng/ml with a GS ≤6 or a PSA ≤10 with a GS ≥7. In this group, 5-year biochemical control (bNED) with or without ADT were 72 and 58 % respectively (Beasley et al. 2008).

Beyer et al., in their retrospective review of 2.378 consecutive PSI cases (33 % intermediate risk, 19.5 % with-ADT) reported a surprising effect of short-course ADT 3–6 months before and 3 months after PSI: at 10 years, overall survival was significantly worse with ADT (20 vs. 44 % in hormone naïve patients, p = 0.02) (Beyer et al. 2005).

In conclusion, the combination of PSI and ADT should be administered with careful consideration, especially in the intermediate risk group.

4.3 High-Risk

The high-risk group is defined as clinical stage T2c or Gleason >7 or PSA >20 ng/ml and has a high probability of microscopic, clinical occult metastases already at diagnosis. Interstitial PSI for these patients is an insufficient monotherapy approach due to the limited dose range of this treatment modality.

According to the guidelines, patients should receive supplemental EBRT ± ADT. In a meta-analysis, this management appears superior to more localized treatment approaches such as surgery, EBRT or PSI alone (Grimm et al. 2012). Results of studies using the SEER Database showed, that treatment approaches including PSI in addition to EBRT in high-risk cancers lead to a significant reduction in 10-year prostate cancer-specific mortality (PCSM) (13.4 % for PSI+EBRT vs. 21.1 % for EBRT alone) (Shen et al. 2012). The key benefit of brachytherapy (also in combination with EBRT) in high-risk cancers is the ability to deliver a higher biological effective dose than with EBRT alone, however, the high effectiveness in this situation can only be achieved when the dose is able to completely enclose clinical occult tumor.

In case of high risk patients: (Gleason Score ≥7 or PSA >10ng/ml or clinical stage ≥T2b) who elect PSI as their treatment component of choice, seminal vesicle biopsy (SVB) can be offered as a further diagnostic step. If positive for tumor invasion (9.9 %), additional seeds can be positioned in the anterior wall of the seminal vesicles (Stone et al. 2012).

The high-risk group may consist of several subgroups. Fang et al. (Fang et al. 2011) described a series of patients (n = 174) with Gleason Score 8–10 tumors and a relative low pretreatment PSA value of ≤15 ng/ml who received PSI. Most of the patients (91.4 %) were additionally treated with EBRT with 45 Gy. Short-term or long-term ADT was administered in 64.9 % of patients. For this group, ten-year-outcomes were surprisingly excellent: biochemically progression free survival (bPFS) was 90 % and overall survival (OS) was 69.4 %. Interestingly, the use of ADT did not significantly impact bPFS, CSS or OS.

Bittner et al. (2012) defined a "very-high risk group" with the following criteria: any Gleason Score 10 or Gleason Score 8–9 with >50 % of positive biopsy cores (PPC) or Gleason Score 8–9 with PSA>20 ng/ml or any T3 or any PSA>40 ng/ml.

At 12 years, bPFS was 86.5 % and OS 60.5 % (all patients received PSI, 91.6 % EBRT and ADT 76.3 %). Remarkably, death from diseases of the heart was still more than twice as likely as death from prostate cancer.

High-risk patients with EBRT ± PSI may profit by additive ADT, when distant microscopic disease is expected. In a prospective, non-randomised data set, Beasley et al. (Beasley et al. 2008) found an increase of biochemical control, when ADT was added to EBRT (55 % vs. 42 % without ADT, p = 0.004).

One retrospective study demonstrated that combined therapy with EBRT and PSI seems to be superior compared to dose-escalated EBRT. Additional use of ADT decreases biochemical failure and prostate cancer specific mortality. The authors report the greatest benefit was observed for long-term ADT (Shilkrut et al. 2012).

In the newest publication of Stone and Stock, the factors influencing 15-year cause-specific and all-cause survival (ACS) of patients treated with PSI were analyzed. In the analyzed patient group, long term ADT (>6 months) has a significant negative impact on ACS in both younger and older men. Therefore long term ADT has to be administered carefully, especially when other risk factors such as cardiovascular comorbidities or diabetes are present (Stone and Stock 2014a).

4.4 Gleason Score 3+4 Versus 4+3

After radical prostatectomy, patients with a higher primary Gleason pattern have higher rates of extracapsular extension or seminal vesicle invasion. Consequently, the risk for biochemical failure is significantly higher (Alenda et al. 2011). It is assumed, that tumors with Gleason 3 pattern are more benign than those with Gleason pattern 4 (Lavery and Droller 2012).

In a survey, the difference in primary Gleason pattern played only a subsidiary role in brachytherapy (Stock et al. 2012a; Herbert et al. 2012), although conflicting results have been reported (Uesugi et al. 2012; Bittner et al. 2013). The authors detected no significant effect on biochemical failure after 10 years independent from supplemental EBRT or ADT (Stock et al. 2012a). Anyhow, patients with Gleason pattern 4+3 deserve careful consideration of additional risk factors (PSA >10 ng/ml, clinical Stage, volume of cancer on biopsy). PSI alone, and a biologically effective dose (BED) ≤160 Gy_2 might lead to increased biochemical failure, while combined therapy (e.g. ADT and PSI or PSI and EBRT) seems to be the treatment of first choice (Stock et al. 2012a).

4.5 Does Age Matter?

Younger men (<50 years) with prostate cancer are more frequent candidates for surgery, because urologists typically recommend surgery as the best chance of long-term cure. Younger patients also feel that radiation is a less aggressive therapy than surgery or they are concerned about difficulties in case of tumor recurrence after radiotherapy (Sidana et al. 2012).

In fact, younger patients (in this study defined as ≤60 years), at average have smaller, better differentiated tumours, with a consequently better prognosis than patients over 60 years (Hinnen et al. 2011). Additionally, younger patients (<50 years) seem to have a lower incidence of extraprostatic extension, seminal vesicle involvement and non-organ-confined disease rate compared with older men aged from 60–69 years (Khan et al. 2003). Therefore, with a higher prevalence of organ-confined disease, all local treatment approaches like radical prostatectomy—but also PSI—may lead to similar survival results in the treatment of younger patients with prostate cancer. Ten years after surgery (PSA <0.2 ng/ml) and PSI (Phoenix, +2 ng/ml above nadir), biochemical free survival of younger patients (<60 years) is about 78–81 and 91.3–95 %, respectively (Khan et al. 2003; Burri et al. 2010; Shapiro et al. 2009). However, this raw comparison does not qualify to deduce any treatment preference.

Merrick et al. presented a data set of 42 consecutive patients ≤50 years with PSI ± supplemental therapies. All risk groups were represented in this cohort. Due to the small patient number in the particular risk groups, they reported the cause-specific survival, bPFS, and OS only for the entire cohort, which was: 100, 97.7, and 100 %, respectively (Merrick et al. 2008). The same group presented a retrospective report of young patients (≤54 years, n = 108) who underwent PSI or EBRT+PSI for clinically localized prostate cancer (cT1c-T2N0M0). At 8 years, biochemical progression-free survival was 96, 100 and 75 % (three of four patients) for the groups with low, intermediate and high-risk tumor, respectively (Merrick et al. 2006).

Another study presented the results of 175 patients (≤55 years) with PSI for T1-3 prostate cancer. Additionally EBRT + ADT was administered to selected low-, intermediate- and high-risk patients. Freedom from biochemical failure (FFBF) after a median follow-up of 4.7 years was

98.7, 97.1 and 89.3 % in the low, intermediate and high risk group, respectively (Boo et al. 2012).

Hinnen et al. presented 10-year outcomes in patients aged ≤60 years with PSI as monotherapy for locally confined, intermediate or well-differentiated tumors: FFBF, disease-specific survival and overall survival were 63, 87 and 81 %, respectively (Hinnen et al. 2011). For low, intermediate and high risk patients, a 10-year freedom from progression was reported from Shapiro et al. as 91.3, 80 and 70.2 %, compared to 91.8, 83.4, and 72.1 % respectively, for men 60 years or older (Shapiro et al. 2009). Similar results were published from other groups (Burri et al. 2010).

Only few studies have analysed survival rates of elderly men, but the data suggest an effective and safe monotherapy in over 75 years old men. In one study, the 5-year FFBF rate was 91.3 % (OS 95 %) with 5 % grade 3 genitourinary toxicity (Chiumento et al. 2013).

In conclusion, young men achieve excellent biochemical control rates with PSI for localized prostate cancer. With regard to comorbidities and adverse effects, administering PSI to elderly patients should be practiced with careful consideration. Patient age alone should not influence treatment decisions.

4.6 Does Size Matter?

Patients with prostate gland size <20 cm^3 are often considered poor candidates for prostate brachytherapy. Some studies have published the association between small glands and inadequate dosimetry, larger 1-month edema, lower D90 and higher intracapsular seed density (Liu et al. 2010; McNeely et al. 2004).

Small prostate sizes seem to be associated with an increased risk of occult higher-grade disease and extracapsular extension. An increased risk for Gleason upgrade was described by Turley and revised later as an effect of the biopsy technique (Turley et al. 2008a, b).

It has to be emphasized, that for high-quality PSI of small sizes, brachytherapy team experience and the achievement of adequate treatment margins is substantial. Under this condition, PSI of smaller glands is at no higher risk of treatment failure than in men with larger prostates (Liu et al. 2010; Taira et al. 2012; Mayadev et al. 2010).

The common recommendation is to be cautious with PSI of large prostates >60 cm^3 at the time of implantation (Davis et al. 2012). Depending on prostate size, but also on individual pelvic anatomy, intraoperative patient position and technique, some prostate glands may be covered by the pubic arch on both lateral or ventral sides ("pubic arch interference"). Thus, these regions can not be punctured with the implantation needles, which may result in insufficient dose coverage.

Larger prostates, up to 100 cm^3 are technically challenging, but toxicity and outcomes are acceptable (Dallas et al. 2012). Despite of conflicting results, there are broad hints for an increased urinary retention after PSI in patients with large gland size (Crook et al. 2002a). A nomogram can be used to predict the risk for acute urinary retention. Besides prostate size, factors such as IPSS and ADT are elements of the scoring system. Prostate protrusion is a substantial predicting factor for post-PSI urinary retention, especially in larger glands (Roeloffzen et al. 2011, 2012).

Larger glands may result in an overdosage of the anterior rectum and the bladder neck, as a result of a broader contact area.

In case of larger glands, several techniques are used to overcome technical issues such as pubic arch interference: exaggeration of intraoperative lithotomy position, downsizing with 5-α reductase inhibitors or angling the rectal probe tip anteriorly. With the use of special equipment, oblique needle guidance supports a more precise implantation approach than free-hand insertion of the needles (Ryu et al. 2012).

Second, conventionally used ultrasound transducers generate an angulated image field in the axial plane. Larger glands tend to "wrap" around the rectum, especially when the ultrasound tip is forced ventrally or the rectal balloon is overfilled with water for better imaging. Some modern ultrasound devices are equipped with a greater image field angle in the axial plane, which is necessary to display dorsolateral regions of very large prostate glands.

Neoadjuvant ADT reduces gland size by an average of approximately 30 % in 3–4 months (Petit et al. 2007), but involves the risk of urinary retention and prolonged catherization (Crook et al. 2002a; Lee et al. 2010).

On the other hand, a survey with a larger patient number didn't confirm this observation. There was no significant increase in urinary retention, although the ADT-group had higher pre-treatment IPS-Scores. Furthermore, IPSS increased less and returned to pre-implantation baseline more rapidly when ADT was used. Only a subgroup of men with an IPSS ≥15 showed beneficial influence of the use of neoadjuvant ADT on the risk of urinary retention. In summary, patients with large glands and minimal urinary symptoms lack the need for neoadjuvant ADT, as long the brachytherapy team has the expertise to treat them (Stone et al. 2010a; Blasko 2004).

In conclusion, no clear relationship exists between large prostate size and increased urinary toxicity. Anyhow, due to existing hints, patients should be informed about the potentially increased risk.

Outcome parameters like PSA failure rate are not influenced by the prostate volume (Aaltomaa et al. 2011; Dallas et al. 2012).

4.7 Does Dose Matter?

Commonly, whole prostate D90, V100 and BED are accepted as dosimetric values for defining PSI implant quality. These metrics can be stratified in different subcategories as explained further below (see "Postplanning") and a lower dose has an obvious impact on biochemical and local control (Miles et al. 2010; Ho et al. 2009; Stock et al. 1998). Nevertheless, this correlation may not be assumed in general. Ash et al. reported that there is only a significant dose response relationship in low risk, but not in intermediate or high risk prostate cancer (Ash et al. 2006). This may be attibuted to different causes. Firstly, there are different criteria for PSA or local failure (ASTRO, Phoenix, post-treatment biopsies), which may result in different statistical outcomes. Secondly, a low whole-prostate D90 is not always associated with treatment failure, when enough dose is delivered to the tumor-affected parts of the prostate (Sidhu et al. 2002). Further on, in intermediate and high risk cancers there might be a higher prevalence of clinical occult microscopic disease outside the prostate which cannot be treated by PSI alone. In this case, an optimal implant with high D90 will possibly result in biochemical failure. At least, data sets regarding intermediate or high risk patient groups with additional ADT need longer follow-up periods to appreciate the impact of higher doses on biochemical control (Stone and Stock 2014b).

In conclusion, there is obvious evidence to regard dosimetric values like D90, V100 or BED as suitable metrics for the estimation of implant quality, but when these metrics are correlated with biochemical treatment failure, multiple aspects have to be taken thoughtfully into account.

5 Indications

Patients with low-, intermediate- and high-risk (Table 1) localized prostate cancer may be candidates for PSI alone or in combination with additional therapy approaches like EBRT and/or ADT.

In short, patients with low-risk disease are ideal candidates for PSI as monotherapy. In intermediate risk, the combination of EBRT and PSI appears equivalent to PSI alone, on the condition that the brachytherapy team provides high expertise and dose margins are selected wide enough. For high-risk patients, combination therapies involving EBRT and PSI ± ADT appear superior to localized approaches (Grimm et al. 2012; Davis et al. 2012).

Before decision-making, patient's life expectancy should be estimated, especially if comorbidities are present. Generally, a life expectancy of >10 years for low-grade and >5 years for intermediate risk patients is suggested (NCCN 2012; Davis et al. 2012; Frank et al. 2011).

Patients with a PSA >50 ng/ml are unlikely to benefit from local treatment due to the high risk for extraprostatic or metastatic disease. Some authors, however, have demonstrated reduction of prostate cancer mortality even in patients with highly elevated PSA-levels (Bittner et al. 2012).

According to the NCCN and German guidelines (NCCN 2012; Deutsche Gesellschaft für Urologie 2011), additional imaging is not mandatory in low-risk disease. A bone scan is indicated if the following factors are present: T1 and PSA >20 ng/ml, T2 and PSA >10 ng/ml, GS >7, T-Stage >T2 or symptomatic skeletal disorders. Pelvic CT or MRI is indicated with a PSA >10 ng/ml, in higher T-stages, or when the nomogram-predicted risk for lymh node involvement is above 20 %.

If brachytherapy is considered as a monotherapy and clinically atypical aspects are present (e.g. 1 positive biopsy core and PSA>10 ng/ml or 100 % positive biopsy cores in T1c), MRI with an endorectal coil and additional sequences, may be helpful. For treatment planning purposes, a standard body array coil MRT is advantageous over endorectal coil MRI, due to its anatomic distortion of the prostate (Albert et al. 2013).

In selected cases, a seminal vesicle biopsy can provide additional information especially if a lesion is detected in MRI that might originate from bleeding after initial prostate biopsy.

PET/CT is not recommended for primary staging, but may help to exclude patients with distant metastases in high-risk groups from local therapy approaches.

6 Contraindications

Several conditions are considered as absolute or relative contra-indications for prostate brachytherapy.

After transurethral resection of the prostate (TUR-P) PSI should be postponed for 6–12 moths. It depends on the size of prostatic defect, whether PSI succeeds with adequate dose distribution, but these patients are at a higher risk for seed loss, urethral necrosis, strictures and incontinence (Ishiyama et al. 2012; McElveen et al. 2004). Limited TUR-P or transurethral incision of the prostate 6 months before PSI for patients with lower urinary tract syndromes (LUTS), elevated IPS-Score or postvoid residual volume >100 ml appears to be safe and doesn't result in retention, urethral necrosis or incontinence (Ivanowicz et al. 2012).

Patients with anticoagulants should stop it at least seven days before implantation. Surprisingly, patients with anticoagulants show a superior biochemical control, since anticoagulants may modulate tumor proliferation, angiogenesis and metastasis (Choe et al. 2010).

The Management of pubic arch interference is discussed elsewhere (see "Does Size Matter?").

The International Prostate Symptom Score (IPSS) is a validated tool of the American Urological Association (AUA) to quantify benign prostatic hyperplasia symptoms.

In short, the use of IPSS is a commonly accepted tool among prostate brachytherapists for scaling acute urinary morbidity due to its simplicity. The preimplant IPSS correlates with the duration of postimplant obstructive symptomatology, patients with a score >20 are reported to be in 29 % risk of retention (IPSS<10: 2 %, IPSS 10–20: 19.11 %) (Terk et al. 1998). Therefore patients with an IPSS above 15, and post-void residual volumes above 100 cm^3 are regarded as poor candidates for PSI (Frank et al. 2011).

Other groups defined a three-tier system: patients with an IPSS of 0–8 do well after PSI, patients with an IPSS of 9–19 do fair, and PSI is not recommended above an IPSS of 20 (Ash et al. 2000).

To predict the risk for acute urinary retention after PSI, a nomogram may be used, which includes the pre-implantation IPS-Score (Roeloffzen et al. 2011).

The flow maximum in uroflowmetry Qmax is another component of treatment decision recommendations. Patients with Qmax >15 ml/s are optimal for PSI. PSI is not recommended for patients with Qmax <10 ml/s (Ash et al. 2000).

This parameter is typically reduced in patients with urethral strictures and higher age, therefore it has a great value in recognising and quantifying existing urinary impairments before PSI, if age is taken into account.

In patients with an IPS-Score ≥7, measurement of uroflow and postvoid residual volume should be carried out when missing (Crook et al. 2002a).

Early voiding disorders after PSI are caused by the traumatic effect of needle implantation and mild swelling of the gland, late disorders are caused by the effects of radioactivity. Therefore, Qmax decreases in the first 1–3 months after PSI, and returns to baseline one year after seed implantation. The changes of IPSS correlate well with the objective parameters Qmax and voided volume (Tanaka et al. 2009; Mallick et al. 2003).

7 Implantation Methods

The technique of permanent seed implantation has been described in many publications. While the basic technique of real-time, rectal ultrasound assisted PSI is similar in all centers (Fig. 1), slight modifications may consist in the type of applicator (Needles vs. Mick-Applicator) and seeds used (stranded vs. single vs. both types used).

7.1 Loose Versus Stranded Seeds

Stranded seeds are fabricated with absorbable spacer material, which fix the distance of 1 cm between the centers of two serial seeds. In some models, loose spacers of different length can be used to build individual designed strands. The main advantage of stranded seeds is the capability of minimizing the risk for seed loss.

Newer studies using free seeds reported about seed loss in about ¼ of patients: 22.8 % (Taussky et al. 2012), 25.6 % (Miyazawa et al. 2012), 24.7 % (Sugawara et al. 2011), and 30 % (Reed et al. 2007).

Loose seeds can migrate through the venous system to the lungs, abdomen and pelvis or are excreted with urine or ejaculate. Rare locations are the coronary artery (risk of myocardial infarction) (Zhu et al. 2006; Davis et al. 2002), the renal artery (Nguyen et al. 2009) or the vertebral venous plexus (Hau et al. 2011; Wagner et al. 2010).

Most of the seeds get lost right after PSI (day 1–day 30), but few patients can loose it up to one year later (Kono et al. 2010; Miyazawa et al. 2012).

Factors predicting seed loss are the number of needles, number of seeds, preoperative prostate volume or expertise of the brachytherapy team (Miyazawa et al. 2012; Kono et al. 2010; Sugawara et al. 2009; Taussky et al. 2012).

Dosimetry is not significantly altered, when only a few seeds are lost (Sugawara et al. 2011; Taussky et al. 2012; Stone and Stock 2005).

Unfortunately, one patient experienced a secondary small cell lung cancer 10 years after PSI with detection of the seed in middle of the pulmonary tumor (Chen et al. 2012).

One study compared stranded seeds versus loose seeds. While loose seeds migrate preferably in the lung, stranded seeds are mostly excreted with urine (Saibishkumar et al. 2009). Surprisingly, overall seed loss was more frequent in the patient group with stranded seeds, which might be biased by low patient number (n = 40) or wrong technique. Another randomized study with 64 patients reported seed loss tendentially twice as often in patients with loose seeds (Reed et al. 2007).

However, it is necessary to distinguish between the implantation of single seeds in "safer" areas, like the centers of both prostate lobes, which can be clearly identified in real time ultrasonography. "Unsafe" areas like the peripheral prostate capsule, periprostatic venous system (Stone and Stock 2005) or the direct adjacent parts of the base of bladder or intraprostatic urethra may lead to a higher risk for seed loss.

As standard, the seed size is approximately 4.5 mm in length and 0.8 mm in diameter. When a thinner seed model is used, the edema after implantation might be reduced, which may result in lower toxicity. On the other hand,

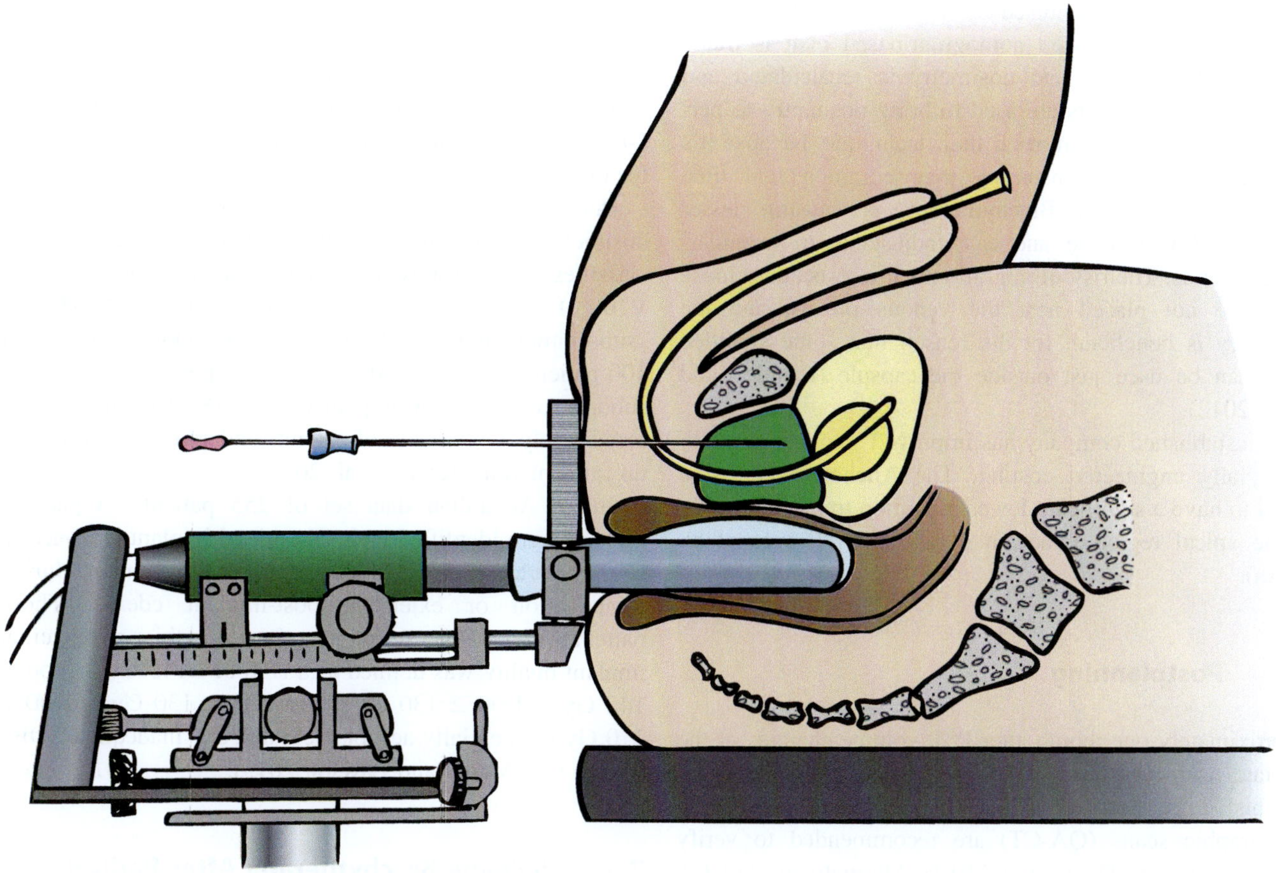

Fig. 1 View of setup for permanent seed implantation. The patient is placed under general anesthesia in exaggerated lithotomy position. A biplane rectal ultrasound system with template (two-directional coordinate system with prefabricated perforations at regular 3–5 mm intervals), stepper (mounting device) and rectal balloon is applied. The urethra may be visualized on the ultrasound images by a urinary catheter or aerated ultrasound gel. Special fixation needles may be used to minimize prostate motion during procedure (not illustrated). After image acquisition of the prostate in 3–5 mm-steps (plus one slice in cranial and caudal direction: "cut above" and "cut below"), brachytherapy planning is performed. During the implantation procedure, the needles with preloaded (stranded) seeds are inserted at the planned coordinates of the template. The precise position of the needle is detected on the real-time ultrasound images (axial plane). Then, in the longitudinal ultrasound plane, the needle is pushed forward to the intended depth. While the wire stylus is fixed, the needle is slowly pulled out, and the seeds are ejected in the tissue of the prostate gland

visibility in ultrasound might be impaired. Roberts et al. demonstrated that the main advantage of thinner seeds is a higher resolution in postplanning-CT, which leads to better visual separation of closely spaced seeds (Roberts et al. 2012). Of notice, seed loss to the lung seems not to depend on seed diameter (Wong and Sylvester 2012).

Some authors compared dosimetrical values of stranded vs. loose seeds. Due to the fact, that the natural prostate length is not a multiple of 1 cm (distance between stranded seeds), differences are to be expected. Therefore stranded seeds have a trend toward lower D90 and V100 values (Reed et al. 2007; Saibishkumar et al. 2009).

Obviously, with loose seeds the isodose contour might enwrap the prostate in a smoother way. But when larger treatment margins are indispensable (e.g. in intermediate-risk groups), this might be achieved easier and safer with stranded seeds in the outer periphery of the prostate gland than with single seeds (or with higher activity). Unfortunately, there are no studies evaluating this issue.

In some areas of the prostate, single seeds are advantageous. Due to the natural bending of the intraprostatic urethra, the use of stranded seeds in the center of the prostate may carry the risk of an overdosage of the middle urethra. In this case, single seeds might be placed in the apical or basal region. To prevent seed lost, single seeds with both-sided attached spacer material may be used.

Langley and Laing (Langley and Laing 2012) presented a new real-time technique called "4D Brachtherapy". This technique uses a combination of stranded seeds around the periphery of the prostate gland and loose seeds within the central area. The planning procedure is based on simple ultrasound based measurements, and the number of stranded and single seeds is calculated by a nomogram. During the implant, the precalculated nomogram-based plan is transferred to the patient, and dosimetry is recalculated and optimized. Single seeds are used to bring dosimetry to perfection. The authors commend their technique, because it's fast and less time consuming than common real time methods. Second, 4D-Brachytherapy is causing lesser edema, and is reliable and easy adjustable to irregular-shaped glands. The risk of migration is lower, because loose seeds are not placed near the venous plexus, and the dosimetry is beneficial, for the reason that some stranded seeds can be used just outside the capsule (Langley and Laing 2012).

An established company has improved single seeds with a specially engineered coating. The AnchorSeeds® were found to have a significant lower migration trend, especially in the apical region (Badwan et al. 2010; Bowes et al. 2012a).

7.2 Postplanning

Approximately one month after PSI, volume changes of the prostate from temporary prostatic edema have diminished. At this time, post-implant quality assurance computed tomographic scans (QA-CT) are recommended to verify proper dosimetry (Davis et al. 2012). Alternatively, QA-CT is performed on day 0 or day 1 after implant.

The ideal moment to perform the CT depends on the type of isotopes as well. For I-125 and Pd-103 implants with longer half-life period, 1 month interval has proven adequate. For Cs-131, with a half-life decay of 9.69 days, the day 14 QA-CT may be most accurate (Smith et al. 2012).

On CT images, prostate gland contours are often obscured by metallic seed artefacts and edema. Accurate prostate contouring is a challenging work, and small inaccuracies may lead to distinct deviation of dosimetry values such as D90 and V100. Experienced brachytherapists may interpret contours of prostate gland more precise, but still interobserver variations in D90 between 9.3 and 30.3 Gy are reported in the literature (Crook et al. 2002b). Another study of the same group revealed a systematic overestimation of CT-contoured prostate volume. Apparently, adjacent normal tissue is erroneously designated as prostate, especially in basal and apical regions (Petrik et al. 2012; Maletz et al. 2012).

When possible, an MRI-CT fusion should be employed to verify prostate contours post implant. But the technique of MRT-CT fusion is also prone to errors, since clear landmarks may be absent (seeds are hardly visible in T2). Special MRT sequences (T2, contrast-enhanced T1-weighted images) should first be established and optimized in close collaboration with the radiologists (Ohashi et al. 2012; Bowes et al. 2013b).

Fortunately, processing seed reconstruction results only in few mistakes and interobserver varability, when CT-MRT fusions are used (De Brabandere et al. 2012).

If MRT is not available, fusion of preimplant TRUS with 1-month postimplant CT appears as a reasonable alternative for the postplanning procedure (Bowes et al. 2013a).

Publications with detailed information about suboptimal dosimetric postplanning results are very rare. Keyes et al. classifies three groups of implant quality: a post-implant-V100 of >85 % is "good", whereas a V100 of 75–85 % is "suboptimal" and a V100 of <75 % is "poor". For the last 400 patients of a vast PSI program, the percentage of good, suboptimal and poor implants were 88, 10, and 2.3 %, respectively. Only 0.7 % of patients underwent a second top-up implantation (Keyes et al. 2004).

In an Australian data set of 255 patients, 6 patients (2.4 %) were identified with suboptimal implant reasoned in equipment/technical problems, patient movement during implantation or extensive post-implant edema. Those patients underwent re-implantation. In this publication, implant quality was defined as a D90 of ≥145 Gy ("good"), 145 Gy > D90 ≥ 130 Gy ("adequate"), 130 Gy > D90 ≥ 110 Gy ("potentially acceptable") and an "inadequate" D90 < 110 Gy (Marcu and Lawson 2013).

7.3 Salvage Brachytherapy After Radical Prostatectomy

Treatment for patients with evidence of local recurrence after radical prostatectomy usually consists of EBRT. There are only few studies with low patient numbers concerning PSI as salvage option. All of them presupposed a biopsy proven local recurrence after radical prostatectomy, which had to be clearly recognizable on ultrasound images. As a first side note, sensitivity and specificity of digital rectal examination (DRE) and TRUS are 72.4 and 64.8 % versus 86.2 and 53.5 %, respectively. Biopsy is most probably negative, when PSA <0.5 ng/ml and TRUS / DRE are unsuspicious (Naya et al. 2005). Second side note, most local recurrences after surgery occur at the anastomotic site (56–76 %), bladder neck (26 %), retrovesical space (4–33 %) and more than one site (14 %) (Leventis et al. 2001; Nguyen et al. 2012; Liauw et al. 2012). In endorectal MRI, recurrence was seen in 37 % of men with a PSA >0.3 ng/ml versus 13 % if the PSA is ≤0.3 ng/ml (Liauw et al. 2012).

In a Spanish survey 42 patients were treated with low dose rate brachytherapy (145 Gy) in the anastomotic region. Five-year biochemical disease free survival was 88.6 % and cancer-specific survival was 97 %. No Grade 3 or 4 gastrointestinal and genitourinary toxicity has been described (Gomez-Veiga et al. 2012). In a case report published by Gaztañaga and Crook, dose escalation with combined external beam (46 Gy) and low-dose (LDR) brachytherapy (115 Gy) was presented as a feasible treatment option (Gaztañaga and Crook 2012).

7.4 Salvage Brachytherapy After EBRT

Radical prostatectomy, cryosurgery and brachytherapy are current salvage treatment options for prostate cancer recurrence after primary radiation therapy.

In a Dutch study, a total of 129 patients with biopsy proven recurrence after primary EBRT or PSI were retrospectively analyzed. Biochemical failure (PSI, cryosurgery: Phoenix, surgery: PSA > 0.1 ng/ml) occurred in 81, 61 and 66 % of men treated with salvage LDR-brachytherapy, salvage cryosurgery, or salvage surgery, respectively. In all salvage therapy groups, 30 % of men suffered from grade >3 genitourinary and gastrointestinal toxicity, therefore patients should be selected with care before offering salvage options (Peters et al. 2012).

High toxicity is expectable, when seeds are placed too close to the rectal wall or the urethra. One method of minimizing these problems is to use an intraoperative dosimetry and planning system (Stock 2004). The poor outcome of local salvage therapy is explainable with a lack of diagnostic tools to discriminate between patients with truly localized recurrence, and those with presence of microscopic disseminated disease.

Aaronson et al. presented a very plausible proceeding. The prescribed dose to the recurrent cancer site (determined by magnetic resonance spectroscopy and biopsy results) was 144 Gy, while 108 Gy were delivered to the remaining prostate gland. With this approach, no notable severe complications were reported, and after 30 months, cancer-free survival was 96 % and biochemical relapse-free survival was 88 % (Aaronson et al. 2009).

A prospective phase II trial of the radiation therapy oncology group (RTOG 0526) was activated in 2007 and closed to accrual on January 2014.

One hundred Patients after primary EBRT of T1-T2c, GS 2-7, PSA ≤20 ng/ml prostate cancer, a local recurrence >30 months after EBRT and a current PSA <10 ng/ml were to be included. The treatment concept involved a PSI with 140 Gy encompassing the PTV, which was defined as the prostate CTV plus margin (anterior, lateral 2–3 mm, posterior 0 mm, cranial and caudal 5 mm) (Crook 2007). The results are expected with attention.

8 Dosimetry

Guidelines for dose selection involve the intraoperative planning and the postplanning procedure. For seed order, the seed number is estimated preoperatively by performing an ultrasound examination with computer planning ("Pre-Plan"), which should give the best results. Alternatively, seed number can be taken from a look-up table based on inhouse analyses or published literature (Cohen et al. 2002).

8.1 Seed Quantity

The number of seeds depends from the size of the prostate and single seed activity used. Usually, nomograms are used to determine the approximate seed count based on prostate volume, and additional 5–10 % are added for uncertainties. When loose seeds are implanted, the used total activity may be 15–23 % higher in comparison to stranded seeds (Kudchadker et al. 2008). Somehow, this effect may be caused by three-dimensional reasons: stranded seeds are allowed to be placed near the surface of the prostate capsule and loose seeds must be placed deeper, while both have to deliver enough dose to the PTV surface.

8.2 Seed Activity and Total Activity

Most centers use low activity of seeds (0.4 mCi per seed), but there is no consensus regarding optimal seed activity. By experience, low activity might beneficial in smaller glands, whereas higher activity (0.6 mCi) reduces the number of needles in larger prostates and possibly the procedure costs. In fact, seed implants with a higher source strength seem to improve the probability of excellent implant quality due a better dose coverage, while there are no differences in the rectal and urethral doses between high- and low activity seeds (Narayana et al. 2005). Another study has shown that neither dose homogenity nor conformality is compromized with a lower source strength (Thomas et al. 2007). However, finally the own experience determines which activity of seed is used.

8.3 EBRT Combined with PSI

If EBRT is combined with PSI (110 Gy), the prescribed dose for EBRT is in the range of 41.4–50.4 Gy (1.8 Gy–2 Gy/d). Neither the optimal sequencing of PSI and EBRT is clear, nor the ideal time interval. PSI before EBRT possibly exposes tissues to radiation simultaneously, but EBRT dose may be adjusted in inadequate dosimetrical results of brachytherapy. Secondly, in times of image guidance, the implant may be used as well-identifiable landmark. Indeed, current practice and clinical trials favor EBRT followed by PSI (RTOG 2011; Bittner et al. 2012; Merrick et al. 2011).

For calculation of the biological effective dose (BED) for EBRT and the low-dose-rate permanent decaying implants the formula in the publication from Stock can be used (Stock et al. 2006).

8.4 CTV and PTV

The clinical target volume (CTV) is defined as the whole prostate as seen in rectal ultrasound. The seminal vesicles are not usually included within the clinical target volume. A margin of 2–3 mm is added to generate the planning target volume (PTV).

In high risk prostate cancer, the PTV may consist of the prostate gland with a 5 mm margin (posteriorly 2 mm). The proximal 1 cm of the seminal vesicles should also be included in the planning target volume (Bittner et al. 2012).

8.5 Intraoperative Planning

The most detailed recommendations are offered by the ESTRO/EAU/EORTC group (Salembier et al. 2007). For reasons of clarity, the abbreviations in the following text obtain prefixes for the particular organ: "p"-D90 for the prostate, "r"-D10 for the rectal or "u"-D90 for the urethral contour.

The dose constraints for the PTV (prostate plus margin) are: pD90 >100 % of prescribed dose (PD), pV100 ≥95 %, pV150 ≤50 %. The primary and secondary parameters for the rectal contour are rD_{2cc} ≤ PD and $rD_{0.1cc}$ <200 Gy, and for the prostatic urethra uD10 <150 % of PD and uD30 <130 % of PD, respectively. The GTV should be encompassed by the 150 % isodose.

8.6 Post-Planning

At first, the actual number of seeds in the target area is detected. This could be obtained using CT scout views. If there are missing seeds, a chest X-ray is recommended.

After contouring of CTV-P (prostate), CTV-PM (prostate + 3mm margin), rectum ("r") and the intraprostatic urethra ("u", as long it is recognizable in CT images by use of urinary catheter), the detection of the seeds in the CT / MRT images is performed by the automatic seed finder feature of the planning software. The primary parameters should be reported for both CTV-P and CTV-PM: D90, V100, V150. Secondary parameters are V200 and D100. For the organs at risk primary parameters are rD_{2cc} and uD10. Secondary parameters are $rD_{0.1cc}$, rV100, $uD_{0.1cc}$, uD30 and uD5 (Salembier et al. 2007). The American Brachytherapy Society (ABS) recommends to determine following postoperative dosimetric parameters: pD90, pV100, pV150, uV150, uV5, uV30 and rV100 (Davis et al. 2012).

pD90 is the minimum dose received by 90 % of the contoured prostate, and is commonly accepted as a prognostic parameter for biochemical outcome. pV100 and the average treatment margin have also shown some correlations with cancer control (Orio et al. 2007) in addition to clinical parameters such as primary Gleason grade 4 (Uesugi et al. 2012), perineural invasion and post-treatment PSA values (Ding et al. 2012).

An acceptable dose range for postimplant pD90 may be 130–180 Gy for I-125 as long as normal structures are not overdosed. High-risk patients may benefit from a pD90 >180 Gy (Davis et al. 2012; Potters et al. 2010).

Regarding BED values, Stock et al. found a significant dose-response relationship between increasing BED and higher biochemical control as well as negative re-biopsy rates. In that paper, the formulas for calculating BED in EBRT and PSI are presented and annotated in detail (Stock et al. 2006). In short, implants that yield BED values less than 150 Gy should be potentially addressed with reimplantation or the addition of supplemental external beam irradiation (Hughes et al. 2005). Stone presented a study with 584 patients receiving PSI and EBRT combined with PSI and found an improved local control with a BED of >200 Gy (α/β=2 Gy) (Stone et al. 2010b). This can be achieved with postimplant pD90 of 188 Gy (I-125) or 110 Gy in combination with EBRT (45 Gy).

8.7 Organs at Risk

Higher dose levels to the prostate correlate with improved tumor control, but this should be balanced with respect to the morbidity of the organs at risk.

Critical organs are the anterior rectum wall and the intraprostatic urethra, which are outlined during intraoperative procedure. It is clear that complications are both dose and volume dependent.

In the ESTRO recommendations for prostate PSI, the rectum dose parameters are rD_{2cc} ≤100 %, $D_{0.1cc}$ (~Dmax) <200 Gy (Salembier et al. 2007). To reduce the probability for rectal toxicity, Merrick et al. recommends that the anterior rectal mucosal point dose should be limited to a maximum of 85 % of the prescribed dose. Only a length of 10 and 5 mm of the anterior rectal mucosa should receive 100 and 120 % of the prescribed dose, respectively (Merrick et al. 1999). The risk of late proctitis remains below 5 %, when the total rectal surface (as seen in the postplanning CT) receiving 100, 150 and 200 Gy is ≤30, ≤20 and ≤10 % (Waterman and Dicker 2003). As the total rectal surface is not seen in intraoperative procedure, absolute volume recommendations are more useful: the 3-year bleeding rate in patients with rV100 ≤1 cm^3 was 14 % (Harada et al. 2012). A 5-year survey in 1006 patients reported a late RTOG ≥2 toxicity of 5.8 %, when less than 0.6cc of outer rectal wall receives 100 % of the prescribed dose (Keyes et al. 2012).

The intraprostatic urethra is usually identified on the rectal ultrasound images due to the typical contrast of an urinary catheter. Some authors discuss the anatomical changings of the urethra when a catheter is used. Without catheter, the urethra can be visualized with aerated gel. Under this condition, the urethra shows a more slit-shaped curved configuration and the real size of the urethra may appear larger when defined by gel. With the use of catheters, the urethra shows a more straight run through the prostate (Anderson et al. 2010). Thus, some brachytherapists recommend the instillation of aerated gel prior to insertion of the catheter or directly inside the lumen of a thinner catheter to visualize the urethra more accurate and to minimize urethral distortion. Defining a margin around the catheter lumen may result in lower urinary toxicity, but might be detrimental to the plan quality. It is uncertain what happens to the position of the seeds relative to the urethra once the catheter is removed. Especially in smaller glands (<30 cm^3), the removal of the catheter may lead to an shrinkage of the prostate contour. This results in higher dosimetric parameters (Shirvani et al. 2011).

In studies concerning urinary morbidity or in published recommendations for dosimetric parameters there is a lack of contouring details for the prostatic urethra. Assuming that the urethral volume is defined by the catheter contour, uD10 should be lower than 150 % of the prescription dose (uD30 < 130 %) (Salembier et al. 2007).

Several series with urethral-sparing techniques (maximal urethral dose of 100–140 % of prescribed dose) have not demonstrated a lower urinary morbidity. In addition, neither individual dose constraints to urethral subsegments such as "base", "midprostate", "apex", or "urogenital diaphragm" segments predict for decrease of lower urinary tract symptoms (Allen et al. 2005). Otherwise, a recent study demonstrated that urinary morbidity is more a consequence of sources placed in the vicinity of the urethra than of dose-volume parameters. The authors recommend a minimum distance of 5 mm between the sources and the urethra (Pinkawa et al. 2012).

The risk for development of urethral strictures is increasing, when the apical and periapical urethra is receiving higher doses (Earley et al. 2012). In a study of 425 patients, Merrick et al. reported on a rate of urethral strictures of 3 %. All strictures involved the membranous urethra and the authors comment, that PSI-induced urethral strictures become less common if seeds are placed more than 5 mm distant from the prostate apex (Merrick et al. 2002a). Therefore these urethral regions require more attention in the implantation procedure.

The neurovascular bundle and penile bulb may play a serious role for conserving long term erectile function, although contrary results have been published (Whaley et al. 2012). Since no dose recommendations can be given at present (Crook et al. 2005), "general" dose sparing for these organs should be taken into consideration (Snyder et al. 2012; Roach 2012). Due to the complex pathophysiology, the early use of PDE5 inhibitors for erectile function preservation should be included into clinical treatment pathways (Stember and Mulhall 2012).

9 Spikes, Bounces and Recurrences

In contrast to surgery, the post-treatment PSA does not reach zero values after brachytherapy. Typically, PSA levels after seed implantation decline over a period of 2–5 years to nadir. In some patients, PSA levels might present transient rises with a following decline to pre-spike level, which are called spikes or bounces (Beriwal et al. 2012). The biological reason for this phenomenon remains unclear, but this PSA rise can be very stressful and may cause unnecessary investigations or salvage treatments. Even in 44–56 % of patients with biochemical failure according to Phoenix (nadir + 2 ng/ml) or ASTRO criteria (3 successive increases), PSA might decrease again (Thompson et al. 2010; Toledano et al. 2006).

Therefore there is a need to define a method or in the simplest way a threshold value, which might be able to distinguish between benign bounces and biochemical relapses.

The absolute rate of bounces among patients after brachytherapy quoted in the in the literature depends on the definition of the PSA bounce magnitude. In recent studies, an increase of 0.2 ng/ml is mostly used to define a PSA-bounce, although different definitions with threshold values of 0.1, 0.4 or 2 ng/ml are used as well (Caloglu and Ciezki 2009). PSA bounces occur 12.5–19 months after brachytherapy with a height of 0.29–1.7 ng/ml and duration of 7–36 months. The frequency is 25–35.9 % of patients, although higher rates are reported (Tanaka et al. 2012; Mazeron et al. 2012a, b; Hinnen et al. 2012; Beriwal et al. 2012; Thompson et al. 2010). In the study by Toledano, the frequency of PSA bounces was 55, 49, 32 and 15 % using a definition of ≥0.1, ≥0.2, ≥0.4 and >1 ng/ml, respectively. 16 % of patients with PSA bounce showed a second PSA spike (Tanaka et al. 2012). 90 % of PSA bounces occur in the first 3 years of follow-up (Hinnen et al. 2012).

PSA bounces seem to occur more frequently in younger men (<65–70 years) and patients with lower body mass index (Mazeron et al. 2012b; Delouya et al. 2012; Thompson et al. 2010; Patel et al. 2004).

In 4.8–15 % of patients high-magnitude bounces can mimic PSA failure (Hinnen et al. 2012; Mazeron et al. 2012a; Crook et al. 2007). In the report of Thompson, 5.3 % of 1,006 patients had reached the Phoenix definition of biochemical failure. But in 44 % of those patients, PSA decreased again and a benign bounce was assumed. These patients were significantly younger (<70 years), tended to meet the Phoenix criteria much sooner (<38 months), had shorter time to reach the nadir (median 6 months) and a shorter PSA doubling time (5.1 months) (Thompson et al. 2010).

Dosimetric parameters predictive of a PSA bounce are controversially discussed. Higher implant dose, the prostate volume receiving 150 % of the prescribed dose (V150) and the minimal percentage of dose received by 90 % of the urethra (%UD90) were associated with higher rates of the bounce phenomenon (Stock et al. 2003; Merrick et al. 2002b; Tanaka et al. 2012). For the prediction of biochemical tumor control after brachytherapy a pD90 >140–160 Gy is an accepted dosimetric predictor as discussed before.

In contrast to EBRT, a PSA bounce of 0.2–0.4 ng/ml is not a predictor of biochemical failure (Bernstein et al. 2012). Moreover, a PSA bounce after PSI is strongly related to better outcome in terms of biochemical failure, disease-specific survival, and overall survival (Hinnen et al. 2012; Patel et al. 2004; Aaltomaa et al. 2011). But with higher bounce amplitudes (≥1 ng/ml), the biochemical failure rate increases (McGrath et al. 2010).

In short, PSA bounce occurs in a substantial percentage of cases, and simple PSA threshold values are not sensitive enough to foresee biochemical relapse after brachytherapy. Some authors were analyzing PSA kinetics after seed implantation and observed characteristic findings in patients with biochemical relapse. First, a PSA percentage of >20 % of pretreatment value 6 months after implant is highly associated with relapse risk with sufficient sensitivity (72.4 %) and specificity (79.8 %). Specificity rises to 91.3 %, when a cutoff value of 30 % of pretreatment value is used (Paoluzzi et al. 2012). Patients achieving post-treatment PSA nadir levels of <0.5 ng/ml in ≤5 years have significantly higher long-term freedom from biochemical failure (Ko et al. 2012; Aaltomaa et al. 2011). Hazard ratios for biochemical relapse were 1, 4.96, 27.57, and 65.10 for PSA levels 12 months after seed implantation at ≤1, 1.01–2, 2.01–3 and >3 ng/ml, respectively (Ding et al. 2012).

The reason of insufficient PSA decrease might be explained by minor radiosensitivity, occult metastatic disease or low-quality treatment (poor dosimetric result).

In conclusion, at suspicion of biochemical failure after 3 years of follow-up (when PSA bounce is less probably), a re-biopsy might be carried out to prove recurrent tumor. When positive, salvage treatment options might be offered to the patient. The probability of positive biopsy rates depends on the biologically effective dose. At BED values of ≤140, 140–180 and >180 Gy, the probability of positive biopsy rate is about 15.1, 6.7 and 2.5 %, respectively (Stock et al. 2006).

In the first 3 years after brachytherapy, the current ASTRO Phoenix definition (Roach et al. 2006) should be commonly used for detection of PSA failure. When the PSA increases <2 ng/ml above the nadir, further follow up is necessary to exclude the presence of a benign PSA increase.

Re-Biopsy should be undertaken only in due consideration of dosimetric BED and D90-values, post treatment PSA kinetics and in awareness of the PSA bounce rate of 15 % triggering failure criteria.

10 Quality Assurance

Quality assurance (QA) is essential in prostate brachytherapy. The American Brachytherapy Society (ABS) recommends to establish a well-documented quality improvement program that assures all staff members are trained and competent. All junior faculty should undergo extensive training and competency review (Davis et al. 2012).

Several Studies investigated the impact of experience on dosimetric data. Some of them found a learning curve with a plateau reached from 10 to 30 patients (Loiselle et al. 2009; Merrick et al. 2007). Other publications demonstrate the effect of the learning curve on the implantation procedure (reduction of operating room time, needles and seeds), toxicity (acute urinary retention, post-implant-IPSS, prostate edema), the decrease in the rectal doses (D0.1cc and R100), while the prostate D90 does not change significantly (Le Fur et al. 2012; Keyes et al. 2006).

Nevertheless, special teaching programs should be established in each institution to guarantee high quality procedures, including all steps in prostate brachytherapy:

- patient selection
- ultrasound simulation
- treatment planning
- implant process
- post-implant dosimetry
- follow-up

Except patient selection and follow up, all terms can be trained in dry runs using an ultrasound training system, which consists of an prostate phantom mounted on a table, an ultrasound device/laptop-system with prostate planning software installed and a stepper unit with a stabilizing table mount.

Proctoring by experienced practitioners is strongly recommended for the first implantations. The follow-up examinations should be conducted in a study-like way. Patients should undergo pre- and post-radiotherapy assessment of toxicity and quality of life using standardized questionnaires (IPSS, IIEF, QLQ-C30 / QLQ-PR-25).

The Radiation Therapy Oncology Group (RTOG) supports a credentialing program by the Radiological Physics Center (MD Anderson). It consists of a facility questionnaires and a knowledge assessment. At least 10 TRUS guided prostate implants should have been performed before a faculty can participate in studies. The credentialing process would be a two-step process: a physics/dosimetry review and a clinical review.

In a newer publication, Zelefsky et al. report a concerted effort of the Quality Research in Radiation Oncology (QRRO). In this survey, postplanning dosimetry of several treating institutions within the United States were re-evaluated by an remote expert reviewer. This approach of independent quality assessment provides an opportunity for self-assessment and might be used for license recertification in the credentialing programs (Zelefsky et al. 2013).

In summary, each brachytherapist needs to insure that his own training is superb and consistently meets high quality standards.

11 Conclusions

In this chapter, recent publications are summarized to give an overview of selected topics of low dose rate brachytherapy of prostate cancer. The effectiveness of this treatment approach has been proven over several decades and is comparable with competing therapies such as surgery or EBRT.

In the United States, the utilization of brachytherapy of prostate cancer decreases significantly.

The reason for declining PSI rates are increasing numbers of prostatectomies. Surgery in patients with localized prostate cancer is accounted for nearly 44 % of treatment before 2000, and about 60 % of patients in 2010. Further reasons for the decline of PSI rates are modern developments of EBRT techniques, reimbursement with IMRT, changing patient/physician preference, or lack of emphasis on brachytherapy during radiation oncology training (Mahmood et al. 2014; Martin et al. 2014). But for the next decades, a dramatic triplication of new prostate cancer cases is forecasted (Quon et al. 2011). It looks doubtful, that this future situation can be managed by institutions offering several weeks lasting EBRT treatments. Therefore international radiotherapy organizations should improve medical education and encouragement of radiooncologists in terms of high-quality, one-day lasting brachytherapy.

References

Aaltomaa SH, Kataja VV, Raty A, Palmgren JE, Lahtinen T (2011) Does the outcome of prostate cancer patients with large prostates differ from small prostate size in permanent seed, low dose-rate brachytherapy? Scand J Urol Nephrol 45(5):339–345. doi:10.3109/00365599.2011.590994

Aaronson DS, Yamasaki I, Gottschalk A, Speight J, Hsu IC, Pickett B, Roach M, 3rd, Shinohara K (2009) Salvage permanent perineal radioactive-seed implantation for treating recurrence of localized prostate adenocarcinoma after external beam radiotherapy. BJU Int 104(5):600–604. doi:BJU8445 [pii] 10.1111/j.1464-410X.2009.08445.x

Albert JM, Swanson DA, Pugh TJ, Zhang M, Bruno TL, Kudchadker RJ, Frank SJ (2013) Magnetic resonance imaging-based treatment planning for prostate brachytherapy. Brachytherapy 12(1):30–37. doi:10.1016/j.brachy.2012.03.009

Alenda O, Ploussard G, Mouracade P, Xylinas E, de la Taille A, Allory Y, Vordos D, Hoznek A, Abbou CC, Salomon L (2011) Impact of the primary Gleason pattern on biochemical recurrence-free survival after radical prostatectomy: a single-center cohort of 1,248 patients with Gleason 7 tumors. World J Urol 29(5):671–676. doi:10.1007/s00345-010-0620-9

Allen ZA, Merrick GS, Butler WM, Wallner KE, Kurko B, Anderson RL, Murray BC, Galbreath RW (2005) Detailed urethral dosimetry in the evaluation of prostate brachytherapy-related urinary morbidity. Int J Radiat Oncol Biol Phys 62(4):981–987. doi:10.1016/j.ijrobp.2004.12.068

Anandadas CN, Clarke NW, Davidson SE, O'Reilly PH, Logue JP, Gilmore L, Swindell R, Brough RJ, Wemyss-Holden GD, Lau MW, Javle PM, Ramani VA, Wylie JP, Collins GN, Brown S, Cowan RA, North West Uro-oncology G (2011) Early prostate cancer–which treatment do men prefer and why? BJU Int 107 (11):1762–1768. doi:10.1111/j.1464-410X.2010.09833.x

Anderson C, Lowe G, Ostler P, Inchley D, Hardiman C, Wills R, Bryant L, Chapman C, Marchant N, Hoskin PJ (2010) I-125 seed planning: an alternative method of urethra definition. Radiother Oncol 94(1):24–29. doi:S0167-8140(09)00615-X [pii] 10.1016/j.radonc.2009.11.003

Ash D, Al-Qaisieh B, Bottomley D, Carey B, Joseph J (2006) The correlation between D90 and outcome for I-125 seed implant monotherapy for localised prostate cancer. Radiother Oncol 79 (2):185–189. doi:10.1016/j.radonc.2006.04.004

Ash D, Flynn A, Battermann J, de Reijke T, Lavagnini P, Blank L (2000) ESTRO/EAU/EORTC recommendations on permanent seed implantation for localized prostate cancer. Radiother Oncol 57 (3):315–321

Badwan HO, Shanahan AE, Adams MA, Shanahan TG, Mueller PW, Markwell SJ, Tarter TH (2010) AnchorSeed for the reduction of source movement in prostate brachytherapy with the Mick applicator implant technique. Brachytherapy 9(1):23–26. doi:10.1016/j.brachy.2009.07.002

Beasley M, Williams SG, Pickles T, Unit BPO (2008) Expanded risk groups help determine which prostate radiotherapy sub-group may benefit from adjuvant androgen deprivation therapy. Radiat Oncol 3:8. doi:10.1186/1748-717X-3-8

Beriwal S, Smith RP, Houser C, Benoit RM (2012) Prostate-specific antigen spikes with (131)Cs brachytherapy. Is there a difference with other radioisotopes? Brachytherapy 11(6):457–459. doi:10.1016/j.brachy.2012.04.004

Bernstein M, Ohri N, Bodner W, Garg M, Dicker A, Guha C (2012) PSA bounce predicts for a favorable prognosis following Brachytherapy, but an unfavorable prognosis after external beam radiation therapy: a meta-analysis. Int J Radiation Oncol Biol Phys 84(3, Supplement):S371. doi:10.1016/j.ijrobp.2012.07.979

Beyer DC, McKeough T, Thomas T (2005) Impact of short course hormonal therapy on overall and cancer specific survival after permanent prostate brachytherapy. Int J Radiat Oncol Biol Phys 61 (5):1299–1305. doi:10.1016/j.ijrobp.2004.08.024

Bittner N, Merrick GS, Butler WM, Galbreath RW, Adamovich E, Wallner KE (2013) Gleason score 7 prostate cancer treated with interstitial brachytherapy with or without supplemental external beam radiation and androgen deprivation therapy: is the primary pattern on needle biopsy prognostic? Brachytherapy 12(1):14–18. doi:10.1016/j.brachy.2012.05.002

Bittner N, Merrick GS, Butler WM, Galbreath RW, Lief J, Adamovich E, Wallner KE (2012) Long-term outcome for very high-risk prostate cancer treated primarily with a triple modality approach to include permanent interstitial brachytherapy. Brachytherapy 11 (4):250–255. doi:10.1016/j.brachy.2012.02.002

Blasko JC (2004) Patient selection for prostate brachytherapy: more myth than fact: Review 1. Oncology (Williston Park) 18(4):452

Boo D, Shasha D, Mourad WF, Salant R, Gorfinkel N, Harrison LB (2012) In Support of Brachytherapy for Young Men With Prostate Cancer. Int J Radiat Oncol Biol Phys 84 (3, Supplement):S409. doi:10.1016/j.ijrobp.2012.07.1082

Bowes D, Crook J, Batchelar D, Araujo C, Parker B, Kim D, Gaztanaga M, Milette M, Rajapakshe R, Petrik D (2012a) A Randomized Trial Comparing Seed Loss and Displacement of Specially Engineered Coated Seeds to Standard Uncoated Loose Seeds. Int J Radiat Oncol Biol Phys 84(3):S402. doi:10.1016/j.ijrobp.2012.07.1061

Bowes D, Crook JM, Araujo C, Batchelar D (2013a) Ultrasound-CT fusion compared with MR-CT fusion for postimplant dosimetry in permanent prostate brachytherapy. Brachytherapy 12(1):38–43. doi:10.1016/j.brachy.2012.03.007

Bowes D, Crook JM, Rajapakshe R, Araujo C, Parker B (2013b) Defining a magnetic resonance scan sequence for permanent seed prostate brachytherapy postimplant assessment. Brachytherapy 12 (1):25–29. doi:10.1016/j.brachy.2012.03.001

Bowes D, Crook JM, Wallace K, Evans A, Toi A, Finelli A, Jewett MA, Fleshner N, Catton C (2012b) Results of a surgically derived nomogram to predict Gleason score upgrading applied to a cohort of patients with "favorable-risk" prostate cancer treated with permanent seed brachytherapy. Urology 80(3):649–655. doi:10.1016/j.urology.2012.03.051

Burri RJ, Ho AY, Forsythe K, Cesaretti JA, Stone NN, Stock RG (2010) Young men have equivalent biochemical outcomes compared with older men after treatment with brachytherapy for prostate cancer. Int J Radiat Oncol Biol Phys 77(5):1315–1321. doi:S0360-3016(09)01000-1 [pii] 10.1016/j.ijrobp.2009.06.052

Caloglu M, Ciezki J (2009) Prostate-specific antigen bounce after prostate brachytherapy: review of a confusing phenomenon. Urology 74(6):1183–1190. doi:10.1016/j.urology.2009.01.043

Chen WC, Katcher J, Nunez C, Tirgan AM, Ellis RJ (2012) Radioactive seed migration after transperineal interstitial prostate brachytherapy and associated development of small-cell lung cancer. Brachytherapy 11(5):354–358. doi:10.1016/j.brachy.2011.12.003

Chiumento C, Fiorentino A, Caivano R, Clemente S, Fusco V (2013) Low-dose rate brachytherapy of the prostate in elderly patients. La Radiologia medica 118(8):1412–1421. doi:10.1007/s11547-012-0872-0

Choe KS, Correa D, Jani AB, Liauw SL (2010) The use of anticoagulants improves biochemical control of localized prostate cancer treated with radiotherapy. Cancer 116(7):1820–1826. doi:10.1002/cncr.24890

Cohen GN, Amols HI, Zelefsky MJ, Zaider M (2002) The Anderson nomograms for permanent interstitial prostate implants: a briefing for practitioners. Int J Radiat Oncol Biol Phys 53(2):504–511

Cooperberg MR, Lubeck DP, Mehta SS, Carroll PR, CaPsure (2003) Time trends in clinical risk stratification for prostate cancer: implications for outcomes (data from CaPSURE). J Urol 170(6 Pt 2):S21–25; discussion S26–27. doi:10.1097/01.ju.0000095025.03331.c6

Crook J (2007) RTOG 0526: A prospective phase II trial of transperineal ultrasound-guided Brachytherapy for locally recurrent prostate adenocarcinoma following external beam radiotherapy

Crook J, Gillan C, Yeung I, Austen L, McLean M, Lockwood G (2007) PSA kinetics and PSA bounce following permanent seed prostate brachytherapy. Int J Radiat Oncol Biol Phys 69(2):426–433. doi:10.1016/j.ijrobp.2007.03.031

Crook J, McLean M, Catton C, Yeung I, Tsihlias J, Pintilie M (2002a) Factors influencing risk of acute urinary retention after TRUS-guided permanent prostate seed implantation. Int J Radiat Oncol Biol Phys 52(2):453–460

Crook J, Milosevic M, Catton P, Yeung I, Haycocks T, Tran T, Catton C, McLean M, Panzarella T, Haider MA (2002b) Interobserver variation in postimplant computed tomography contouring affects quality assessment of prostate brachytherapy. Brachytherapy 1 (2):66–73

Crook JM, Gomez-Iturriaga A, Wallace K, Ma C, Fung S, Alibhai S, Jewett M, Fleshner N (2011) Comparison of health-related quality of life 5 years after SPIRIT: surgical prostatectomy versus interstitial radiation intervention trial. J Clin Oncol 29 (4):362–368. doi:10.1200/JCO.2010.31.7305

Crook JM, Potters L, Stock RG, Zelefsky MJ (2005) Critical organ dosimetry in permanent seed prostate brachytherapy: defining the organs at risk. Brachytherapy 4(3):186–194. doi:10.1016/j.brachy.2005.01.002

D'Amico AV, Whittington R, Malkowicz SB, Schultz D, Blank K, Broderick GA, Tomaszewski JE, Renshaw AA, Kaplan I, Beard CJ, Wein A (1998) Biochemical outcome after radical prostatectomy, external beam radiation therapy, or interstitial radiation therapy for clinically localized prostate cancer. JAMA 280(11):969–974

Dallas NL, Malone PR, Jones A, Doggart AJ, McConway KJ, Rogers PB (2012) The results of real-time brachytherapy for the management of low- and intermediate-risk prostate cancer in patients with prostate volumes up to 100 mL. BJU Int 110(3):383–390. doi:10.1111/j.1464-410X.2012.10931.x

Davis BJ, Bresnahan JF, Stafford SL, Karon BL, King BF, Wilson TM (2002) Prostate brachytherapy seed migration to a coronary artery found during angiography. J Urol 168(3):1103

Davis BJ, Horwitz EM, Lee WR, Crook JM, Stock RG, Merrick GS, Butler WM, Grimm PD, Stone NN, Potters L, Zietman AL, Zelefsky MJ (2012) American Brachytherapy Society consensus guidelines for transrectal ultrasound-guided permanent prostate brachytherapy. Brachytherapy 11(1):6–19. doi:10.1016/j.brachy.2011.07.005

De Brabandere M, Hoskin P, Haustermans K, Van den Heuvel F, Siebert FA (2012) Prostate post-implant dosimetry: interobserver variability in seed localisation, contouring and fusion. Radiother Oncol 104(2):192–198. doi:10.1016/j.radonc.2012.06.014

Delouya G, Taussky D, Ji CR, Sylvestre MP, Donath D (2012) Relationship between prostate-specific antigen bounce body fat distribution and body mass index in permanent seed brachytherapy for prostate cancer. Brachytherapy 11(3):214–218. doi:10.1016/j.brachy.2011.05.009

Deutsche Gesellschaft für Urologie (2011) Interdisziplinäre Leitlinie der Qualität S3 zur Früherkennung, Diagnose und Therapie der verschiedenen Stadien des Prostatakarzinoms (Version 2.0 - 1. Aktualisierung 2011). 2.0 edn. Leitlinienprogramm Onkologie der AWMW, Deutschen Krebsgesellschaft e.V. und Deutschen Krebshilfe e.V., Berlin

Ding W, Lee J, Chamberlain D, Cunningham J, Yang L, Tay J (2012) Twelve-month prostate-specific antigen values and perineural invasion as strong independent prognostic variables of long-term biochemical outcome after prostate seed brachytherapy. Int J Radiat Oncol Biol Phys 84(4):962–967. doi:10.1016/j.ijrobp.2012.01.043

Earley JJ, Abdelbaky AM, Cunningham MJ, Chadwick E, Langley SE, Laing RW (2012) Correlation between prostate brachytherapy-related urethral stricture and peri-apical urethral dosimetry: a matched case-control study. Radiother Oncol 104(2):187–191. doi:10.1016/j.radonc.2012.06.001

Eastham JA (2004) Comparing radical prostatectomy and brachytherapy for localized prostate cancer, Discussion1. Oncology (Williston Park) 18(10):1302–1304

Fang LC, Merrick GS, Butler WM, Galbreath RW, Murray BC, Reed JL, Adamovich E, Wallner KE (2011) High-risk prostate cancer with Gleason score 8-10 and PSA level </=15 ng/mL treated with permanent interstitial brachytherapy. Int J Radiat Oncol Biol Phys 81(4):992–996. doi:10.1016/j.ijrobp.2010.07.006

Fisher CM, Troncoso P, Swanson DA, Munsell MF, Kuban DA, Lee AK, Yeh SF, Frank SJ (2012) Knife or needles? A cohort analysis of outcomes after radical prostatectomy or brachytherapy for men with low- or intermediate-risk adenocarcinoma of the prostate. Brachytherapy 11(6):429–434. doi:10.1016/j.brachy.2012.04.009

Frank SJ, Arterbery VE, Hsu IC, Abdel-Wahab M, Ciezki JP, Hahn NM, Mohler JL, Moran BJ, Rosenthal SA, Rossi CJ, Yamada Y, Merrick G (2011) American College of Radiology Appropriateness Criteria permanent source brachytherapy for prostate cancer. Brachytherapy 10(5):357–362. doi:10.1016/j.brachy.2011.01.014

Gaztañaga M, Crook JM (2012) Permanent seed brachytherapy for locally recurrent prostate cancer after radical prostatectomy: a case report and review of the literature. Brachytherapy. doi:10.1016/j.brachy.2012.04.006

Gomez-Veiga F, Marino A, Alvarez L, Rodriguez I, Fernandez C, Pertega S, Candal A (2012) Brachytherapy for the treatment of recurrent prostate cancer after radiotherapy or radical prostatectomy. BJU Int 109(Suppl 1):17–21. doi:10.1111/j.1464-410X.2011.10826.x

Graham J, Baker M, Macbeth F, Titshall V, Guideline Development G (2008) Diagnosis and treatment of prostate cancer: summary of NICE guidance. Bmj 336(7644):610–612. doi:10.1136/bmj.39498.525706.AD

Grimm P, Billiet I, Bostwick D, Dicker AP, Frank S, Immerzeel J, Keyes M, Kupelian P, Lee WR, Machtens S, Mayadev J, Moran BJ, Merrick G, Millar J, Roach M, Stock R, Shinohara K, Scholz M, Weber E, Zietman A, Zelefsky M, Wong J, Wentworth S, Vera R, Langley S (2012) Comparative analysis of prostate-specific antigen free survival outcomes for patients with low, intermediate and high risk prostate cancer treatment by radical therapy. Results from the Prostate Cancer Results Study Group. BJU Int 109Suppl 1:22–29. doi:10.1111/j.1464-410X.2011.10827.x

Hansen EK, Roach M III (2010) Handbook of Evidence-Based Radiation Oncology, 2nd edn. Springer, New York

Harada K, Ishikawa H, Saito Y, Nakamoto S, Kawamura H, Wakatsuki M, Etsunaga T, Takezawa Y, Kobayashi M, Nakano T (2012) Risk factors for rectal bleeding associated with I-125 brachytherapy for prostate cancer. J Radiat Res 53(6):923–929. doi:10.1093/jrr/rrs059

Hau EK, Oborn BM, Bucci J (2011) An unusual case of radioactive seed migration to the vertebral venous plexus and renal artery with nerve root compromise. Brachytherapy 10(4):295–298. doi:10.1016/j.brachy.2010.08.006

Heidenreich A, Bolla M, Joniau S, Mason MD, Matveev V, Mottet N, Schmid H-P, van der Kwast TH, Wiegel T, Zattoni F (2011) Guidelines on prostate cancer. Eur Assoc Urol http://www.uroweb.org/gls/pdf/08_Prostate_Cancer.pdf

Henry AM, Al-Qaisieh B, Gould K, Bownes P, Smith J, Carey B, Bottomley D, Ash D (2010) Outcomes following iodine-125 monotherapy for localized prostate cancer: the results of leeds 10-year single-center brachytherapy experience. Int J Radiat Oncol Biol Phys 76(1):50–56. doi:S0360-3016(09)00191-6 [pii] 10.1016/j.ijrobp.2009.01.050

Herbert C, Morris WJ, Keyes M, Hamm J, Lapointe V, McKenzie M, Pickles T, Spadinger I (2012) Outcomes following iodine-125 brachytherapy in patients with Gleason 7, intermediate risk prostate cancer: a population-based cohort study. Radiother Oncol 103 (2):228–232. doi:10.1016/j.radonc.2012.01.006

Hinnen KA, Battermann JJ, van Roermund JG, Moerland MA, Jurgenliemk-Schulz IM, Frank SJ, van Vulpen M (2010) Long-term biochemical and survival outcome of 921 patients treated with I-125 permanent prostate brachytherapy. Int J Radiat Oncol Biol Phys 76(5):1433–1438. doi:10.1016/j.ijrobp.2009.03.049

Hinnen KA, Monninkhof EM, Battermann JJ, van Roermund JG, Frank SJ, van Vulpen M (2012) Prostate specific antigen bounce is related to overall survival in prostate brachytherapy. Int J Radiat Oncol Biol Phys 82(2):883–888. doi:10.1016/j.ijrobp.2010.11.049

Hinnen KA, Roeloffzen EM, Battermann JJ, Van Moorselaar RJ, van Roermund JG, van Vulpen M (2011) Survival after prostate brachytherapy in patients aged 60 years and younger. BJU Int 107 (12):1906–1911. doi:10.1111/j.1464-410X.2010.09769.x

Ho AY, Burri RJ, Cesaretti JA, Stone NN, Stock RG (2009) Radiation dose predicts for biochemical control in intermediate-risk prostate cancer patients treated with low-dose-rate brachytherapy. Int J Radiat Oncol Biol Phys 75(1):16–22. doi:S0360-3016(08)03870-4 [pii] 10.1016/j.ijrobp.2008.10.071

Hoeks CM, Barentsz JO, Hambrock T, Yakar D, Somford DM, Heijmink SW, Scheenen TW, Vos PC, Huisman H, van Oort IM, Witjes JA, Heerschap A, Futterer JJ (2011) Prostate cancer: multiparametric MR imaging for detection, localization, and staging. Radiology 261(1):46–66. doi:10.1148/radiol.11091822

Holmes JA, Wang AZ, Hoffman KE, Hendrix LH, Rosenman JG, Carpenter WR, Godley PA, Chen RC (2012) Is primary prostate cancer treatment influenced by likelihood of extraprostatic disease? A surveillance, epidemiology and end results patterns of care study. Int J Radiat Oncol Biol Phys 84(1):88–94. doi:10.1016/j.ijrobp.2011.10.076

Horwich A, Parker C, Bangma C, Kataja V, Group EGW (2010) Prostate cancer: ESMO Clinical Practice Guidelines for diagnosis, treatment and follow-up. Ann Oncol 21(Suppl 5):v129–133. doi:10.1093/annonc/mdq174

Huang J, Vicini FA, Williams SG, Ye H, McGrath S, Ghilezan M, Krauss D, Martinez AA, Kestin LL (2012) Percentage of positive biopsy cores: a better risk stratification model for prostate cancer? Int J Radiat Oncol Biol Phys 83(4):1141–1148. doi:10.1016/j.ijrobp.2011.09.043

Hughes L, Waterman FM, Dicker AP (2005) Salvage of suboptimal prostate seed implantation: Reimplantation of underdosed region of prostate base. Brachytherapy 4(2):163–170. doi:10.1016/j.brachy.2005.03.002

Ishiyama H, Hirayama T, Jhaveri P, Satoh T, Paulino AC, Xu B, Butler EB, Teh BS (2012) Is There an Increase in Genitourinary Toxicity in Patients Treated With Transurethral Resection of the Prostate and Radiotherapy?: A Systematic Review. Am J Clin Oncol (in press). doi:10.1097/COC.0b013e3182546821

Ivanowicz AN, Wakeman CM, Hubbard RT, Devoe WB, Haake MR, Teigland CM (2012) Two-step transurethral surgery of the prostate and permanent implant brachytherapy for patients with lower urinary tract symptoms and low- to intermediate-risk prostate cancer. Brachytherapy 11(6):483–488. doi:10.1016/j.brachy.2011.08.006

Kaplan A, German L, Chen J, Matzkin H, Mabjeesh NJ (2012) Validation and comparison of the two Kattan nomograms in patients with prostate cancer treated with (125) iodine brachytherapy. BJU Int 109(11):1661–1665. doi:10.1111/j.1464-410X.2011.10748.x

Katz MH, Shikanov S, Sun M, Abdollah F, Budaeus L, Gong EM, Eggener SE, Steinberg GD, Zagaja GP, Shalhav AL, Karakiewicz PI, Zorn KC (2011) Gleason 6 prostate cancer in one or two biopsy cores can harbor more aggressive disease. J Endourol/Endourological Soc 25(4):699–703. doi:10.1089/end.2010.0425

Keyes M, Pickles T, Agranovich A, Kwan W, Morris WJ (2004) 125I reimplantation in patients with poor initial dosimetry after prostate brachytherapy. Int J Radiat Oncol Biol Phys 60(1):40–50. doi:10.1016/j.ijrobp.2004.02.011

Keyes M, Schellenberg D, Moravan V, McKenzie M, Agranovich A, Pickles T, Wu J, Liu M, Bucci J, Morris WJ (2006) Decline in urinary retention incidence in 805 patients after prostate brachytherapy: the effect of learning curve? Int J Radiat Oncol Biol Phys 64(3):825–834. doi:10.1016/j.ijrobp.2005.04.056

Keyes M, Spadinger I, Liu M, Pickles T, Pai H, Hayden A, Moravan V, Halperin R, McKenzie M, Kwan W, Agranovic A, Lapointe V, Morris WJ (2012) Rectal toxicity and rectal dosimetry in low-dose-rate (125)I permanent prostate implants: a long-term study in 1006 patients. Brachytherapy 11(3):199–208. doi:10.1016/j.brachy.2011.05.007

Khan MA, Han M, Partin AW, Epstein JI, Walsh PC (2003) Long-term cancer control of radical prostatectomy in men younger than 50 years of age: update 2003. Urology 62(1):86–91 (discussion 91–82)

Ko EC, Stone NN, Stock RG (2012) PSA nadir of <0.5 ng/mL following brachytherapy for early-stage prostate adenocarcinoma is associated with freedom from prostate-specific antigen failure. Int J Radiat Oncol Biol Phys 83(2):600–607. doi:10.1016/j.ijrobp.2011.07.009

Kono Y, Kubota K, Aruga T, Ishibashi A, Morooka M, Ito K, Itami J, Kanemura M, Minowada S, Tanaka T (2010) Swelling of the prostate gland by permanent brachytherapy may affect seed migration. Japan J Clin Oncol 40(12):1159–1165. doi:10.1093/jjco/hyq118

Kudchadker RJ, Swanson DA, Kuban DA, Lee AK, Bruno TL, Frank SJ (2008) Is a loose-seed nomogram still valid for prostate brachytherapy in a stranded-seed era? Int J Radiat Oncol Biol Phys 72(2):623–627. doi:10.1016/j.ijrobp.2008.03.001

Langley SE, Laing RW (2012) 4D Brachytherapy, a novel real-time prostate brachytherapy technique using stranded and loose seeds. BJU Int 109(Suppl 1):1–6. doi:10.1111/j.1464-410X.2011.10824.x

Lavery HJ, Droller MJ (2012) Do Gleason patterns 3 and 4 prostate cancer represent separate disease States? J Urol 188(5):1667–1675. doi:10.1016/j.juro.2012.07.055

Lawton CA, Yan Y, Lee WR, Gillin M, Firat S, Baikadi M, Crook J, Kuettel M, Morton G, Sandler H (2012) Long-term results of an RTOG Phase II trial (00-19) of external-beam radiation therapy combined with permanent source brachytherapy for intermediate-risk clinically localized adenocarcinoma of the prostate. Int J Radiat Oncol Biol Phys 82(5):e795–801. doi:10.1016/j.ijrobp.2011.11.040

Le Fur E, Malhaire JP, Baverez D, Delage F, Perrouin-Verbe MA, Schlurmann F, Guerif S, Fournier G, Pradier O, Valeri A (2012) Impact of learning curve and technical changes on dosimetry in low-dose brachytherapy for prostate cancer. Strahlenther Onkol. doi:10.1007/s00066-012-0242-9

Lee HK, Adams MT, Shi Q, Basillote J, Lamonica J, Miranda L, Motta J (2010) Seed implant retention score predicts the risk of prolonged urinary retention after prostate brachytherapy. Int J Radiat Oncol Biol Phys 76(5):1445–1449. doi:10.1016/j.ijrobp.2009.04.008

Lee LN, Stock RG, Stone NN (2002) Role of hormonal therapy in the management of intermediate- to high-risk prostate cancer treated with permanent radioactive seed implantation. Int J Radiat Oncol Biol Phys 52(2):444–452

Leventis AK, Shariat SF, Slawin KM (2001) Local recurrence after radical prostatectomy: correlation of US features with prostatic fossa biopsy findings. Radiology 219(2):432–439

Liauw SL, Pitroda SP, Eggener SE, Stadler WM, Pelizzari CA, Vannier MW, Oto A (2012) Evaluation of the Prostate Bed for Local Recurrence After Radical Prostatectomy Using Endorectal Magnetic Resonance Imaging. Int J Radiat Oncol Biol Phys. doi:10.1016/j.ijrobp.2012.05.015

Liu HW, Malkoske K, Sasaki D, Bews J, Demers A, Nugent Z, Ong A, Bashir B, Dufan T, Cho P, Drachenberg D, Chowdhury A (2010) The dosimetric quality of brachytherapy implants in patients with small prostate volume depends on the experience of the brachytherapy team. Brachytherapy 9(3):202–207. doi:10.1016/j.brachy.2009.07.009

Loiselle CR, Waheed M, Sylvester J, Allen ZA, Grimm PD, Eulau S, Butler WM, Merrick GS (2009) Analysis of the Pro-Qura Database: rectal dose, implant quality, and brachytherapist's experience. Brachytherapy 8(1):34–39. doi:10.1016/j.brachy.2008.09.003

Mahmood U, Pugh T, Frank S, Levy L, Walker G, Haque W, Koshy M, Graber W, Swanson D, Hoffman K, Kuban D, Lee A (2014) Declining use of brachytherapy for the treatment of prostate cancer. Brachytherapy 13(2):157–162. doi:10.1016/j.brachy.2013.08.005

Maletz KL, Ennis RD, Ostenson J, Pevsner A, Kagen A, Wernick I (2012) Comparison of CT and MR-CT fusion for prostate post-implant dosimetry. Int J Radiat Oncol Biol Phys 82(5):1912–1917. doi:10.1016/j.ijrobp.2011.01.064

Mallick S, Azzouzi R, Cormier L, Peiffert D, Mangin PH (2003) Urinary morbidity after 125I brachytherapy of the prostate. BJU Int 92(6):555–558

Marcu LG, Lawson JM (2013) Technical and dosimetric aspects of iodine-125 seed reimplantation in suboptimal prostate implants. Br J Radiol 86(1026):20130058. doi:10.1259/bjr.20130058

Martin JM, Handorf EA, Kutikov A, Uzzo RG, Bekelman JE, Horwitz EM, Smaldone MC (2014) The rise and fall of prostate brachytherapy: Use of brachytherapy for the treatment of localized prostate cancer in the National Cancer Data Base. Cancer. doi:10.1002/cncr.28697

Mayadev J, Merrick GS, Reed JR, Butler WM, Galbreath RW, Allen ZA, Wallner KE (2010) Permanent prostate brachytherapy in prostate glands <20 cm(3). Int J Radiat Oncol Biol Phys 76(5):1450–1455. doi:10.1016/j.ijrobp.2009.04.014

Mazeron R, Bajard A, Montbarbon X, Gassa F, Malet C, Rocher F, Clippe S, Bringeon G, Desmettre O, Pommier P (2012a) Permanent 125I-seed prostate brachytherapy: early prostate specific antigen value as a predictor of PSA bounce occurrence. Radiat Oncol 7:46. doi:10.1186/1748-717X-7-46

Mazeron R, Bajard A, Pommier P (2012b) Prostate-specific antigen bounce after permanent seed prostate brachytherapy: A literature review. Cancer Radiother 16(8):702–710. doi:10.1016/j.canrad.2012.09.004

McElveen TL, Waterman FM, Kim H, Dicker AP (2004) Factors predicting for urinary incontinence after prostate brachytherapy. Int J Radiat Oncol Biol Phys 59(5):1395–1404. doi:10.1016/j.ijrobp.2004.01.050

McGrath SD, Antonucci JV, Fitch DL, Ghilezan M, Gustafson GS, Vicini FA, Martinez AA, Kestin LL (2010) PSA bounce after prostate brachytherapy with or without neoadjuvant androgen deprivation. Brachytherapy 9(2):137–144. doi:10.1016/j.brachy.2009.07.005

McNeely LK, Stone NN, Presser J, Chircus JH, Stock RG (2004) Influence of prostate volume on dosimetry results in real-time 125I seed implantation. Int J Radiat Oncol Biol Phys 58(1):292–299

Merrick GS, Butler WM, Dorsey AT, Lief JH, Walbert HL, Blatt HJ (1999) Rectal dosimetric analysis following prostate brachytherapy. Int J Radiat Oncol Biol Phys 43(5):1021–1027

Merrick GS, Butler WM, Galbreath RW, Lief J, Bittner N, Wallner KE, Adamovich E (2011) Prostate cancer death is unlikely in high-risk patients following quality permanent interstitial brachytherapy. BJU Int 107(2):226–232. doi:10.1111/j.1464-410X.2010.09486.x

Merrick GS, Butler WM, Lief JH, Dorsey AT (2001) Is brachytherapy comparable with radical prostatectomy and external-beam radiation for clinically localized prostate cancer? Tech Urol 7(1):12–19

Merrick GS, Butler WM, Tollenaar BG, Galbreath RW, Lief JH (2002a) The dosimetry of prostate brachytherapy-induced urethral strictures. Int J Radiat Oncol Biol Phys 52(2):461–468

Merrick GS, Butler WM, Wallner KE, Galbreath RW, Anderson RL (2002b) Prostate-specific antigen spikes after permanent prostate brachytherapy. Int J Radiat Oncol Biol Phys 54(2):450–456

Merrick GS, Butler WM, Wallner KE, Galbreath RW, Lief JH, Allen Z, Adamovich E (2005) Impact of supplemental external beam radiotherapy and/or androgen deprivation therapy on biochemical outcome after permanent prostate brachytherapy. Int J Radiat Oncol Biol Phys 61(1):32–43. doi:10.1016/j.ijrobp.2004.05.003

Merrick GS, Grimm PD, Sylvester J, Blasko JC, Butler WM, Allen ZA, Chaudhry UU, Mazza A, Sitter M (2007) Initial analysis of Pro-Qura: a multi-institutional database of prostate brachytherapy dosimetry. Brachytherapy 6(1):9–15. doi:10.1016/j.brachy.2006.10.002

Merrick GS, Wallner KE, Butler WM, Galbreath RW, Allen ZA, Adamovich E, True L (2006) Brachytherapy in men aged < or = 54 years with clinically localized prostate cancer. BJU Int 98 (2):324–328. doi:BJU6248 [pii] 10.1111/j.1464-410X.2006.06248.x

Merrick GS, Wallner KE, Galbreath RW, Butler WM, Brammer SG, Allen ZA, Lief JH, Adamovich E (2008) Biochemical and functional outcomes following brachytherapy with or without supplemental therapies in men < or = 50 years of age with clinically organ-confined prostate cancer. Am J Clin Oncol 31 (6):539–544. doi:10.1097/COC.0b013e318172dcb7

Miles EF, Nelson JW, Alkaissi AK, Das S, Clough RW, Broadwater G, Anscher MS, Chino JP, Oleson JR (2010) Biologically effective dose (BED) correlation with biochemical control after low-dose rate prostate brachytherapy for clinically low-risk prostate cancer. Int J Radiat Oncol Biol Phys 77(1):139–146. doi:10.1016/j.ijrobp.2009.04.052

Miyazawa K, Matoba M, Minato H, Morita N, Chikazawa I, Ota K, Tokunaga K, Tonami H, Nojima T, Suzuki K (2012) Seed migration after transperineal interstitial prostate brachytherapy with I-125 free seeds: analysis of its incidence and risk factors. Japan J Radiol 30(8):635–641. doi:10.1007/s11604-012-0102-7

Mohler JL, Armstrong AJ, Bahnson RR, Boston B, Busby JE, D'Amico AV, Eastham JA, Enke CA, Farrington T, Higano CS, Horwitz EM, Kantoff PW, Kawachi MH, Kuettel M, Lee RJ, MacVicar GR, Malcolm AW, Miller D, Plimack ER, Pow-Sang JM, Roach M, 3rd, Rohren E, Rosenfeld S, Srinivas S, Strope SA, Tward J, Twardowski P, Walsh PC, Ho M, Shead DA (2012) Prostate cancer, Version 3.2012: featured updates to the NCCN guidelines. J Nat Compr Cancer Netw : JNCCN 10(9):1081–1087

Narayana V, Troyer S, Evans V, Winfield RJ, Roberson PL, McLaughlin PW (2005) Randomized trial of high- and low-source strength (125)I prostate seed implants. Int J Radiat Oncol Biol Phys 61(1):44–51. doi:10.1016/j.ijrobp.2004.05.001

Naya Y, Okihara K, Evans RB, Babaian RJ (2005) Efficacy of prostatic fossa biopsy in detecting local recurrence after radical prostatectomy. Urology 66(2):350–355. doi:10.1016/j.urology.2005.03.014

NCCN (2012) NCCN clinical practice guidelines in oncology (National comprehensive cancer network guideline) prostate cancer. National comprehensive cancer network. http://www.nccn.org/professionals/physician_gls/pdf/prostate.pdf

Nguyen BD, Schild SE, Wong WW, Vora SA (2009) Prostate brachytherapy seed embolization to the right renal artery. Brachytherapy 8(3):309–312. doi:10.1016/j.brachy.2008.11.011

Nguyen DP, Giannarini G, Seiler R, Schiller R, Thoeny HC, Thalmann GN, Studer UE (2012) Local recurrence after retropubic radical prostatectomy for prostate cancer does not exclusively occur at the anastomotic site. BJU Int. doi:10.1111/j.1464-410X.2012.11506.x

Ohashi T, Momma T, Yamashita S, Nagatsuma K, Kanai K, Kitagawa K, Takahashi S, Hanada T, Yorozu A, Shigematsu N (2012) Impact of MRI-based postimplant dosimetric assessment in prostate brachytherapy using contrast-enhanced T1-weighted images. Brachytherapy 11(6):468–475. doi:10.1016/j.brachy.2011.12.010

Orio P, Wallner K, Merrick G, Herstein A, Mitsuyama P, Thornton K, Butler W, Sutlief S (2007) Dosimetric parameters as predictive factors for biochemical control in patients with higher risk prostate cancer treated with Pd-103 and supplemental beam radiation. Int J Radiat Oncol Biol Phys 67(2):342–346. doi:10.1016/j.ijrobp.2006.09.010

Paoluzzi M, Mignogna M, Lorenzini E, Valent F, Fontana N, Pinzi N, Repetti F, Ponchietti R (2012) Is prostate-specific antigen percentage decrease predictive of clinical outcome after permanent iodine-125 interstitial brachytherapy for prostate cancer? Brachytherapy 11 (4):277–283. doi:10.1016/j.brachy.2011.08.008

Patel C, Elshaikh MA, Angermeier K, Ulchaker J, Klein EA, Chehade N, Wilkinson DA, Reddy CA, Ciezki JP (2004) PSA bounce predicts early success in patients with permanent iodine-125 prostate implant. Urology 63(1):110–113

Peters M, Moman MR, van der Poel HG, Vergunst H, de Jong IJ, Vijverberg PL, Battermann JJ, Horenblas S, van Vulpen M (2012) Patterns of outcome and toxicity after salvage prostatectomy, salvage cryosurgery and salvage brachytherapy for prostate cancer recurrences after radiation therapy: a multi-center experience and literature review. World J Urol. doi:10.1007/s00345-012-0928-8

Petit JH, Gluck C, Kiger WS, 3rd, Laury Henry D, Karasiewicz C, Talcott JA, Berg S, Holupka EJ, Kaplan ID (2007) Androgen deprivation-mediated cytoreduction before interstitial brachytherapy for prostate cancer does not abrogate the elevated risk of urinary morbidity associated with larger initial prostate volume. Brachytherapy 6(4):267–271. doi:10.1016/j.brachy.2007.08.007

Petrik D, Araujo C, Kim D, Halperin R, Crook JM (2012) Implications of CT imaging for postplan quality assessment in prostate brachytherapy. Brachytherapy 11(6):435–440. doi:10.1016/j.brachy.2012.05.001

Petros JA (2004) Comparing radical prostatectomy and brachytherapy for localized prostate cancer, Discussion2. Oncology (Williston Park) 18(10):1309

Pickett B, Kurhanewicz J, Pouliot J, Weinberg V, Shinohara K, Coakley F, Roach M 3rd (2006) Three-dimensional conformal external beam radiotherapy compared with permanent prostate implantation in low-risk prostate cancer based on endorectal magnetic resonance spectroscopy imaging and prostate-specific antigen level. Int J Radiat Oncol Biol Phys 65(1):65–72. doi:10.1016/j.ijrobp.2005.11.037

Pickett B, Ten Haken RK, Kurhanewicz J, Qayyum A, Shinohara K, Fein B, Roach M 3rd (2004) Time to metabolic atrophy after permanent prostate seed implantation based on magnetic resonance spectroscopic imaging. Int J Radiat Oncol Biol Phys 59 (3):665–673. doi:10.1016/j.ijrobp.2003.11.024

Pickles T, Keyes M, Morris WJ (2010) Brachytherapy or conformal external radiotherapy for prostate cancer: a single-institution matched-pair analysis. Int J Radiat Oncol Biol Phys 76(1):43–49. doi:S0360-3016(09)00421-0 [pii] 10.1016/j.ijrobp.2009.01.081

Pinkawa M, Holy R, Piroth MD, Klotz J, Pfister D, Heidenreich A, Eble MJ (2012) Urinary morbidity after permanent prostate brachytherapy—impact of dose to the urethra vs. sources placed in close vicinity to the urethra. Radiother Oncol 103(2):247–251. doi:10.1016/j.radonc.2011.12.011

Potters L, Roach M, 3rd, Davis BJ, Stock RG, Ciezki JP, Zelefsky MJ, Stone NN, Fearn PA, Yu C, Shinohara K, Kattan MW (2010) Postoperative nomogram predicting the 9-year probability of prostate cancer recurrence after permanent prostate brachytherapy using radiation dose as a prognostic variable. Int J Radiat Oncol Biol Phys 76(4):1061–1065. doi:S0360-3016(09)00469-6 [pii] 10.1016/j.ijrobp.2009.03.031

Quon H, Loblaw A, Nam R (2011) Dramatic increase in prostate cancer cases by 2021. BJU Int 108(11):1734–1738. doi:10.1111/j.1464-410X.2011.10197.x

Reed DR, Wallner KE, Merrick GS, Arthurs S, Mueller A, Cavanagh W, Butler WB, Ford E, Sutlief SG (2007) A prospective randomized comparison of stranded vs. loose 125I seeds for prostate brachytherapy. Brachytherapy 6(2):129–134. doi:S1538-4721(07)00006-2 [pii] 10.1016/j.brachy.2007.01.003

Reese AC, Sadetsky N, Carroll PR, Cooperberg MR (2011) Inaccuracies in assignment of clinical stage for localized prostate cancer. Cancer 117(2):283–289. doi:10.1002/cncr.25596

Roach M (2012) Editorial Comment: Long-Term Potency Preservation Following Brachytherapy For Prostate Cancer. BJU Int (in press)

Roach M 3rd, Hanks G, Thames H Jr, Schellhammer P, Shipley WU, Sokol GH, Sandler H (2006) Defining biochemical failure following radiotherapy with or without hormonal therapy in men with clinically localized prostate cancer: recommendations of the RTOG-ASTRO Phoenix Consensus Conference. Int J Radiat Oncol Biol Phys 65(4):965–974. doi:10.1016/j.ijrobp.2006.04.029

Roberts G, Al-Qaisieh B, Bownes P (2012) Evaluation of the visibility of a new thinner (125)I radioactive source for permanent prostate brachytherapy. Brachytherapy 11(6):460–467. doi:10.1016/j.brachy.2012.01.009

Rodrigues G, Warde P, Pickles T, Crook J, Brundage M, Souhami L, Lukka H (2012) Pre-treatment risk stratification of prostate cancer patients: A critical review. Can Urol Assoc J, Journal de l'Association des urologues du Canada 6(2):121–127. doi:10.5489/cuaj.11085

Roeloffzen EM, Crook J, Monninkhof EM, McLean M, van Vulpen M, Saibishkumar EP (2012) External validation of the pretreatment nomogram to predict acute urinary retention after (125)I prostate brachytherapy. Brachytherapy 11(4):256–264. doi:10.1016/j.brachy.2011.12.011

Roeloffzen EM, van Vulpen M, Battermann JJ, van Roermund JG, Saibishkumar EP, Monninkhof EM (2011) Pretreatment nomogram to predict the risk of acute urinary retention after I-125 prostate brachytherapy. Int J Radiat Oncol Biol Phys 81(3):737–744. doi:10.1016/j.ijrobp.2010.06.009

Rosenthal SA, Bittner NH, Beyer DC, Demanes DJ, Goldsmith BJ, Horwitz EM, Ibbott GS, Lee WR, Nag S, Suh WW, Potters L (2011) American Society for Radiation Oncology (ASTRO) and American College of Radiology (ACR) practice guideline for the transperineal permanent brachytherapy of prostate cancer. Int J Radiat Oncol Biol Phys 79(2):335–341. doi:10.1016/j.ijrobp.2010.08.045

RTOG (2011) RTOG 0232: A phase III study comparing combined external beam radiation and transperineal interstitial permanent Brachytherapy with Brachytherapy alone for selected patients with intermediate risk prostatic Carcinoma

Ryu B, Bax J, Edirisinge C, Lewis C, Chen J, D'Souza D, Fenster A, Wong E (2012) Prostate brachytherapy with oblique needles to treat large glands and overcome pubic arch interference. Int J Radiat Oncol Biol Phys 83(5):1463–1472. doi:10.1016/j.ijrobp.2011.10.012

Saibishkumar EP, Borg J, Yeung I, Cummins-Holder C, Landon A, Crook J (2009) Sequential comparison of seed loss and prostate dosimetry of stranded seeds with loose seeds in 125I permanent implant for low-risk prostate cancer. Int J Radiat Oncol Biol Phys 73(1):61–68. doi:10.1016/j.ijrobp.2008.04.009

Salembier C, Lavagnini P, Nickers P, Mangili P, Rijnders A, Polo A, Venselaar J, Hoskin P (2007) Tumour and target volumes in permanent prostate brachytherapy: a supplement to the ESTRO/EAU/EORTC recommendations on prostate brachytherapy. Radiother Oncol 83(1):3–10. doi:10.1016/j.radonc.2007.01.014

Schmedders M, Janatzek S, Zimmer B (2011) Benefit assessment by the Federal Joint Committee: assessment of treatment strategies for low risk prostate cancer. Der Urologe Ausg A 50(8):938–943. doi:10.1007/s00120-011-2545-3

Shapiro EY, Rais-Bahrami S, Morgenstern C, Napolitano B, Richstone L, Potters L (2009) Long-term outcomes in younger men following permanent prostate brachytherapy. J Urol 181(4):1665–1671 (discussion 1671). doi:10.1016/j.juro.2008.11.122

Shen X, Keith SW, Mishra MV, Dicker AP, Showalter TN (2012) The impact of brachytherapy on prostate cancer-specific mortality for definitive radiation therapy of high-grade prostate cancer: a population-based analysis. Int J Radiat Oncol Biol Phys 83(4):1154–1159. doi:10.1016/j.ijrobp.2011.09.055

Shilkrut M, Merrick GS, McLaughlin PW, Stenmark MH, Abu-Isa E, Vance SM, Sandler HM, Feng FY, Hamstra DA (2012) The addition of low-dose-rate brachytherapy and androgen-deprivation therapy decreases biochemical failure and prostate cancer death compared with dose-escalated external-beam radiation therapy for high-risk prostate cancer. Cancer. doi:10.1002/cncr.27784

Shirvani SM, Kudchadker RJ, Bruno TL, Likhacheva A, Swanson DA, Frank SJ (2011) Impact of urinary catheterization on dosimetry after prostate implant brachytherapy with palladium-103 or iodine-125. Brachytherapy 10(4):269–274. doi:10.1016/j.brachy.2010.12.001

Sidana A, Hernandez DJ, Feng Z, Partin AW, Trock BJ, Saha S, Epstein JI (2012) Treatment decision-making for localized prostate cancer: what younger men choose and why. The Prostate 72(1):58–64. doi:10.1002/pros.21406

Sidhu S, Morris WJ, Spadinger I, Keyes M, Hilts M, Harrison R, Otto K, McKenzie M, Agranovich A (2002) Prostate brachytherapy postimplant dosimetry: a comparison of prostate quadrants. Int J Radiat Oncol Biol Phys 52(2):544–552

Smith RP, Flickinger JC, Kehwar TS, Benoit RM, Beriwal S (2012) Prediction of true dosimetric parameters over the life of the implant in prostate Brachytherapy. Int J Radiat Oncol Biol Phys 84(3, Supplement):S394–S395. doi:10.1016/j.ijrobp.2012.07.1041

Snyder KM, Stock RG, Buckstein M, Stone NN (2012) Long-term potency preservation following brachytherapy for prostate cancer. BJU Int 110(2):221–225. doi:10.1111/j.1464-410X.2011.10800.x

Stember DS, Mulhall JP (2012) The concept of erectile function preservation (penile rehabilitation) in the patient after brachytherapy for prostate cancer. Brachytherapy 11(2):87–96. doi:10.1016/j.brachy.2012.01.002

Stephenson AJ, Kattan MW (2006) Nomograms for prostate cancer. BJU Int 98(1):39–46. doi:10.1111/j.1464-410X.2006.06173.x

Stock R, Stone N, Tabert A, Iannuzzi C, DeWyngaert JK (1998) A dose-response study for I-125 prostate implants. Int J Radiat Oncol Biol Phys 41(1):101–108

Stock RG (2004) Salvage brachytherapy after external-beam irradiation for prostate cancer: Review 2. Oncology (Williston Park) 18(2):151–158 (discussion 158–160, 163–154)

Stock RG, Berkowitz J, Blacksburg SR, Stone NN (2012a) Gleason 7 prostate cancer treated with low-dose-rate brachytherapy: lack of impact of primary Gleason pattern on biochemical failure. BJU Int. doi:10.1111/j.1464-410X.2012.11057.x

Stock RG, Liu JT, Blacksburg SR, Stone NN (2012b) The Relative Effects of Biologically Effective Dose (BED) Versus Adjuvant Androgen Suppression (AS) on Biochemical Control and Post-treatment Biopsy Results Following the Brachytherapy Management of Prostate Cancer. Int J Radiat Oncol Biol Phys 84(3, Supplement):S384–S385. doi:10.1016/j.ijrobp.2012.07.1013

Stock RG, Stone NN, Cesaretti JA (2003) Prostate-specific antigen bounce after prostate seed implantation for localized prostate cancer: descriptions and implications. Int J Radiat Oncol Biol Phys 56(2):448–453

Stock RG, Stone NN, Cesaretti JA, Rosenstein BS (2006) Biologically effective dose values for prostate brachytherapy: effects on PSA failure and posttreatment biopsy results. Int J Radiat Oncol Biol Phys 64 (2):527-533. doi:S0360-3016(05)02372-2 [pii] 10.1016/j.ijrobp.2005.07.981

Stone NN, Marshall DT, Stone JJ, Cesaretti JA, Stock RG (2010a) Does neoadjuvant hormonal therapy improve urinary function when given to men with large prostates undergoing prostate brachytherapy? J Urol 183 (2):634-639. doi:S0022-5347(09)02625-1 [pii] 10.1016/j.juro.2009.09.084

Stone NN, Skouteris VM, Stock RG (2012) Biopsy and implantation of the seminal vesicles. Brachytherapy 11(5):334–340. doi:10.1016/j.brachy.2011.12.008

Stone NN, Stock RG (2005) Reduction of pulmonary migration of permanent interstitial sources in patients undergoing prostate brachytherapy. Urology 66 (1):119-123. doi:S0090-4295(05)00146-9 [pii] 10.1016/j.urology.2005.01.047

Stone NN, Stock RG (2014a) 15-Year Cause Specific and All-Cause Survival Following Brachytherapy for Prostate Cancer: Negative Impact of Long-term Hormonal Therapy. J Urol. doi:10.1016/j.juro.2014.03.094

Stone NN, Stock RG (2014b) Does dose matter? Editorial comments to Morris et al. Whole prostate D90 and V100: a dose-response analysis of 2000 consecutive (125)I monotherapy cases. Brachytherapy 13 (1):42-43. doi:10.1016/j.brachy.2013.11.009

Stone NN, Stock RG, Cesaretti JA, Unger P (2010b) Local control following permanent prostate brachytherapy: effect of high biologically effective dose on biopsy results and oncologic outcomes. Int J Radiat Oncol Biol Phys 76 (2):355-360. doi:S0360-3016(09)00339-3 [pii] 10.1016/j.ijrobp.2009.01.078

Stone NN, Stone MM, Rosenstein BS, Unger P, Stock RG (2011) Influence of pretreatment and treatment factors on intermediate to long-term outcome after prostate brachytherapy. J Urol 185 (2):495–500. doi:10.1016/j.juro.2010.09.099

Sugawara A, Nakashima J, Kunieda E, Nagata H, Mizuno R, Seki S, Shiraishi Y, Kouta R, Oya M, Shigematsu N (2011) Incidence of seed migration to the chest, abdomen, and pelvis after transperineal interstitial prostate brachytherapy with loose (125)I seeds. Radiat Oncol 6:130. doi:10.1186/1748-717X-6-130

Sugawara A, Nakashima J, Shigematsu N, Kunieda E, Kubo A (2009) Prediction of seed migration after transperineal interstitial prostate brachytherapy with I-125 free seeds. Brachytherapy 8(1):52–56. doi:10.1016/j.brachy.2008.10.003

Sylvester JE, Blasko JC, Grimm PD, Meier R, Malmgren JA (2003) Ten-year biochemical relapse-free survival after external beam radiation and brachytherapy for localized prostate cancer: the Seattle experience. Int J Radiat Oncol Biol Phys 57(4):944–952

Sylvester JE, Grimm PD, Blasko JC, Millar J, Orio PF, 3rd, Skoglund S, Galbreath RW, Merrick G (2007) 15-Year biochemical relapse free survival in clinical Stage T1-T3 prostate cancer following combined external beam radiotherapy and brachytherapy; Seattle experience. Int J Radiat Oncol Biol Phys 67 (1):57-64. doi:S0360-3016(06)02774-X [pii] 10.1016/j.ijrobp.2006.07.1382

Sylvester JE, Grimm PD, Wong J, Galbreath RW, Merrick G, Blasko JC (2011) Fifteen-year biochemical relapse-free survival, cause-specific survival, and overall survival following i(125) prostate brachytherapy in clinically localized prostate cancer: Seattle experience. Int J Radiat Oncol Biol Phys 81(2):376–381. doi:10.1016/j.ijrobp.2010.05.042

Taira AV, Merrick GS, Butler WM, Galbreath RW, Lief J, Adamovich E, Wallner KE (2011) Long-term outcome for clinically localized prostate cancer treated with permanent interstitial brachytherapy. Int J Radiat Oncol Biol Phys 79(5):1336–1342. doi:10.1016/j.ijrobp.2010.01.005

Taira AV, Merrick GS, Galbreath RW, Butler WM, Adamovich E, Wallner KE (2012) Prognostic importance of small prostate size in men receiving definitive prostate brachytherapy. Int J Radiat Oncol Biol Phys 84(2):396–401. doi:10.1016/j.ijrobp.2011.11.068

Tanaka N, Asakawa I, Anai S, Hirayama A, Hasegawa M, Konishi N, Fujimoto K (2013) Periodical assessment of genitourinary and gastrointestinal toxicity in patients who underwent prostate low-dose-rate brachytherapy. Radiat Oncol 8(1):25. doi:10.1186/1748-717X-8-25

Tanaka N, Asakawa I, Fujimoto K, Anai S, Hirayama A, Hasegawa M, Konishi N, Hirao Y (2012) Minimal percentage of dose received by 90% of the urethra (%UD90) is the most significant predictor of PSA bounce in patients who underwent low-dose-rate brachytherapy (LDR-brachytherapy) for prostate cancer. BMC urology 12:28. doi:10.1186/1471-2490-12-28

Tanaka N, Fujimoto K, Hirao Y, Asakawa I, Hasegawa M, Konishi N (2009) Variations in international prostate symptom scores, uroflowmetric parameters, and prostate volume after (125)I permanent brachytherapy for localized prostate cancer. Urology 74(2):407–411. doi:10.1016/j.urology.2008.12.062

Taussky D, Moumdjian C, Larouche R, Beliveau-Nadeau D, Boudreau C, Hervieux Y, Donath D (2012) Seed migration in prostate brachytherapy depends on experience and technique. Brachytherapy 11(6):452–456. doi:10.1016/j.brachy.2012.03.003

Terk MD, Stock RG, Stone NN (1998) Identification of patients at increased risk for prolonged urinary retention following radioactive seed implantation of the prostate. J Urol 160 (4):1379-1382. doi:S0022-5347(01)62542-4 [pii]

Thomas CW, Kruk A, McGahan CE, Spadinger I, Morris WJ (2007) Prostate brachytherapy post-implant dosimetry: a comparison between higher and lower source density. Radiother Oncol 83 (1):18–24. doi:10.1016/j.radonc.2007.02.004

Thompson A, Keyes M, Pickles T, Palma D, Moravan V, Spadinger I, Lapointe V, Morris WJ (2010) Evaluating the Phoenix definition of biochemical failure after (125)I prostate brachytherapy: Can PSA kinetics distinguish PSA failures from PSA bounces? Int J Radiat Oncol Biol Phys 78(2):415–421. doi:10.1016/j.ijrobp.2009.07.1724

Thompson I, Thrasher JB, Aus G, Burnett AL, Canby-Hagino ED, Cookson MS, D'Amico AV, Dmochowski RR, Eton DT, Forman JD, Goldenberg SL, Hernandez J, Higano CS, Kraus SR, Moul JW, Tangen CM (2007) Guideline for the management of clinically localized prostate cancer: 2007 update. J Urol 177(6):2106–2131. doi:10.1016/j.juro.2007.03.003

Toledano A, Chauveinc L, Flam T, Thiounn N, Solignac S, Timbert M, Rosenwald JC, Cosset JM (2006) PSA bounce after permanent implant prostate brachytherapy may mimic a biochemical failure: a study of 295 patients with a minimum 3-year followup. Brachytherapy 5(2):122–126. doi:10.1016/j.brachy.2006.02.003

Turley RS, Hamilton RJ, Terris MK, Kane CJ, Aronson WJ, Presti JC, Jr., Amling CL, Freedland SJ, Group SDS (2008a) Small transrectal ultrasound volume predicts clinically significant Gleason score upgrading after radical prostatectomy: results from the SEARCH database. J Urol 179 (2):523-527; discussion 527-528. doi:10.1016/j.juro.2007.09.078

Turley RS, Terris MK, Kane CJ, Aronson WJ, Presti JC, Jr., Amling CL, Freedland SJ, Group SDS (2008b) The association between prostate size and Gleason score upgrading depends on the number of biopsy cores obtained: results from the Shared Equal Access Regional Cancer Hospital Database. BJU Int 102(9):1074–1079. doi:10.1111/j.1464-410X.2008.08015.x

Uesugi T, Saika T, Edamura K, Nose H, Kobuke M, Ebara S, Abarzua F, Katayama N, Yanai H, Nasu Y, Kumon H (2012) Primary Gleason grade 4 impact on biochemical recurrence after permanent interstitial brachytherapy in Japanese patients with low- or intermediate-risk prostate cancer. Int J Radiat Oncol Biol Phys 82 (2):e219–223. doi:10.1016/j.ijrobp.2011.04.018

Wagner W, Bolling T, Hambruegge C, Hartlapp J, Krukemeyer MG (2011) Patients' satisfaction with different modalities of prostate cancer therapy–a retrospective survey among 634 patients. Anticancer Res 31(11):3903–3908

Wagner W, Willich N, Radmard A, Christ A, Fleig PW, Krukemeyer MG (2010) Seed migration to the vertebral venous plexus after prostate brachytherapy. Der Urologe Ausg A 49(11):1390–1392. doi:10.1007/s00120-010-2382-9

Waterman FM, Dicker AP (2003) Probability of late rectal morbidity in 125I prostate brachytherapy. Int J Radiat Oncol Biol Phys 55 (2):342–353

Whaley JT, Levy LB, Swanson DA, Pugh TJ, Kudchadker RJ, Bruno TL, Frank SJ (2012) Sexual function and the use of medical devices or drugs to optimize potency after prostate brachytherapy. Int J Radiat Oncol Biol Phys 82(5):e765–771. doi:10.1016/j.ijrobp.2011.11.004

Williams SG, Duchesne GM, Gogna NK, Millar JL, Pickles T, Pratt GR, Turner S (2006) An international multicenter study evaluating the impact of an alternative biochemical failure definition on the judgment of prostate cancer risk. Int J Radiat Oncol Biol Phys 65 (2):351–357. doi:10.1016/j.ijrobp.2005.12.007

Wong JC, Sylvester J (2012) First Report on Seed Migration to the Lung With the Use of a Thinner I125 Radioactive Seed Within 20 Gauge Needles for Permanent Seed Prostate Brachytherapy. Int J Radiat Oncol Biol Phys 84 (3, Supplement):S380. doi:10.1016/j.ijrobp.2012.07.1002

Zelefsky MJ, Chou JF, Pei X, Yamada Y, Kollmeier M, Cox B, Zhang Z, Schechter M, Cohen GN, Zaider M (2012) Predicting biochemical tumor control after brachytherapy for clinically localized prostate cancer: The Memorial Sloan-Kettering Cancer Center experience. Brachytherapy 11(4):245–249. doi:10.1016/j.brachy.2011.08.003

Zelefsky MJ, Cohen GN, Bosch WR, Morikawa L, Khalid N, Crozier CL, Lee WR, Zietman A, Owen J, Wilson JF, Devlin PM (2013) Results from the Quality Research in Radiation Oncology (QRRO) survey: Evaluation of dosimetric outcomes for low-dose-rate prostate brachytherapy. Brachytherapy 12(1):19–24. doi:10.1016/j.brachy.2012.04.001

Zelefsky MJ, Leibel SA, Gaudin PB, Kutcher GJ, Fleshner NE, Venkatramen ES, Reuter VE, Fair WR, Ling CC, Fuks Z (1998) Dose escalation with three-dimensional conformal radiation therapy affects the outcome in prostate cancer. Int J Radiat Oncol Biol Phys 41(3):491–500

Zelefsky MJ, Nedelka MA, Arican ZL, Yamada Y, Cohen GN, Shippy AM, Park JJ, Zaider M (2008) Combined brachytherapy with external beam radiotherapy for localized prostate cancer: reduced morbidity with an intraoperative brachytherapy planning technique and supplemental intensity-modulated radiation therapy. Brachytherapy 7(1):1–6. doi:10.1016/j.brachy.2007.12.002

Zhu AX, Wallner KE, Frivold GP, Ferry D, Jutzy KR, Foster GP (2006) Prostate brachytherapy seed migration to the right coronary artery associated with an acute myocardial infarction. Brachytherapy 5(4):262–265. doi:10.1016/j.brachy.2006.08.004

High-Dose-Rate Brachytherapy in the Treatment of Clinically Localized Prostate Cancer

Nikolaos Tselis and Nikolaos Zamboglou

Contents

Abstract

Recent radiobiological findings support that the α/β-ratio for prostate adenocarcinoma is less than that for the normal organs that ordinarily constrain the delivery of radiation therapy. As a result, hypofractionation has attracted greatly renewed interest and during the last 15 years a special interest in the implementation of brachytherapy (BRT) has evolved for the treatment of localized prostate cancer. Especially high-dose-rate (HDR) BRT is recently gaining momentum as an alternative to low-dose-rate and technological improvements in image guidance and real-time treatment planning place this interventional radiooncological modality at the forefront of innovation in radiotherapy. This chapter will explore the rationale for HDR BRT as a highly conformal method of dose delivery and safe biologic dose escalation through hypofractionation. Oncological outcome data and toxicity profiles will be discussed for the combination with external beam radiotherapy and in the monotherapy setting. In addition to clinical results of primary and salvage treatment protocols, dose-fractionation schedules and normal tissue dose constraints used by various centres are also reported.

1 Introduction

In patients with clinically localized prostate cancer, permanent low-dose-rate (LDR) brachytherapy (BRT) (Potters et al. 2005; Zelefsky et al. 2007; Battermann et al. 2004), external beam radiotherapy (EBRT) (Kupelian and Meyer 2011; Kuban et al. 2008; Dearnaley et al. 2007; Zelefsky et al. 2008) and interstitial (IRT) high-dose-rate (HDR) BRT alone (Zamboglou et al. 2012; Demanes et al. 2011; Hoskin et al. 2012) or in combination with EBRT (Galalae et al. 2004; Pistis et al. 2010; Kotecha et al. 2013; Prada et al. 2012; Deutsch et al. 2010; Martinez et al. 2002; Demanes et al. 2005) are commonly used treatment options.

N. Tselis (✉) · N. Zamboglou
Sana Klinikum Offenbach Strahlenklinik, 63069 Offenbach, Germany
e-mail: ntselis@hotmail.com

H. Geinitz et al. (eds.), *Radiotherapy in Prostate Cancer*, Medical Radiology. Radiation Oncology,
DOI: 10.1007/174_2014_1020,

Published Online: 10 June 2014

These modalities have shown biochemical control (BC) rates comparable to those of patients treated with radical prostatectomy D'Amico et al. (1998, 2002). In the absence of randomized clinical trials of sufficient size, however, the optimal therapeutic strategy for organ-confined prostate cancer remains controversial and treatment assignment appears influenced by physician bias and patient preference (Harlan et al. 2001). Notwithstanding, during the last 15 years a special interest in the implementation of BRT has evolved and a large body of literature corroborates the efficacy of both permanent LDR and temporary HDR BRT in the treatment of localized prostate cancer. Especially, HDR is recently gaining momentum as an alternative to LDR BRT and technological improvements in image guidance and real-time treatment planning place this interventional radiooncological modality at the forefront of innovation in radiotherapy (RT).

2 Background

2.1 Rationale for HDR Brachytherapy

A large body of literature corroborates that radiation dose escalation for organ-confined prostate cancer improves local (LC) and biochemical disease control (Kuban et al. 2008; Dearnaley et al. 2007; Zelefsky et al. 2008; Peeters et al. 2006; Kupelian et al. 2008). In addition, persistence of local disease has shown to be associated not only with a higher incidence of biochemical failure, but also increased rates of distant metastasis (Kupelian et al. 2008; Coen et al. 2002; Zelefsky et al. 2008). Recent research suggests that eradication of locally confined disease by dose-escalated radical RT results not only in improved metastasis-free survival (MFS), but also improved prostate cancer-specific mortality (Zelefsky et al. 2008, 2011; Kim et al. 2012; Nguyen et al. 2013; Pahlajani et al. 2012). In this context, emerging radiobiological data indicate that prostate adenocarcinoma has a low α/β-ratio, 1.2–3.0 Gy, suggesting that biological dose escalation can be achieved by hypofractionated treatment schemes (Brenner et al. 2002; Nath et al. 2009; Fowler et al. 2001; Brenner and Hall 1999; Ritter et al. 2009). High-dose-rate BRT optimally exploits the radiobiological advantage of large fraction sizes while ensuring superior conformality. It enables the anatomy-based optimization of the spatial dose distribution by accurately controlling radiation source positions and modulating source dwell times (Mavroidis et al. 2010; Karabis et al. 2005). This permits an active partitioning of radiation between the prostate and healthy organs without unacceptable dosimetric changes caused by source migration and tissue deformity as can be the case with LDR implants (Kono et al. 2010; Knaup et al. 2012; Franca et al. 2009) or due to significant intrafraction motion occurring frequently during treatment delivery times encountered in intensity-modulated external beam radiotherapy (IMRT) (Shah et al. 2011; Algan et al. 2012; Mutanga et al. 2012). Temporary HDR BRT is not limited by positioning uncertainties as the target is immobilized by the implanted catheters and treated within very short treatment times. Since there is no permanent implant with HDR, no long-term radiation protection issues exist as in the case of LDR BRT. In addition, the precise dosimetry allows the technique to be used in combination with EBRT. This is of particular relevance when it may be necessary to extend the treatment volume to include areas of extraprostatic extension or pelvic lymphadenopathy to a moderate dose whilst administering a high-dose boost to the prostate. Surgical and RT series have led to the identification of several clinical pathologic factors associated with extraprostatic extension, presence of regional lymphadenopathy, or development of metastatic disease (D'Amico et al. 2002; Sung et al. 2007; Davis et al. 1999; Han et al. 2001, 2003; Zelefsky et al. 2007; Hanks et al. 2001; Briganti et al. 2009). These include serum prostate-specific antigen (PSA), Gleason score (GS), and clinical tumor (T) stage, allowing the classification of patients into risk group categories of low-, intermediate- and high-risk according to stratification schemes as described by D'Amico et al. (1998), Zelefsky et al. (1998), or the National Comprehensive Cancer Network (Mohler et al. 2010). Consequently, patients are aimed to be treated according to their risk of local recurrence or progression after radical treatment. Although no direct prospective comparison with EBRT or BRT has been made, surgical series have demonstrated that following radical prostatectomy, a considerable proportion of patients will relapse, particularly where surgical margin positivity or extraprostatic disease extension are present (Aydin et al. 2004; Chuang et al. 2007). This therapeutic crux from a surgical point of view is reflected in a unique comparative study by Grimm et al. looking at all modern treatment outcomes based on the different risk group stratifications in more than 52,000 patients with localized prostate cancer (Grimm et al. 2012). According to the findings, BRT alone or in combination with EBRT, depending on the risk stratification category, appear superior to surgery alone or definitive EBRT in terms of long-term BC. The comparatively high clinical efficacy is causally explicable by the higher dose that can be prescribed when IRT BRT is used for treatment and by virtue of a higher dose within the implant. Therefore, it is reasonable to assume that further improvements in the therapeutic ratio of prostate RT can be generated by escalating the treatment dose using image-guided hypofractionated HDR BRT.

2.2 Radiobiological Considerations

Radiobiological research demonstrates that the probabilities of acute and late radiation reactions vary between normal tissues and tumors and between different RT dose-fractionation schedules. The α/β-ratio, a means of expressing the sensitivity of a particular tissue to altered fraction size, is used to estimate the impact of a given schedule on tumor control and toxicity while enabling comparisons between different treatment schedules. Tissues and tumors with a low α/β-ratio have a higher sensitivity to changes in fraction size than those with a high α/β-ratio. The attractiveness of HDR BRT over LDR BRT and conventional EBRT is explained particularly by the fact that radiobiological evidence supports a low α/β-ratio, 1.2–3.0 Gy, for prostate adenocarcinoma, which is lower than the α/β-ratio of acutely and late reacting normal tissues (Brenner et al. 2002; Nath et al. 2009; Fowler et al. 2001; Brenner and Hall 1999; Tucker et al. 2011; Brenner 2004; Miralbell et al. 2012). For prostate cancer, this implies that a hypofractionated dose regimen is favored for optimal tumor control with a reduction in late sequelae. Image-guided hypofractionated HDR BRT with anatomy-based dose optimization is an excellent method for conformal dose escalation in terms of both radiation biology and physics (Lee 2009). In order to compare HDR regimes with EBRT treatment schemes, the linear-quadratic formula as described by Fowler at al. (2001) is usually used:

$$\mathrm{BED} = \mathrm{nd}\left(1 + \frac{d}{(\alpha/\beta)}\right)$$

where *BED* is the biologically effective dose as a measure of the true biological dose delivered by a particular RT regime, *n* the number of treatment fractions and *d* the dose per fraction. To understand by intuition, the comparison of schedules consisting of different total doses or doses per fraction is also possible by converting each RT schedule into an equivalent schedule in 2Gy-fractions, which would give the same biological effect:

$$\mathrm{EQD}_2 = \mathrm{nd}\frac{\left(1 + \frac{d}{(\alpha/\beta)}\right)}{\left(1 + \frac{2}{(\alpha/\beta)}\right)}$$

where *D* is the total treatment dose and *d* the dose per fraction. Based on those formulae for calculating isoeffect relationships, when comparing HDR BRT with definitive conventional EBRT (including dose-escalated IMRT), the clinically delivered doses with HDR BRT regimens are up to 50 % higher compared to conventional EBRT schemes (Hoskin et al. 2012; Kotecha et al. 2013; Fatyga et al. 2009; Masson et al. 2012; Bolla and Poppel 2012; Hoskin 2008; Martinez et al. 2011; Yoshioka et al. 2013a, b; Zaorsky et al. 2013).

2.3 Patient Selection for HDR Brachytherapy

Based on the assumption that failure to eradicate organ-confined prostate cancer may lead to the development of metastatic disease, patients without advanced disease may benefit most from dose-escalated RT in terms of improved LC, BC, and MFS (Zelefsky et al. 2008a, b, 2011; Kupelian et al. 2008; Coen et al. 2002; Kim et al. 2012; Nguyen et al. 2013; Pahlajani et al. 2012). Accordingly, the main indication for HDR treatment is histologically proven localized prostate cancer in patients considered otherwise suitable for radical treatment (Yamada et al. 2012; Hoskin et al. 2013). Mature results exist for the application of HDR BRT as a boost modality in combination with EBRT for intermediate- and high-risk disease. In addition, evolving clinical evidence implicates its effective use as monotherapy with encouraging results reported for mainly low—and intermediate—but also selected cases of high-risk disease. However, monotherapy with curative intent for high-risk disease should still be considered investigational and more mature data are needed to confirm its role. In the clinical setting of regional lymphadenopathy with or without distant disease spread, HDR BRT may be implemented combined with EBRT in individualized treatment schemes in order to avoid increased toxicity where conventional conformal EBRT is employed with the goal of LC.

Pre-treatment investigations for HDR BRT should be no different from those for other forms of radical treatment and should follow the EAU guidelines (Hoskin et al. 2013; Heidenreich et al. 2011). All patients considered for IRT irradiation should have histological confirmation of malignancy. Staging tests for evaluation of prostatic disease burden and of any extraprostatic extension should include digital rectal examination, transrectal ultrasound (TRUS) and, if indicated, computed tomography (CT) and/or magnetic resonance imaging (MRI) and bone scintigraphy. In equivocal cases of regional lymphadenopathy, laparoscopic pelvic lymphadenectomy (Touijer et al. 2011) or choline positron emission tomography (Evangelista et al. 2013) may be considered. Even though functional outcome is predicted by the baseline urinary function (Eid et al. 2013), neither larger gland size nor previous transurethral resection of the prostate (TURP) are absolute contraindications for treatment. Transperineal implantation in lithotomy position enables the complete and safe coverage of prostate volumes appreciably greater than 60 ccm provided a sufficiently broad pelvic inlet and freedom from lower urinary tract symptoms (LUTS) requiring treatment (Yamada et al. 2012; Le et al. 2013; White et al. 2013; Monroe et al. 2008; Rogers et al. 2012). In addition, temporary IRT implantation with HDR irradiation is safely feasible at >3 months after TURP given freedom from persistent LUTS and provided a sufficient amount of

Table 1 Patient selection criteria for image-guided high-dose-rate brachytherapy in the treatment of clinically localized or locally-advanced prostate cancer

Inclusion criteria
Stages T1–T3b[a]
Any GS
Any PSA level
Exclusion criteria
TURP within 3 months
Urinary flow rate <10 ml/s
IPSS > 20
Pubic arch interference[b]
Lithotomy position not possible[c]
Anesthesia not possible
Rectal fistula

[a] T4 included with curative intent in the protocols of selected centers (Kotecha et al. 2013; Yoshioka et al. 2011, 2013; Sakamoto et al. 2011)

[b, c] relevant for TRUS-guided techniques, not relevant for MRI-guided implantation (Ménard et al. 2004; Lakosi et al. 2011)

PSA prostate-specific antigen, *TURP* transurethral resection of the prostate, *IPSS* international prostate symptom score, *TRUS* transrectal ultrasound, *MRI* magnetic resonance imaging, *GS* Gleason score

residual gland volume for image-based three-dimensional (3D) treatment planning including precise organs at risk identification (Luo et al. 2009, 2013; Peddada et al. 2007; Ishiyama et al. 2012). However, limited resection-TURP may also be part of an interdisciplinary patient management prior to planned HDR BRT when a prominent median lobe is encountered during staging. Selection criteria for HDR BRT combined with EBRT or as monotherapy are shown in Table 1. Unlike for permanent LDR implants, in temporary HDR BRT the IRT catheters can be placed next to extracapsular lesions or the seminal vesicles also into the bladder pouch, if necessary. Therefore, the indication for HDR BRT is by various groups extended to even T4 tumors (Kotecha et al. 2013; Yoshioka et al. 2011, 2013; Sakamoto et al. 2011). Nevertheless, in cases of previous pelvic EBRT or surgery resulting in anatomical changes of the organs of the small pelvis, a very careful evaluation of the potential risks and benefits should be performed.

3 Brachytherapy Techniques

Interstitial catheter insertion is usually performed under spinal or general anesthesia with various catheter placement patterns being described. Extensive experience exists for the technique of real-time TRUS-guided implantation (Zamboglou et al. 2012; Demanes et al. 2009, 2011; Hoskin et al. 2012; Martinez et al. 2002; Lee 2009; Corner et al. 2008; Ghilezan et al. 2011), however, MRI-based techniques have also been implemented in clinical practice (Ménard et al. 2004; Lakosi et al. 2011).

In general, implant dosimetry is based on 3D image data sets for definition and delineation of the target volume (prostate gland = planning target volume, PTV) and the organs at risk (OAR's, i.e., intraprostatic urethra, anterior rectal wall, and urinary bladder). The clinical workflow includes the creation of virtual volumes prior to implantation for inverse treatment pre-planning and volume studies after catheter insertion for treatment planning prior to irradiation (Mavroidis et al. 2010; Karabis et al. 2005). Treatment planning after TRUS-guided implantation is most commonly performed using either CT- (Martinez et al. 2002; Demanes et al. 2005; Galalae et al. 2002; Hoskin et al. 2007) or TRUS-imaging (Zamboglou et al. 2012; Demanes et al. 2011; Hoskin et al. 2012; Ghilezan et al. 2011). For CT-based planning, the image data set should be contiguous with no more than 3 mm slice thickness in the axial plane. Imaging should extend the prostate in the craniocaudal extension and should include sufficient normal anatomy for meaningful normal tissue dosimetry (Yamada et al. 2012). When more than one implantation is performed, it is not uncommon for the prostate to have varying volumes between the procedures. This has to be taken into account by planning each BRT fraction separately. In contrary to the totally TRUS-based clinical workflow with intraoperative real-time treatment planning, CT-based planning bears an additional risk for catheter re-arrangement and target volume changes due to transferring of the patient to a CT-scanner, which constitutes a deviation of the patient setup (Whitaker et al. 2011; Holly et al. 2011; Seppenwoolde et al. 2008). From this perspective, the totally TRUS-based technique illustrates the standard of care in prostate BRT ensuring improved 3D implant stability (Milickovic et al. 2011).

Representatively described, transperineal implantation is performed under TRUS-guidance using a continuous probe movement technique and a perineal template to aid catheter placement (Martin et al. 2004). For pre-planning, transversal ultrasound images of the prostate, urethra, and anterior rectal wall are acquired in real-time and 3D volumes are reconstructed based on 1.0 mm image distance. The PTV is defined as the entire prostate gland without margins. Contour definition for the rectum extends 10 mm cranially from the prostatic base and 10 mm caudally from the prostatic apex. Urethra contouring encounters the intraprostatic urethra marked by the insertion of a radiopaque three-way Foley catheter and extends by 5 mm caudally to include the apical membranous urethra. The urinary bladder is contoured based on the TRUS-based visible volume. Based on the acquired 3D anatomy, the appropriate virtual needle positions are generated, the needle source dwell positions located within the PTV are activated, and the radioactive source dwell

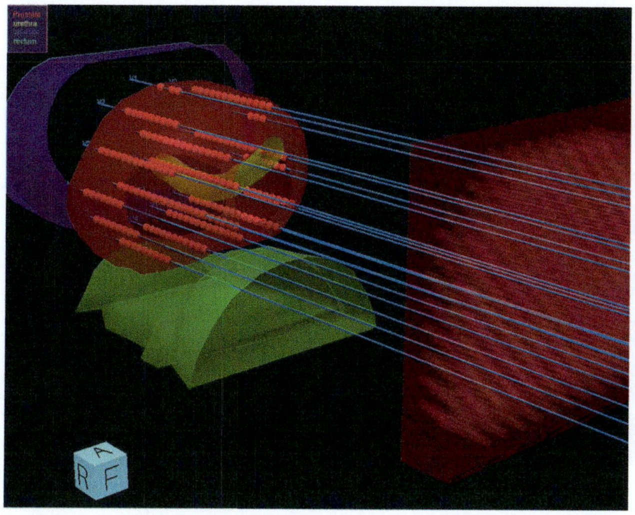

Fig. 1 Three-dimensional reconstruction of the prostate, urethra, rectum, and bladder with ideal template needle trajectories for TRUS-guided implantation as calculated for pre-planning by the real-time treatment planning system SWIFT/Oncentra Prostate (Nucletron B.V., Veenendaal, The Netherlands). The virtual perineal template is displayed on the *right side*

times are calculated using an intraoperative treatment planning system (Fig. 1). Dose volume histograms (DVH's) for the PTV and OAR's are calculated for evaluation of the anatomy-based dose optimisation. If the pre-planning dosimetry parameters fulfill the dosimetric protocol, TRUS-guided implantation of catheters is performed at the previously determined positions (Fig. 2). After completion of implantation, a final 3D TRUS data set is acquired for intraoperative real-time treatment planning. Planning target volume and OAR's contouring is checked and updated according to the new image set. Real needle positions are reconstructed and dwell positions located within the PTV are activated ensuring the 3D dose distribution fulfills the dosimetric protocol (Fig. 3). The prescribed dose is the intended minimum dose delivered to the PTV surface.

Given the extreme heterogeneity in clinically implemented dose-fractionation schedules, it is difficult to establish absolute dose guidelines for total physical prescription doses and normal tissue dose constraints. For comparison, Table 2 lists dose-fractionation schedules and normal tissue dose constraints used by various centers. For example, the William Beaumont Hospital monotherapy protocol consists of one IRT implant that delivers four fractions of 9.5 Gy in 2 days under spinal anesthesia with an interfractional interval of at least 6 h (Demanes et al. 2011). The current Offenbach Hospital monotherapy protocol consists of three implants each delivering one fraction of 11.5 Gy under spinal anesthesia with all implants separated by 21 days (Zamboglou et al. 2012). The Mount Vernon Cancer Center combined treatment protocol

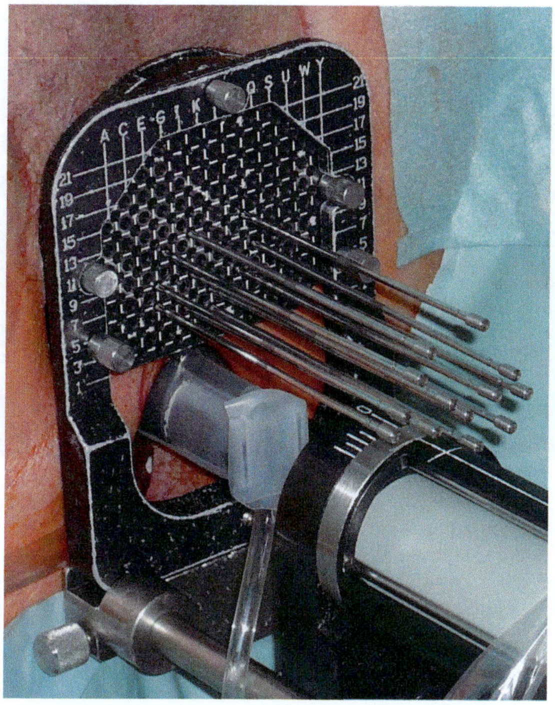

Fig. 2 High-resolution template with implanted interstitial steel needles (200 mm length, 1.9 mm diameter). The transducer probe for TRUS-guidance is attached to a floor-mounted stepping unit and inserted into the rectum. A thin intestinal tube for the discharge of intestinal gases is inserted laterally to the probe and is partly visible behind the *lower right angle* of the template

consists of 35.75 Gy EBRT delivered in 13 fractions followed within 6 days by an HDR boost. Interstitial implantation is performed under general anesthesia with one implant delivering a total dose of 17 Gy in two fractions within 24 h (Hoskin et al. 2007). At the Catalan Institute of Oncology, combined treatment is delivered with 60 Gy conventionally-fractionated EBRT followed within 21 days by a single-fraction HDR boost of 9 Gy under spinal anesthesia (Pistis et al. 2010).

In MRI-based techniques, catheter placement is performed transperineally and maximum insertion depth, direction, and positional control of the implanted catheters are estimated by interactive MR-scanning (Ménard et al. 2004; Lakosi et al. 2011). Number, geometrical alignment, and distance between the catheters depend on the size/shape of the prostate and the alignment of the intraprostatic urethra. Total physical prescription doses and dose restrictions for OAR's are in accordance with the protocols listed in Table 3. Irrespective of the imaging modality for interventional guidance or treatment planning, IRT HDR irradiation is performed using a remote afterloading system. Iridium 192 is the most commonly used isotope with an average energy of 380 keV, a half-life of 73.8 days and a half value layer of 2.5 mm of lead (Nag et al. 2003).

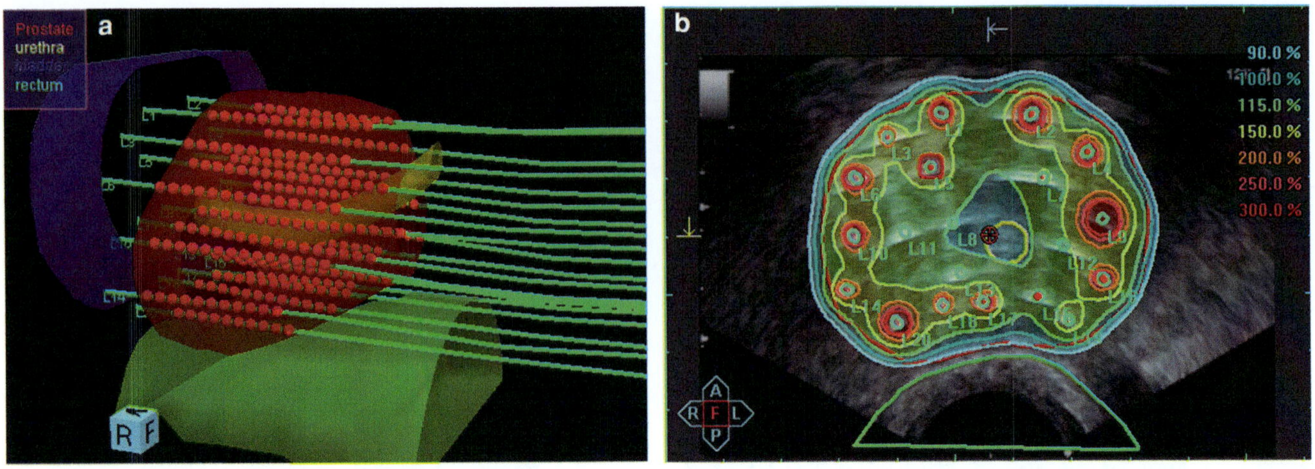

Fig. 3 Intraoperative real-time TRUS-based treatment planning. **a** Three-dimensional reconstruction of the prostate, organs at risk (i.e., rectum, urethra, bladder), in situ needles and the intraprostatic source dwell positions as calculated using the real-time treatment planning system SWIFT/Oncentra Prostate for the final treatment plan; **b** Isodose distribution after anatomy-based dose optimisation. The isodose color code convention is: *dark red* 300 % {isodose = 28.5 Gy}; *orange* 200 % {isodose = 19.0 Gy}; *yellow* 150 % {isodose = 14.25 Gy}; *turquoise* 100 % {isodose = 9.5 Gy}. The 100 % isodose was set to encompass the red delineated prostate capsule

Table 2 Total physical prescription doses and normal tissue dose constraints (as percent of prescribed high-dose-rate brachytherapy reference dose or absolute dose value) of various brachytherapy schemes

Treatment protocol	PTV	Rectum	Bladder	Urethra	D_{90} (%)	V_{100} (%)	V_{150} (%)
Demanes et al. (2011)[a]							
CET	7.0 Gy × 6 (42 Gy)	$D_{0.1\ ccm} \leq 80\ \%$	$D_{0.1\ ccm} \leq 80\ \%$	$D_{0.1\ ccm} \leq 110\ \%$	>100	>97	–
WBH	9.5 Gy × 4 (38 Gy)	$D_{0.1\ ccm} \leq 75\ \%$	$D_{0.1\ ccm} \leq 80\ \%$	$D_{0.1\ ccm} \leq 120\ \%$	>100	>96	–
Zamboglou et al. (2012)[a]	9.5 Gy × 4 (38 Gy)	$D_{0.1\ ccm} \leq 80\ \%$	$D_{0.1\ ccm} \leq 80\ \%$	$D_{0.1\ ccm} \leq 120\ \%$	≥100	≥90	≤35
	11.5 Gy × 3 (34.5 Gy)	$D_{0.1\ ccm} \leq 80\ \%$	$D_{0.1\ ccm} \leq 80\ \%$	$D_{0.1\ ccm} \leq 120\ \%$	≥100	≥90	≤35
Prada et al. (2012)[a]	19 Gy × 1 (19 Gy)	$D_{0.1\ ccm} \leq 75\ \%$	–	$D_{0.1\ ccm} \leq 110\ \%$	–	–	–
Hoskin et al. (2007)[b]	37.7 Gy EBRT + 2 × 8.5 Gy (17 Gy) BRT	$D_{2.0\ ccm} < 6.7$ Gy	–	$D_{10} < 10$ Gy	–	–	–
Kotecha et al. (2013)[b]	45–50.4 Gy EBRT + 3 × (5.5–7.5 Gy) BRT	$D_{0.1\ ccm} \leq 100\ \%$	–	$D_{0.1\ ccm} \leq 120\ \%$	–	≥100	–
Pistis et al. (2010)[b]	60 Gy EBRT + 1 × 9 Gy BRT	$D_{2.0\ ccm} \leq 75\ \%$	–	$D_{2\ \%} < 120\ \%$	≥105	≥98	≤50

PTV planning target volume, *EBRT* external beam radiotherapy, *BRT* brachytherapy, *HDR* high-dose-rate, D_{10} HDR dose delivered to 10 % of the organ, $D_{0.1}$ ccm minimum HDR dose to the most exposed 0.1 ccm of the organ, $D_{2.0}$ ccm minimum HDR dose to the most exposed 2.0 ccm of the organ, D_2 % minimum HDR dose to the most exposed 2 % of the organ, V_{100}, V_{150} percent of PTV receiving 100 % and 150 % of the HDR prescription dose, *CET* California Endocurietherapy Cancer Center, *WBH* William Beaumont Hospital.

[a] HDR monotherapy

[b] Combined treatment with additional EBRT

Table 3 Literature results of high-dose-rate brachytherapy as boost modality to external beam radiotherapy for localized prostate cancer

		Treatment scheme				
Study	n	Total EBRT dose (Gy/fx)	Total HDR dose (Gy/fx)	Total BED/ EQD2 (Gy)	Follow-up (y)	Biochemical control[a]
Galalae et al. (2002)	144	40/20	18/2	219/94	Median 8.2	74 %/69 % all risk groups at 5 years/ 8 years
Pistis et al. (2010)	114	60/20	9/1	203/87	Mean 2.7	97.4 % IR and HR at 4 years
Kotecha et al. (2013)	229	45–50.4/25–28	16.5–22.5/3	171–226/74–97	Median 5.1	95 % LR at 7 years, 90 % IR at 7 years, 57% HR at 7 years (81 % HR with BED > 190 Gy)
Martin et al. (2004)	102	45/25	20–28/4	191–251/82–108	Median 2.6	100 % LR/IR at 3 years, 79 % HR at 3 years
Prada et al. (2012)	252	46/23	21–23/2	292–366/109–137	Median 6.1	84 %/78 % HR at 5 years/10 years
Åström et al. (2005)	214	50/25	20/2	269/116	Median 4	82 % all risk groups at 5 years
Martinez et al. (2002)	207	46/23	16.5–23/2–3	184–306/79–131	Mean 4.4	52 % all risk groups for EQD2 < 93 Gy and 87 % all risk groups for EQD2 > 93 Gy at 5 years
Noda et al. (2011)	59	50/25	15–18/2	191–243/82–104	Median 5.1	100 % LR at 5 years, 92 % IR at 5 years, 72 % HR at 5 years
Hoskin et al. (2007)	220	35.75/13	17/2	214/92	Median 2.5	Mean PSA relapse-free survival for all risk groups 4.3 years

LR low-risk group, *IR* intermediate-risk group, *HR* high-risk group, *y* years, *BED* biologically effective dose considering an α/β-ratio for prostate cancer of 1.5 Gy, *EQD2* biologically effective dose administered in 2 Gy-fractions considering an α/β-ratio for prostate cancer of 1.5 Gy, *EBRT* external beam radiotherapy, *BRT* brachytherapy, *HDR* high-dose-rate, *fx* fraction(s)

[a] Biochemical failure defined by the *Phoenix* definition (absolute nadir plus 2 ng/ml)

4 Clinical Data

4.1 HDR Boost in Combination with EBRT

In patients with organ-confined prostate cancer, radiation dose escalation has shown to improve both LC and BC (Kuban et al. 2008; Dearnaley et al. 2007; Zelefsky et al. 2008, 2011; Peeters et al. 2006; Kupelian et al. 2008; Kim et al. 2012; Nguyen et al. 2013; Pahlajani et al. 2012; Pollack et al. 2002; Zietman et al. 2010). However, the benefits of local dose escalation must be weighed against the risks of toxicity to the surrounding healthy tissues. The combination of EBRT and HDR BRT allows the safe delivery of high biologic equivalent doses to the prostate not achievable in terms of conformality even by adaptive image-guided IMRT (Kupelian and Meyer 2011).

Two randomized trials have helped to show the superiority of HDR BRT combined with EBRT over EBRT alone in the radical treatment of localized prostate cancer. In the mid-1990s, Sathya et al. (Sathya et al. 2005) assigned 104 patients to conventional EBRT of 66 Gy in 33 fractions or to 35 Gy HDR BRT to the prostate with supplemental conventional EBRT of 40 Gy in 20 fractions. At a median follow-up of 8.2 years, the authors reported biochemical failure in 17 patients of the combined arm compared with 33 patients in the EBRT alone arm ($P = 0.0024$). Overall survival was 94 % in the combined arm versus 92 % in the EBRT arm without statistically significant differences in acute and late toxicity. The authors reported 2.0 % Grade 3–4 genitourinary (GU) and 3.9 % Grade 3–4 gastrointestinal (GI) adverse events at 18 months for the combined arm compared to 3.8 and 1.9 %, respectively, for the EBRT arm. Almost a decade later, Hoskin et al. (2007) randomized 220 patients to receive either hypofractionated EBRT alone or hypofractionated EBRT plus HDR BRT. The EBRT group ($n = 111$) received 55 Gy in 20 fractions, whereas the combined treatment group ($n = 109$) was given 35.75 Gy EBRT in 13 fractions plus a 17-Gy HDR boost applied in two fractions within a single implant. With a median follow-up of 30 months, a significant improvement in actuarial biochemical relapse-free survival was seen in favor of the combined treatment schedule. The mean biochemical failure-free survival in the BRT arm was 5.1 versus 4.3 years in the EBRT only group ($p = 0.03$) with no significant difference in late bowel or bladder reactions between the two arms when considering Grade 2 and greater severity. The results of these randomized trials are in line with the oncological outcomes in large retrospective series reporting promising long-term biochemical relapse-free survival rates (Pistis et al. 2010; Kotecha et al. 2013; Prada et al. 2012). Pistis et al. (2010) treated 114 patients with intermediate- and high-risk prostate cancer using a treatment schedule consisting of mean 60 Gy conventional EBRT, followed 3 weeks later by a single-fraction 9 Gy HDR boost yielding a total combined $BED_{1.5}$ of 203 Gy. The generated overall BC at 4 years was 97.4 % with no higher grade acute or late GI and GU adverse events. Kotecha et al. (2013) treated 229 patients with an HDR BRT boost followed 3 weeks later by supplemental EBRT. The boost consisted of three fractions BRT of 5.5–7.5 Gy per fraction and supplemental EBRT of conventionally fractionated IMRT delivering 45.0–50.4 Gy. The generated $BED_{1.5}$ levels ranged from 171 to 226 Gy with a median value of 191.5 Gy. The 7-year biochemical relapse-free survival rates were 95, 90, and 57 % for low-, intermediate-, and high-risk patients, respectively, with a 7-year BC of 81 % among high-risk patients with $BED_{1.5}$ values >190 Gy. The reported incidence of late Grade 3 GU and GI toxicity was 3.1 and 0.4 %, respectively. In a scheme consisting of EBRT interdigitated with BRT, Prada et al. (2012) reported on 252 high-risk patients treated with 46 Gy EBRT and two fractions HDR BRT (on day 5 and 15 of EBRT) of 10.5–11.5 Gy yielding total combined $BED_{1.5}$ doses ranging from 292 to 366 Gy. The accomplished 5- and 10-year BC rate was 84 and 78 %, respectively, with 2.7 % late Grade 3 GU and no late GI toxicity.

Even though a variety of clinically implemented dose schedules make uniform recommendations concerning the optimal combined dose regime difficult, the literature data on HDR BRT with supplemental EBRT are consistent and reproducible (Table 3). The high clinical efficacy of the so-called “combined treatment protocols” is explicable by the higher dose that can be prescribed when BRT is used for treatment and by virtue of a higher dose within the implant. Most authors use BRT fractions ranging from 6 to 10 Gy yielding total physical HDR doses of 12–20 Gy applied in two to four fractions. The supplemental EBRT doses range from 45 to 54 Gy, generating total $BED_{1.5}$ and EQD2 doses in the range of 171–366 Gy and 74–137 Gy, respectively (Galalae et al. 2002, 2004, 2006; Pistis et al. 2010; Kotecha et al. 2013; Prada et al. 2012; Martinez et al. 2002, 2003, 2005, 2011; Demanes et al. 2005; Sathya et al. 2005; Vargas et al. 2006; Martin et al. 2004; Aström et al. 2005; Hiratsuka et al. 2004; Noda et al. 2011; Deger et al. 2005; Morton et al. 2010; Agoston et al. 2011; Izard et al. 2006; Pellizzon et al. 2008; Phan et al. 2007; Viani et al. 2009). The reported rates of late Grade 3 GU adverse events are far less than 5 % in the majority of HDR boost series comparing favorably with high-grade late GU toxicity rates in modern dose-escalating EBRT series (Peeters et al. 2006; de Meerleer et al. 2004; Hanks et al. 2000).

Overall, HDR BRT with supplemental EBRT enables the highly conformal administration of escalated biological doses to the prostate while ensuring favorable toxicity profiles. At this point, there is no consensus about the role of androgen deprivation therapy (ADT) in combination with HDR BRT for the treatment of locally-confined prostate cancer. Temporary hormonal ablative treatment may not be of additional advantage since it has not shown to be associated with improved oncological outcomes (Galalae et al. 2004; Demanes et al. 2009; Hoskin et al. 2007; Martinez et al. 2003, 2005).

4.2 HDR Monotherapy

Mature results from different institutions demonstrate HDR monotherapy to be an excellent option for the definitive treatment of organ-confined disease. Constant and reproducible 5-year BC rates have been reported for patients with low-risk (85–97 %), intermediate-risk (93–97 %), and high-risk (79–88 %) prostate cancer (Zamboglou et al. 2012; Demanes et al. 2011; Hoskin et al. 2012; Yoshioka et al. 2011, 2013; Rogers et al. 2012; ; Corner et al. 2008; Ghilezan et al. 2011; Martin et al. 2004; Mark et al. 2010; Barkati et al. 2012; Grills et al. 2004; Martinez et al. 2001, 2010; Komiya et al. 2013; Ghadjar et al. 2009; Prada et al. 2012) using a variety of dose-fractionation regimes. Table 4 lists dose-fractionation schemes and associated BEDs of monotherapy protocols from the literature.

Even though direct comparisons are difficult, the clinical outcomes yielded with single- or multiple implant regimes are consistent. Martinez et al. (2010) treated 248 low- and intermediate-risk patients employing one implant at 3 fractions of 9.5 Gy ($n = 171$) or two implants at 3 fractions of 7.0 Gy ($n = 77$). Their reported overall BC was 88 % at 5 years. Mark et al. (2010) reported an actuarial BC rate of 88 % at 8 years in 301 patients for all risk groups utilising two implants at 3 fractions of 7.5 Gy. Similarly, Rogers et al. (2012) reported a BC rate of 94 % at 5 years in 284 intermediate-risk patients treated with two implants at three fractions of 6.5 Gy. Both Mark et al. (2010) and Rogers et al. (2012) included clinical stages ≥T2b with no exclusions for any GS or pre-treatment PSA in the series by Mark et al. (2010). These recently published data corroborate the experience of other groups (Zamboglou et al. 2012; Hoskin et al. 2012; Yoshioka et al. 2011) indicating that HDR BRT is applicable for monotherapy over a range of risk groups including intermediate and carefully selected high-risk cases. In line with this experience, large monotherapy series failed to verify GS, pre-treatment PSA, or clinical T-stage as significant predictors of risk of biochemical failure (Hoskin et al. 2012; Rogers et al. 2012; Yoshioka et al.

Table 4 Literature results of high-dose-rate brachytherapy as monotherapy for localized prostate cancer

Study	n	Treatment protocol Gy/fx	Fractions (Implants)	Total	Median f/u (y)	Biochemical control[a]	BED (Gy)	EQD2 (Gy)
Yoshioka et al. (2011)	111	6.0 Gy	9 (1 Implant)	54 Gy	5.4	93 % IR at 3 years, 85 % HR at 3 years	270	116
Yoshioka et al. (2013)	63	6.5 Gy	7 (1 Implant)	45.5 Gy	3.5	96 % IR at 3 years, 90 % HR at 3 years	243	104
Hoskin et al. (2012)	197	8.5–9.0 Gy	4 (1 Implant)	34–36 Gy	4.5–5	95 % IR at 4 years, 87 % HR at 4 years	227–252	97–108
		10.5 Gy	3 (1 Implant)	31.5 Gy	3			
		13.0 Gy	2 (1 Implant)	26 Gy	0.5			
Rogers et al. (2012)	284	6.5 Gy	6 (2 Implants)	39 Gy	3	94 % IR at 5 years	208	89
Mark et al. (2010)	301	7.5 Gy	6 (2 Implants)	45 Gy	8	88 % all risk groups at 8 years	270	117
Prada et al. (2012)	40	19.0 Gy	1 (1 Implant)	19 Gy	1.6	100 % LR at 32 months, 88 % IR at 32 months	260	111
Demanes et al. (2011)	298	7.0 Gy	6 (2 Implants)	42 Gy	5.2	97 % LR/IR at 5 years	238–279	102–119
		9.5 Gy	4 (1 Implant)	38 Gy				
Zamboglou et al. (2012)	718	9.5 Gy	4 (1 Implant)	38 Gy	4.4	95 % LR at 5 years, 93 % IR at 5 years, 93 % HR at 5 years	279–299	119–128
		9.5 Gy	4 (2 Implants)	38 Gy				
		11.5 Gy	3 (3 Implants)	34.5 Gy				

LR low-risk group; *IR* intermediate-risk group; *HR* high-risk group; *f/u* follow-up; *y* years; *BED* biologically effective dose considering an α/β-ratio for prostate cancer of 1.5 Gy, *EQD2* biologically effective dose administered in 2 Gy-fractions considering an α/β-ratio for prostate cancer of 1.5 Gy, *fx* fraction

[a] Biochemical failure defined by the *Phoenix* definition (absolute nadir plus 2 ng/ml)

2011; Tselis et al. 2013). Hoskin et al. (2012) reported on a group of 197 patients with a 4-year BC rate of 87 % in 86 high risk cases. Those included stages ≥T3 in 21 %, GS ≥ 8 in 10 %, and PSA > 20 in 25 % of cases with 92 % of high-risk patients receiving temporary ADT of median 6.3 months duration. In the series by Tselis et al. (2013), the BC at 80 months for low-risk, intermediate-risk and high-risk patients was 90, 92, and 82 %, respectively. There was no statistically significant difference between these risk groups. However, 60 % of the high-risk patients received for median 9 months ADT including all patients with PSA ≥ 20 ng/ml, 93 % of patients with GS ≥ 7b (4 + 3), and 52 % of all cases staged >T2b. Nonetheless, the potential advantage of temporary ADT for patients treated with HDR monotherapy remains an issue of ongoing discussion as no corroborative evidence exclusive to this modality exists (Krauss et al. 2011).

Gastrointestinal and GU morbidity of monotherapy series has been shown to be low with consistent toxicity incidences across all scales. Hoskin et al. (2012) reported up to 16 % late Grade 3 GU adverse events with 7 % urethral strictures requiring surgery. Ghilezan et al. (2011), however, only documented 1.1 % late Grade 3 toxicity with no strictures requiring urethrotomy and overall 23 % Grade 2 adverse events. Zamboglou et al. (2012) encountered 3.5 % late Grade 3 GU morbidity with 1.8 % of patients developing urethral strictures requiring surgical intervention. Data on erectile dysfunction after HDR monotherapy have been rarely reported using various multidimensional or ordinal scales for assessment. However, potency preservation rates of 75–90 % are documented in the recent literature (Zamboglou et al. 2012; Rogers et al. 2012; Ghadjar et al. 2009; Prada et al. 2012). Late rectal toxicity rates following HDR monotherapy have also been reported to be low. Hoskin et al. (2012) encountered 14.6 % Grade 2 adverse events with 1 % Grade 3 toxicity. Ghilezan et al. (2011) documented 4 % Grade 2 and overall 1.1 % Grade 3 adverse events. In the analysis by Zamboglou et al. (2012), 1.6 % of patients experienced Grade 3 rectal morbidity with 0.6 % of patients requiring rectal surgery for Grade 3 radiogenic mucositis. So far, no randomized trial has ever compared LDR and HDR monotherapy, but nonrandomized evaluations have confirmed that both acute and late high-grade toxicities are less frequent after HDR than LDR monotherapy (Grills et al. 2004; Martinez et al. 2010). This may reflect the accuracy and reproducibility of the HDR dosimetry, which eliminates uncertainties in the spatial accuracy of dose delivery (Yamada et al. 2012).

Overall, the clinical outcome data of HDR monotherapy reflect current radiobiological considerations for optimal tumor control through hypofractionation. The BED in Table 4 ranges from 208 to 299 Gy, with a median value of 256 Gy, considering an a/β-ratio of 1.5 Gy. However, even for an a/β-ratio of 3.0 Gy, the BED would be in the range of 123–167 Gy. In comparison with LDR implants, where attempts are made to attain a $BED_{2.0} > 200$ Gy by mainly adding EBRT (Stone et al. 2007, 2010), HDR monotherapy can generate $BED_{2.0}$ values far higher than 200 Gy in a significant part of the fractionation schedules listed in Table 4. The values for EQD2 in Table 4 range from 89 to 128 Gy for an a/β-ratio of 1.5 Gy (77–104 Gy for an a/β-ratio of 3.0 Gy), which may be mostly impossible to administer with conventional EBRT.

4.3 HDR Salvage for Locally Recurrent Disease

Up to 60 % of prostate cancer patients that underwent radical therapy for clinically localized disease will harbor a biochemical recurrence (BCR) within 10 years after treatment (Djavan et al. 2003; Brachman et al. 2000; Bruce et al. 2012). The ideal management of these patients remains a controversial clinical issue (Bruce et al. 2012). Despite the primary treatment-related variation in the definition of BCR and the difficulty to differentiate between local or distant relapse based on PSA follow-up, clinical data suggest that up to 70 % of patients with a rising PSA will have local disease as the only demonstrable site of recurrent disease (Chen et al. 2013; Ahmed et al. 2007; Pound et al. 1999). Others, however, cite that most patients with BCR will experience micrometastatic disease and will therefore not benefit from local salvage treatment modalities (Chen et al. 2013; Nguyen et al. 2007). However, new promising molecular imaging approaches are evolving in order to improve accurate patient selection and provide more precise localization possibilities that can be used for optimization of salvage therapy modalities (Ahmed et al. 2007; Ward et al. 2005).

Different therapeutic options such as salvage ADT or local procedures, such as salvage radical prostatectomy, salvage cryosurgical ablation, salvage photodynamic therapy, salvage thermal ablation, salvage high-intensity focused ultrasound and salvage radiation therapy (RT), including all forms of salvage EBRT and/or salvage BRT are currently clinically practiced (Ward et al. 2008). For pathologically proven local failure after previous definitive treatment, salvage HDR BRT (sHDR BRT) with or without ADT appears to be an effective, well-tolerated approach with a curative potential in accurately selected patients (Chen et al. 2013; Lee et al. 2007; Scala et al. 2009; Pellizzon et al. 2009). Even though most clinical data are derived from small retrospective studies, the disease control and toxicity rates using sHDR BRT compare favorably with those reported using other treatment modalities (Chen et al. 2013; Pellizzon et al. 2009). Lee et al. (2007) treated 21 patients (median pre-salvage PSA of 3.8 ng/ml with median pre-salvage GS of 7) after primary EBRT of median 66.6 Gy with 36 Gy sHDR BRT in 6 fractions using two TRUS-guided implants separated by 1 week. The reported BC at median 18.7 months of follow-up was 89 % with 86 % Grade 2 and 14 % Grade 3 GU adverse events at 3 months after BRT. Pellizzon et al. (2009) treated 17 patients after median 68 Gy primary EBRT with a HDR BRT dose ranging from 34–36 Gy, achieving long-term (median follow-up of 47 months) BC of 70.5 % associated with a 47 % incidence of acute Grade 2 rectal toxicity and 6 % incidence of Grade 3 late rectal toxicity. The rate of symptomatic urethral strictures was 17. 6 %. Scala et al. (2009) reported a short-term (median follow-up of 18.5 months) BC rate of 70 % in a series of 10 patients (median pre-salvage PSA 5.8 ng/ml), who underwent sHDR BRT after either primary EBRT or LDR BRT. All patients received 36 Gy HDR BRT in 6 fractions using two TRUS-guided temporary implants separated by 2 weeks. The authors reported 70 % Grade 2 or greater late GU toxicity and 0 % Grade 2 or greater late GI toxicity. Similarly, Oliai et al. (2013) reported on a group of 22 patients, who underwent sHDR BRT with or without ADT after primary treatment with EBRT, LDR BRT, or HDR BRT with supplemental EBRT, receiving 36 Gy HDR BRT in 6 fractions using two TRUS-guided implants. At a median follow-up of 45 months, the generated BC rate was 75 %. Urethral strictures requiring TURP developed in 32 % of patients and Grade 2 hematuria manifested in 18 % of patients. In the series by Chien et al. (2013), which is the largest series of patients treated with sHDR BRT after previous definitive RT, 52 patients were analyzed. After pathologic confirmation of locally recurrent disease, patients received 36 Gy HDR BRT in 6 fractions. Median follow-up was 59.6 months with an actuarial BC rate of 51 % at 5 years. Acute and late Grade 3 GU adverse events were observed in only 2 % and 2 % of patients, respectively. No Grade 2 or higher acute GI adverse events and 4 % Grade 2 late GI toxicity were documented. In summary, sHDR BRT with or without ADT for locally recurrent disease after initial radical treatment, compared with other salvage modalities, is a promising radiotherapeutic approach with an acceptable acute and late toxicity profile. However, more research and longer follow-up are needed to evaluate this salvage modality in comparison with other existing treatment alternatives.

References

Agoston P, Major T, Fröhlich G et al (2011) Moderate dose escalation with single-fraction high-dose-rate brachytherapy boost for clinically localized intermediate- and high-risk prostate cancer: 5-year outcome of the first 100 consecutively treated patients. Brachytherapy 10(5):376–384

Ahmed HU, Pendse D, Illing R et al (2007) Will focal therapy become a standard of care for men with localized prostate cancer? Nat Clin Pract Oncol 4(11):632–642

Algan O, Jamgade A, Ali I et al (2012) The dosimetric impact of daily setup error on target volumes and surrounding normal tissue in the treatment of prostate cancer with intensity-modulated radiation therapy. Med Dosim 37(4):406–411

Aström L, Pedersen D, Mercke C et al (2005) Long-term outcome of high dose rate brachytherapy in radiotherapy of localized prostate cancer. Radiother Oncol 74(2):157–161

Aydin H, Tsuzuki T, Hernandez D et al (2004) Positive proximal (bladder neck) margin at radical prostatectomy confers greater risk of biochemical progression. Urology 64(3):551–555

Barkati M, Williams SG, Foroudi F et al (2012) High-dose-rate brachytherapy as a monotherapy for favorable-risk prostate cancer: a phase II trial. Int J Radiat Oncol Biol Phys 82(5): 1889–1896

Battermann JJ, Boon TA, Moerland MA (2004) Results of permanent prostate brachytherapy, 13 years of experience at a single institution. Radiother Oncol 71(1):23–28

Bolla M, Poppel HV (2012) Management of prostate cancer. A multidisciplinary approach. Springer, Berlin

Brachman DG, Thomas T, Hilbe J et al (2000) Failure-free survival following brachytherapy alone or external beam irradiation alone for T1-2 prostate tumors in 2,222 patients: results from a single practice. Int J Radiat Oncol Biol Phys 48(1):111–117

Brenner DJ (2004) Fractionation and late rectal toxicity. Int J Radiat Oncol Biol Phys 60(4):1013–1015

Brenner DJ, Hall EJ (1999) Fractionation and protraction for radiotherapy of prostate carcinoma. Int J Radiat Oncol Biol Phys 43(5):1095–1101

Brenner DJ, Martinez AA, Edmundson GK et al (2002) Direct evidence that prostate tumors show high sensitivity to fractionation (low alpha/beta ratio), similar to late-responding normal tissue. Int J Radiat Oncol Biol Phys 52(1):6–13

Briganti A, Blute ML, Eastham JH et al (2009) Pelvic lymph node dissection in prostate cancer. Eur Urol 55(6):1251–1265

Bruce JY, Lang JM, McNeel DG et al (2012) Current controversies in the management of biochemical failure in prostate cancer. Clin Adv Hematol Oncol 10(11):716–722

Chen CP, Weinberg V, Shinohara K et al (2013) Salvage HDR brachytherapy for recurrent prostate cancer after previous definitive radiation therapy: 5-year outcomes. Int J Radiat Oncol Biol Phys 86(2):324–329

Chuang A, Nielsen ME, Hernandez DJ et al (2007) The significance of positive surgical margin in areas of capsular incision in otherwise organ-confined disease at radical prostatectomy. J Urol 178:1306–1310

Coen JJ, Zietman AL, Thakral H et al (2002) Radical radiation for localized prostate cancer: local persistence of disease results in a late wave of metastases. J Clin Oncol 20(15):3199–3205

Corner C, Rojas AM, Bryant L et al (2008) A Phase II study of high-dose-rate afterloading brachytherapy as monotherapy for the treatment of localized prostate cancer. Int J Radiat Oncol Biol Phys 72(2):441–446

D'Amico AV, Whittington R, Malkowicz SB et al (1998) Biochemical outcome after radical prostatectomy, external beam radiation therapy, or interstitial radiation therapy for clinically localized prostate cancer. JAMA 280(11):969–974

D'Amico AV, Whittington R, Malkowicz SB et al (2002) Biochemical outcome after radical prostatectomy or external beam radiation therapy for patients with clinically localized prostate carcinoma in the prostate specific antigen era. Cancer 95(2):281–286

Davis BJ, Pisansky TM, Wilson TM et al (1999) The radial distance of extraprostatic extension of prostate carcinoma: implications for prostate brachytherapy. Cancer 85(12):2630–2637

de Meerleer G, Vakaet L, Meersschout S et al (2004) Intensity-modulated radiotherapy as primary treatment for prostate cancer: acute toxicity in 114 patients. Int J Radiat Oncol Biol Phys 60(3):777–787

Dearnaley DP, Sydes MR, Graham JD et al (2007) Escalated-dose versus standard-dose conformal radiotherapy in prostate cancer: first results from the MRC RT01 randomised controlled trial. Lancet Oncol 8(6):475–487

Deger S, Boehmer D, Roigas J et al (2005) High dose rate (HDR) brachytherapy with conformal radiation therapy for localized prostate cancer. Eur Urol 47(4):441–448

Demanes DJ, Rodriguez RR, Schour L et al (2005) High-dose-rate intensity-modulated brachytherapy with external beam radiotherapy for prostate cancer: california endocurietherapy's 10-year results. Int J Radiat Oncol Biol Phys 61(5):1306–1316

Demanes DJ, Brandt D, Schour L et al (2009) Excellent results from high dose rate brachytherapy and external beam for prostate cancer are not improved by androgen deprivation. Am J Clin Oncol 32(4):342–347

Demanes DJ, Martinez AA, Ghilezan M et al (2011) High-dose-rate monotherapy: safe and effective brachytherapy for patients with localized prostate cancer. Int J Radiat Oncol Biol Phys 81(5):1286–1292

Deutsch I, Zelefsky MJ, Zhang Z et al (2010) Comparison of PSA relapse-free survival in patients treated with ultra-high-dose IMRT versus combination HDR brachytherapy and IMRT. Brachytherapy 9(4):313–318

Djavan B, Moul JW, Zlotta A et al (2003) PSA progression following radical prostatectomy and radiation therapy: new standards in the new Millennium. Eur Urol 43(1):12–27

Eid K, Krughoff K, Stoimenova D et al (2013) Validation of the urgency, weak stream, incomplete emptying, and nocturia (uwin) score compared with the american urological association symptoms score in assessing lower urinary tract symptoms in the clinical setting. Urology. 83(1):181–185

Evangelista L, Guttilla A, Zattoni F et al (2013) Utility of choline positron emission tomography/computed tomography for lymph node involvement identification in intermediate- to high-risk prostate cancer: a systematic literature review and meta-analysis. Eur Urol 63(6):1040–1048

Fatyga M, Williamson JF, Dogan N et al (2009) A comparison of HDR brachytherapy and IMRT techniques for dose escalation in prostate cancer: a radiobiological modeling study. Med Phys 36(9): 3995–4006

Fowler J, Chappell R, Ritter M (2001) Is alpha/beta for prostate tumors really low? Int J Radiat Oncol Biol Phys 50(4):1021–1031

Franca CAS, Vieira SL, Carvalho ACP, et al (2009) Radioactive seed migration after prostate brachytherapy with iodine-125 using loose seeds versus stranded seeds. Int Braz J Urol 35(5):573–579 (discussion 579–580)

Galalae RM, Kovács G, Schultze J et al (2002) Long-term outcome after elective irradiation of the pelvic lymphatics and local dose escalation using high-dose-rate brachytherapy for locally advanced prostate cancer. Int J Radiat Oncol Biol Phys 52(1):81–90

Galalae RM, Martinez A, Mate T et al (2004) Long-term outcome by risk factors using conformal high-dose-rate brachytherapy (HDR-BT) boost with or without neoadjuvant androgen suppression for localized prostate cancer. Int J Radiat Oncol Biol Phys 58(4):1048–1055

Galalae RM, Martinez A, Nuernberg N et al (2006) Hypofractionated conformal HDR brachytherapy in hormone naïve men with localized prostate cancer. Is escalation to very high biologically equivalent dose beneficial in all prognostic risk groups? Strahlenther Onkol 182(3):135–141

Ghadjar P, Keller T, Rentsch CA et al (2009) Toxicity and early treatment outcomes in low- and intermediate-risk prostate cancer managed by high-dose-rate brachytherapy as a monotherapy. Brachytherapy 8(1):45–51

Ghilezan M, Martinez A, Gustason G et al (2011) High-dose-rate brachytherapy as monotherapy delivered in two fractions within one day for favorable/intermediate-risk prostate cancer: preliminary toxicity data. Int J Radiat Oncol Biol Phys 83(3):927–932
Grills IS, Martinez AA, Hollander M et al (2004) High dose rate brachytherapy as prostate cancer monotherapy reduces toxicity compared to low dose rate palladium seeds. The Journal of Urology 171(3):1098–1104
Grimm P, Billiet I, Bostwick D et al (2012) Comparative analysis of prostate-specific antigen free survival outcomes for patients with low, intermediate and high risk prostate cancer treatment by radical therapy. results from the prostate cancer results study group. BJU Int. 109(Suppl 1):22–29
Han M, Partin AW, Pound CR et al (2001) Long-term biochemical disease-free and cancer-specific survival following anatomic radical retropubic prostatectomy. The 15-year Johns Hopkins experience. Urol Clin North Am 28(3):555–565
Han M, Partin AW, Zahurak M et al (2003) Biochemical (prostate specific antigen) recurrence probability following radical prostatectomy for clinically localized prostate cancer. J Urol 169(2):517–523
Hanks GE, Hanlon AL, Pinover WH et al (2000) Dose selection for prostate cancer patients based on dose comparison and dose response studies. Int J Radiat Oncol Biol Phys 46(4):823–832
Hanks GE, Hanlon AL, Horwitz EM (2001) Evidence for cure of 'young' men with prostate cancer. Oncology (Williston Park, N.Y.) 15(5):563–567 (discussion 571–574)
Harlan LC, Potosky A, Gilliland FD et al (2001) Factors associated with initial therapy for clinically localized prostate cancer: prostate cancer outcomes study. JNCI Journal of the National Cancer Institute 93(24):1864–1871
Heidenreich A, Bellmunt J, Bolla M et al (2011) EAU guidelines on prostate cancer. Part 1: screening, diagnosis, and treatment of clinically localized disease. Eur Urol 59(1):61–71
Hiratsuka J, Jo Y, Yoshida K et al (2004) Clinical results of combined treatment conformal high-dose-rate iridium-192 brachytherapy and external beam radiotherapy using staging lymphadenectomy for localized prostate cancer. Int J Radiat Oncol Biol Phys 59(3): 684–690
Holly R, Morton GC, Sankreacha R et al (2011) Use of cone-beam imaging to correct for catheter displacement in high dose-rate prostate brachytherapy. Brachytherapy 10(4):299–305
Hoskin P (2008) High dose rate brachytherapy for prostate cancer. Cancer Radiother 12(6–7):512–514
Hoskin PJ, Motohashi K, Bownes P et al (2007) High dose rate brachytherapy in combination with external beam radiotherapy in the radical treatment of prostate cancer: initial results of a randomised phase three trial. Radiother Oncol 84(2):114–120
Hoskin P, Rojas A, Lowe G et al (2012) High-dose-rate brachytherapy alone for localized prostate cancer in patients at moderate or high risk of biochemical recurrence. Int J Radiat Oncol Biol Phys 82(4):1376–1384
Hoskin PJ, Colombo A, Henry A et al (2013) GEC/ESTRO recommendations on high dose rate afterloading brachytherapy for localized prostate cancer: an update. Radiother Oncol 107(3):325–332
Ishiyama H, Hirayama T, Jhaveri P, et al (2012) Is there an increase in genitourinary toxicity in patients treated with transurethral resection of the prostate and radiotherapy?: A systematic review. Am J Clin Oncol 37(3):297–304
Izard MA, Haddad RL, Fogarty GB et al (2006) Six year experience of external beam radiotherapy, brachytherapy boost with a 1 Ci (192)Ir source, and neoadjuvant hormonal manipulation for prostate cancer. Int J Radiat Oncol Biol Phys 66(1):38–47
Karabis A, Giannouli S, Baltas D (2005) HIPO: A hybrid inverse treatment planning optimization algorithm in HDR brachytherapy. Radiother Oncol 76(Suppl. 2):29
Kim MM, Hoffman KE, Levy LB et al (2012) Prostate cancer-specific mortality after definitive radiation therapy: who dies of disease? Eur J Cancer 48(11):1664–1671
Knaup C, Mavroidis P, Esquivel C et al (2012) Investigating the dosimetric and tumor control consequences of prostate seed loss and migration. Med Phys 39(6):3291–3298
Komiya A, Fujiuchi Y, Ito T et al (2013) Early quality of life outcomes in patients with prostate cancer managed by high-dose-rate brachytherapy as monotherapy. Int J Urol 20(2):185–192
Kono Y, Kubota K, Aruga T et al (2010) Swelling of the prostate gland by permanent brachytherapy may affect seed migration. Jpn J Clin Oncol 40(12):1159–1165
Kotecha R, Yamada Y, Pei X et al (2013) Clinical outcomes of high-dose-rate brachytherapy and external beam radiotherapy in the management of clinically localized prostate cancer. Brachytherapy 12(1):44–49
Krauss D, Kestin L, Ye H et al (2011) Lack of benefit for the addition of androgen deprivation therapy to dose-escalated radiotherapy in the treatment of intermediate- and high-risk prostate cancer. Int J Radiat Oncol Biol Phys 80(4):1064–1071
Kuban D, Tucker S, Dong L et al (2008) Long-term results of the M. D. Anderson randomized dose-escalation trial for prostate cancer. Int J Radiat Oncol Biol Phys 70(1):67–74
Kupelian P, Meyer JL (2011) Image-guided, adaptive radiotherapy of prostate cancer: toward new standards of radiotherapy practice. Front Radiat Ther Oncol 43:344–368
Kupelian PA, Ciezki J, Reddy CA et al (2008) Effect of increasing radiation doses on local and distant failures in patients with localized prostate cancer. Int J Radiat Oncol Biol Phys 71(1):16–22
Lakosi F, Antal G, Vandulek C et al (2011) Open MR-guided high-dose-rate (HDR) prostate brachytherapy: feasibility and initial experiences open MR-guided high-dose-rate (HDR) prostate brachytherapy. Pathol. Oncol. Res. 17(2):315–324
Le H, Rojas A, Alonzi R et al (2013) The influence of prostate volume on outcome after high-dose-rate brachytherapy alone for localized prostate cancer. Int J Radiat Oncol Biol Phys 87(2):270–274
Lee WR (2009) Extreme hypofractionation for prostate cancer. Expert Rev Anticancer Ther 9(1):61–65
Lee B, Shinohara K, Weinberg V et al (2007) Feasibility of high-dose-rate brachytherapy salvage for local prostate cancer recurrence after radiotherapy: the University of California-San Francisco experience. Int J Radiat Oncol Biol Phys 67(4):1106–1112
Luo HL, Fang FM, Chuang YC et al (2009) Previous transurethral resection of the prostate is not a contraindication to high-dose rate brachytherapy for prostate cancer. BJU Int 104(11):1620–1623
Luo HL, Fang FM, Kang CH et al (2013) Can high-dose-rate brachytherapy prevent the major genitourinary complication better than external beam radiation alone for patients with previous transurethral resection of prostate? Int Urol Nephrol 45(1): 113–119
Mark R, Anderson P, Akins R (2010) Interstitial high-dose-rate brachytherapy as monotherapy for early stage prostate cancer: median 8-year results in 301 patients (Abstract). Brachytherapy 9:76
Martin T, Baltas D, Kurek R et al (2004a) 3-D conformal HDR brachytherapy as monotherapy for localized prostate cancer. A pilot study. Strahlenther Onkol 180(4):225–232
Martin T, Röddiger S, Kurek R et al (2004b) 3D conformal HDR brachytherapy and external beam irradiation combined with temporary androgen deprivation in the treatment of localized prostate cancer. Radiother Oncol 71(1):35–41
Martinez AA, Pataki I, Edmundson G et al (2001) Phase II prospective study of the use of conformal high-dose-rate brachytherapy as monotherapy for the treatment of favorable stage prostate cancer: a feasibility report. Int J Radiat Oncol Biol Phys 49(1):61–69

Martinez AA, Gustafson G, Gonzalez J et al (2002) Dose escalation using conformal high-dose-rate brachytherapy improves outcome in unfavorable prostate cancer. Int J Radiat Oncol Biol Phys 53(2):316–327

Martinez A, Gonzalez J, Spencer W, et al (2003) Conformal high dose rate brachytherapy improves biochemical control and cause specific survival in patients with prostate cancer and poor prognostic factors. J. Urol. 169(3):974–979 (discussion 979–980)

Martinez A, Galalae R, Gonzalez J et al (2003b) No apparent benefit at 5 years from a course of neoadjuvant/concurrent androgen deprivation for patients with prostate cancer treated with a high total radiation dose. J Urol 170:2296–2301

Martinez AA, Demanes DJ, Galalae R et al (2005) Lack of benefit from a short course of androgen deprivation for unfavorable prostate cancer patients treated with an accelerated-hypofractionated regime. Int J Radiat Oncol Biol Phys 62(5):1322–1331

Martinez AA, Demanes J, Vargas C et al (2010) High-dose-rate prostate brachytherapy: an excellent accelerated-hypofractionated treatment for favorable prostate cancer. Am J Clin Oncol 33(5): 481–488

Martinez AA, Gonzalez J, Ye H et al (2011) Dose escalation improves cancer-related events at 10 years for intermediate- and high-risk prostate cancer patients treated with hypofractionated high-dose-rate boost and external beam radiotherapy. Int J Radiat Oncol Biol Phys 79(2):363–370

Masson S, Persad R, Bahl A (2012) HDR Brachytherapy in the Management of High-Risk Prostate Cancer. Adv Urol 2012:980841

Mavroidis P, Katsilieri Z, Kefala V et al (2010) Radiobiological evaluation of the influence of dwell time modulation restriction in HIPO optimized HDR prostate brachytherapy implants. J Contemp Brachyther 2(3):117–128

Ménard C, Susil RC, Choyke P et al (2004) MRI-guided HDR prostate brachytherapy in standard 1.5T scanner. Int J Radiat Oncol Biol Phys 59(5):1414–1423

Milickovic N, Mavroidis P, Tselis N et al (2011) 4D analysis of influence of patient movement and anatomy alteration on the quality of 3D U/S-based prostate HDR brachytherapy treatment delivery. Med Phys 38(9):4982–4993

Miralbell R, Roberts SA, Zubizarreta E et al (2012) Dose-fractionation sensitivity of prostate cancer deduced from radiotherapy outcomes of 5,969 patients in seven international institutional datasets: $\alpha/\beta = 1.4$ (0.9–2.2) Gy. Int J Radiat Oncol Biol Phys 82(1):17–24

Mohler J, Bahnson RR, Boston B et al (2010) NCCN clinical practice guidelines in oncology: prostate cancer. J Natl Compr Canc Netw 8(2):162–200

Monroe AT, Faricy PO, Jennings SB et al (2008) High-dose-rate brachytherapy for large prostate volumes ($\geq$50 cc)—Uncompromised dosimetric coverage and acceptable toxicity. Brachytherapy 7(1):7–11

Morton GC, Loblaw DA, Sankreacha R et al (2010) Single-fraction high-dose-rate brachytherapy and hypofractionated external beam radiotherapy for men with intermediate-risk prostate cancer: analysis of short- and medium-term toxicity and quality of life. Int J Radiat Oncol Biol Phys 77(3):811–817

Mutanga TF, de Boer HCJ, Rajan V et al (2012) Day-to-day reproducibility of prostate intrafraction motion assessed by multiple kV and MV imaging of implanted markers during treatment. Int J Radiat Oncol Biol Phys 83(1):400–407

Nag S, Dobelbower R, Glasgow G et al (2003) Inter-society standards for the performance of brachytherapy: a joint report from ABS, ACMP and ACRO. Crit Rev Oncol Hematol 48(1):1–17

Nath R, Bice WS, Butler WM et al (2009) AAPM recommendations on dose prescription and reporting methods for permanent interstitial brachytherapy for prostate cancer: report of Task Group 137. Med Phys 36(11):5310–5322

Nguyen PL, Chen M, D'Amico AV et al (2007) Magnetic resonance image-guided salvage brachytherapy after radiation in select men who initially presented with favorable-risk prostate cancer: a prospective phase 2 study. Cancer 110(7):1485–1492

Nguyen Q, Levy LB, Lee AK et al (2013) Long-term outcomes for men with high-risk prostate cancer treated definitively with external beam radiotherapy with or without androgen deprivation. Cancer 119(18):3265–3271

Noda Y, Sato M, Shirai S et al (2011) Efficacy and safety of high-dose-rate brachytherapy of single implant with two fractions combined with external beam radiotherapy for hormone-naïve localized prostate cancer. Cancers (Basel) 3(3):3585–3600

Oliai C, Yang L, Lee JY (2013) Prospective quality of life and efficacy of high-dose-rate brachytherapy salvage for recurrent prostate cancer. Int J Radiat Oncol Biol Phys 87(2):396

Pahlajani N, Ruth KJ, Buyyounouski MK et al (2012) Radiotherapy doses of 80 Gy and higher are associated with lower mortality in men with Gleason score 8 to 10 prostate cancer. Int J Radiat Oncol Biol Phys 82(5):1949–1956

Peddada AV, Jennings SB, Faricy PO et al (2007) Low morbidity following high dose rate brachytherapy in the setting of prior transurethral prostate resection. J Urol 178(5):1963–1967

Peeters STH, Heemsbergen WD, Koper PCM et al (2006) Dose-response in radiotherapy for localized prostate cancer: results of the dutch multicenter randomized phase III trial comparing 68 Gy of radiotherapy with 78 Gy. J Clin Oncol 24(13):1990–1996

Pellizzon ACA, Salvajoli J, Novaes P et al (2008) The relationship between the biochemical control outcomes and the quality of planning of high-dose rate brachytherapy as a boost to external beam radiotherapy for locally and locally advanced prostate cancer using the RTOG-ASTRO Phoenix definition. Int J Med Sci 5(3):113–120

Pellizzon A, Miziara MC. Neviani C (2009) Long-term results of salvage interstitial high-dose brachytherapy for local-only recurrent prostate cancer treated with definitive conventional external beam radiotherapy. http://meetinglibrary.asco.org/content/20049-64

Phan TP, Syed AMN, Puthawala A, et al (2007) High dose rate brachytherapy as a boost for the treatment of localized prostate cancer. J Urol 177(1):123–127 (discussion 127)

Pistis F, Guedea F, Pera J et al (2010) External beam radiotherapy plus high-dose-rate brachytherapy for treatment of locally advanced prostate cancer: the initial experience of the Catalan Institute of Oncology. Brachytherapy 9(1):15–22

Pollack A, Zagars GK, Starkschall G et al (2002) Prostate cancer radiation dose response: results of the M. D. Anderson phase III randomized trial. Int J Radiat Oncol Biol Phys 53(5):1097–1105

Potters L, Morgenstern C, Calugaru E et al (2005) Twelve-year outcomes following permanent prostate brachytherapy in patients with clinically localized prostate cancer. J Urol 173(5):1562–1566

Pound CR, Partin AW, Eisenberger MA et al (1999) Natural history of progression after PSA elevation following radical prostatectomy. JAMA 281(17):1591–1597

Prada PJ, Mendez L, Fernández J et al (2012a) Long-term biochemical results after high-dose-rate intensity-modulated brachytherapy with external beam radiotherapy for high risk prostate cancer. Radiat Oncol 7:31

Prada PJ, Jimenez I, González-Suárez H et al (2012b) High-dose-rate interstitial brachytherapy as monotherapy in one fraction and transperineal hyaluronic acid injection into the perirectal fat for the treatment of favorable stage prostate cancer: treatment description and preliminary results. Brachytherapy 11(2):105–110

Ritter M, Forman J, Kupelian P et al (2009) Hypofractionation for prostate cancer. Cancer J 15(1):1–6

Rogers CL, Alder SC, Rogers RL et al (2012) High dose brachytherapy as monotherapy for intermediate-risk prostate cancer. J Urol 187(1):109–116

Sakamoto N, Akitake M, Ikoma S et al (2011) Clinical outcome in prostate cancer patients undergoing high-dose-rate brachytherapy with external beam radiotherapy in our institute. Nippon Hinyokika Gakkai Zasshi 102(4):621–627

Sathya JR, Davis IR, Julian JA et al (2005) Randomized trial comparing iridium implant plus external-beam radiation therapy with external-beam radiation therapy alone in node-negative locally advanced cancer of the prostate. J Clin Oncol 23(6):1192–1199

Scala L, Page PN, Lee JW (2009) Salvage high dose rate brachytherapy for locally recurrent prostate cancer after primary radiotherapy. Int J Radiat Oncol Biol Phys 75(3):322

Seppenwoolde Y, Kolkman-Deurloo I, Sipkema D et al (2008) HDR prostate monotherapy: dosimetric effects of implant deformation due to posture change between TRUS- and CT-imaging. Radiother Oncol 86(1):114–119

Shah AP, Kupelian PA, Willoughby TR et al (2011) An evaluation of intrafraction motion of the prostate in the prone and supine positions using electromagnetic tracking. Radiother Oncol 99(1):37–43

Stone NN, Potters L, Davis BJ et al (2007) Customized dose prescription for permanent prostate brachytherapy: insights from a multicenter analysis of dosimetry outcomes. Int J Radiat Oncol Biol Phys 69(5):1472–1477

Stone NN, Stock RG, Cesaretti JA et al (2010) Local control following permanent prostate brachytherapy: effect of high biologically effective dose on biopsy results and oncologic outcomes. Int J Radiat Oncol Biol Phys 76(2):355–360

Sung M, Lin H, Koch MO et al (2007) Radial distance of extraprostatic extension measured by ocular micrometer is an independent predictor of prostate-specific antigen recurrence: A new proposal for the substaging of pT3a prostate cancer. Am J Surg Pathol 31(2):311–318

Touijer K, Fuenzalida RP, Rabbani F et al (2011) Extending the indications and anatomical limits of pelvic lymph node dissection for prostate cancer: improved staging or increased morbidity? BJU Int 108(3):372–377

Tselis N, Tunn UW, Chatzikonstantinou G et al (2013) High dose rate brachytherapy as monotherapy for localized prostate cancer: a hypofractionated two-implant approach in 351 consecutive patients. Radiat Oncol 8:115

Tucker SL, Thames HD, Michalski JM et al (2011) Estimation of α/β for late rectal toxicity based on RTOG 94–06. Int J Radiat Oncol Biol Phys 81(2):600–605

Vargas CE, Martinez AA, Boike TP et al (2006) High-dose irradiation for prostate cancer via a high-dose-rate brachytherapy boost: results of a phase I to II study. Int J Radiat Oncol Biol Phys 66(2):416–423

Viani GA, Pellizzon AC, Guimarães FS et al (2009) High dose rate and external beam radiotherapy in locally advanced prostate cancer. Am J Clin Oncol 32(2):187–190

Ward JF, Sebo TJ, Blute ML et al (2005) Salvage surgery for radiorecurrent prostate cancer: contemporary outcomes. J Urol 173(4):1156–1160

Ward JF, Pagliaro LC, Pisters LL (2008) Salvage therapy for radiorecurrent prostate cancer. Curr Probl Cancer 32(6):242–271

Whitaker M, Hruby G, Lovett A et al (2011) Prostate HDR brachytherapy catheter displacement between planning and treatment delivery. Radiother Oncol 101(3):490–494

White EC, Kamrava MR, Demarco J et al (2013) High-dose-rate prostate brachytherapy consistently results in high quality dosimetry. Int J Radiat Oncol Biol Phys 85(2):543–548

Yamada Y, Rogers L, Demanes DJ et al (2012) American Brachytherapy Society consensus guidelines for high-dose-rate prostate brachytherapy. Brachytherapy 11(1):20–32

Yoshioka Y, Konishi K, Sumida I et al (2011) Monotherapeutic high-dose-rate brachytherapy for prostate cancer: five-year results of an extreme hypofractionation regimen with 54 Gy in nine fractions. Int J Radiat Oncol Biol Phys 80(2):469–475

Yoshioka Y, Yoshida K, Yamazaki H et al (2013a) The emerging role of high-dose-rate (HDR) brachytherapy as monotherapy for prostate cancer. J Radiat Res 54(5):781–788

Yoshioka Y, Konishi K, Suzuki O et al (2013b) Monotherapeutic high-dose-rate brachytherapy for prostate cancer: a dose reduction trial. Radiother Oncol 110(1):114–119

Zamboglou N, Tselis N, Baltas D, et al (2012) High-dose-rate interstitial brachytherapy as monotherapy for clinically localized prostate cancer: treatment evolution and mature results. Int J Radiat Oncol Biol Phys 85(3):672–678

Zaorsky NG, Doyle LA, Yamoah K et al (2013) High dose rate brachytherapy boost for prostate cancer: A systematic review. Cancer Treat Rev 40(3):414–425

Zelefsky MJ, Leibel SA, Gaudin PB et al (1998) Dose escalation with three-dimensional conformal radiation therapy affects the outcome in prostate cancer. Int J Radiat Oncol Biol Phys 41(3):491–500

Zelefsky MJ, Kuban DA, Levy LB et al (2007a) Multi-institutional analysis of long-term outcome for stages T1-T2 prostate cancer treated with permanent seed implantation. Int J Radiat Oncol Biol Phys 67(2):327–333

Zelefsky MJ, Kattan MW, Fearn P et al (2007b) Pretreatment nomogram predicting ten-year biochemical outcome of three-dimensional conformal radiotherapy and intensity-modulated radiotherapy for prostate cancer. Urology 70(2):283–287

Zelefsky MJ, Yamada Y, Fuks Z et al (2008a) Long-term results of conformal radiotherapy for prostate cancer: impact of dose escalation on biochemical tumor control and distant metastases-free survival outcomes. Int J Radiat Oncol Biol Phys 71(4):1028–1033

Zelefsky MJ, Reuter VE, Fuks Z, et al (2008b) Influence of local tumor control on distant metastases and cancer-related mortality after external beam radiotherapy for prostate cancer. J. Urol. 179(4): 1368–1373 (discussion 1373)

Zelefsky MJ, Pei X, Chou JF et al (2011) Dose escalation for prostate cancer radiotherapy: predictors of long-term biochemical tumor control and distant metastases-free survival outcomes. Eur Urol 60(6):1133–1139

Zietman AL, Bae K, Slater JD et al (2010) Randomized trial comparing conventional-dose with high-dose conformal radiation therapy in early-stage adenocarcinoma of the prostate: long-term results from proton radiation oncology group/american college of radiology 95-09. J Clin Oncol 28(7):1106–1111

Part VII

Adjuvant Treatment and Salvage Treatment

Target Volume Definition in Postoperative Radiotherapy

Martin Stuschke

Contents

Abstract

Randomized trials on postoperative radiotherapy for prostate were reviewed. Target volume consensus guidelines were compared and discussed with respect to inter-observer variability, normal tissue exposure and size of the target volume.

1 Randomized Trials on Early Postoperative Radiotherapy

Early postoperative radiotherapy after radical prostatectomy to a dose of 60–64 Gy with conventional fractionation can reduce the hazard of biochemical relapse of high-risk prostate cancer by a hazard ratio of about 0.5. This long-term effect has been shown by three randomized trials (Bolla et al. 2012; Thompson et al. 2009; Wiegel et al. 2009). These randomized trials were heterogeneous by the various postoperative risk groups of patients included. All trials included patients with pT3a or pT3b tumors with or without positive resection margins. The EORTC trial included also patients with pT2 tumors and positive resection margins, the ARO/AUO trial patients with pT4 tumors. All trials required a pN0 status. Postoperative PSA serum levels had to achieve undetectable values in the ARO/AUO trial with assays having PSA detection limits of 0.1 ng/ml or lower. Therefore, patients in this trial got adjuvant radiotherapy according to the strict definition of undetectable PSA values at the time of radiotherapy. In the SWOG and EORTC trial, 66–70 % of patients had postoperative PSA serum levels below 0.2 ng/ml. Early postoperative radiotherapy started within 18 weeks after surgery in all these trials. PSA relapses at 5 years were found in 58, 46, and 46 % of patients in the control arms of the SWOG, ARO/AUO, and EORTC trials. The cancer-specific mortality rate was only 4 % in the EORTC trial at 10 years. Therefore, it is difficult to detect a significant effect of postoperative radiotherapy on survival within this time span

M. Stuschke (✉)
Direktor der Klinik und Poliklinik für Strahlentherapie, Universitätsklinikum Essen, Hufelandstr. 55, 45147 Essen, Germany
e-mail: martin.stuschke@uk-essen.de

H. Geinitz et al. (eds.), *Radiotherapy in Prostate Cancer*, Medical Radiology. Radiation Oncology,
DOI: 10.1007/174_2014_959, © Springer-Verlag Berlin Heidelberg 2014
Published Online: 20 March 2014

despite the large effect on biochemical relapse. In addition, 56 % of patients in the control arm of the EORTC study received salvage radiotherapy after PSA-progression diminishing differences between treatment arms on the survival endpoint. In the EORTC trial, no effect of postoperative radiotherapy on the cumulative risk of distant metastases was found and the cumulative risk at 10 years was 11 % in both ams. On the other hand, the crude rates of distant metastases were 35/211 in the control and 17/214 in the postoperative radiotherapy group in the SWOG trial at a median follow-up of 10.9 years, indicating a certain effect of postoperative radiotherapy on the development of distant metastases (Thompson et al. 2006). If one assumes that the effect of postoperative radiotherapy on the development of distant metastases is smaller than the local effect and given that the hazard ratio on freedom from biochemical relapse is 0.5, then the hazard ratio on local tumor control should be even smaller than 0.5. The treated prostate bed volumes in the EORTC trial were rather large. The mean 95 % isodose volume in the initial series treated up to 50 Gy was 930 cm^3 and in the second series 535 cm^3, as known from a dummy run for quality assurance (Davis et al. 2002). Similar large volumes were treated in SWOG trial. Here a four field or an arch technique was allowed. For the four-field approach 9×9 cm^2 or 10×10 cm^2 anterior or posterior fields were used. As an additional requirement, parts of the rectum have to be blocked in the lateral beams (Swanson et al. 2007). Some toxicity of postoperative radiotherapy was reported from these three trials. The risk of late grade 2+ gastrointestinal toxicity attributable to radiotherapy was $\leq$4 %, the risk of late grade 2+ genitourinary toxicity was $\leq$12 % in all trials. In addition, late grade 3 side effects were below 3 % in the EORTC and ARO/AUO trials.

2 Postoperative Salvage Radiotherapy

Salvage radiotherapy is an alternative to postoperative adjuvant radiotherapy and should be performed early at PSA serum levels < 0.5 ng/ml having a postoperative PSA rise or a PSA persistence in patients after prostatectomy with a pN0 or pNx lymph node status. Analyses of retrospective studies showed a 2.6 % loss of biochemical relapse-free survival for an incremental PSA level of 0.1 ng/ml after salvage prostate bed radiotherapy (King 2012). In addition, there are hints for a dose response in the range of total dose between 60 and 70 Gy (King 2012). When starting salvage RT at a PSA level below 0.2 ng/ml, long-term biochemical relapses-free survival approaches 65 %, which is similar to the results of the randomized trials with early or adjuvant postoperative radiotherapy (King 2012). Additional prognostic factors for biochemical relapse after postoperative radiotherapy are prostatectomy Gleason score, PSA doubling time, and androgen deprivation during salvage therapy (Stephenson et al. 2007). However, mature randomized data on salvage therapy are missing. Randomized trials on dose-response (e.g., SAKK 09/10), target volume (e.g., RTOG 0534 with whole pelvic versus prostate bed alone of salvage radiotherapy), or additional androgen deprivation and salvage radiotherapy (e.g., RTOG 0543), or comparison with adjuvant postoperative radiotherapy (Radicals, GETUG-17/0702, Raves) are under way. Until these data are available, the highest evidence for postoperative radiotherapy comes from the above three randomized trials on early postoperative radiotherapy (Bolla et al. 2012; Thompson et al. 2009; Wiegel et al. 2009). As a consequence of these trials, adjuvant prostate bed radiotherapy has gained the status of a standard treatment option after prostatectomy with the highest grade of recommendation for patients with pT3 pN0 tumors and positive surgical margins. But what are the optimal target volumes for postoperative radiotherapy and are they clearly defined?

3 Target Volume Definitions of Prostate Bed Radiotherapy, Inter-Observer Variability, Prostate Bed Coverage, and Associated Normal Tissue Dose–Volume Exposure

Four target volume delineation consensus guidelines were published for post-prostatectomy prostate bed radiotherapy based on different strategies (Michalski et al. 2010a; Postmanns et al. 2007; Sidhom et al. 2008; Wiltshire et al. 2007). The Toronto Group and the Australian/New Zealand Radiation Oncology Genito-Urinary Group described the anatomic boundaries of the prostate bed (Sidhom et al. 2008; Wiltshire et al. 2007). The EORTC consensus started with analyses of the locations of local recurrences after radical prostatectomy and the extents of extracapsular tumor extensions found in surgical series (Postmanns et al. 2007). The RTOG consensus tried to estimate the clinical target volume by a statistical simultaneous truth and performance level estimation method from contour datasets created by 11 experts for two exemplary cases (Michalski et al. 2010a). Contouring protocols can reduce inter-observer variation in the target volumes (Mitchell et al. 2009). Remaining variabilities in prostate bed delineation following the EORTC guidelines were analyzed by Ost et al. (2011). The mean intersection volume for the prostate bed and seminal vesicles volumes delineated by six physicians was only 5.0 and 0.9 ml, respectively, for 10 cases. The mean union volumes were 41 and 25 ml for the prostate bed and seminal vesicles, respectively. The highest variability of the target volumes was observed in the posterior and superior directions.

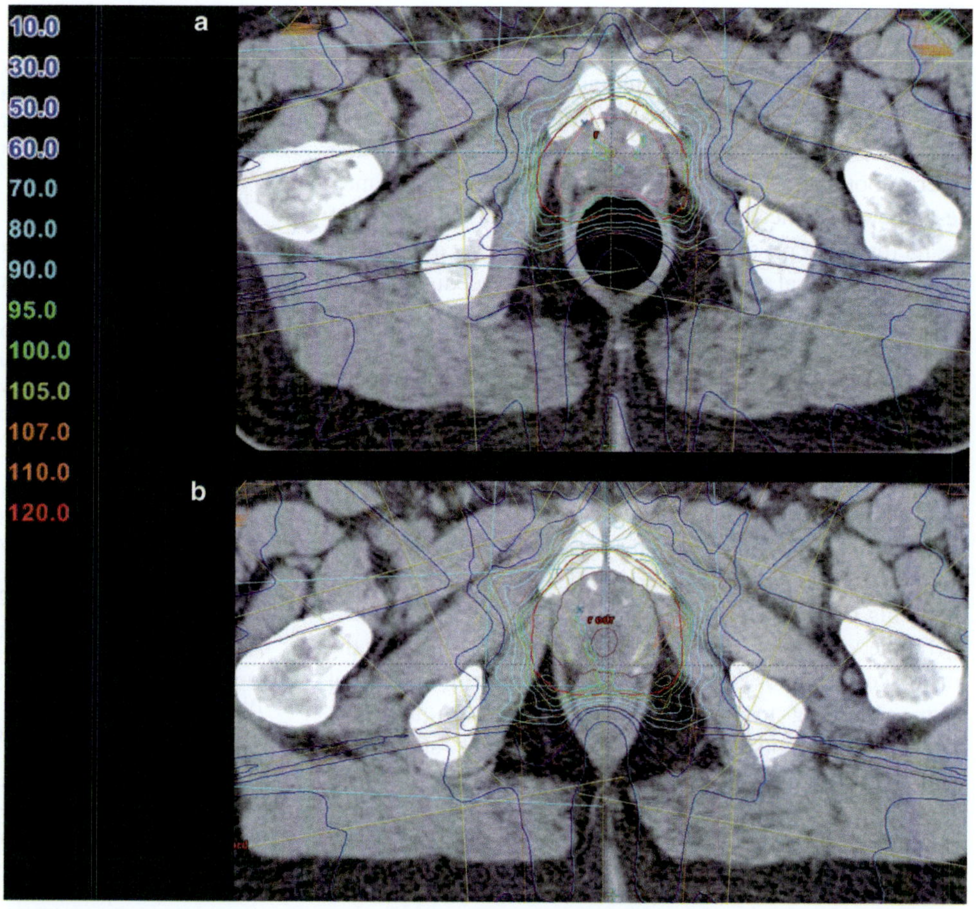

Fig. 1 Axial dose distribution of prostate bed 7-field IMRT **a** with and **b** without an endorectal balloon

In conclusion, contouring following the EORTC guideline gives room for considerable residual inter-observer variability. Croke et al. (2012) analyzed the agreement of the clinical target volumes for 20 postoperative prostate cancer patients contoured according to the four mentioned guidelines and found that the clinical target volumes according to the EORTC guideline were significantly smaller than those according to the other guidelines. In comparison with the macroscopic tumor volumes on preoperative MRI, the clinical target volumes did not cover the gross tumor in $\geq$16 of 18 patients by a varying extent, irrespectively on the guideline used. The whole prostate on preoperative MRI was covered by the clinical target volume according to the different guidelines in none of the patients. Especially, the base and the posterior aspects of the prostate capsule were poorly covered. While preoperative imaging might not be highly predictive for the location of postoperative recurrences, these data should caution not to choose too small target volumes in the superior and posterior directions where anatomic boundaries are less defined than in the lateral, anterior, and inferior directions. Malone et al. analyzed the dose–volume exposures of the rectum and bladder by treatment plans based on the four contouring guidelines (Malone et al. 2012). The restrictive Quantec dose–volume constraints for the rectum were only met in 1 of 20 cases with 3D-conformal treatment plans for target volumes according to each of the guidelines (Michalski et al. 2010b; Malone et al. 2012). Highly conformal tomotherapy IMRT plans allowed maintaining Quantec rectal constraints in 5 of 20 patients in that study. The fact, that rectum dose–volume exposure can be reduced by IMRT has also been shown in other series in the postoperative situation (Koontz et al. 2009). An endorectal balloon is used in some institutions in the postoperative situation after prostatectomy to reduce the dose to the rectum (Ishiyama et al. 2013). In our institution, we use rectal balloons filled with 100 ml air together with IMRT in most patients in the postoperative situation. The endorectal balloon allows to spare parts of the dorsal aspect of the rectum and can reduce the high dose volume in the rectum substantially (Fig. 1).

In order to be well protected against too small clinical target volume, it is useful to consider the anatomy-based target volume definition of the Toronto group (Wiltshire et al. 2007) and in addition to use the RTOG consensus definition (Michalski et al. 2010a). The RTOG consensus decreased the inferior border of the CTV from 8 mm in the guideline from Toronto to at least 8–12 mm below the vesicourethral anastomosis. The superior boundary was defined by the superior surgical clips if present or 5 mm above the inferior border of the vas deferens by the Toronto consensus.

The RTOG guideline modified that border so that the CTV usually had not to extend more than 3–4 cm above the level of the symphysis in general. Seminal vesicles remnants have to be included in the clinical target volume according to the RTOG consensus. The posterior caudal boundary is the anterior border of the rectal wall and the levator ani and may be somewhat concave around the anterior–lateral aspect of the rectum. The posterior cranial boundary is the mesorectal fascia. The lateral caudal boundaries are the medial borders of the levator ani and obturator internus muscles. The lateral cranial borders are defined by the sacrorectogenitopubic fascia. The anterior borders are the posterior edges of the pubic bones inferiorly. Above the superior aspect of the pubic bone, the CTV retracts posteriorly and encompasses the 1–2 cm of the posterior bladder wall at the minimum. With that definition, more than 1,000 patients were treated within the RTOG-0534 trial to the prostate bed alone or to the prostate bed in the second series after pelvic radiotherapy including pelvic nodal stations.

In the case of gross residual or recurrent disease, the macroscopic tumor has to be included with a margin of 1 cm according to the Toronto guidelines. In addition, surgical clips outside the above boundaries should be included excluding high lymphadenectomy vessel clips.

4 Conclusion

Postoperative adjuvant or salvage radiotherapy can offer a substantial chance of long-term freedom from PSA progression. The risk of severe late effects of this treatment modality is usually low, as found in the randomized trials on early postoperative radiotherapy using 3D techniques. Modern IMRT radiotherapy techniques can reduce the rectum and bladder exposure further. Care has to be taken to cover the posterior and superior aspects of the prostate bed.

References

Bolla M, van Poppel H, Tombal B et al (2012) Postoperative radiotherapy after radical prostatectomy for high-risk prostate cancer: long-term results of a randomized controlled trial (EORTC trial 22911). Lancet 380:2018–2027

Croke J, Malone S, Roustan-Delatour N et al (2012) Postoperative radiotherapy in prostate cancer: the case of the missing target. Int J Radiat Oncol Biol Phys 83:1160–1168

Davis JB, Reiner B, Dusserre A et al (2002) Quality assurance of the EORTC trial 2291. A phase III study of post-operative external radiotherapy in pathological stage T3N0 prostatic carcinoma: the dummy run. Radiother Oncol 64:65–73

Ishiyama H, The BS, Blanco AI et al (2013) Salvage intensity modulated radiotherapy using endorectal balloon after radical prostatectomy: clinical outcomes. Int J Urol 20:1178–1183

King CR (2012) The timing of salvage radiotherapy after radical prostatectomy: a systematic review. Int J Radiat Oncol Biol Phys 84:104–111

Koontz BF, Das S, Temple K et al (2009) Dosimetric and radiobiologic comparison of 3D conformal versus intensity modulated planning techniques for prostate bed radiotherapy. Med Dosim 34:256–260

Malone S, Croke J, Roustan-Delatour N et al (2012) Postoperative radiotherapy for prostate cancer: a comparison of four consensus guidelines and dosimetric evaluation of 3D-CRT versus tomotherapy IMRT. Int J Radiat Oncol Biol Phys 84:725–732

Michalski JM, Lawton C, El Naqa I et al (2010a) Development of RTOG consensus guidelines for the definition of the clinical target volume for postoperative conformal radiation therapy for prostate cancer. Int J Radiat Oncol Biol Phys 76:361–368

Michalski JM, Gay H, Jackson A et al (2010b) Radiation dose-volume effects in radiation-induced rectal injury. Int J Radiat Oncol Biol Phys 76(Suppl. 3):S123–S129

Mitchell DM, Perry L, Smith S et al (2009) Assessing the effect of a contouring protocol on postprostatectomy radiotherapy clinical target volumes and interphysician variation. Int J Radiat Oncol Biol Phys 75:990–993

Ost P, De Meerleer G, Vercauteren T et al (2011) Delineation of the postprostatectomy prostate bed using computed tomography: interobserver variability following the EORTC delineation guidelines. Int J Radiat Oncol Biol Phys 81:e143–e149

Postmanns P, Bossi A, Vandeputte K et al (2007) Guidelines for target volume definition in post-operative radiotherapy for prostate cancer, on behalf of the EORTC radiation oncology group. Radiother Oncol 84:121–127

Sidhom MA, Kneebone AB, Lehman M et al (2008) Post-prostatectomy radiation therapy: consensus guidelines of the Australian and NW Zealand radiation oncology genito-urinary group. Radiother Oncol 88:10–19

Swanson GP, Hussey MA, Tangen CM et al (2007) Predominant treatment failure in prostatectomy patients is local: analysis of patterns of treatment failure in SWOG 8794. J Clin Oncol 25:2225–2229

Stephenson AJ, Scardino PT, Kattan MW et al (2007) Predicting the outcome of salvage radiation therapy for recurrent prostate cancer after radical prostatectomy. J Clin Oncol 25:2035–2041

Thompson IM, Tangen CM, Paradelo J et al (2009) Adjuvant radiotherapy for pathological T3N0M0 prostate cancer significantly reduces risk of metastases and improves survival: long-term follow up of a randomized clinical trial. J Urol 181:956–962

Thompson IM, Tangen CM, Paradelo J et al (2006) Adjuvant radiotherapy for pathologically advanced prostate cancer. JAMA 296(19):2329–2335

Wiltshire KL, Brock KK, Haider MA et al (2007) Anatomic boundaries of the clinical target volume (prostate bed) after radical prostatectomy. Int J Radiat Oncol Biol Phys 69:1090–1999

Wiegel T, Bottke D, Steiner U et al (2009) Phase III postoperative adjuvant radiotherapy after radical prostatectomy alone in pT3 prostate cancer with postoperative undetectable prostate-specific antigen: ARO 96-02/AUO AP 09/95. J Clin Oncol 27:2924–2930

Randomized Trials for Adjuvant Radiotherapy

Dirk Bottke and Thomas Wiegel

Contents

Abstract

The optimal management of patients with adverse clinical and pathologic features concerning the risk of a biochemical recurrence after radical prostatectomy is still under discussion. The two treatment approaches for patients with undetectable PSA are immediate adjuvant radiotherapy or observation followed by early salvage radiation therapy in case of PSA increase out of the undetectable range. The purpose of this chapter is to review the rationale, results, and possible side effects of adjuvant radiotherapy with main focus on the three randomized phase III trials: Southwest Oncology Group (SWOG) 8794, the European Organization for Research and Treatment of Cancer (EORTC 22911), and the German Cancer Society (ARO 96-96/AUOAP 09/95). All three trials demonstrated a benefit in terms of bNED (biochemically no evidence of disease) after adjuvant radiotherapy compared to a "wait-and-see" policy. The greatest benefit was achieved in patients with positive margins and pT3 tumors. The rate of side effects was comparably low. It remains unknown if early salvage radiation therapy initiated after PSA failure is equivalent to adjuvant radiotherapy. At the present time, there are no published randomized trials to compare adjuvant radiotherapy versus salvage radiation therapy.

1 Introduction

For patients with low-risk prostate cancer/localized disease and/or higher age active surveillance or watchful waiting are suitable options regarding side effects and quality of life (Kyrdalen et al. 2013; McVey et al. 2010; Cooperberg et al. 2011; Budaus et al. 2012). Alternatively, and for more advanced stages, radical prostatectomy (RP) and radiation therapy are the two major first-line therapeutic options. There are multiple established risk factors for recurrence of prostate cancer after RP such as infiltration of the seminal

D. Bottke (✉)
Department of Radiotherapy and Radiation Oncology, University Hospital Ulm, Albert-Einstein-Allee 23, 89081 Ulm, Germany
e-mail: dirk.bottke@uniklinik-ulm.de

T. Wiegel
Klinik für Strahlentherapie und Radioonkologie, Universitätsklinikum Ulm, Albert-Einstein-Allee 23, 89081 Ulm, Germany

H. Geinitz et al. (eds.), *Radiotherapy in Prostate Cancer*, Medical Radiology. Radiation Oncology,
DOI: 10.1007/174_2013_948,

Published Online: 11 January 2014

vesicles, advanced tumor stage, positive surgical margins, a high Gleason score, and a high pre-RP PSA level (Chun et al. 2006; Salomon et al. 2003; Swindle et al. 2005; Pfitzenmaier et al. 2008; Pinto et al. 2006). However, recurrences do even occur with a favorable pattern of risk parameters; their overall absolute rates in terms of biochemical relapse are 15–30 % (Cooperberg et al. 2005; Stephenson et al. 2007, 2012; Bianco et al. 2005), while with adverse features, figures greater than 60 % have been reported (Kawamorita et al. 2009; Swanson et al. 2007).

Post-RP PSA should fall below detection threshold within 4–6 weeks (biochemically no evidence of disease; bNED), as its serum half-life is only 2–3 days (Lotan and Roehrborn 2002). Measurable PSA levels after RP indicate residual prostatic tissue, either malignant or benign (BPH). In the former case, persisting PSA levels predate clinically evident disease and do correlate well with disease progression.

A PSA value of ≥0.2 ng/ml is a widely accepted threshold to state biochemical relapse if confirmed in a second measurement, while minimum detectable concentrations are approximately 1 pg/ml or less (Chikkaveeraiah et al. 2011; Triroj et al. 2011), (Stephenson et al. 2007; Wiegel et al. 2009b; Freedland et al. 2005; Heidenreich et al. 2011; Wenz et al. 2010).

Vital tumor tissue is histopathologically proven by biopsies form the vesicourethral anastomosis in up to 53 % of all patients with rising PSA after RP without clinical correlates suggestive of recurrent tumor (Shekarriz et al. 1999).

Rising PSA values serve as a surrogate marker of recurrence after primary therapy, as they precede metastatic progression and tumor-specific death by several years (Stephenson et al. 2006). However, patients with (slowly) rising PSA values do not coercively develop distant metastases. Although there is no fixed relation between PSA level and risk of metastasis, bone scintigrams at a PSA <7 ng/ml are mostly negative, while at >20 ng/ml they are quite likely to be positive (Gomez et al. 2004; Mottet et al. 2011).

The optimal management of patients with adverse clinical and pathologic features concerning the risk of a biochemical recurrence after RP continues to be a source of controversy. The two treatment approaches for the postoperative management of these patients are immediate adjuvant radiation therapy in men with an undetectable PSA or observation followed by early salvage radiation therapy in case of PSA persistence or increase after initially postoperative undetectable values.

The purpose of this chapter is to review the rationale, results, and possible side effects of adjuvant radiotherapy with main focus on the three phase III randomized trials SWOG 8794, EORTC 22911 and ARO 96-02/AUO AP 09/95.

2 Adjuvant Radiotherapy

Adjuvant radiotherapy (ART) implies that the patient has achieved an undetectable post-RP PSA level and, despite this apparent success, is irradiated. Evidently, a dilemma results from the unavoidable overtreatment by ART, which must be justified by clinical advantage.About 40–50 % percentage of the patients are presumably overtreated, which is the percentage of bNED 5 years after RP alone (King 2012; Briganti et al. 2012). Furthermore, in patients with tumor spread beyond the pelvis, ART is useless and thus 30 % of ART patients are expected to develop progression or die despite treatment (King 2012; Richaud et al. 2010). Such concern probably causes low ART application rates (Tyldesley et al. 2012; Showalter et al. 2012; Hoffman et al. 2011). On the other hand, ART might be superior to (delayed) salvage radiation therapy for those patients who are at higher risk of post-RP recurrence and who could profit from early initiation of radiotherapy.

3 Randomized Clinical Trials

Definitive evidence that adjuvant radiotherapy improves the outcome of men with pathologically advanced prostate cancer is available from three phase III randomized trials: Southwest Oncology Group (SWOG) 8794, the European Organization for Research and Treatment of Cancer (EORTC) 22911, and the German Cancer Society (ARO 96-02/AUO AP 09/95).

All three trials demonstrated a benefit in terms of bNED after adjuvant radiation therapy (60–64 Gy) compared to a "wait-and-see" policy, mostly for pT3 cN0 or pN0 tumors (Table 1).

3.1 Southwest Oncology Group (SWOG) 8794

The SWOG 8794 was a randomized multi-institutional prospective trial of ART with 60–64 Gy versus observation alone for locally advanced prostate cancer following RP. Between 1988 and 1997, the study enrolled 425 patients with pathological stage T2 or T3 tumors who met at least one of the following pathological criteria: extracapsular extension, positive surgical margin, or seminal vesicle invasion. Pelvic lymph node dissection was obligatory, an undetectable PSA level before study entry was not mandatory. Thirty-three percentage of men in both arms had a serum PSA level >0.2 ng/ml at the time of randomization. A total 8 % of patients received pre-RP androgen deprivation therapy (ADT) (Thompson et al. 2006, 2009; van der Kwast et al. 2007).

Table 1 Overview of all three randomized trials for adjuvant radiation therapy after radical prostatectomy

Reference	n	Inclusion criteria	Randomization	Definition of biochemical recurrence	Median follow-up	Biochemical progression-free survival (bNED)	Overall survival
Thompson et al. (2009), SWOG 8794	431	pT3 pN0 ± involved SM	60–64 Gy versus "wait and see"	>0.4	152 mo.	10 years: 53 versus 30 % ($p < 0.05$)	10 years: 74 versus 66 % Median time: 15.2 versus 13.3 years $p = 0.023$
Bolla et al. (2012), EORTC 22911	1005	pT3 ± involved SM pN0 pT2 involved SM	60 Gy versus "wait and see"	>0.2	127 mo.	10 years: 61 versus 38 % ($p < 0.001$)	81 versus 77 % n.s.
Wiegel et al. (2013b), ARO 96-02	388	pT3 (± involved SM) pN0 PSA post RP undetectable	60 Gy versus "wait and see"	>0.05 + confirmation	112 mo.	10 years: 56 versus 35 % ($p < 0.0001$)	82 versus 86 % n.s.

n.s. not significant, *PSA* Prostate Specific Antigen, *SM* surgical margins

Patients randomized to the ART arm began radiotherapy within 18 weeks after surgery. Treatment delivery was done utilizing 2D-based planning aimed at the prostatic fossa and paraprostatic tissues.

The primary end point in this study was metastasis-free survival. bNED was a secondary end point. A biochemical failure was defined as PSA level >0.4 ng/ml.

At the time of initial publication of the study (median follow-up 10.6 years), there was a significant benefit for patients treated with ART in terms of PSA relapse-free survival (median time to PSA relapse 10.3 vs. 3.3 years; $p < 0.001$) and recurrence-free survival (median time 13.8 vs. 9.9 years; $p = 0.001$).

In the observation arm, the use of salvage radiotherapy was not mandated by protocol. Ultimately a total of 70 men (33 %) received postoperative radiotherapy, mostly for a rising serum PSA level. The median PSA level at the time of salvage radiotherapy in these patients was 1.0 ng/ml, which would be considered 'late' salvage therapy by current standards.

By 5 years, twice as many men in the observation arm had received hormonal therapy versus in the ART arm (21 vs. 10 %; $p < 0.001$).

The initial report did not reveal advantage for ART concerning metastasis-free survival or overall survival. However, after a median follow-up of 12.5 years, a subsequent publication demonstrated a significant improvement in metastasis-free survival (12.9 years for the observation arm vs. 14.7 years for the ART arm; $p = 0.016$) as well as in overall survival in favor of ART (59 % for the ART arm vs. 48 %, observation arm; $p = 0.023$). The authors calculated that, on average, 12.2 patients had to be treated with ART to prevent one case of metastatic disease and 9.1 patients to prevent one death. It is interesting to note that the differences between the treatment groups become measurable not before 10 years, highlighting the importance of long-term follow-up in these patients.

However, the rate of observed distant metastasis was low (37 men in the observation arm and 20 men in the radiotherapy arm) and the majority of events in the analysis of metastasis-free survival and overall survival in both groups were deaths without evidence of metastatic prostate cancer (77 of 114 men in the observation arm and 73 of 93 men in the radiotherapy arm). Consequently, it has been argued that the survival benefit after ART was largely due to a lower rate of competing-cause deaths without evidence of distant metastasis, and that the impact of ART on metastatic disease and cancer-specific death was still uncertain.

3.2 European Organization for Research and Treatment of Cancer (EORTC) 22911

The EORTC 22911 was a phase III clinical trial of ART versus no immediate further treatment for patients with pN0 M0 prostate cancer with non-organ-confined disease (extracapsular extension or seminal vesicle invasion) or positive margins. All patients had ilio-obturator lymphadenectomy. A total of 1,005 men <75 years were accrued to the trial between 1992 and 2001. An undetectable PSA following prostatectomy was not mandatory for study enrollment. In total, 69.5 % of the patients had an undetectable PSA following RP. A total of 10 % of the patients received pre-RP ADT (Bolla et al. 2005, 2012).

For patients randomized to the ART arm, radiotherapy was initiated within 16 weeks following surgery, after recovery of urinary function. RT was delivered using 2D-based treatment planning to a total dose of 60 Gy over a period of 6 weeks.

The 'revised primary end point' of the study was PSA progression (initially it was metastasis-free survival), defined as an increase of more than 0.2 ng/ml over the lowest post-RP value measured on three occasions at least 2 weeks apart.

Overall, 301 (30 %) of men had a serum PSA level >0.2 ng/ml at the time of randomization (157 in the observation arm, 144 in the radiotherapy arm). In the observation arm, patients with biochemical or local recurrence were recommended to receive salvage radiotherapy. However, only 113 (51 %) of men with recurrent cancer after RP in the control arm received salvage radiotherapy, and 45 % of these received 'late' radiotherapy on the basis of clinically evident locoregional recurrence.

After a median follow-up of 5 years, biochemical progression-free survival (bPFS), clinical progression-free survival, and the cumulative rate of locoregional failures were significantly improved in the ART group (74 vs. 56 %; $p < 0.0001$ for bPFS). In total, 22.5 % of men in the observation arm subsequently underwent pelvic RT and 9 % eventually required hormonal treatment. Overall, the rates of distant metastasis (seen in 18 men in the observation arm and 19 in the radiotherapy arm) and deaths from prostate cancer (15 in the observation arm and 8 in the radiotherapy arm) as secondary endpoints in both arms were low and not significant different as well as in overall survival ($p = 0.7$).

Updated results with 10 -year follow-up data showed a continued bPFS advantage in favor of ART (61 vs. 41 %; $p < 0.001$) and a nonsignificant trend toward improved overall survival in the ART group (81 vs. 77 %; $p > 0.1$).

3.3 German Study Group (ARO 96-02/AUO AP 09/95)

The third phase III trial of ART versus a wait-and-see policy for patients with non-organ-confined prostate cancer (pathological stage pT3 pN0) with or without positive margins enrolled a total of 385 patients between 1994 and 2004. Approximately 11 % of patients received pre-RP ADT. All patients were required to have undergone a pelvic lymph node dissection. Unlike the SWOG and EORTC trials, patients were required to have an undetectable PSA following RP. Seventy-eight patients did not achieve an undetectable PSA and were excluded from treatment according to random assignment. Of the remaining 307 patients, 34 patients on the RT arm did not receive RT and five patients on the wait-and-see arm received RT. Therefore, 114 patients underwent RT and 154 patients were treated with a wait-and-see policy (Wiegel et al. 2009a, 2013b).

The primary end point of the study was bPFS. A biochemical failure was defined as a PSA increase out of the undetectable range with a consecutive confirmation.

Unlike the prior two studies, patients in this trial were treated with more modern 3D conformal RT. RT was prescribed to a dose of 60 Gy and initiated within 6–12 weeks following RP.

Over a median follow-up duration of 54 months, 67 progression events were observed in the observation arm and 38 in the radiotherapy arm, most of which were due to biochemical recurrence. Five-year progression-free survival was 54 and 72 % in the observation and radiotherapy arms, respectively ($p = 0.0015$). The benefit in favor of adjuvant radiotherapy was also observed when the 78 patients with persistent serum PSA elevation after radical prostatectomy were included in the analysis ($p = 0.05$), and persisted across all subgroups, with the exception of those with negative surgical margins. There was no benefit for metastasis-free survival or overall survival.

In the meantime, an update with data of 10-year follow-up was presented at the 2013 Genitourinary Cancers Symposium in Orlando, Florida. At 10 years, freedom from biochemical failure was achieved in 56 % of the adjuvant radiotherapy arm versus 35 % of the wait-and-see arm, for an absolute difference of 21 % favoring adjuvant treatment ($p = 0.00002$). No significant benefit was observed for adjuvant radiotherapy regarding metastasis-free survival or overall survival, though the trial was not powered to show this.

For patients with positive surgical margins, adjuvant radiotherapy had a clear advantage: Biochemical control was achieved in 55 versus 27 % of those in the wait-and-see arm, for an absolute difference of 28 %. Baseline factors associated with greater efficacy of adjuvant radiotherapy included higher Gleason scores, higher PSA levels, and more aggressive tumors. In a multivariate analysis, adjuvant radiotherapy reduced the risk of biochemical failure by 54 %. The relative risk of biochemical failure was reduced for patients with positive surgical margins, higher PSA level, stage T3a/b, and higher Gleason scores.

3.4 Clinical Trials Overview

Patients with pT3 tumors and positive margins have been demonstrated to benefit most from ART (30 % bNED after 5 years) (Bolla et al. 2005; Thompson et al. 2006; Van der Kwast et al. 2007; Wiegel et al. 2009a). The 10-year follow-up data of all three trials confirm these results (Bolla et al. 2012; Wiegel et al. 2013b). In the prospective study of the South Western Oncology Group (SWOG), overall survival was improved from 13.5 years without to 15.2 years with ART (Thompson et al. 2009).

It is notable that the three randomized studies have used different definitions of biochemical progression: SWOG: PSA >0.4 ng/ml, EORTC: PSA >0.2 ng/ml, ARO/AUO: PSA >0.05 ng/ml.

Consequently biochemical recurrences (as an increase of PSA over the detection threshold) were detected earlier in the latter two studies, which explains the apparently worse results of the ARO study including patients with more favorable risk profile (undetectable PSA after RP) (Table 1).

In the EORTC and SWOG trials radiation was based on 2D treatment planning, where the prostatic fossa and paraprostatic tissue were targeted by using large treatment portals. Obviously, precise definition of target volumes was not essential, which is in great contrast to modern 3D conformal radiation treatment techniques such as IMRT. Compared to 2D-based planning, IMRT provides significant normal tissue sparing, but also demands exact definition of target volume.

Due to more precise techniques in treatment delivery, the Radiation Therapy Oncology Group (RTOG) (Michalski et al. 2010), the EORTC Radiation Oncology Group (Poortmans et al. 2007), and other cooperative groups (Wiltshire et al. 2007) have created consensus guidelines for delineation of target volumes for post-prostatectomy patients.

In 2011, Daly et al. reported the results of a meta-analysis of the three randomized clinical trials comparing radical prostatectomy alone to radical prostatectomy plus adjuvant radiation therapy for the treatment of men with prostate cancer and at least one of the following adverse pathologic features: extracapsular tumor extension, positive surgical margins, or seminal vesicle invasion. In total, 1,815 men were studied (385 from ARO, 1005 from EORTC, and 425 from SWOG). Analysis of oncological outcome was performed at 5- and 10-year time points. At this date, 10-year follow-up data were only available from the SWOG trial. An improved bPFS after ART could be demonstrated at 5 and 10 years with risk differences (RDs, risk difference is the risk in the treated group minus the risk in the control group) of 0.16 (95 % confidence interval [CI], 0.21–0.11) and 0.29 (95 % CI, 0.39–0.19), respectively. Furthermore, at 10 years, adjuvant radiation improved overall survival (RD: 0.11; 95 % CI, 0.20–0.02) and reduced the risk of metastatic disease (RD: 0.11; 95 % CI, 0.20–0.01) (Daly et al. 2011).

3.5 The Role of Positive Margins

Notably, central pathological review on the outcome at 5 years in the EORTC trial demonstrated positive surgical margins interacting statistically significantly with the treatment effect, to such an extent that the treatment benefit in patients with negative margins did not remain significant. The hazard ratio for the treatment benefit in the group with negative surgical margins was 0.87 ($p = 0.601$), compared to 0.38 ($p < 0.0001$) in the group with positive surgical margins according to the review pathology. Excluding the patients with a PSA of >0.2 ng/ml after prostatectomy, the hazard ratio for postoperative irradiation was 1.11 ($p = 0.740$) and 0.29 ($p < 0.0001$) for the patients with negative and positive margins, respectively (Van der Kwast et al. 2007). This benefit was also seen in the real adjuvant situation with the undetectable PSA before the start of radiation therapy (Wiegel et al. 2009a, b). After a median follow-up of nearly 5 years, there was a significant benefit from adjuvant radiation therapy for bNED: 72 versus 54 % ($p < 0.03$). In the subgroup of pT3 R1-tumors this benefit increased from 18 to 28 % (Wiegel et al. 2009a).

The location, the extent and the number of positive surgical margins after radical prostatectomy are significant predictors of biochemical progression after radical prostatectomy. The investigators of the Cleveland Clinic/Ohio found in their retrospective multi-institutional series of 7,160 patients treated with radical prostatectomy 1,540 patients with positive margins. The 7-year progression-free probability was 60 % in those patients, resulting in a hazard ratio for biochemical recurrence of 2.3 in the case of positive surgical margins compared with negative margins. The risk of biochemical recurrence was increased in patients with multiple versus solitary positive surgical margins (HR 1.4) and extensive versus focal positive surgical margins (adjusted HR 1.3) (Stephenson et al. 2009). Summing up the data from randomized trials and large retrospective series patients with positive margins and pT3-tumors have the largest profit from postoperative radiation therapy.

3.6 pT2 R1 Tumors

In the EORTC trial, when the data of patients with pT2 tumors and positive surgical margins were analyzed, there was a significant benefit with regard to 5-year biochemical progression-free survival rate in the irradiated group (76.4 vs. 52.2 % in the wait-and-see group) (Bolla et al. 2005). However, these data come from a subgroup analysis and biochemical progression-free survival was not the primary end point of this study. Therefore, the results must be interpreted with caution. The possible benefit of radiotherapy must be weighed out carefully in consideration of potential late effects as impaired erectile dysfunction.

4 The Impact of Pathology Review

The precise histologic assessment of RP specimens in patients with prostate cancer is of major importance for an accurate risk assessment of disease recurrence. The three histopathologic parameters of greatest prognostic importance are pathologic stage, Gleason score, and surgical margin status, where pathologic stage includes assessment for seminal vesicle invasion and extraprostatic extension. Several studies have previously evaluated interobserver variability between local pathologists and review pathologists in Gleason score in both the settings of needle biopsy and RP specimens (Allsbrook et al. 2001a, b; Glaessgen et al. 2004a, b; Oyama et al. 2005). In contrast, only five studies have evaluated interobserver variability in pathologic staging and margin status after RP (Van der Kwast et al. 2006; Ekici et al. 2003; Evans et al. 2008; Kuroiwa et al. 2010; Netto et al. 2011).

It is well known that pathology review has a significant impact on the results of randomized studies of definitive treatment of prostate cancer (Lawton et al. 2001). The RTOG trial 8531 randomized patients with locally advanced prostate cancer to either androgen suppression therapy (AST) or no AST after the administration of RT. In a subgroup of patients with pathologically reviewed biopsy specimens with Gleason score 8–10, there was a significant difference in overall survival (Lawton et al. 2001). However, comparable information is scarce concerning the postoperative treatment of prostate cancer.

The first published results came from the EORTC 22911 trial: 552 radical prostatectomy specimens (approximately 50 % of the patients) were retrospectively reviewed by a single pathologist with experience in urogenital pathology who examined all slides of the sample series (Van der Kwast et al. 2006, 2007). While there was a close concordance between local and review pathology regarding seminal vesicle invasion (94 %), less agreement was reached for extraprostatic extension (58 %) and for surgical margin status (69 %). An agreement rate cannot be given for the Gleason score, because it was not determined by the local pathologists in the EORTC trial (van der Kwast et al. 2006).

Biochemical progression was significantly delayed in all subgroups of men treated with adjuvant radiotherapy in EORTC 22911 ($p \leq 0.02$ for all comparisons) (Bolla et al. 2005). However, the subsequent retrospective study involving central pathology review found that only surgical margin status was significantly associated with a benefit of adjuvant radiotherapy treatment ($p < 0.01$), and that the treatment benefit in patients with negative margins was not significant, irrespective of other risk factors ($p = 0.6$) (Van der Kwast et al. 2007). Among patients with positive surgical margins, a beneficial effect on biochemical recurrence was seen with adjuvant radiotherapy treatment in men with high Gleason score cancers and those with seminal vesicle invasion.

In the German ARO/AUO study, a prospective pathology review was performed on 85 % of RP specimen of 307 patients with undetectable PSA to investigate the influence of pathology review on the analysis. There was a fair concordance between pathology review and local pathologists for seminal vesicle invasion (91 %), surgical margin status (84 %), and for extraprostatic extension (75 %). Agreement was much less for Gleason score (47 %), whereby the review pathology resulted in a shift to Gleason score seven. In contrast to the analysis of progression-free survival with local pathology, the multivariate analysis including review pathology reveals positive surgical margins and Gleason score >6 as significant prognostic factors (Bottke et al. 2013b). The authors conclude, that phase 3 studies of postoperative treatment of prostate cancer should be accomplished in the future with a pathology review. In daily practice, a second opinion by a pathologist experienced in urogenital pathology would be desirable, in particular, for high-risk patients after RP.

This is why the PREFERE study has included pathology review as a mandatory step for study inclusion in the design of the nationwide German prostate cancer trial Evaluation of Four Treatment Modalities in Prostate Cancer with Low or "Early Intermediate" Risk (PREFERE), which has just opened (Wiegel et al. 2013a; Bottke et al. 2013a). PREFERE is a prospective randomized multicenter trial developed to compare the four possible treatment options currently recommended by the European guidelines (Heidenreich et al. 2011) for favorable risk prostate cancer (radical prostatectomy, external beam radiotherapy, permanent seed implantation, and active surveillance) (Wiegel et al. 2013a).

5 Optimal Radiation Dose

To date there is no established consensus regarding the optimal prescription dose for adjuvant radiotherapy. Petrovich et al. have indicated that even low doses in the range of 45–50 Gy are beneficial in terms of local control and disease-free survival (Petrovich et al. 1991, 2002). The findings of the three randomized studies have been obtained with a prescription dose of 60 Gy with conventional irradiation over 6 weeks.

Based on American Society of Therapeutic Radiation Oncology recommendations, a dose of 64 Gy or higher (with conventional fractionation) should be prescribed (Thompson et al. 2013). Valicenti and Gomella have demonstrated evidence of improved biochemical outcomes using higher radiation doses. Despite higher doses, in fact, treatment is generally well tolerated with minimal late severe toxicity (Valicenti and Gomella 2000).

6 Adjuvant RT of Pelvic Lymph Nodes?

The three randomized trials included only patients with cN0 or pN0-disease. The effect of adjuvant RT in node-positive prostate cancer has not yet been prospectively assessed. However, there are interesting retrospective data raising the question whether men with nodal involvement confirmed during prostatectomy could benefit from adjuvant RT. A recent retrospective study reported a significant positive impact of RT in combination with hormonal therapy in patients with nodal metastases treated with RP and pelvic lymph node dissection (Da Pozzo et al. 2009). However, this study was limited by a potential patient selection bias mainly due to its retrospective and unmatched design. In fact, patients treated with adjuvant RT were those affected by more aggressive disease. For this reason, no effect of adjuvant RT on cancer-specific survival was demonstrated on univariate survival analyses. There was significant gain in predictive accuracy when adjuvant RT was included in multivariable models predicting biochemical recurrence-free and cancer-specific survival (gain: 3.3 and 3 %, respectively; all $p < 0.001$).

In a huge retrospective series, Briganti et al. assessed the effect of adjuvant RT in node-positive prostate cancer including two homogeneous matched patient cohorts exposed to either adjuvant RT plus HT or adjuvant HT alone after surgery. In this series from Milan and Jacksonville a total of 703 patients were treated, with a median follow-up of 95 months. Patients were matched for age at surgery, pathologic T stage and Gleason score, number of nodes removed, surgical margin status, and length of follow-up. The overall survival advantage was 19 % in favor of adjuvant radiation therapy plus hormonal treatment compared with hormonal treatment alone. Similarly, higher survival rates associated with the combination of HT plus RT were found when patients were stratified according to the extent of nodal invasion (namely, ≤2 vs. >2 positive nodes; all $p \leq 0.006$) (Briganti et al. 2011). Because of the retrospective nature of this series with no standardized definition of target volumes, radiation dose and duration of hormonal treatment, these results should be interpreted with caution. However, it provides support for this treatment in selected cases, whereas it should be validated in prospective clinical trials.

7 Additional Use of Hormone Therapy to ART

It is now clearly established that the standard nonoperative management for patients with locally advanced prostate adenocarcinoma includes long-term ADT. Two previous cooperative group trials have demonstrated an overall survival advantage for high-risk patients with an intact prostate treated with 2–3 years of ADT as compared to patients treated with short-term ADT (Bolla et al. 2009; Horwitz et al. 2008). It remains unknown if there is a benefit for the addition of adjuvant ADT for men with high-risk, node negative prostate adenocarcinoma initially treated with RP and pelvic lymph node dissection. The primary rationale for use of ADT post-RP is to (1) improve local control by eradicating disease in a hypoxic scar that may be radioresistant; (2) address micrometastatic disease which may have spread to the lymph nodes or distant sites; and (3) alter PSA kinetics in patients who will eventually relapse (Hanlon et al. 2004; Kaminski et al. 2003; Rossi et al. 2011).

Previous studies have indicated a potential benefit for men at high risk of recurrence treated with combination therapy. A secondary analysis of patients status-post an RP enrolled on Radiation Therapy Oncology Group (RTOG) 85-31 (Corn et al. 1999), a phase III trial comparing standard external beam RT plus immediate ADT versus RT alone for patients with nonbulky prostate cancer, found a biochemical control advantage for patients who received combination therapy as compared to men treated with RT alone. With a median follow-up of 5 years, the progression-free survival for men treated with combination therapy was estimated to be 65 % as compared to 42 % for men treated with RT alone ($p = 0.002$). Similar results were seen in a retrospective study performed at Stanford University (King et al. 2004). A subsequent RTOG study (P-0011) was designed to determine the benefit of combination therapy for man with unfavorable prognostic factors and an undetectable PSA treated with ART. This trial was unfortunately closed due to poor accrual (Elshaikh et al. 2011).

Recently, Abdollah et al. evaluated the long-term survival of prostate cancer patients who have experienced biochemical recurrence after RP and ART. Patients with a short time to biochemical recurrence, a Gleason score of ≥8 and ≥2 positive lymph nodes had lower survival rates than other patients (Abdollah et al. 2013).

In ongoing EORTC trial 22043, patients with Gleason score 5–10, undetectable PSA and pathological stage pT2R1 or pT3a-b will be randomized within 3 months after radical prostatectomy between postoperative irradiation alone or postoperative irradiation and short-term adjuvant androgen deprivation for 6 months. The primary trial endpoint is 5-year biochemical progression-free survival.

Another large randomized study is underway; RADICALS aims to recruit >4,000 patients and addresses both the comparison of ART versus SRT and the question of additional hormone treatment (using a gonadotropin-releasing hormone analog) and its appropriate timing after RP (Parker et al. 2007).

8 Side Effects and Toxicity

The three randomized clinical trials included prospective collection of data on gastrointestinal or genitourinary toxicity in the two cohorts (ART vs. observation). However, it should be mentioned that in the EORTC and SWOG trials radiation was based on 2D treatment planning which did not enable significant normal tissue sparing. In contrast, modern

3D-based radiation treatment techniques such as IMRT allow for minimization of dose to the rectum and bladder.

In the SWOG 8794 study, 3.3 % of postoperative irradiated patients developed grade 3 or higher adverse events such as rectal bleeding or proctitis as compared to 0 % of patients in the observation group ($p = 0.002$). The incidence of urethral strictures was significantly higher in the immediate postoperative RT group (17.8 vs. 9.5 %. RR 1.9, $p = 0.02$). Total urinary incontinence occurred in 6.5 % of men in the RT group as compared to 2.8 % of men in the observation group (RR 2.3, $p = 0.11$) (Thompson et al. 2006).

In the EORTC trial, there was no significant difference in high-grade (grade 3 or higher) toxicity between both arms, ART and observation. At 5 years, the cumulative incidence of late grade 3 events was 4.3 % versus 2.6 % ($p = 0.0726$). Though, in the ART cohort all late grade 2 and 3 toxicity events combined were more prominent ($p = 0.0005$). Unlike the SWOG trial, the EORTC trial did not assess total urinary incontinence, however in an interim analysis there was no significant difference concerning urinary incontinence between the two treatment arms (Bolla et al. 2005).

In the German study, which utilized 3-D-based radiation treatment planning, the incidence of late grade 3 or higher adverse events was only 0.3 % (Wiegel et al. 2009a). One patient developed a urethral stricture in the observation arm, compared to two patients in the ART arm. Urinary incontinence was not assessed in this trial.

In the EORTC study, 100 randomized patients were evaluated concerning the continence situation. There was no difference in the number of fully continent patients after 24 months between the group receiving 60 Gy and the group under observation (Van Cangh 1998).

It may be difficult to differentiate side effects of RT from pre-existing disabilities and sequelae of RP. At least equivalent rates of severe genitourinary complications following RP alone have been reported in a SEER data base analysis of 11,522 patients (Begg et al. 2002). Formenti et al. investigated the rate and degree of incontinence and erectile dysfunction after nerve-sparing RP with or without adjuvant RT. Unfortunately, follow-up examinations only comprised a questionnaire with inherent weaknesses. No difference was found between 72 patients who underwent both RP and RT and 138 patients who underwent RP only when total doses of 45–54 Gy were applied (Formenti et al. 1996).

9 Adjuvant Versus Salvage Radiation Therapy

PubMed shows >250 entries between 2008 and 2012 for a search of adjuvant radiotherapy, radical prostatectomy and just under 200 entries for salvage radiotherapy. While prospective randomized trials are underway to compare ART and SRT, many retrospective/indirect analyses into that question have been conducted (Thompson et al. 2006; Bolla et al. 2005; Wiegel et al. 2009a, b; Stephenson et al. 2007; Neuhof et al. 2007; Trock et al. 2008; Loeb et al. 2008; Bernard et al. 2010; Siegmann et al. 2011; King and Kapp 2008). Some are nonrandomized retrospective series comparing ART and SRT or ART and surveillance with delayed treatment. A consistently higher improvement in local control and freedom from biochemical failure (FFBF) has been observed in adjuvant radiation therapy compared with salvage radiation therapy patients. The 5-yr FFBF rates are approximately 69–89 % after adjuvant radiation therapy. Local control is 96–100 % after adjuvant radiation therapy and 79–93 % after salvage radiation therapy (Bottke et al. 2007, 2012; Bartkowiak et al. 2013a, b). Recently, Trabulsi and colleagues studied a group of patients undergoing adjuvant radiation therapy with a matched control group undergoing salvage radiation therapy after biochemical failure. Using a multi-institutional database of 2,299 patients, 449 patients with pT3–4 N0 disease were eligible, including 211 patients receiving adjuvant radiation therapy and 238 patients receiving salvage radiation therapy. Adjuvant radiation therapy significantly reduced the risk of long-term biochemical progression after radical prostatectomy compared with salvage radiation therapy (5-yr FFBF was 73 % after adjuvant radiation therapy compared with 50 % after salvage radiation therapy; $p = 0.007$). Gleason score eight was a significant predictor of FFBF (Trabulsi et al. 2008). These results were confirmed by others (Budiharto et al. 2010), but Ost et al. reported a better outcome after salvage radiation therapy compared with adjuvant radiation therapy (Ost et al. 2011). For all of these reasons, the best choice for treatment (adjuvant radiation therapy vs. salvage radiation therapy) has to be discussed individually with each patient, taking into account the possible risk for overtreatment with immediate postoperative irradiation.

In 2007, a prospective randomized study was initiated to address this question as well as the potential role of concomitant androgen deprivation (Parker et al. 2007). The RADICALS (Radiotherapy and Androgen Deprivation in Combination After Local Surgery) trial is an effort to evaluate adjuvant versus salvage radiation therapy. Patients are randomized after surgery to early or delayed radiation. Delayed radiation will be given when there are either two consecutive PSA rises and a final PSA >0.1 ng/ml or three consecutive PSA rises. The planned accrual is 2,600 patients with cause-specific survival being the primary outcome. There is a second randomization regarding androgen deprivation therapy.

In the meantime, the American Society for Radiation Oncology (ASTRO) and the American Urological Association (AUA) has published "The Adjuvant and Salvage

Radiotherapy After Prostatectomy: ASTRO/AUA Guideline," a comprehensive review of 324 research articles of English-language publications within the Pubmed, Embase, and Cochrane databases, published from January 1, 1990 through December 15, 2012 (Thompson et al. 2013). According to this guideline, physicians should offer adjuvant radiotherapy to patients with adverse pathologic findings at prostatectomy (i.e., seminal vesicle invasion, positive surgical margins, extraprostatic extension) and should offer salvage radiotherapy to patients with PSA or local recurrence after RP in whom there is no evidence of distant metastatic disease. The decision to administer radiotherapy should be made by the patient and the multidisciplinary treatment team with full consideration of the patient's history, values, preferences, quality of life, and functional status (Thompson et al. 2013).

10 Second Malignancies

One point that was not included in the above model is the risk of second malignancies. This is an issue of growing concern specifically with modern multiportal radiation techniques (Bartkowiak et al. 2012). Presumably, the risk is most prominent after first cancer therapy at a younger age. After prostate cancer treatment with definitive IMRT ($n = 897$) or brachytherapy ($n = 413$), no significantly increased rates of second cancer were observed within or out the treatment field compared with the general population extracted from the National Cancer Institute's Surveillance, Epidemiology, and End Results dataset combined with the 2000 census data (Zelefsky et al. 2012). While the cohorts were small and follow-up was comparably short regarding the potentially long latency of radiation induced tumors, there was a positive trend toward early diagnosis, resulting from routine surveillance and increased awareness of patients after the first malignancy.

11 Conclusions

Treatment decisions after prostatectomy require risk assessment. Adjuvant radiotherapy (ART) provides improved biochemical relapse-free survival, and potentially, overall survival for patients at high-risk following prostatectomy compared to a wait-and-see policy. The long-term results of the completed randomized trials will identify subgroups of patients who profit from ART. For others, such as pN + with ≤ 2 involved nodes, new randomized trials are planned.

It remains unknown if early salvage radiation therapy (SRT) initiated after a PSA failure is equivalent to ART. At the present time, there are no published randomized trials to compare ART versus SRT. Until the ongoing trials hopefully settle this question ART should be regarded as an option at least in the case of positive surgical margins.

Modern radiation therapy techniques like intensity-modulated radiation therapy (IMRT) or arc radiation therapy and image-guided radiotherapy (IGRT) are going to become standards. The resulting reduction of toxicity may influence the decision about how and when to apply radiotherapy in post-RP prostate cancer patients.

References

Abdollah F, Boorjian S, Cozzarini C (2013) Survival following biochemical recurrence after radical prostatectomy and adjuvant radiotherapy in patients with prostate cancer: the impact of competing causes of mortality and patient stratification. Eur Urol 64:557–564

Allsbrook WC Jr, Mangold KA, Johnson MH et al (2001a) Interobserver reproducibility of Gleason grading of prostatic carcinoma: urologic pathologists. Hum Pathol 32:74–80

Allsbrook WC Jr, Mangold KA, Johnson MH et al (2001b) Interobserver reproducibility of Gleason grading of prostatic carcinoma: general pathologist. Hum Pathol 32:81–88

Bartkowiak D, Bottke D, Wiegel T (2013a) Adjuvant radiotherapy or early salvage radiotherapy in pT3R0 or pT3R1 prostate cancer. Curr Opin Urol 23:360–365

Bartkowiak D, Bottke D, Wiegel T (2013b) Radiotherapy in the management of prostate cancer after radical prostatectomy. Future Oncol 9:669–679

Bartkowiak D, Humble N, Suhr P et al (2012) Second cancer after radiotherapy, 1981–2007. Radiother Oncol 105:122–126

Begg CB, Riedel ER, Bach PB et al (2002) Variations in morbidity after radical prostatectomy. N Engl J Med 346:1138–1144

Bernard JR Jr, Buskirk SJ, Heckman MG et al (2010) Salvage radiotherapy for rising prostate-specific antigen levels after radical prostatectomy for prostate cancer: dose-response analysis. Int J Radiat Oncol Biol Phys 76:735–740

Bianco FJ Jr, Scardino PT, Eastham JA (2005) Radical prostatectomy: long-term cancer control and recovery of sexual and urinary function ("trifecta"). Urology 66:83–94

Bolla M, De Reijke TM, Van Tienhoven G et al (2009) Duration of androgen suppression in the treatment of prostate cancer. N Engl J Med 360:2516–2527

Bolla M, Van Poppel H, Collette L et al (2005) Postoperative radiotherapy after radical prostatectomy: a randomised controlled trial (EORTC trial 22911). Lancet 366:572–578

Bolla M, Van Poppel H, Tombal B et al (2012) Postoperative radiotherapy after radical prostatectomy for high-risk prostate cancer: long-term results of a randomised controlled trial (EORTC trial 22911). Lancet 380:2018–2027

Bottke D, Abrahamsson PA, Welte B et al (2007) Adjuvant radiotherapy after radical prostatectomy. Eur J Cancer Suppl 5:171–176

Bottke D, Bartkowiak D, Schrader M et al (2012) Radiotherapy after radical prostatectomy: immediate or early delayed? Strahlenther Onkol 188:1096–1101

Bottke D, Kristiansen G, Golz R et al (2013a) Central pathology review: a must for prostate cancer studies and an option for selected patients in daily practise. Eur Urol 64:202–203

Bottke D, Golz R, Störkel S et al (2013b) Phase 3 study of adjuvant radiotherapy versus wait and see in pT3 prostate cancer: Impact of pathology review on analysis. Eur Urol 64:193–198

Briganti A, Karnes RJ, Da Pozzo LF et al (2011) Combination of adjuvante hormonal and radiation therapy significantly prolongs survival of patients with pT2-4 pN + prostate cancer: results of a matched analysis. Eur Urol 59:832–840

Briganti A, Wiegel T, Joniau S et al (2012) Early salvage radiation therapy does not compromise cancer control in patients with pT3N0 prostate cancer after radical prostatectomy: results of a match-controlled multi-institutional analysis. Eur Urol 62:472–487

Budaus L, Bolla M, Bossi A et al (2012) Functional outcomes and complications following radiation therapy for prostate cancer: a critical analysis of the literature. Eur Urol 61:112–127

Budiharto T, Perneel C, Haustermans K et al (2010) A multi-institutional analysis comparing adjuvant and salvage radiation therapy for high-risk prostate cancer patients with undetectable PSA after prostatectomy. Radiother Oncol 97:474–479

Chikkaveeraiah BV, Mani V, Patel V et al (2011) Microfluidic electrochemical immunoarray for ultrasensitive detection of two cancer biomarker proteins in serum. Biosens Bioelectron 26:4477–4483

Chun FK, Graefen M, Zacharias M et al (2006) Anatomic radical retropubic prostatectomy-long-term recurrence-free survival rates for localized prostate cancer. World J Urol 24:273–280

Cooperberg MR, Carroll PR, Klotz L (2011) Active surveillance for prostate cancer: progress and promise. J Clin Oncol 29:3669–3676

Cooperberg MR, Pasta DJ, Elkin EP et al (2005) The University of California, San Francisco cancer of the prostate risk Assessment score: a straightforward and reliable preoperative predictor of disease recurrence after radical prostatectomy. J Urol 173:1938–1942

Corn BW, Winter K, Pilepich MV (1999) Does androgen suppression enhance the efficacy of postoperative irradiation? A secondary analysis of RTOG 85-31. Radiat Ther Oncol Group Urol 54:495–502

Da Pozzo LF, Cozzarini C, Briganti A et al (2009) Long-term follow-up of patients with prostate cancer and nodal metastases treated by pelvic lymphadenectomy and radical prostatectomy: the positive impact of adjuvant radiotherapy. Eur Urol 55:1003–1011

Daly T, Hickey BE, Lehman M et al (2011) Adjuvant radiotherapy following radical prostatectomy for prostate cancer. Cochrane Database Syst Rev 12:CD007234

Ekici S, Ayhan A, Erkan I et al (2003) The role of the pathologist in the evaluation of radical prostatectomy specimens. Scand J Urol Nephrol 37:387–391

Elshaikh MA, Ibrahim DR, Stricker H et al (2011) Adjuvant radiation treatment after prostatectomy. Where do we stand? Can J Urol 18:5592–5600

Evans AJ, Henry PC, Van der Kwast TH et al (2008) Interobserver variability between expert urologic pathologists for extraprostatic extension and surgical margin status in radical prostatectomy specimens. Am J Surg Pathol 32:1503–1512

Formenti SC, Lieskovsky G, Simoneau AR et al (1996) Impact of moderate dose of postoperative radiation on urinary continence and potency in patients with prostate cancer treated with nerve sparing prostatectomy. J Urol 155:616–619

Freedland SJ, Humphreys EB, Mangold LA et al (2005) Risk of prostate cancer-specific mortality following biochemical recurrence after radical prostatectomy. JAMA 294:433–439

Glaessgen A, Hamberg H, Pihl CG et al (2004a) Interobserver reproducibility of modified Gleason score in radical prostatectomy specimens. Virchows Arch 445:17–21

Glaessgen A, Hamberg H, Pihl CG et al (2004b) Interobserver reproducibility of percent Gleason grade 4/5 in prostate biopsies. J Urol 171:664–667

Gomez P, Manoharan M, Kim SS et al (2004) Radionuclide bone scintigraphy in patients with biochemical recurrence after radical prostatectomy: when is it indicated? BJU Int 94:299–302

Hanlon AL, Horwitz EM, Hanks GE et al (2004) Short-term androgen deprivation and PSA doubling time: their association and relationship to disease progression after radiation therapy for prostate cancer. Int J Radiat Oncol Biol Phys 58:43–52

Heidenreich A, Bellmunt J, Bolla M et al (2011) EAU guidelines on prostate cancer. Part 1: screening, diagnosis, and treatment of clinically localised disease. Eur Urol 59:61–71

Hoffman KE, Nguyen PL, Chen MH et al (2011) Recommendations for post-prostatectomy radiation therapy in the United States before and after the presentation of randomized trials. J Urol 185:116–120

Horwitz EM, Bae K, Hanks GE et al (2008) Ten-year follow-up of radiation therapy oncology group protocol 92-02: a phase III trial of the duration of elective androgen deprivation in locally advanced prostate cancer. J Clin Oncol 26:2497–2504

Kaminski JM, Hanlon AL, Joon DL et al (2003) Effect of sequencing of androgen deprivation and radiotherapy on prostate cancer growth. Int J Radiat Oncol Biol Phys 57:24–28

Kawamorita N, Saito S, Ishidoya S et al (2009) Radical prostatectomy for high-risk prostate cancer: biochemical outcome. Int J Urol 16:733–738

King CR (2012) Adjuvant versus salvage radiotherapy after prostatectomy: the apple versus the orange. Int J Radiat Oncol Biol Phys 82:1045–1046

King CR, Kapp DS (2008) Radiotherapy after prostatectomy: is the evidence for dose escalation out there? Int J Radiat Oncol Biol Phys 71:346–350

King CR, Presti JC Jr, Gill H et al (2004) Radiotherapy after radical prostatectomy: does transient androgen suppression improve outcomes? Int J Radiat Oncol Biol Phys 59:341–347

Kyrdalen AE, Dahl AA, Hernes E et al (2013) A national study of adverse effects and global quality of life among candidates for curative treatment for prostate cancer. BJU Int 111:221–232

Kuroiwa K, Shiraishi T, Ogawa O et al (2010) Discrepancy between local and central pathological review of radical prostatectomy specimens. J Urol 183:952–957

Lawton CA, Winter K, Murray K et al (2001) Updated results of the phase III radiation therapy oncology group (RTOG) trial 85-31 evaluating the potential benefit of androgen suppression following standard radiation therapy for unfavorable prognosis carcinoma of the prostate. Int J Radiat Oncol Biol Phys 49:937–946

Loeb S, Roehl KA, Viprakasit DP et al (2008) Long-term rates of undetectable PSA with initial observation and delayed salvage radiotherapy after radical prostatectomy. Eur Urol 54:88–94

Lotan Y, Roehrborn CG (2002) Clearance rates of total prostate specific antigen (PSA) after radical prostatectomy in African-Americans and Caucasians. Prostate Cancer Prostatic Dis 5:111–144

McVey GP, McPhail S, Fowler S et al (2010) Initial management of low-risk localized prostate cancer in the UK: analysis of the British association of urological surgeons cancer registry. BJU Int 106:1161–1164

Michalski JM, Lawton C, El Naqa I et al (2010) Development of RTOG consensus guidelines for the definition of the clinical target volume for postoperative conformal radiation therapy for prostate cancer. Int J Radiat Oncol Biol Phys 76:361–368

Mottet N, Bellmunt J, Bolla M et al (2011) EAU guidelines on prostate cancer. Part II: treatment of advanced, relapsing, and castration-resistant prostate cancer. Eur Urol 59:572–583

Netto GJ, Eisenberger M, Epstein JI (2011) Interobserver variability in histologic evaluation of radical prostatectomy between central and local pathologists: findings of TAX 3501 multinational clinical trial. Urology 77:1155–1157

Neuhof D, Hentschel T, Bischof M et al (2007) Long-term results and predictive factors of three-dimensional conformal salvage radiotherapy for biochemical relapse after prostatectomy. Int J Radiat Oncol Biol Phys 67:1411–1417

Ost P, De Troyer B, Fonteyne V et al (2011) A matched control analysis of adjuvant and salvage high-dose postoperative intensity-modulated radiotherapy for prostate cancer. Int J Radiat Oncol Biol Phys 80:1316–1322

Oyama T, Allsbrook WC Jr, Kurokawa K et al (2005) A comparison of interobserver reproducibility of Gleason grading of prostatic carcinoma in Japan and the United States. Arch Pathol Lab Med 129:1004–1010

Parker C, Sydes MR, Catton C et al (2007) Radiotherapy and androgen deprivation in combination after local surgery (RADICALS): a new medical research council/national cancer institute of Canada phase III trial of adjuvant treatment after radical prostatectomy. BJU Int 99:1376–1379

Petrovich Z, Lieskovsky G, Langholz B (2002) Postoperative radiotherapy in 423 patients with pT3N0 prostate cancer. Int J Radiat Oncol Biol Phys 53:600–609

Petrovich Z, Lieskovsky G, Langholz B (1991) Radiotherapy following radical prostatectomy in patients with adenocarcinoma of the prostate. Int J Radiat Oncol Biol Phys 21:949–954

Pfitzenmaier J, Pahernik S, Tremmel T et al (2008) Positive surgical margins after radical prostatectomy: do they have an impact on biochemical or clinical progression? BJU Int 102:1413–1418

Pinto F, Prayer-Galetti T, Gardiman M et al (2006) Clinical and pathological characteristics of patients presenting with biochemical progression after radical retropubic prostatectomy for pathologically organ-confined prostate cancer. Urol Int 76:202–208

Poortmans P, Bossi A, Vandeputte K et al (2007) Guidelines for target volume definition in post-operative radiotherapy for prostate cancer, on behalf of the EORTC radiation oncology group. Radiother Oncol 84:121–127

Richaud P, Sargos P, Henriques de Figueiredo B et al (2010) Postoperative radiotherapy of prostate cancer. Cancer Radiother 14:500–503

Rossi CJ Jr, Joe Hsu IC, Abdel-Wahab M et al (2011) ACR appropriateness criteria postradical prostatectomy irradiation in prostate cancer. Am J Clin Oncol 34:92–98

Salomon L, Anastasiadis AG, Antiphon P et al (2003) Prognostic consequences of the location of positive surgical margins in organ-confined prostate cancer. Urol Int 70:291–296

Shekarriz B, Upadhyay J, Wood DP Jr et al (1999) Vesicourethral anastomosis biopsy after radical prostatectomy: predictive value of prostate-specific antigen and pathologic stage. Urology 54:1044–1048

Showalter TN, Ohri N, Teti KG et al (2012) Physician beliefs and practices for adjuvant and salvage radiation therapy after prostatectomy. Int J Radiat Oncol Biol Phys 82:e233–e238

Siegmann A, Bottke D, Faehndrich J et al (2011) Dose escalation for patients with decreasing PSA during radiotherapy for elevated PSA after radical prostatectomy improves biochemical progression-free survival: results of a retrospective study. Strahlenther Onkol 187:467–472

Stephenson AJ, Bolla M, Briganti A et al (2012) Postoperative radiation therapy for pathologically advanced prostate cancer after radical prostatectomy. Eur Urol 61:443–451

Stephenson AJ, Kattan MW, Eastham JA et al (2006) Defining biochemical recurrence of prostate cancer after radical prostatectomy: a proposal for a standardized definition. J Clin Oncol 24:3973–3978

Stephenson AJ, Scardino PT, Kattan MW et al (2007) Predicting the outcome of salvage radiation therapy for recurrent prostate cancer after radical prostatectomy. J Clin Oncol 25:2035–2041

Stephenson AJ, Wood DP, Kattan MW et al (2009) Location, extent and number of positive surgical margins do not improve accuracy of predicting prostate cancer recurrence after radical prostatectomy. J Urol 182:1357–1363

Swanson GP, Hussey MA, Tangen CM et al (2007) Predominant treatment failure in postprostatectomy patients is local: analysis of patterns of treatment failure in SWOG 8794. J Clin Oncol 25:2225–2229

Swindle P, Eastham JA, Ohori M et al (2005) Do margins matter? The prognostic significance of positive surgical margins in radical prostatectomy specimens. J Urol 174:903–907

Thompson IM Jr, Tangen CM, Paradelo J et al (2006) Adjuvant radiotherapy for pathologically advanced prostate cancer: a randomized clinical trial. JAMA 296:2329–2335

Thompson IM, Tangen CM, Paradelo J et al (2009) Adjuvant radiotherapy for pathological T3N0M0 prostate cancer significantly reduces risk of metastases and improves survival: long-term followup of a randomized clinical trial. J Urol 181:956–962

Thompson IM, Valicenti RK, Albertsen P et al (2013) Adjuvant and salvage radiotherapy after prostatectomy: AUA/ASTRO guideline. J Urol 190:441–449

Trabulsi EJ, Valicenti RK, Hanlon AL et al (2008) A multi-institutional matched-control analysis of adjuvant and salvage postoperative radiation therapy for pT3-4N0 prostate cancer. Urology 72:1298–1302; discussion 1302–1294

Triroj N, Jaroenapibal P, Shi H et al (2011) Microfluidic chip-based nanoelectrode array as miniaturized biochemical sensing platform for prostate-specific antigen detection. Biosens Bioelectron 26:2927–2933

Trock BJ, Han M, Freedland SJ et al (2008) Prostate cancer-specific survival following salvage radiotherapy vs observation in men with biochemical recurrence after radical prostatectomy. JAMA 299:2760–2769

Tyldesley S, Peacock M, Morris JW et al (2012) The need for, and utilization of prostate-bed radiotherapy after radical prostatectomy for patients with prostate cancer in British Columbia. Can Urol Assoc J 6:89–94

Valicenti RK, Gomella LG (2000) Durable efficacy of adjuvant radiation therapy for prostate cancer: will the benefit last? Semin Urol Oncol 18:115–120

Van Cangh PJ, Richard F, Lorge F et al (1998) Adjuvant radiation therapy does not cause urinary incontinence after radical prostatectomy: results of a prospective randomized study. J Urol 159:164–166

Van der Kwast TH, Collette L, Van Poppel H et al (2006) Impact of pathology review of stage and margin status of radical prostatectomy specimens (EORTC trial 22911). Virchows Arch 449:428–434

Van der Kwast TH, Bolla M, van Poppel H et al (2007) Identification of patients with prostate cancer who benefit from immediate postoperative radiotherapy: EORTC 22911. J Clin Oncol 25:4178–4186

Wenz F, Martin T, Böhmer D et al (2010) The German S3 guideline prostate cancer: aspects for the radiation oncologist. Strahlenther Onkol 186:531–534

Wiegel T, Albers P, Bussar-Maatz R et al (2013a) PREFERE—the German prostatic cancer study: questions and claims surrounding study initiation in January 2013. Urol A 52:576–579

Wiegel T, Bottke D, Bartkowiak D et al (2013b) Phase III results of adjuvant radiotherapy versus wait-and-see in patients with pT3 prostate cancer following radical prostatectomy (ARO96-02/AUO AP 9/95). In: Genitourinary Cancers Symposium, Abstract 4. Presented, 14 Feb 2013

Wiegel T, Bottke D, Steiner U et al (2009a) Phase III postoperative adjuvant radiotherapy after radical prostatectomy compared with radical prostatectomy alone in pT3 prostate cancer with postoperative undetectable prostate-specific antigen: ARO 96-02/AUO AP 09/95. J Clin Oncol 27:2924–2930

Wiegel T, Lohm G, Bottke D et al (2009b) Achieving an undetectable PSA after radiotherapy for biochemical progression after radical prostatectomy is an independent predictor of biochemical outcome–results of a retrospective study. Int J Radiat Oncol Biol Phys 73:1009–1016

Wiltshire KL, Brock KK, Haider MA et al (2007) Anatomic boundaries of the clinical target volume (prostate bed) after radical prostatectomy. Int J Radiat Oncol Biol Phys 69:1090–1099

Zelefsky MJ, Housman DM, Pei X et al (2012) Incidence of secondary cancer development after high-dose intensity-modulated radiotherapy and image-guided brachytherapy for the treatment of localized prostate cancer. Int J Radiat Oncol Biol Phys 83:953–959

Salvage Radiotherapy After Radical Prostatectomy

Alexandros Papachristofilou, Pirus Ghadjar, and Frank Zimmermann

Contents

Abstract

Salvage radiation therapy is the sole curative treatment for patients experiencing biochemical relapse after radical surgical treatment of prostate cancer. The main dilemma in salvage radiation therapy is, whether or not biochemical relapse represents purely localized recurrent disease in the prostatic fossa or systemic micrometastasis. Initiating salvage radiation therapy at an early time point raises its chances of success, but may lead to overtreatment of patients. Target volume definition and treatment techniques are a matter of current research, with still many questions unanswered. Strategies of treatment escalation either by increasing the treatment dose or combining radiation therapy with androgen deprivation therapy are being addressed in clinical trials.

1 Introduction

Within 5 years after radical prostatectomy (RP) 15–40 % (Han et al. 2003; Ward and Moul 2005) of the patients experience a biochemical relapse, defined as rising prostate specific antigen (PSA). The risk may be even higher with longer follow-up (Amling et al. 2000) and in patients with an initial PSA value higher than 10 ng/ml and a Gleason Score $\geq$7 (Kupelian et al. 1997). Histopathologic risk factors for recurrent disease include higher Gleason Score, extracapsular extension (pT3a), invasion of the seminal vesicles (pT3b), and positive resection margins (R1).

Asymptomatic biochemical relapse evolves to bone metastasis after a median time of 8 years (Pound et al. 1999). Systemic disease progression is more pronounced with PSA-doubling time of <12 months, resulting in a 5-year-metastatic progression-free survival of less than 20 % (Slovin et al. 2005).

Salvage radiotherapy (RT) is the only potentially curative treatment in this situation, with the aim to eradicate local recurrence, prevent metastasis, and provide a durable

A. Papachristofilou · F. Zimmermann (✉)
Department of Radiation Oncology,
University Hospital Basel, Basel, Switzerland
e-mail: fzimmermann@uhbs.ch; radioonkologie@uhbs.ch

P. Ghadjar
Department of Radiation Oncology, Inselspital,
Bern University Hospital, Bern, Switzerland

H. Geinitz et al. (eds.), *Radiotherapy in Prostate Cancer*, Medical Radiology. Radiation Oncology,
DOI: 10.1007/174_2013_939,
Published Online: 10 December 2013

freedom from further disease progression. The risk of biochemical relapse is particularly high in patients, who were eligible for adjuvant RT directly after surgery due to risk factors such as pT3a-stage and/or R1-resection, but who did not receive this therapy due to patient's and/or physician's preference.

The main argument for omitting adjuvant radiotherapy and resorting to salvage radiotherapy in case of biochemical relapse is the avoidance of overtreating patients, who may have been cured by surgery alone. Three randomized controlled trials compared adjuvant RT versus observation in patients with risk factors (pT3a/R1) after RP and demonstrated improved biochemical control rates (Bolla et al. 2005; Thompson et al. 2006; Wiegel et al. 2009) through adjuvant RT, whereas metastasis-free survival and overall survival was improved in one of these trials after 12.7 years of follow-up (Thompson et al. 2009). However, despite having high-risk factors for local recurrence after RP, approximately 45–54 % of the patients on the control arms of these studies did not experience biochemical relapse (Bolla et al. 2005; Thompson et al. 2006; Wiegel et al. 2009). Thus, overtreatment with adjuvant radiotherapy is an issue and selective (early) salvage treatment for patients with biochemical relapse might be an alternative strategy. Salvage RT has only been studied in retrospective studies with doses ranging from 64 to 72 Gy. The dose level has often been guided by the absence or presence of macroscopic tumor recurrence and the preirradiation PSA. The level of evidence concerning the effectiveness and tolerability of salvage RT is thus not as high as in the adjuvant setting.

Randomized trials are currently investigating the role of adjuvant and salvage RT, focusing on timing of treatment initiation, interaction with androgen deprivation therapy (ADT), and efficacy of different radiation dose levels.

2 Definition of Biochemical Relapse

Approximately 15–40 % of prostate cancer patients experience a rise in PSA after RP. The definition of biochemical relapse after RP remains a matter of controversy, with several definitions found in the literature.

The current National Comprehensive Cancer Network (NCCN)-guidelines (NCCN 2012) define biochemical relapse after RP as either *"failure of PSA to fall to undetectable levels"* or *"PSA detectable and rising at 2 or more subsequent determinations"*. The Guidelines of the European Association of Urology (EAU) (European Urology Association 2012) state that *"after RP, a serum PSA level of more than 0.2 ng/mL can be associated with residual or recurrent disease"*.

At least one study has demonstrated, that a postoperative PSA of 0.1 ng/ml does not necessarily translate into a high risk of subsequent biochemical relapse (Schild et al. 1996). Several surgical series (Paul et al. 2004; Shah et al. 2001; Tongco et al. 2001) have shown residual normal prostate tissue remains after RP, especially in the bladder neck and apex regions, which may be responsible for low, yet detectable postsurgical PSA values.

Stephenson et al. carried out a systematic analysis on 3,125 patients to define appropriate PSA thresholds for disease progression (Stephenson et al. 2007). A PSA of 0.2 ng/ml and rising was found as adequate for selection of patients to undergo salvage RT, while a PSA of 0.4 ng/ml followed by another rise was deemed most appropriate to define patients in high risk to develop metastatic disease. Ultra-sensitive PSA-testing may allow to detect multiple, consecutive PSA-rises highly suggestive of biochemical relapse, despite the highest PSA-value being $\leq$0.2 ng/ml.

The authors believe that biochemical relapse after RP should be defined as a PSA >0.2 ng/ml confirmed by a second measurement.

3 Filtering Out the Patients with a Pure Local Tumor Recurrence

Salvage RT provides the sole curative option after RP in case of biochemical relapse. However, a sizable amount of patients undergoing salvage RT will not respond to treatment, showing a continuous PSA rise after therapy or only a short-lasting PSA remission.

Predictive factors for a long-lasting biochemical progression-free survival (bPFS) after salvage RT include (Stephenson et al. 2007; Meng et al. 2002; Wiegel et al. 2009; Pazona et al. 2005; Buskirk et al. 2006; Ward et al. 2004; Macdonald et al. 2008):

(a) A slow slope of PSA, defined as: a rise >1 year after surgery, PSA-doubling time >12 months, PSA-increase within 12 months (PSA-velocity/year) <0.75 ng/ml
(b) A better differentiated cancer (Gleason Score <8)
(c) Positive resection margins
(d) Negative pelvic lymph nodes.

Diagnostic procedures can help to detect local recurrence and rule out distant metastasis. Magnetic resonance imaging (MRI) of the pelvis using a 3 tesla machine or an endorectal coil combined with dynamic contrast-enhanced or diffusion-weighted techniques may have a higher sensitivity than standard MRI or computed tomography (CT). This maybe even further increased by adding MR-spectroscopy in cases with previous negative biopsies of the prostatic fossa (Huch Böni et al. 1996; Sciarra et al. 2008, 2010; Giannarini et al. 2012). The accuracy of detecting tumor cells may be around

90 %, but is not conclusively agreed by all authors (Liauw et al. 2012). However, solely endorectal coils and 3 tesla MRI have so far been introduced into widespread clinical practice, partially due to reimbursement issues with more advanced and expensive techniques.

Choline positron emission tomography (C-PET) has the major advantage over MRI in its ability to detect not only local recurrent disease, but also to rule out systemic metastasis. The sensitivity of C-PET increases with PSA and with increasing PSA-velocity, with a detection rate of 50 % and higher for PSA-doubling times of less than 3 months (Picchio et al. 2011); a current review suggests to consider C-PET as a diagnostic procedure in case of PSA >1 ng/ml, whereas others describe a sensitivity of more than 80 % only for PSA-levels beyond 1.7 ng/ml (Picchio et al. 2011; Graute et al. 2012). In summary, results are heterogeneous, with the sensitivity depending on PSA-magnitude and velocity of 38–98 %, and a detection rate of 15–91 % for PSA-values between 1 and 3 ng/ml.

Routine radionuclide bone scans cannot be recommended for patients with rising PSA after RP, who are being considered for salvage RT. Both the sensitivity and negative predictive value are too low to guide clinical management (Cher et al. 1998).

Perhaps the most pragmatic approach to identify patients profiting from salvage RT may be to measure PSA immediately before commencing treatment and again at a dose level of 50 or 60 Gy (Wiegel et al. 2002). Patients will most probably not benefit from salvage RT, if the PSA continues to rise during treatment at these dose levels. These patients may be spared of treatment-related toxicity by early termination of salvage RT between 50 and 60 Gy. This strategy can only be followed in patients receiving pure salvage RT without ADT. Although this strategy cannot be generally recommended due to its low level of evidence, it could be considered for patients being treated for rising PSA with adverse prognostic features indicative of systemic disease (high Gleason score, short PSA-doubling time and high PSA velocity).

4 Timing of Treatment

A critical question in the management of patients with biochemical relapse, who are planned to undergo salvage RT, is when to start treatment.

Retrospective analyses demonstrated enhanced bPFS in patients with low PSA before treatment (Stephenson et al. 2007; Meng et al. 2002; Wiegel et al. 2009; Pazona et al. 2005; Buskirk et al. 2006; Ward et al. 2004; Macdonald et al. 2008). On the other hand, early salvage RT can lead to earlier treatment-related toxicity or interfere with the post-surgical recovery of the patient, including bladder control and sexual function. The NCCN guidelines (NCCN 2012) do not state at which PSA-threshold salvage RT should be initiated and merely suggest administering salvage RT before the PSA exceeds 1.5 ng/ml. The guidelines of the EAU (European Urology Association 2012) suggest to initiate salvage RT at PSA-levels <0.5 ng/ml.

A radiobiological model to predict bPFS according to PSA prior to salvage RT was developed by pooling in the data from numerous published patient series. For every additional 1 ng/ml of PSA prior to salvage RT a drop in bPFS was estimated at 18.3 % (Ohri et al. 2012). This is in good accordance with another recent publication, emphasizing the early onset of salvage RT, while losing bPFS of even 2.6 % for each incremental 0.1 ng/ml (King 2012).

The introduction of ultra-sensitive PSA-testing may lead to overtreatment of patients with low, yet detectable and rising PSA-levels <0.2 ng/ml. These patients may have never experienced a true biochemical relapse without any treatment, so that ultra-sensitive PSA-testing must be used with caution (European Urology Association 2012).

The authors believe, that salvage RT should preferably be initiated at PSA-levels of >0.2 ng/ml and <0.5 ng/ml, provided that the patient has completed his postsurgical recovery and his life expectancy beyond prostatic cancer is still respectable and above 5 years. Patients undergoing ultra-sensitive PSA-testing as follow-up may show multiple consecutive PSA rises. Advising treatment at PSA <0.2 ng/ml is legitimate in these cases, following a throughout discussion with the patient about the pros and cons of early salvage RT including the possibility of overtreatment.

5 Target Volume Definition

Target volume definition for prostate cancer can be more challenging than in the primary treatment setting. Both the European Organisation for Research and Treatment of Cancer (EORTC) and the Radiation Therapy Oncology Group (RTOG) have developed consensus guidelines for the postoperative clinical target volume (CTV) delineation of the prostatic fossa (Poortmans et al. 2007; Michalski et al. 2010). These guidelines define the boundaries of the CTV by anatomical structures visible in the RT planning CT. It does, however, seem prudent to take into account the initial size of the prostate and delineate the CTV accordingly, if preoperative imaging is available. Imaging studies describe the majority of the tumor recurrences at the urethral anastomosis and also in the previous seminal vesicle area. It seems appropriate, with missing initial preoperative imaging, to calculate the extension of the prostate based on the pathologists report, with the apex usually being located at the inferior junction of the pubical arch. The location of the rectum has to be taken into account as well, usually

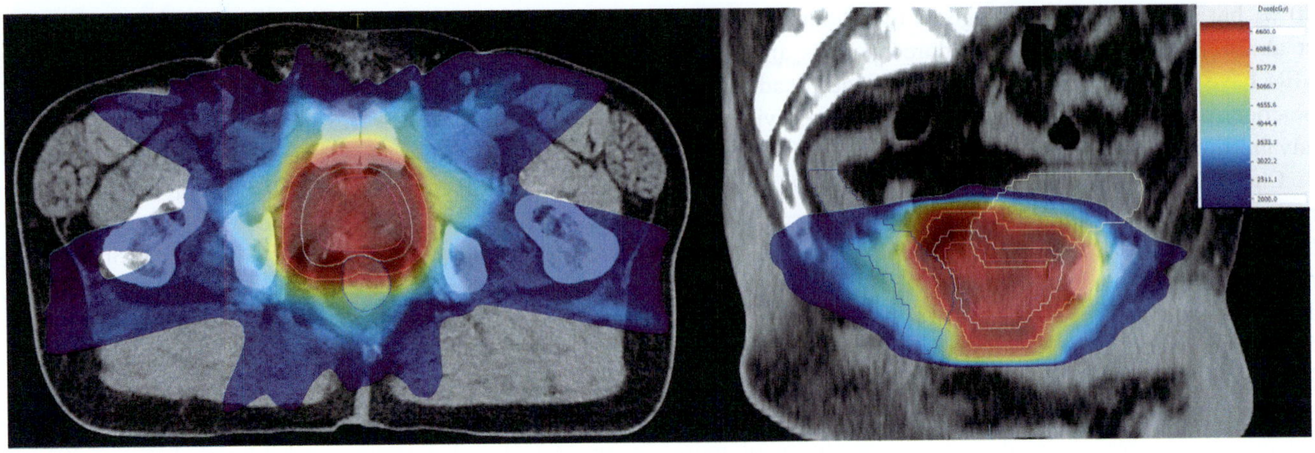

Fig. 1 Dose distribution with an IMRT plan for salvage RT of the prostatic fossa, prescribed dose 66 Gy, 7 beams (XIO®, Elekta). *Pink* prostatic fossa, *white* clinical target volume, *orange* planning target volume, *yellow* bladder, *blue* rectum

being shifted ventrally between the former seminal vesicle region and lymphatic drainage of the small pelvis.

The question of elective treatment of the pelvic lymph nodes in the postoperative setting remains open. All three randomized studies on adjuvant RT (Bolla et al. 2005; Thompson et al. 2006; Wiegel et al. 2009) defined only the prostatic fossa as CTV. One retrospective study has demonstrated superior bPFS through pelvic nodal irradiation over only prostatic fossa RT in high-risk patients (pT3a/b, Gleason Score ≥8, initial PSA >20 ng/ml) (Spiotto et al. 2007). However, 17 % of patients in that study had pathologic pelvic nodes (pN1) found during RP. A retrospective study in pN1 patients compared adjuvant ADT with or without pelvic irradiation and showed superior bPFS and cancer-specific survival (CSS) through adjuvant pelvic irradiation (Da Pozzo et al. 2009). Finally, the efficacy of elective nodal irradiation in the setting of primary prostate RT is still highly debatable; as shown in the RTOG-9413 and GETUG-01 studies (Lawton et al. 2007; Pommier et al. 2007). An appropriate guideline for delineation of pelvic lymph nodes to be contoured in prostate RT has been published by the RTOG (2012).

The authors believe, that salvage RT for the majority of patients should only target the prostatic fossa, according to international published guidelines. Some patients may profit from elective nodal irradiation, particularly those harboring high-risk tumor features (≥T3a, Gleason score ≥8, initial PSA >20 ng/ml), especially if an adequate pathologic staging of the pelvic lymph nodes has not been performed during RP. In patients experiencing biochemical relapse after RP and with a known pN1-stage disease, it seems advisable to include the pelvic lymph nodes in the RT volumes too. On the other hand, pelvic RT should be withheld from patients bearing typical risk factors for clinically relevant late sequela as severe enteritis.

6 Radiation Therapy Techniques

Conformal RT techniques have been widely employed in the primary treatment of prostate cancer. 3D-conformal RT (CRT) has replaced conventional RT, allowing for dose escalation without greater risk for genitourinary (GU) and gastrointestinal (GI) toxicity (Dearnaley et al. 1999). The attempt to safely escalate the total dose delivered to the prostate has led to the introduction of intensity modulated RT (IMRT, Fig. 1). High-dose IMRT has replaced CRT in many centers, demonstrating so far a favorable toxicity profile (Sheets et al. 2012).

The role of modern RT techniques in the post-prostatectomy setting is not well defined, due to the lack of prospective studies in this area. Some recent trials have compared the dose distribution of CRT and IMRT, with a superiority of IMRT regarding the coverage of the prostate bed and the reduction of radiation dose to the organs at risk (Riou et al. 2012).

Most published retrospective clinical studies have included patients treated over decades with different RT techniques. In the past couple of years, evidence from single institution experiences has emerged on the role of modern techniques in the salvage RT setting. A retrospective study from the Memorial Sloan-Kettering Cancer Center has demonstrated lower rates of late GI toxicity with IMRT than with CRT. Late GU-toxicity was not influenced by the RT technique. It is important to note, that the majority of the patients in this study were treated with doses ≥70 Gy (Goenka et al. 2011). An Italian retrospective study demonstrated lower rates of acute upper GI toxicity with IMRT than with CRT, probably because of better sparing of small bowel through IMRT (Alongi et al. 2009). Quite favorable acute and late GU/GI toxicity rates have been reported in a single institution study of image-guided IMRT (Nath et al.

2010). IMRT is particularly attractive in the case of pelvic nodal irradiation from the dosimetric point of view (Digesú et al. 2011).

The authors believe that the use of highly conformal techniques for salvage RT is justified. Whether IMRT and image-guided RT (IGRT) lead to a better outcome or limit treatment-related toxicity, cannot be definitely answered based on current evidence. However, the so far published results from small retrospective trials seem promising. Therefore IMRT and IGRT should be used, whenever they are available.

7 Treatment Outcome

Treatment outcome after salvage RT for biochemical relapse is defined as:

(a) response to treatment
(b) bPFS
(c) incidence of acute and late treatment related toxicity.

Response to treatment describes the percentage of patients, who will experience a PSA drop after salvage RT. This measure indicates how many patients had—at least in part—a biochemical relapse because of a microscopic local recurrence. The range of possible PSA response differs from study to study, due to differences in patient characteristics and the proportion of patients also receiving concomitant ADT. Published series have shown PSA-response rates of 80–95 % (Pazona et al. 2005; Buskirk et al. 2006; Pisansky et al. 2000; Neuhof et al. 2007; Stephenson et al. 2004).

The biggest published series reported bPFS at 5-year post-treatment in the range of 35–45 % (Buskirk et al. 2006; Ward et al. 2004; Pisansky et al. 2000; Neuhof et al. 2007; Stephenson et al. 2004; Geinitz et al. 2012). Interestingly the Kaplan–Meier-plots show a continuous drop in bPFS even beyond 5 years after treatment. These late relapses could be indicative of secondary tumor relapse in the prostatic fossa rather than activated micrometastatic disease because of the long interval following primary treatment.

The incidence of acute and late treatment-related toxicity has been inconsistently reported in published trials. Late treatment-related toxicity seems to be in the range known from adjuvant RT trials. In a large review late Grade 2 GU and GI toxicity was evident in 10 and 4 % of all patients respectively, while less than 1 % of all patients experienced Grade 3 toxicity (Feng et al. 2007). Compromising urinary continence is a major concern in salvage RT. Patients with incomplete continence before salvage RT are almost four times more likely to suffer from urinary incontinence at 3 years after treatment, than those who had complete urinary continence before salvage RT (Pearse et al. 2008).

Nevertheless, in the majority of the retrospective trials, the applied total doses have been below 70 Gy, and may in the near future be considered too low. With increasing dose, increasing toxicities might result, especially while the urinary tract cannot be spared even with modern RT techniques. Dose escalation trials are necessary, and have to be carried out carefully.

One critical point concerning the value of salvage RT in prostate cancer is the potential influence of a prolonged bPFS on CSS and overall survival. Data from retrospective studies provide conflicting evidence. One study found no decreased mortality with salvage RT despite a large benefit in bPFS (Boorjian et al. 2009). On the other hand, two studies provide retrospective evidence in larger patient populations, that CSS can be increased through salvage RT in patients having both a short (<6 months) and long (≥6 months) PSA-doubling time (Trock et al. 2008; Cotter et al. 2011).

8 Treatment Escalation: Radiation Dose

Average salvage RT doses given in most retrospective studies ranged from 64 to 70 Gy. The NCCN and EAU guidelines (NCCN 2012; European Urology Association Guidelines on Prostate Cancer 2012) recommend a salvage RT dose of 64–68 Gy and 64–66 Gy, respectively. In fact these recommendations seem reasonable, considering there are no prospective dose-comparing studies for salvage RT and that higher doses may potentially lead to treatment-related toxicities. On the other hand, some authors advocate dose escalation in salvage RT as well (King 2012; King and Spiotto 2008; King and Kapp 2008), based on the experience of dose escalation in primary RT for prostate cancer (Viani et al. 2009). The interesting dose level seems to be in the direction of 70 Gy, within the steep part of the dose–effect curve and a projected 2–3 % absolute gain in bPFS per additional Gy of RT dose (King 2012; King and Kapp 2008). Higher doses of salvage RT, however, may be associated with late treatment-related toxicity, as for example shown in an IMRT-study with 75 Gy to the prostatic fossa leading to 30 % Grade 2 GU-toxicity (Meerleer et al. 2008). Recently, a radiobiological model has been proposed to predict the impact of dose escalation in salvage RT on terms of bPFS and GI/GU-toxicity (Ohri et al. 2012).

The authors recommend a salvage RT dose of 64–66 Gy for the majority of patients undergoing salvage RT. Selected patients with intact urinary continence may benefit from a dose escalation to 70 Gy. In patients with macroscopic disease recurrence in the prostatic fossa it seems plausible to prescribe higher RT doses (70–74 Gy).

9 Treatment Escalation: Androgen Deprivation Therapy (ADT)

Randomized trials have shown that ADT given concomitantly to primary RT for prostate cancer can improve overall survival (Nguyen et al. 2011). This effect is attributed both to absolute tumor cell kill within the prostate as well as battling micrometastatic disease. The absolute number of tumor cells in the prostatic fossa in case of a biochemical relapse should be rather low (provided a macroscopic recurrence is excluded and treatment started at an early timepoint). Thus, the main target for ADT additional to salvage RT should be micrometastatic disease. On the other hand, if dose escalated salvage RT leads to higher bPFS (King and Spiotto 2008; King and Kapp 2008), the concomitant use of ADT in patients with only low risk of systemic disease may only be beneficial when standard dose salvage RT (64–66 Gy) is prescribed.

Two prospective trials have combined salvage RT with LHRH-analog either for 2 years within a phase-II—or until tumor progression within a randomized phase-III-trial, demonstrating excellent results in terms of bPFS (78 % at 7 years and 65 % at 5 years), far superior to those reported by retrospective trials on salvage RT alone (Choo et al. 2009; Corn et al. 1999). Both trials could not demonstrate a better local control, metastasis-free survival or overall survival, questioning the real value of immediate androgen suppression instead of delayed use of hormonal treatment if deemed necessary (Corn et al. 1999).

Small retrospective studies also show a trend for better bPFS through combined modality treatment, the interpretation of these results hampered however due to limited follow-up and possible selection bias (Katz et al. 2003; Tiguert et al. 2003; Taylor et al. 2003; King et al. 2004). Preliminary results of the randomized RTOG 9601 trial comparing salvage RT with or without 24 months of bicalutamide show a superior bPFS and a decreased cumulative incidence of distant metastasis in the combined modality arm. The effect of combined treatment on the primary trial endpoint overall survival is however not yet visible at 7 years of follow-up (Shipley et al. 2011).

Since ADT is the standard treatment following biochemical failure after salvage RT, one must question whether bPFS and MFS are eligible endpoints when comparing the outcome after salvage RT or combined salvage RT and ADT. Overall survival may not be influenced, if ADT is given at first upon further disease progression after salvage RT and may therefore represent a more appropriate endpoint. The possible impairment of quality of life through ADT (especially if given over a longer period of time, like in the RTOG 9601 trial) should also be considered.

The authors believe, that salvage RT for biochemical relapse should be given without ADT, until definite results from randomized trials are available showing an improved overall survival while preserving a high quality of life in those men. Patients with macroscopic recurrence can be treated with combined RT and ADT, because of the higher local tumor load. This strategy is based on the favorable results of combined RT and ADT in primary prostate cancer treatment (Nguyen et al. 2011).

10 Future Directions: Running Trials

A considerable number of randomized trials (Table 1) are currently underway, seeking answers to important questions in the field of postoperative RT for prostate cancer.

The RTOG 0534 trial is randomizing patients to salvage RT of the prostatic fossa with or without ADT, while in the third study arm patients are receiving additional RT of the pelvic lymph nodes (Prostate radiation therapy 2012). A UK-led trial is testing multiple questions by randomizing patients to immediate postoperative or salvage RT with or without ADT of different durations (Radiation therapy and androgen deprivation therapy 2012). A similar approach is being followed in an EORTC-trial, randomizing patients to adjuvant or salvage RT with or without ADT (Radiation therapy with or without hormone therapy 2012). Adjuvant versus salvage treatment with a combination of RT and ADT is the focus of an active French trial (Radiation therapy with or without Goserelin 2012). A Japanese randomized trial has completed accrual testing salvage ADT with or without RT (Trial to evaluate radiotherapy 2012). The Trans-Tasman Radiation Oncology Group (TROG) is randomizing patients to adjuvant or early salvage RT (Radiotherapy—Adjuvant Versus Early Salvage (RAVES 2012). The MAPS-study is looking at focal dose escalation through integrated boost techniques based on dynamic contrast-enhanced MRI (Radiation therapy in treating patients 2012). A more straightforward approach is being followed by a Swiss-German trial, which is testing dose escalation (64 vs. 70 Gy) to the prostatic fossa with special interest to modern RT techniques (Radiation therapy in treating 2012).

It is expected, that these trials will shed light in the field of postoperative RT by directly answering critical questions on timing of treatment as well as necessity of RT dose escalation and value of ADT. Further retrospective analyses of the large groups of patients to be included in these trials in combination with tissue analysis may help us to clarify which groups of patients are served the best with more or less aggressive treatment approaches.

Table 1 Overview of active studies on postoperative RT

Title	Setting	Randomization	Inclusion criteria	Primary endpoint	Status
RTOG 0534 (Shipley et al. 2011)	Salvage	1. Prostatic fossa RT 2. Prostatic fossa RT + ADT (4–6 months) 3. Prostatic and pelvic node RT + ADT (4–6 months)	PSA $\geq$ 0.1 < 2.0 ng/ml R0-1 GS $\leq$ 8	Freedom from progression	Active since 02/08
RADICALS (Radiation therapy and androgen deprivation therapy 2012)	Adjuvant versus early salvage	*First randomization* 1. Adjuvant RT 2. Early salvage RT *Second randomization* 1. RT 2. RT + ADT (6 months) 3. RT + ADT (24 months)	*First randomization* PSA $\leq$ 0.2 ng/ml *one or more* – pT3/4 – GS 7–10 – pre-RP PSA > 10 ng/ml – R1	Disease specific survival	Active since 10/07
EORTC 22043 (Radiation therapy with or without hormone therapy 2012)	Adjuvant and early salvage	*Adjuvant setting* 1. RT 2. RT + ADT (6 months) *Early salvage setting* 1. RT 2. RT + ADT (6 months)	pT2 R1 or pT3 R0-1 GS 5–10 *Adjuvant setting* PSA < 0.2 ng/ml *Early salvage setting* PSA < 0.5 or 3 rises	bPFS at 5 years	Active since 05/09
GETUG 17/0702 (Radiation therapy with or without Goserelin 2012)	Adjuvant versus early salvage	1. Adjuvant ADT + RT 2. Early salvage ADT + RT	PSA 0.2–2 ng/ml pT3a-pT4 R0-1 GS < 8	Event free survival at 5 years	Active since 12/07
JCOG0401 (Trial to evaluate radiotherapy 2012)	Salvage	1. ADT (until progression) 2. RT + ADT (until progression)	PSA 0.4–1.0 ng/ml pT1-2	Time to treatment failure	Accrual complete (2004–2011)
RAVES TROG 08.03 (Radiotherapy - Adjuvant Versus Early Salvage (RAVES) 2012)	Adjuvant versus early salvage	1. Adjuvant RT 2. Early salvage RT	PSA $\leq$ 0.1 ng/ml *one or more* – pT3a/b – R1	Biochemical failure	Active since 03/09
MAPS (A phase III randomized trial 2012)	Salvage	1. Standard salvage RT 2. Mapped tumor salvage RT with integrated boost	PSA 0.1–3.0 ng/ml detectable lesion in the prostatic fossa	Biochemical control at 5 years	Active since 06/11
SAKK 09/10 (Radiation therapy in treating patients 2012)	Salvage	1. 64 Gy RT 2. 70 Gy RT	PSA < 2.0 ng/ml pT2a-pT3b R0-1	Freedom from biochemical progression	Active since 01/11

RT radiotherapy; *ADT* androgen deprivation therapy; *PSA* prostate specific antigen; *bPFS* biochemical progression-free survival; *RP* radical prostatectomy; *GS* Gleason Score

11 Conclusions

Salvage RT is the sole potentially curative treatment for biochemical relapse after RP in patients with prostate cancer. Salvage RT should be performed as early as possible, ideally with a PSA-value between 0.2 and 0.5 ng/ml. Since it is not clear, which groups of patients will not benefit from such a potentially curative treatment, salvage RT should not be withheld from any subgroup of patients with biochemical relapse. The optimal timing and dose of postoperative RT as well as its combination with ADT are currently being tested in phase-III trials. Patients with biochemical relapse after RP should be treated whenever possible within clinical trials in order to answer these open questions as soon as possible.

Outside clinical trials 64–72 Gy are the standard dose of salvage RT, the exact dose to be defined by absence or presence of macroscopic recurrence and the urinary continence status of the patient prior to treatment.

Conflict of Interest Notification The authors have no actual or potential conflict of interest related to this review. There are no financial disclosures from any author.

References

A phase III randomized trial of MRI-mapped dose-escalated salvage radiotherapy post-prostatectomy: the MAPS trial. http://www.clinicaltrials.gov/ct2/show/NCT01411345. Accessed 26 Nov 2012

Alongi F, Fiorino C, Cozzarini C et al (2009) IMRT significantly reduces acute toxicity of whole-pelvis irradiation in patients treated with post-operative adjuvant or salvage radiotherapy after radical prostatectomy. Radiother Oncol 93(2):207–212

Amling CL, Blute ML, Bergstralh EJ et al (2000) Long-term hazard of progression after radical prostatectomy for clinically localized prostate cancer: continued risk of biochemical failure after 5 years. J Urol 164:101–105

Bolla M, van Poppel H, Collette L et al (2005) Postoperative radiotherapy after radical prostatectomy: a randomised controlled trial (EORTC trial 22911). Lancet 366:572–578

Boorjian SA, Karnes RJ, Crispen PL et al (2009) Radiation therapy after radical prostatectomy: impact on metastasis and survival. J Urol 182(6):2708–2714

Buskirk SJ, Pisansky TM, Schild SE et al (2006) Salvage radiotherapy for isolated prostate specific antigen increase after radical prostatectomy: evaluation of prognostic factors and creation of a prognostic scoring system. J Urol 176(3):985–990

Cher ML, Bianco FJ Jr, Lam JS et al (1998) Limited role of radionuclide bone scintigraphy in patients with prostate specific antigen elevations after radical prostatectomy. J Urol 160(4):1387

Choo R, Danjoux C, Gardner S et al (2009) Efficacy of salvage radiotherapy plus 2-year androgen suppression for postradical prostatectomy patients with PSA relapse. Int J Radiat Oncol Biol Phys 75(4):983–989

Corn BW, Winter K, Pilepich MV (1999) Does androgen suppression enhance the efficacy of postoperative irradiation? A secondary analysis of RTOG 85-31 Radiation Therapy Oncology Group. Urology 54(3):495–502

Cotter SE, Chen MH, Moul JW (2011) Salvage radiation in men after prostate-specific antigen failure and the risk of death. Cancer 117(17):3925–3932

Da Pozzo LF, Cozzarini C, Briganti A et al (2009) Long-term follow-up of patients with prostate cancer and nodal metastases treated by pelvic lymphadenectomy and radical prostatectomy: the positive impact of adjuvant radiotherapy. Eur Urol 55(5):1003–1011

Dearnaley DP, Khoo VS, Norman AR et al (1999) Comparison of radiation side-effects of conformal and conventional radiotherapy in prostate cancer: a randomised trial. Lancet 353(9149):267–272

Digesú C, Cilla S, De Gaetano A et al. (2011) Postoperative intensity modulated radiation therapy in high risk prostate cancer: a dosimetric comparison. Med Dosim 36(3):231–239 (Autumn)

European Urology Association Guidelines on Prostate Cancer (2012). http://www.uroweb.org/gls/pdf/08%20Prostate%20Cancer_LR%20March%2013th%202012.pdf. Accessed 26 Nov 2012

Feng M, Hanlon AL, Pisansky TM (2007) Predictive factors for late genitourinary and gastrointestinal toxicity in patients with prostate cancer treated with adjuvant or salvage radiotherapy. Int J Radiat Oncol Biol Phys 68(5):1417–1423

Geinitz H, Riegel MG, Thamm R et al (2012) Outcome after conformal salvage radiotherapy in patients with rising prostate-specific antigen levels after radical prostatectomy. Int J Radiat Oncol Biol Phys 82(5):1930–1937

Giannarini G, Nguyen DP, Thalmann GN et al (2012) Diffusion-weighted magnetic resonance imaging detects local recurrence after radical prostatectomy: initial experience. Eur Urol 61(3):616–620

Goenka A, Magsanoc JM, Pei X et al (2011) Improved toxicity profile following high-dose post prostatectomy salvage radiation therapy with intensity-modulated radiation therapy. Eur Urol 60(6):1142–1148

Graute V, Jansen N, Ubleis C et al (2012) Relationship between PSA kinetics and (18F) fluorocholine PET/CT detection rates of recurrence in patients with prostate cancer after total prostatectomy. Eur J Nucl Med Mol Imag 39(2):271–282

Han M, Partin AW, Zahurak M et al (2003) Biochemical (prostate specific antigen) recurrence probability following radical prostatectomy for clinically localized prostate cancer. J Urol 169:517–523

Huch Böni RA, Meyenberger C, Pok Lundquist J et al. (1996) Value of endorectal coil versus body coil MRI for diagnosis of recurrent pelvic malignancies. Abdom Imag 21(4):345–352

Katz MS, Zelefsky MJ, Venkatraman ES et al (2003) Predictors of biochemical outcome with salvage conformal radiotherapy after radical prostatectomy for prostate cancer. J Clin Oncol 21(3):483–489

King CR (2012) The timing of salvage radiotherapy after radical prostatectomy: a systematic review. Int J Radiat Oncol Biol Phys 84(1):104–111

King CR, Kapp DS (2008) Radiotherapy after prostatectomy: is the evidence for dose escalation out there? Int J Radiat Oncol Biol Phys 71:346–350

King CR, Spiotto MT (2008) Improved outcomes with higher doses for salvage radiotherapy after prostatectomy. Int J Radiat Oncol Biol Phys 71:23–27

King CR, Presti JC Jr, Gill H et al (2004) Radiotherapy after radical prostatectomy: does transient androgen suppression improve outcomes? Int J Radiat Oncol Biol Phys 59(2):341–347

Kupelian PA, Katcher J, Levin HS, Klein EA (1997) Stage T1-prostate cancer: a multivariate analysis of factors affecting biochemical and clinical failures after radical prostatectomy. Int J Radiat Oncol Biol Phys 37:1043–1052

Lawton CA, DeSilvio M, Roach M 3rd et al (2007) An update of the phase III trial comparing whole pelvic to prostate only radiotherapy and neoadjuvant to adjuvant total androgen suppression: updated analysis of RTOG 94-13, with emphasis on unexpected hormone/radiation interactions. Int J Radiat Oncol Biol Phys 69(3):646–655

Liauw SL, Pitroda SP, Eggener SE et al. (2012) Evaluation of the prostate bed for local recurrence after radical prostatectomy using endorectal magnetic resonance imaging. Int J Radiat Oncol Biol Phys 85:378–384

Macdonald OK, D'Amico AV, Sadetsky N et al. (2008) Predicting PSA failure following salvage radiotherapy for a rising PSA post-prostatectomy: from the CaPSURE database. Urol Oncol 26(3):271–275

Meerleer GD, Fonteyne V, Meersshout S et al (2008) Salvage intensity-modulated radiotherapy for rising PSA after radical prostatectomy. Radiother Oncol 89:205–213

Meng MV, Shinohara K, Grossfeld GD, Carroll PR (2002) Local therapy for recurrent prostate cancer. In: Kantoff PW, Carroll PR,

D'Amico AV (eds) Prostate cancer: principles and practice, pp 307–316. Lippincott Williams and Wilkins, Philadelphia
Michalski J, Lawton C, El Naqa I et al (2010) Development of RTOG consensus guidelines for the definition of the clinical target volume for postoperative conformal radiation therapy for prostate cancer. Int J Radiat Oncol Biol Phys 76(2):361–368
Nath SK, Sandhu AP, Rose BS et al (2010) Toxicity analysis of postoperative image-guided intensity-modulated radiotherapy for prostate cancer. Int J Radiat Oncol Biol Phys 78(2):435–441
NCCN (2012) Clinical practice guidelines in oncology: prostate cancer version 3.2012. http://www.nccn.org/professionals/physician_gls/pdf/prostate.pdf. Accessed on 26 Nov 2012
Neuhof D, Hentschel T, Bischof M et al (2007) Long-term results and predictive factors of three-dimensional conformal salvage radiotherapy for biochemical relapse after prostatectomy. Int J Radiat Oncol Biol Phys 67:1411–1417
Nguyen PL, Je Y, Schutz FA et al (2011) Association of androgen deprivation therapy with cardiovascular death in patients with prostate cancer: a meta-analysis of randomized trials. JAMA 306(21):2359–2366
Ohri N, Dicker AP, Trabulsi EJ et al (2012a) Can early implementation of salvage radiotherapy for prostate cancer improve the therapeutic ratio? A systematic review and regression meta-analysis with radiobiological modelling. Eur J Cancer 48(6):837–844
Ohri N, Dicker AP, Trabulsi EJ et al (2012b) Can early implementation of salvage radiotherapy for prostate cancer improve the therapeutic ratio? A systematic review and regression meta-analysis with radiobiological modelling. Eur J Cancer 48(6):837–844
Paul R, Hoppmann M, van Randenborgh H et al (2004) Residual benign prostatic glands at the urethrovesical anastomosis after radical retropubic prostatectomy: prediction and impact on disease outcome. Eur Urol 46(3):321–326
Pazona JF, Han M, Hawkins SA et al (2005) Salvage radiation therapy for prostate specific antigen progression following radical prostatectomy: 10-year outcome estimates. J Urol 174(4 Pt 1):1282–1286
Pearse M, Choo R, Danjoux C et al (2008) Prospective assessment of gastrointestinal and genitourinary toxicity of salvage radiotherapy for patients with prostate-specific antigen relapse or local recurrence after radical prostatectomy. Int J Radiat Oncol Biol Phys 72(3):792–798
Picchio M, Briganti A, Fanti S et al (2011) The role of choline positron emission tomography/computed tomography in the management of patients with prostate-specific antigen progression after radical treatment of prostate cancer. Eur Urol 59(1):51–60
Pisansky TM, Kozelsky TF, Myers RP et al (2000) Radiotherapy for isolated serum prostate specific antigen elevation after prostatectomy for prostate cancer. J Urol 163(3):845–850
Pommier P, Chabaud S, Lagrange JL et al (2007) Is there a role for pelvic irradiation in localized prostate adenocarcinoma? Preliminary results of GETUG-01. J Clin Oncol 25(34):5366–5373
Poortmans P, Bossi A, Vandeputte K et al (2007) Guidelines for target volume definition in post-operative radiotherapy for prostate cancer, on behalf of the EORTC Radiation Oncology Group. Radiother Oncol 84(2):121–127
Pound CR, Partin AW, Eisenberger MA et al (1999) Natural history of progression after PSA elevation following radical prostatectomy. JAMA 281:1591–1597
Prostate radiation therapy or short-term androgen deprivation therapy and pelvic lymph node radiation therapy with or without prostate radiation therapy in treating patients with a rising PSA after surgery for prostate cancer. http://clinicaltrials.gov/show/NCT00567580 Accessed 26 Nov 2012
Radiation therapy and androgen deprivation therapy in treating patients who have undergone surgery for prostate cancer (RADICALS). http://clinicaltrials.gov/show/NCT00541047. Accessed 26 Nov 2012
Radiation therapy in treating patients with relapsed prostate cancer after surgery. http://clinicaltrials.gov/show/NCT01272050. Accessed 26 Nov 2012
Radiation therapy with or without Goserelin in treating patients who have undergone surgery for recurrent or refractory prostate cancer. http://clinicaltrials.gov/show/NCT00423475. Accessed 26 Nov 2012
Radiation therapy with or without hormone therapy in treating patients who have undergone surgery for stage I, stage II, or stage III prostate cancer. http://www.clinicaltrials.gov/ct2/show/NCT00949962. Accessed 26 Nov 2012
Radiotherapy—Adjuvant Versus Early Salvage (RAVES). http://www.clinicaltrials.gov/ct2/show/NCT00860652. Accessed 26 Nov 2012
Riou O, Laliberte B, Azria D et al. (2012) Implementing intensity modulated radiotherapy to the prostate bed: dosimetric study and early clinical results. Med Dosim pii: S0958-3947 (12) 00167-7
RTOG (2012) Pelvic lymph node volumes for prostate cancer atlas. http://www.rtog.org/LinkClick.aspx?fileticket=glmTGKHTmr0%3d&tabid=234. Accessed 26 Nov 2012
Schild SE, Wong WW, Novicki DE et al (1996) Detection of residual prostate cancer after radical prostatectomy with the Abbott IMx PSA assay. Urology 47(6):878–881
Sciarra A, Panebianco V, Salciccia S et al (2008) Role of dynamic contrast-enhanced magnetic resonance (MR) imaging and proton MR spectroscopic imaging in the detection of local recurrence after radical prostatectomy for prostate cancer. Eur Urol 54(3):589–600
Sciarra A, Panebianco V, Ciccariello M et al (2010) Value of magnetic resonance spectroscopy imaging and dynamic contrast-enhanced imaging for detecting prostate cancer foci in men with prior negative biopsy. Clin Cancer Res 16(6):1875–1883
Shah O, Melamed J, Lepor H (2001) Analysis of apical soft tissue margins during radical retropubic prostatectomy. J Urol 165(6 Pt 1):1943–1948
Sheets NC, Goldin GH, Meyer AM et al (2012) Intensity-modulated radiation therapy, proton therapy, or conformal radiation therapy and morbidity and disease control in localized prostate cancer. JAMA 307(15):1611–1620
Shipley WU, Hunt D, Lukka HR et al. (2011) Initial report of RTOG 9601, a phase III trial in prostate cancer: effect of anti-androgen therapy (AAT) with bicalutamide during and after radiation therapy (RT) on freedom from progression and incidence of metastatic disease in patients following radical prostatectomy (RP) with pT2-3, N0 disease and elevated PSA levels. J Clin Oncol 29 (suppl 7; abstr 1)
Slovin SF, Wilton AS, Heller G, Scher HI (2005) Time to detectable metastatic disease in patients with rising prostate-specific antigen values following surgery or radiation therapy. Clin Cancer Res 11:8669–8673
Spiotto MT, Hancock SL, King CR (2007) Radiotherapy after prostatectomy: improved biochemical relapse-free survival with whole pelvic compared with prostate bed only for high-risk patients. Int J Radiat Oncol Biol Phys 69(1):54–61
Stephenson AJ, Shariat SF, Zelefsky MJ et al (2004) Salvage radiotherapy for recurrent prostate cancer after radical prostatectomy. JAMA 291:1325–1332
Stephenson AJ, Scardino PT, Kattan MW et al (2007) Predicting the outcome of salvage radiation therapy for recurrent prostate cancer after radical prostatectomy. J Clin Oncol 25:2035–2041
Taylor N, Kelly JF, Kuban DA et al (2003) Adjuvant and salvage radiotherapy after radical prostatectomy for prostate cancer. Int J Radiat Oncol Biol Phys 56(3):755–763
Thompson IM Jr, Tangen CM, Paradelo J et al (2006) Adjuvant radiotherapy for pathologically advanced prostate cancer: a randomized clinical trial. JAMA 296:2329–2335
Thompson IM, Tangen CM, Paradelo J et al (2009) Adjuvant radiotherapy for pathological T3N0M0 prostate cancer

significantly reduces risk of metastases and improves survival: long-term followup of a randomized clinical trial. J Urol 181:956–962

Tiguert R, Rigaud J, Lacombe L et al (2003) Neoadjuvant hormone therapy before salvage radiotherapy for an increasing post-radical prostatectomy serum prostate specific antigen level. J Urol 170(2 Pt 1):447–450

Tongco WP, Wehner MS, Basler JW (2001) Does urethral-sparing prostatectomy risk residual prostate cancer? Urology 57(3):495–498

Trial to evaluate radiotherapy followed by endocrine therapy vs endocrine therapy alone for PSA failure after radical prostatectomy. http://clinicaltrials.gov/show/NCT00138008. Accessed on 26 Nov 2012

Trock BJ, Han M, Freedland SJ et al (2008) Prostate cancer-specific survival following salvage radiotherapy vs observation in men with biochemical recurrence after radical prostatectomy. JAMA 299(23):2760–2769

Viani GA, Stefano EJ, Afonso SL (2009) Higher-than-conventional radiation doses in localized prostate cancer treatment: a meta-analysis of randomized, controlled trials. Int J Radiat Oncol Biol Phys 74:1405–1418

Ward JF, Moul JW (2005) Rising prostate-specific antigen after primary prostate cancer therapy. Nat Clin Pract Urol 2:174–182

Ward JF, Zincke H, Bergstralh EJ et al (2004) Prostate specific antigen doubling time subsequent to radical prostatectomy as a prognosticator of outcome following salvage radiotherapy. J Urol 172(6 Pt 1):2244–2248

Wiegel T, Bottke D, Bandlow P et al (2002) The value of PSA measurements at 30 Gy, 50 Gy and 60 Gy for dose limitation in patients with radiotherapy for PSA increase after radical prostatectomy. Strahlenther Onkol 178(8):422–425

Wiegel T, Bottke D, Steiner U et al (2009a) Phase III postoperative adjuvant radiotherapy after radical prostatectomy compared with radical prostatectomy alone in pT3 prostate cancer with postoperative undetectable prostate-specific antigen: ARO 96-02/AUO AP 09/95. J Clin Oncol 27:2924–2930

Wiegel T, Lohm G, Bottke D et al (2009b) Achieving an undetectable PSA after radiotherapy for biochemical progression after radical prostatectomy is an independent predictor of biochemical outcome–results of a retrospective study. Int J Radiat Oncol Biol Phys 73(4):1009–1016

Salvage Prostatectomy After Radiotherapy

Hubert Kübler, Tobias Maurer, Thomas Horn,
and Jürgen E. Gschwend

Contents

Abstract

Radiotherapy is widely utilized as primary therapy for clinically localized prostate cancer. Biochemical recurrence after external radiotherapy or brachytherapy occurs in up to 60 % of patients treated for prostate cancer within 10 years. Salvage radical prostatectomy represents a secondary local treatment with curative intent in patients with organ confined prostate cancer recurrences following radiation therapy. Patients most likely to benefit from salvage prostatectomy have low-risk disease, a pretreatment PSA velocity <2.0 ng/ml per year at the time of initial presentation, an interval to PSA failure >3 years, and a PSA doubling time >12 months. In experienced hands, morbidity is low with a continence rate of approximately 80 % depending on the type of previous radiation therapy. Long-term oncological control can be achieved in more than 75 % of the patients. Despite these well-established oncological outcomes, salvage radical prostatectomy is infrequently performed or reported.

1 Introduction

Prostate cancer is the second most commonly diagnosed and the sixth leading cause of death in men worldwide (Jemal et al. 2011). Despite improved methods of delivery (ultrasound-guided brachytherapy, three-dimensional conformal techniques, and intensity-modulated radiotherapy) that have permitted the administration of higher radiation doses with fewer side effects, up to one-third of patients treated with radiation therapy for clinically localized prostate cancer will have evidence of treatment failure (Zietman et al. 2005; Zelefsky et al. 2002). However, data from Cancer of the Prostate Strategic Urologic Research Endeavor (CaPSURE) identified that 63 % of patients have an increase in their serum PSA level within 10 years after radiotherapy (Agarwal et al. 2008). Apart from expectant

H. Kübler (✉) · T. Maurer · T. Horn · J. E. Gschwend
Department of Urology, Klinikum rechts der Isar,
Technische Universität München, Ismaninger Str. 22,
81675 Munich, Germany
e-mail: h.kuebler@lrz.tum.de

H. Geinitz et al. (eds.), *Radiotherapy in Prostate Cancer*, Medical Radiology. Radiation Oncology,
DOI: 10.1007/174_2013_950,
Published Online: 11 January 2014

management and systemic therapy, there are four available local treatment options for radio-recurrent prostate cancer: salvage radical prostatectomy, salvage cryoablation, salvage brachytherapy, and salvage high-intensity focused ultrasound HIFU (Kimura et al. 2010). The role of salvage radical prostatectomy has evolved, with recent series showing improved results for the treatment of radiation-recurrent prostate cancer. In this chapter, we review the current status of salvage radical prostatectomy after failure of radiotherapy with regard to patient selection, oncological efficacy, functional outcomes, and complications.

2 Diagnosis of Radiation-Recurrent Prostate Cancer

The vast majority of patients with local recurrence of prostate cancer after radiation therapy are identified by an elevated and rising serum PSA level. Biochemical recurrence after radiotherapy is defined by the American Society for Therapeutic Radiation and Oncology (ASTRO) as a rise in serum PSA by $\geq$2 ng/ml from the nadir PSA after radiotherapy ("Phoenix definition," Roach et al. 2006). The challenge for the clinician is to determine whether the PSA-level elevation originates from local persistence of cancer or from distant metastases or both. Currently, there is no consensus on when and how to detect and cure local recurrence of prostate cancer after failed radiotherapy. Overall, 60–72 % of patients with a rising PSA level and a negative metastatic evaluation after external beam radiotherapy have biopsy-confirmed local persistence of disease (Bianco et al. 2005). When a prostate cancer recurrence is diagnosed by rising PSA-values, most current guidelines recommend a confirmatory prostate biopsy in case local salvage therapy is considered (Mottet et al. 2011; Mohler et al. 2010).

3 Patient Selection for Salvage Prostatectomy

Careful patient selection for effective salvage therapy with curative intent implies that some patients will not fulfill the criteria for local salvage treatment and will require palliative or systemic salvage treatment strategies. According to current guidelines, a candidate for salvage radical prostatectomy should fulfill the following requirements: surgically curable disease at initial radiation, no evidence of metastatic disease, a postradiation biopsy confirming prostate cancer, and a live expectancy long enough to benefit from intervention (Mohler et al. 2010; Mottet et al. 2011). Patients most likely to benefit from salvage prostatectomy have

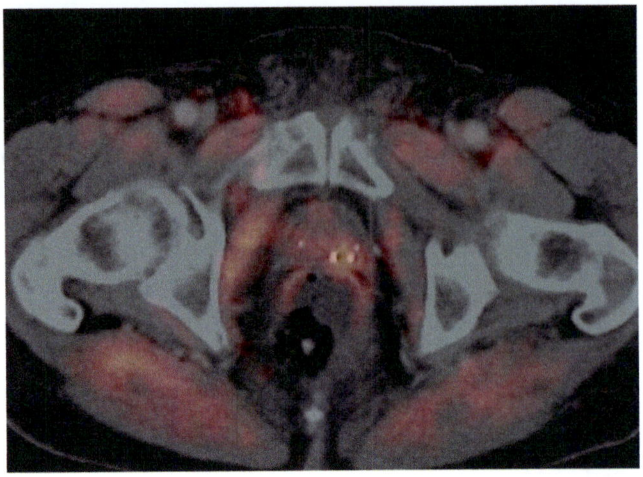

Fig. 1 11C-Choline PET/CT showing increased uptake on the *left side* corresponding to radio-recurrent prostate cancer

low-risk diseases (PSA <10 ng/ml, Gleason-Score $\leq$6, and clinical T1c or T2a tumor status), pretreatment PSA velocity <2.0 ng/ml per year at the time of initial presentation, interval to PSA failure >3 years, PSA doubling time >12 months. In addition, men with pre-salvage PSA levels >10 ng/ml, pre-salvage T3/T4 disease, or pre-salvage Gleason scores $\geq$7 on a rebiopsy sample without significant radiotherapy effects are unlikely to be cured by salvage prostatectomy (Nguyen et al. 2007). Imaging evaluation of locally recurrent prostate cancer to plan salvage therapy remains challenging (Jadvar and Alavi 2009). In one study, 11C-Choline (Fig. 1) was determined to localize recurrence in a higher percentage of men after primary radiation therapy than after radical prostatectomy (78 % vs. 38 %, respectively) (de Jong et al. 2003). Nevertheless, the role of PET/CT imaging in localizing radio-recurrent prostate cancer remains unclear and needs further evaluation.

4 Surgical Technique of Salvage Prostatectomy

Radical prostatectomy is the local salvage treatment modality with the longest history. Several authors described salvage radical prostatectomy to be a challenging procedure with a high probability of encountering locally advanced disease at surgery and corresponding surgical complications. Carson et al. showed the feasibility of prostatic surgery after radiotherapy with 18 patients who underwent radical prostatectomy as an adjuvant therapy after radiotherapy with acceptable surgical morbidity (Carson et al. 1980). Salvage radical prostatectomy (Fig. 2) is performed with the same technical steps described for anatomic radical prostatectomy

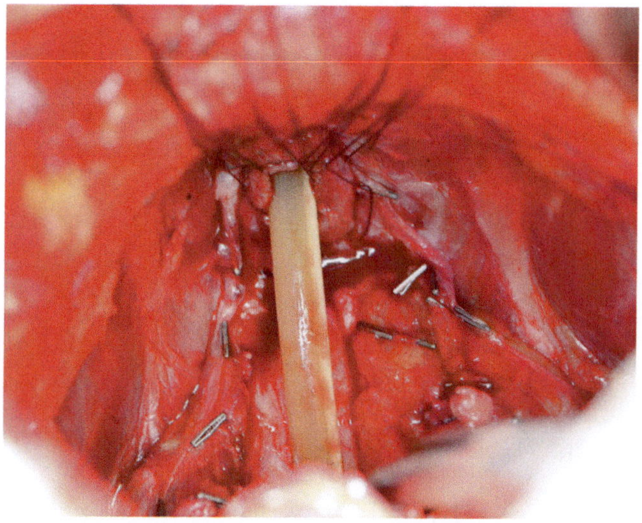

Fig. 2 Intraoperative aspect after salvage radical prostatectomy with a catheter and anastomotic sutures in the urethral stump. On the *right side* there are brachytherapy seeds in the Denonvilliers fascia. On the *left side* the neurovascular bundle could partly be preserved

(Walsh 1998), despite expected technical difficulties such as unclear plane of dissection and adherences, especially in the posterior aspect of the prostate, where rectal injury is a major concern (Chade et al. 2012). Yet, several authors describe that salvage prostatectomy as currently performed is similar in its degree of difficulty to standard radical prostatectomy and not as challenging as previously reported (Rogers et al. 1995; Zincke 1992; Pontes et al. 1993). However, these surgeons are usually experienced in radical prostatectomy and pelvic surgery, and none has reported an analysis of his or her learning curve with salvage prostatectomy. Moreover, there has been no report specifically addressing and comparing critical aspects of the procedure, allowing a more comprehensible evidence-based guideline (Chade et al. 2012). The feasibility of salvage prostatectomy after EBRT alone is frequently described as the same as primary radical prostatectomy (Rogers et al. 1995). Although there is no evidence to confirm any difference in complications according to the method of radiotherapy (EBRT vs. brachytherapy), authors eventually describe greater difficulty and surgical complexity at salvage prostatectomy after brachytherapy because of increased adhesions (Gotto et al. 2010).

5 Oncologic Outcomes of Salvage Prostatectomy

As salvage radical prostatectomy is technically demanding, experienced surgeons are needed to optimize outcomes. Accordingly, relatively few centers have reported on salvage radical prostatectomy. The study with the largest number of patients is a recently published multi-institutional collaboration project that included high volume referral centers (Chade et al. 2011). In a systematic review of salvage prostatectomy the median follow-up of the reported studies ranged from 18 to 84 months, which may explain the wide variation in findings of oncologic outcomes across those studies with less biochemical control in studies with longer follow-up. Thus critical analyses should be limited to those studies with longer follow-up periods (Chade et al. 2012). None of the published studies on salvage prostatectomy adequately studied potential oncologic differences between salvage prostatectomy after external beam radiotherapy and after brachytherapy or between distinct radiotherapy techniques (three-dimensional conformal radiotherapy, intensity-modulated radiotherapy) or radiotherapy doses (Chade et al. 2012).

Table 1 summarizes the specimen characteristics of some of the largest salvage prostatectomy series. Positive surgical margin rate varied from 11 to 36 %. Pathologic organ confined disease was reported in 25–71 % of studies. Lymph node dissection was reported infrequently in the studies and was not standardized among different institutions. Also, no studies were able to analyze the impact of pelvic lymph node dissection on cancer-specific survival.

The 5-year biochemical recurrence-free survival rates typically range from 50 to 60 % in most salvage prostatectomy series. At 10 years, the biochemical recurrence-free probability ranges from 37 to 47 %. The definition of biochemical-free recurrence after salvage prostatectomy was different in almost each publication. Table 2 summarizes the oncologic outcomes of some of the largest salvage prostatectomy series. Series from single centers reported probabilities of cancer-specific survival from 65 to 77 % at 10 years (Bianco et al. 2005; Ward et al. 2005; Sanderson et al. 2006), while the multi-institutional collaboration study reported an 83 % cancer-specific survival at 10 years (Chade et al. 2011). Overall survival varied from 54 to 89 % at 10 years (Chade et al. 2012).

In the series from Mayo Clinic and Memorial Sloan-Kettering Cancer Center/Baylor Medical Center, men who had PSA levels <10 ng/ml at the time of salvage prostatectomy had significantly lower estimates of PSA failure compared with men who had PSA levels ≥ 10 ng/ml (Bianco et al. 2005; Ward et al. 2005).

Oncologic outcome was worse for patients who underwent salvage cystoprostatectomy compared with patients who underwent salvage prostatectomy, with a 5-year biochemical disease-free survival rate of 19 % versus 63 %, respectively, in the Mayo Clinic series and 30 % versus 50 %, respectively, in the Wayne State series (Ward et al. 2005; Gheiler et al. 1998).

Table 1 Specimen characteristics of contemporary open salvage prostatectomy series

Series	Number of patients	PSA (ng/ml)	pT2 (%)	≥pT3 (%)	pT3b (%)	PSM (%)	Gleason-score			Lymph node metastasis (%)
							≤6	7	≥8	
Multicenter (Chade et al. 2011)	404	4.5	45	53	30	25	14	37	24	16
MSKCC/Baylor (Bianco et al. 2005)	100	5.9	35	23	33	21	17	62	13	9
Mayo Clinic (Ward et al. 2005)	121	8.5	N/A	61	N/A	21	14	59	27	N/A
USC (Sanderson et al. 2006)	51	8.0	25	59	N/A	36	20	36	44	16
Aachen (Heidenreich et al. 2010)	45	7.8	71	11	18	11	33	47	20	20
Wayne State (Gheiler et al. 1998)	38	14	39	61	29	13	N/A	N/A	N/A	16
Rome (Leonardo et al. 2009)	32	2.3	53	47	N/A	34	38	N/A	N/A	0

PSM positive surgical margin, *N/A* not available

Table 2 Oncologic outcomes of contemporary open salvage prostatectomy series

Series	Number of patients	Follow-up (years)	PSA > 10 ng/ml (%)	Time to RP (months)	pT2 (%)	Disease-free rate (%)		Cancer-specific survival	
						5 years	10 years	5 years	10 years
Multicenter (Chade et al. 2011)	404	4.4	N/A	41	45	48	37	92	83
MSKCC/Baylor (Bianco et al. 2005)	100	5	29	40	39	65	43	93	73
Mayo Clinic (Ward et al. 2005)	138	6.4	29	40	39	65	43	90	77
USC (Sanderson et al. 2006)	51	7.2	36	62	25	47	47	85	65
Aachen (Heidenreich et al. 2010)	55	1.9	47.3	32	73.3	87 (2 years)	N/A	N/A	N/A
Wayne State (Gheiler et al. 1998)	40	3	48	58	43	47	N/A	N/A	N/A
Rome (Leonardo et al. 2009)	32	2.9	N/A	31	53	75 (35 months)	N/A	N/A	N/A

RP radical prostatectomy *N/A* not available

The neoadjuvant androgen deprivation before salvage prostatectomy was poorly reported, or patients were analyzed in mixed cohorts. Prospective data to support the use of neoadjuvant androgen deprivation in the salvage prostatectomy setting are missing. Retrospective data from the Mayo Clinic and the Netherlands Cancer Institute series showed no reduction in positive margin rate or improvement in outcome with neoadjuvant androgen deprivation, although it is possible that the selection of men with more advanced disease to receive androgen deprivation obscured any potential benefit (Ward et al. 2005; van der Poel et al. 2007).

Table 3 Surgical complications of contemporary open salvage prostatectomy series

Series	Year	Number of patients	Perioperative complications (%)	Rectal injury (%)	Urinary incontinence (%)	Anastomotic stricture (%)
MSKCC (Stephenson et al. 2004)	1993–2003	60	13	2	32	32
Mayo Clinic (Ward et al. 2005)	1990–2000	89	27	3	44	23
USC (Ward et al. 2005)	1983–2002	51	N/A	2	27	41
Aachen (Heidenreich et al. 2010)	2004–2008	55	27.3	3.6	20	10.9
Wayne State (Gheiler et al. 1998)	1992–1997	30	17	3	50	17
Rome (Leonardo et al. 2009)	2001–2004	32	N/A	0	16	12.5

N/A not available

Table 4 Functional outcomes of contemporary open salvage prostatectomy series

Series	Number of patients	Continence		Preservation of erectile function	
		0–1 pad (%)	0 pads (%)		+PDE5-Is
MSKCC (Stephenson et al. 2004)	100	68	39	45 %	N/A
Aachen (Heidenreich et al. 2010)	55	80	68	4/15	10/15
Rome (Leonardo et al. 2009)	32	84	22	N/A	9 %

PDE5-Is PDE-5 inhibitors, *N/A* not available

6 Surgical Complications of Salvage Prostatectomy

Salvage prostatectomy has not been widely accepted for the treatment of radiation-recurrent prostate cancer because of a historical concern that most men will recur and fear of the procedure's associated surgical morbidity. Radiotherapy-induced cystitis, fibrosis, and tissue plane obliteration have been factors leading to significant complications, such as rectal injuries, anastomosis strictures, and urinary incontinence. In the MSKCC early experience, surgeons reported an incontinence rate of 58 % and a major complication rate of 33 %, including a 15 % risk of rectal injury (Rogers et al. 1995). These complications are associated with extensive fibrosis between the bladder, prostate, and rectum. In contemporary open salvage prostatectomy series, rectal injury occurred in 0–3.6 % of patients, and anastomotic stricture varied from 12.5 to 41 % (Table 3). Major complications (Clavien 3–5) occurred in 0–25 % of patients, and estimated blood loss varied between 119 and 1000 ml. Except for the early series that reported high rates of blood loss because of locally advanced and challenging procedures, most authors thereafter showed blood transfusion rates similar to the standard radical prostatectomy procedure in their institutions (Chade et al. 2012).

7 Functional Outcomes of Salvage Prostatectomy

The potential for cure with salvage radical prostatectomy must be balanced against the risks of substantial potential toxicities. Postoperative development of sexual and urinary dysfunction represents the mainstay limitations for preserving quality of life, when tumor burden becomes a less important issue. These risks are greater in the salvage prostatectomy setting than in the de novo setting because of radiation changes in the operation field that may cause fibrosis and merging of tissue planes used for dissection. In open salvage prostatectomy series, urinary continence defined by zero pads after salvage prostatectomy, ranged from 22 to 68 % (Table 4). This seems to be related, in part, to radiation-induced sphincteric dysfunction, as published continence rates have not improved markedly over time despite better patient selection, less pelvic fibrosis, and changes in surgical technique (Kimura et al. 2010). Erectile dysfunction was previously thought to be an inevitable consequence of salvage prostatectomy. However, cavernous nerve preservation is feasible in selected patients with good preoperative erectile function, who might recover potency after bilateral nerve-sparing salvage prostatectomy (Masterson et al. 2005).

References

Agarwal PK, Sadetsky N, Konety BR, Resnick MI, Carroll PR (2008) Treatment failure after primary and salvage therapy for prostate cancer: likelihood, patterns of care, and outcomes. Cancer 112(2):307–314. doi:10.1002/cncr.23161

Bianco FJ Jr, Scardino PT, Stephenson AJ, Diblasio CJ, Fearn PA, Eastham JA (2005) Long-term oncologic results of salvage radical prostatectomy for locally recurrent prostate cancer after radiotherapy. Int J Radiat Oncol Biol Phys 62(2):448–453. doi:10.1016/j.ijrobp.2004.09.049

Carson CC 3rd, Zincke H, Utz DC, Cupps RE, Farrow GM (1980) Radical prostatectomy after radiotherapy for prostatic cancer. J Urol 124(2):237–239

Chade DC, Eastham J, Graefen M, Hu JC, Karnes RJ, Klotz L, Montorsi F, van Poppel H, Scardino PT, Shariat SF (2012) Cancer control and functional outcomes of salvage radical prostatectomy for radiation-recurrent prostate cancer: a systematic review of the literature. Eur Urol 61(5):961–971. doi:10.1016/j.eururo.2012.01.022

Chade DC, Shariat SF, Cronin AM, Savage CJ, Karnes RJ, Blute ML, Briganti A, Montorsi F, van der Poel HG, Van Poppel H, Joniau S, Godoy G, Hurtado-Coll A, Gleave ME, Dall'Oglio M, Srougi M, Scardino PT, Eastham JA (2011) Salvage radical prostatectomy for radiation-recurrent prostate cancer: a multi-institutional collaboration. Eur Urol 60(2):205–210. doi:10.1016/j.eururo.2011.03.011

de Jong IJ, Pruim J, Elsinga PH, Vaalburg W, Mensink HJ (2003) 11C-choline positron emission tomography for the evaluation after treatment of localized prostate cancer. Eur Urol 44(1):32–38 (discussion 38–39)

Gheiler EL, Tefilli MV, Tiguert R, Grignon D, Cher ML, Sakr W, Pontes JE, Wood DP Jr (1998) Predictors for maximal outcome in patients undergoing salvage surgery for radio-recurrent prostate cancer. Urology 51(5):789–795

Gotto GT, Yunis LH, Vora K, Eastham JA, Scardino PT, Rabbani F (2010) Impact of prior prostate radiation on complications after radical prostatectomy. J Urol 184(1):136–142. doi:10.1016/j.juro.2010.03.031

Heidenreich A, Richter S, Thuer D, Pfister D (2010) Prognostic parameters, complications, and oncologic and functional outcome of salvage radical prostatectomy for locally recurrent prostate cancer after 21st-century radiotherapy. Eur Urol 57(3):437–443. doi:10.1016/j.eururo.2009.02.041

Jadvar H, Alavi A (2009) Role of imaging in prostate cancer. PET clinics 4(2):135–138. doi:10.1016/j.cpet.2009.05.003

Jemal A, Bray F, Center MM, Ferlay J, Ward E, Forman D (2011) Global cancer statistics. CA Cancer J Clin 61(2):69–90. doi:10.3322/caac.20107

Kimura M, Mouraviev V, Tsivian M, Mayes JM, Satoh T, Polascik TJ (2010) Current salvage methods for recurrent prostate cancer after failure of primary radiotherapy. BJU international 105(2):191–201. doi:10.1111/j.1464-410X.2009.08715.x

Leonardo C, Simone G, Papalia R, Franco G, Guaglianone S, Gallucci M (2009) Salvage radical prostatectomy for recurrent prostate cancer after radiation therapy. Int J Urol Official J Jpn Urol Assoc 16(6):584–586. doi:10.1111/j.1442-2042.2008.02209.x

Masterson TA, Stephenson AJ, Scardino PT, Eastham JA (2005) Recovery of erectile function after salvage radical prostatectomy for locally recurrent prostate cancer after radiotherapy. Urology 66(3):623–626. doi:10.1016/j.urology.2005.04.002

Mohler J, Bahnson RR, Boston B, Busby JE, D'Amico A, Eastham JA, Enke CA, George D, Horwitz EM, Huben RP, Kantoff P, Kawachi M, Kuettel M, Lange PH, Macvicar G, Plimack ER, Pow-Sang JM, Roach M 3rd, Rohren E, Roth BJ, Shrieve DC, Smith MR, Srinivas S, Twardowski P, Walsh PC (2010) NCCN clinical practice guidelines in oncology: prostate cancer. J Natl Comprehensive Cancer Netw JNCCN 8(2):162–200

Mottet N, Bellmunt J, Bolla M, Joniau S, Mason M, Matveev V, Schmid HP, Van der Kwast T, Wiegel T, Zattoni F, Heidenreich A (2011) EAU guidelines on prostate cancer. Part II: treatment of advanced, relapsing, and castration-resistant prostate cancer. Eur Urol 59(4):572–583. doi:10.1016/j.eururo.2011.01.025

Nguyen PL, D'Amico AV, Lee AK, Suh WW (2007) Patient selection, cancer control, and complications after salvage local therapy for postradiation prostate-specific antigen failure: a systematic review of the literature. Cancer 110(7):1417–1428. doi:10.1002/cncr.22941

Pontes JE, Montie J, Klein E, Huben R (1993) Salvage surgery for radiation failure in prostate cancer. Cancer 71(3 Suppl):976–980

Roach M 3rd, Hanks G, Thames H Jr, Schellhammer P, Shipley WU, Sokol GH, Sandler H (2006) Defining biochemical failure following radiotherapy with or without hormonal therapy in men with clinically localized prostate cancer: recommendations of the RTOG-ASTRO Phoenix consensus conference. Int J Radiat Oncol Biol Phys 65(4):965–974. doi:10.1016/j.ijrobp.2006.04.029

Rogers E, Ohori M, Kassabian VS, Wheeler TM, Scardino PT (1995) Salvage radical prostatectomy: outcome measured by serum prostate specific antigen levels. J Urol 153(1):104–110. doi:10.1097/00005392-199501000-00037

Sanderson KM, Penson DF, Cai J, Groshen S, Stein JP, Lieskovsky G, Skinner DG (2006) Salvage radical prostatectomy: quality of life outcomes and long-term oncological control of radiorecurrent prostate cancer. J Urol 176(5):2025–2031 (discussion 2031–2022). doi:10.1016/j.juro.2006.07.075

Stephenson AJ, Scardino PT, Bianco FJ Jr, DiBlasio CJ, Fearn PA, Eastham JA (2004) Morbidity and functional outcomes of salvage radical prostatectomy for locally recurrent prostate cancer after radiation therapy. J Urol 172(6 Pt 1):2239–2243

van der Poel HG, Beetsma DB, van Boven H, Horenblas S (2007) Perineal salvage prostatectomy for radiation resistant prostate cancer. Eur Urol 51(6):1565–1571 (discussion 1572). doi:10.1016/j.eururo.2006.08.011

Walsh PC (1998) Anatomic radical prostatectomy: evolution of the surgical technique. J Urol 160(6 Pt 2):2418–2424

Ward JF, Sebo TJ, Blute ML, Zincke H (2005) Salvage surgery for radiorecurrent prostate cancer: contemporary outcomes. J Urol 173(4):1156–1160. doi:10.1097/01.ju.0000155534.54711.60

Zelefsky MJ, Fuks Z, Hunt M, Yamada Y, Marion C, Ling CC, Amols H, Venkatraman ES, Leibel SA (2002) High-dose intensity modulated radiation therapy for prostate cancer: early toxicity and biochemical outcome in 772 patients. Int J Radiat Oncol Biol Phys 53(5):1111–1116

Zietman AL, DeSilvio ML, Slater JD, Rossi CJ Jr, Miller DW, Adams JA, Shipley WU (2005) Comparison of conventional-dose vs high-dose conformal radiation therapy in clinically localized adenocarcinoma of the prostate: a randomized controlled trial. JAMA J Am Med Assoc 294(10):1233–1239. doi:10.1001/jama.294.10.1233

Zincke H (1992) Radical prostatectomy and exenterative procedures for local failure after radiotherapy with curative intent: comparison of outcomes. J Urol 147(3 Pt 2):894–899

Part VIII

Use of Protons and Heavy Ions

Proton Therapy for Prostate Cancer: Technological and Clinical Aspects

Ralf A. Schneider

Contents

R. A. Schneider (✉)
Center for Proton Therapy, Paul Scherrer Institute, Villigen, Switzerland
e-mail: ralf.Schneider@psi.ch

Abstract

Proton beam therapy (PBT) is an up-coming technology within the framework of radiation oncology. To date, patients with low to intermediate prostate cancer represent the largest group of patients treated with protons. This patient group was of special interest because of expected low toxicity and high tumor control rates. However, there is no published data demonstrating a benefit for protons compared to other radiation modalities. Therefore, prospective randomized phase III trials comparing photon radiation (RT) with that of PBT are needed including evaluation of quality of life after treatment. On the other hand, PBT might be superior to other radiation techniques for advanced prostate cancer where there is a need for pelvic lymph node irradiation, especially in younger patients with a long life expectancy. Also for this subgroup of prostate cancer patients prospective randomized phase III trials comparing RT and PBT are needed. The significance of PBT within the framework of modern radiation oncology in general will be dependent on accrual of scientific data of treated patients. Smaller and less cost-intensive facility layouts with faster beam application are needed. Permanent establishment of protons in radiation therapy will also be dependent on financial resources provided by healthcare systems. That will be finally a political discussion in most countries.

1 Introduction

Proton radiation therapy (PT) has become an increasing factor in high-tech medicine in the field of oncology. A small number of companies in the global market offer $100 million PT facilities with all-inclusive packages. High numbers of patients with short-term treatments are needed to reimburse these projects. Because of localization and size of tumor as well as planned therapy volumes, prostate cancer promises

H. Geinitz et al. (eds.), *Radiotherapy in Prostate Cancer*, Medical Radiology. Radiation Oncology,
DOI: 10.1007/174_2014_1018,
Published Online: 22 May 2014

fast treatments with expected low incidences of severe side effects. Therefore prostate cancer patients increasingly wish to undergo PT instead of established treatment modalities. Even the name PROton leads to positive associations in comparison to X-ray therapy. Several patients expect PT as a treatment option without any side effects.

On the other hand, recently there was a first publication comparing intensity-modulated radiation therapy, proton therapy, or conformal radiation therapy and morbidity and disease control in localized prostate cancer. IMRT compared with PT was associated with less gastrointestinal morbidity (Sheets et al. 2012).

The main problem of the study was a comparison after propensity matching of a multi-center IMRT database of 9,437 patients with a single institution database of 685 PT patients, based on the Surveillance, Epidemiology, and Results (SEER)-Medicare-linked database. The results were inconsistent with follow-up data of several studies' patients including also prospective trials of PT (see below).

Nevertheless, the scientific evidence of PT for prostate cancer in the framework of radiation oncology has to be questioned, especially regarding the fact that even at high ranked university-based PT facilities in the U.S., up to 70 % of treated patients get a therapy for their low-risk prostate cancer. This chapter gives a short but comprehensive overview of the technological and clinical aspects in PT for prostate cancer.

2 Development of Proton Radiation Therapy (PT)

The principal technology of PT is well known and is in use since the 1950s. Hence, it is as old as photon radiation therapy (RT) with linear accelerators. But because of its technological complexity as well as the uncertainty to verify its targets and doses, PT was limited to a few research centers treating low numbers of patients. Only with the development of 3-D planning systems based on data of first computer tomographs, exact calculations of a proton beam in a patient could have been realized for PT. It was the beginning of modern PT using its physical characteristics of improved dose distribution in tumor and reduced radiation dose to surrounding normal tissues. Harvard Cyclotron (HCL) research center in Boston became the first PT facility using CT planning in the mid-1970s. Table 1 summarizes patients treated worldwide by the end of 2013. Of 108,066 patients treated worldwide with particle therapy, proton therapy has been applied in 95,325 patients (88.2 %), and carbon ion therapy in 12,741 patients (11.8 %) (Table 1). Taking into account all facilities (in operation and out of operation), these numbers increase to 122,399 patients (total), 105,631 treated with protons (86.3 %) and 16,768 with C-ions or other heavy ions (13.7 %) (frequent updates at PTCOG website). Hence, a large series of patients have been treated with proton therapy, while treatment with C-ions can be still considered experimental. Although proton radiation therapy has been available for many decades, until recently it was only applied in a relatively small number of approximately 20 centers worldwide. Increased clinical experience with protons, as well as extensive research in the physics, biology, and clinical aspects of proton therapy have led to increasing acceptance and interest in proton therapy among radiation oncologists. Numerous proton therapy facilities are currently being built and planned worldwide. The number of patients treated with protons will increase substantially in the near future.

Nowadays, protons are an accepted treatment modality for tumors in difficult to treat locations, i.e., in the area of the skull base or along the spinal axis, also including sarcomas involving the thoracic chest wall, as well as malignancies in pediatric patients, where minimizing normal tissue radiation exposure is of paramount importance. Outcome analyses demonstrate very satisfying tumor control rates and at the same time low incidence of radiation-induced toxicities (Hug and Slater 2000; DeLaney et al. 2009; Rutz et al. 2008).

3 Physical Characteristics of Protons

PT with its physical characteristics of superior dose deposition in a given tumor and reduced radiation dose to surrounding normal tissues offers an inherent geometric advantage. Lower entrance doses as well as sharp dose falloff at the distal edge of the beam result in a significant higher conformality in comparison to photons. The main disadvantage of the proton beam is the worse lateral dose falloff and the range of uncertainties when treating tissues of different densities especially if there are inter- and intra-fractional changes during treatment (Fig. 1).

4 Radio-Biological Effectiveness (RBE) of Protons

According to the International Commission on Radiation Units and Measurements (ICRU) report 78 (ICRU 2007) the radio-biological effectiveness (RBE) of protons is comparable with the RBE of photons. Dose units expressed as physical dose have a difference of about 10 % in favor of protons (Paganetti et al. 2002). The usually constant RBE of 1.1 in comparison to photons is an advantage of the proton beam. Nevertheless, one has to estimate a higher RBE at the distal edge of the proton beam. Also, the intensity of the linear energy transfer (LET) influences the RBE (see also the following chapter "There is Evidence of the Superiority of Protons or Heavy Ions, Pro"). Comparable proton or photon doses have a similar cell-killing effect on tumors and

Table 1 Patient statistics for facilities in operation (by end of 2013): 95,326 proton treatments and 12,741 carbon ion treatments

Country	Who, where	Particle	S/C/SC[a] Max. energy (MeV)	Beam directions	Start of treatment	Total patients treated	Date of total
Canada	TRIUMF, Vancouver	p	C 72	1 horiz.	1995	175	Dec-13
Czech Republic	PTC Czech r.s.o., Prague	p	C 230	3 gantries, 1 horiz.	2012	140	Dec-13
China	WPTC, Wanjie/Zibo	p	C 230	2 gantries, 1 horiz.	2004	1,078	Dec-13
China	IMP-CAS, Lanzhou	C-ion	S 400/u	1 horiz.	2006	213	Dec-13
England	Clatterbridge	p	C 62	1 horiz.	1989	2,446	Dec-13
France	CAL, Nice	p	C165	1 horiz.	1991	4,936	Dec-13
France	CPO, Orsay	p	S 250	1 gantry, 2 horiz.	1991	6,432	Dec-13
Germany	HZB, Berlin	p	C 250	1 horiz.	1998	2,312	Dec-13
Germany	RPTC, Munich	p	C 250	4 gantries, 1 horiz.	2009	1,811	Dec-13
Germany	HIT, Heidelberg	p	S 250	2 horiz., 1 gantry[b]	2009, 2012	503	Dec-13
Germany	HIT, Heidelberg	C-ion	S 430/u	2 horiz., 1 gantry[b]	2009, 2012	1,368	Dec-13
Germany	WPE, Essen	p	C 230	4 gantries[c], 1 horiz.	2013	32	Dec-13
Italy	INFN-LNS, Catania	p	C 60	1 horiz.	2002	350	Dec-13
Italy	CNAO, Pavia	p	S 250	3 horiz., 1 vertical	2011	76	Dec-13
Italy	CNAO, Pavia	C-ion	S 480/u	3 horiz., 1 vertical	2012	105	Dec-13
Japan	HIMAC, Chiba	C-ion	S 800/u	horiz.[c], vertical[c]	1994	8,073	Dec-13
Japan	NCC, Kashiwa	p	C 235	2 gantries[c]	1998	1,226	Mar-13
Japan	HIBMC, Hyogo	p	S 230	1 gantry	2001	4,223	Dec-13
Japan	HIBMC, Hyogo	C-ion	S 320/u	horiz.,vertical	2002	1,935	Dec-13
Japan	PMRC 2, Tsukuba	p	S 250	2 gantries	2001	2,967	Dec-13
Japan	Shizuoka Cancer Center	p	S 235	3 gantries, 1 horiz.	2003	1,590	Dec-13
Japan	STPTC, Koriyama-City	p	S 235	2 gantries, 1 horiz.	2008	2,306	Dec-13
Japan	GHMC, Gunma	C-ion	S 400/u	3 horiz., 1 vertical	2010	985	Dec-13
Japan	MPTRC, Ibusuki	p	S 250	3 gantries	2011	919	Dec-13
Japan	Fukui Prefectural Hospital PTC, Fukui City	p	S 235	2 gantries, 1 horiz.	2011	428	Dec-13
Japan	Nagoya PTC, Nagoya City, Aichi	p	S 250	2 gantries, 1 horiz.	2013	199	Dec-13
Japan	SAGA-HIMAT, Tosu	C-ion	S 400/u	3 horiz., vertical, 45 deg.	2013	62	Dec-13
Poland	IFJ PAN, Krakow	p	C 60	1 horiz.	2011	39	Dec-13
Russia	ITEP, Moscow	p	S 250	1 horiz.	1969	4,320	Dec-13
Russia	St. Petersburg	p	S 1000	1 horiz.	1975	1,386	Dec-12
Russia	JINR 2, Dubna	p	C 200[d]	1 horiz.	1999	995	Dec-13
South Africa	NRF—iThemba Labs	p	C 200	1 horiz.	1993	521	Dec-13
South Korea	NCC, Ilsan	p	C 230	2 gantries, 1 horiz.	2007	1,158	Dec-13
Sweden	Uppsala	p	C 200	1 horiz.	1989	1,356	Dec-13
Switzerland	PSI, Villigen	p	C 250	2 gantries[e], 1 horiz.	1984, 1996, 2013	7,045	Dec-13
USA, CA	Loma Linda	p	S 250	3 gantries, 1 horiz.	1990	17,829	Dec-13
USA, CA	UCSF	p	C 60	1 horiz.	1994	1,621	Dec-13
USA, MA	NPTC, MGH Boston	p	C 235	2 gantries[c], 1 horiz.	2001	7,345	Dec-13
USA, IN	IU Health PTC, Bloomington	p	C 200	2 gantries[c], 1 horiz.	2004	1,927	Dec-13

(continued)

Table 1 (continued)

Country	Who, where	Particle	S/C/SC[a] Max. energy (MeV)	Beam directions	Start of treatment	Total patients treated	Date of total
USA, TX	MD Anderson Cancer Center, Houston	p	S 250	3 gantries[c], 1 horiz.	2006	4,746	Dec-13
USA, FL	UFPTI, Jacksonville	p	C 230	3 gantries, 1 horiz.	2006	5,085	Dec-13
USA, OK	ProCure PTC, Oklahoma City	p	C 230	1 gantry, 1 horiz, 2 horiz/60 deg.	2009	1,364	Dec-13
USA, PA	UPenn, Philadelphia	p	C 230	4 gantries, 1 horiz.	2010	1,744	Dec-13
USA, IL	CDH Proton Center, Warrenville	p	C 230	1 gantry, 1 horiz, 2 horiz/60 deg.	2010	1,329	Dec-13
USA, VA	HUPTI, Hampton	p	C 230	4 gantries, 1 horiz.	2010	767	Dec-13
USA, NY	ProCure Proton Therapy Center, New Jersey	p	C 230	4 gantries	2012	512	Dec-13
USA, WA	SCCA ProCure Proton Therapy Center, Seattle	p	C 230	4 gantries	2013	86	Dec-13
USA, MO	S. Lee Kling PTC, Barnes Jewish Hospital, St. Louis	p	SC 250	1 gantry	2013	1	Dec-13
USA, CA	Scripps Proton Therapy Center, San Diego	p	C 250	3 gantries, 2 horiz.	2014	1	Feb-14

Particle therapy facilities in operation: Information about technical equipment and patient statistics. Last update: 24 March 2014

[a] *S/C/SC* = Synchrotron (S) or Cyclotron (C) or SynchroCyclotron (SC)

[b] With beam scanning

[c] With spread beam and beam scanning

[d] Degraded beam

[e] With beam scanning, Gantry 1 since 1996, Gantry 2 since 2013

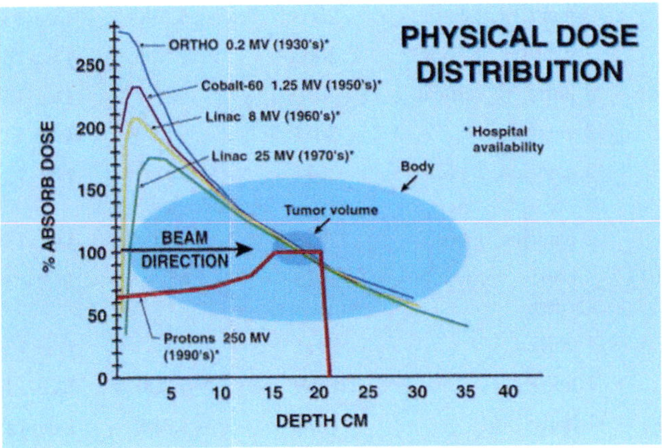

Fig. 1 Dose distribution of different beam qualities

similar toxic effects on normal healthy tissues (Paganetti et al. 2004). This results in an excellent estimation of expected toxicities in comparison to applied doses during the treatment planning process. Established tolerance doses in RT are generally transferable to PT. All available publications on treatments with protons confirmed it. No publication has raised the issue of unexpected acute or late toxicity. Any described incidence of late toxicity was related to high dose escalation rather than use of protons. The initial concept of physical dose distribution and effectiveness has not been called into question by clinical results. However, no phase III trials were available comparing protons and photons. Most proton radiation therapy data were based on retrospective reviews and only for a few indications data were based on phase I/II trials of single institution experiences. Multi-institutional collaboration was very limited.

5 Technological Innovations

Common passive scattering systems (Fig. 2) will be replaced by developed scanning systems in the medium term. Activities of most vendors are going into this direction. Spot scanning-based PT has been pioneered at Paul Scherrer Institute (PSI) and is in routine clinical use since 1996. Presently, PSI remains the only facility with long-term experience (Fig. 3).

Spot scanning will be the preferred technology, because of its excellent dose distribution and the planning option to use intensity modulated proton therapy (IMPT) (Fig. 4). IMPT is routinely used in patient treatments at PSI, if the dose can be safely applied because several uncertainties need to be taken into account when working with spot scanning

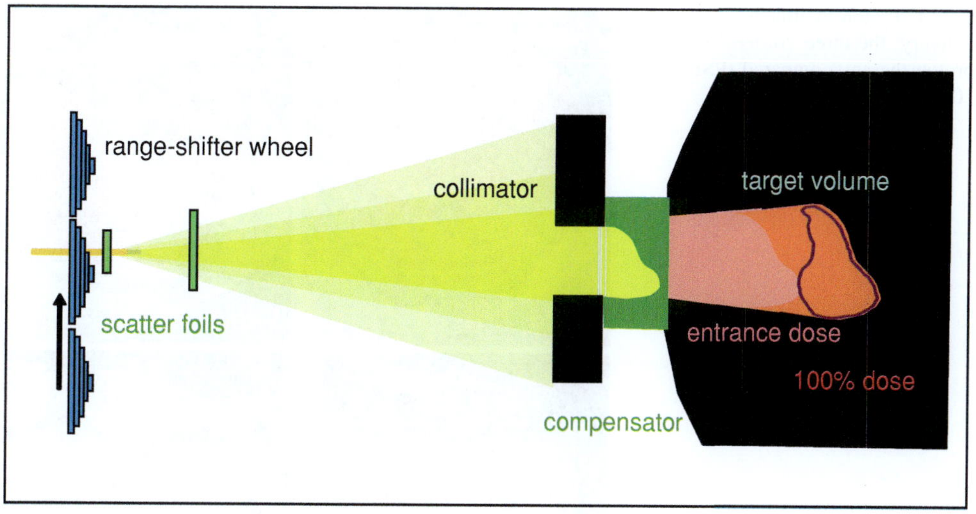

Fig. 2 Technique of scattered proton radiation therapy

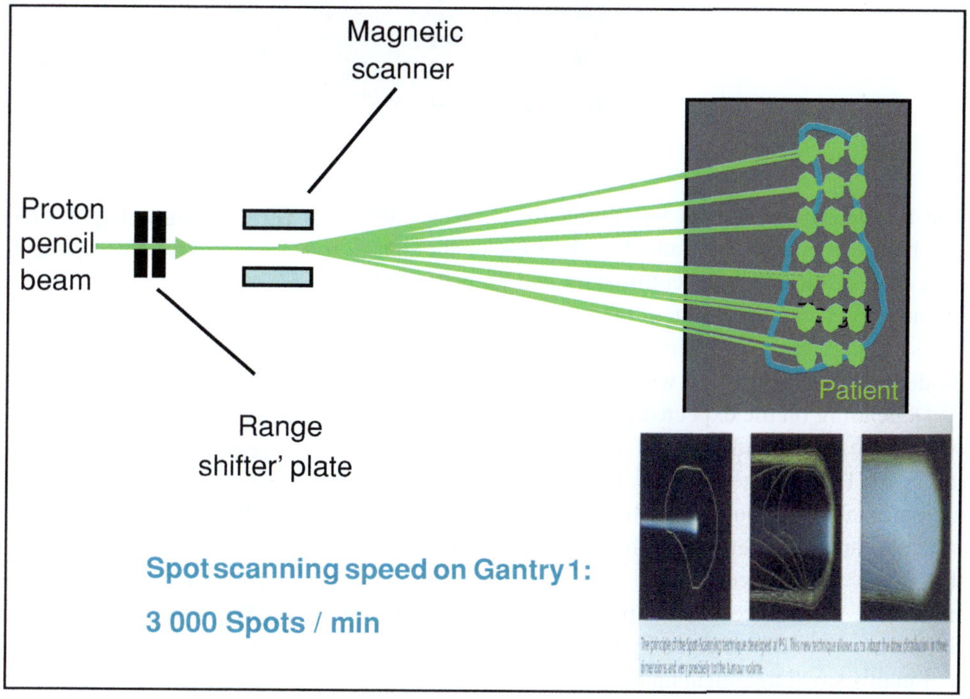

Fig. 3 Spot scanning technique: developed at Paul Scherrer Institute (PSI) and in clinical practice since 1996

technology. Especially, limits of the innovative IMPT have yet not been reached aside from its well-known less robustness to movements of the patient or target. Density uncertainties in the treatment volumes can decrease as well the robustness of IMPT plans (Lomax 2008a, b). To treat moving targets with spot scanning posed already a challenge, how to use IMPT in these cases will be one of the most interesting and important scientific projects for the next years.

Faster scanning techniques will enable to apply multiple target repainting (Gantry 2 at PSI). This implies a fast double magnetic scanning with speeds of 1 and 2 cm/ms, fast dynamic energy variations with the beam line, and degrader before the gantry (100 ms for changes of 5 mm in proton range). Beam analyses at Gantry 2 are promising, also as the potential of the intensity modulation at the ion source for dose painting. Fast target repainting may enable to treat moving tumors with conformal scanning in all situations.

Other technological innovations as multileaf collimators, in-room CT for positioning, and 4-D images as well as beam-eye-view (BEV) X-ray images at the nozzle will increase the precision and quality assurance especially when treating moving targets and will be implemented into new facility layouts.

Nozzles will be designed with minimal material in the beam, in order to keep the size of the scanning beam small at all energies (<3–4 mm sigma between 100–230 MeV).

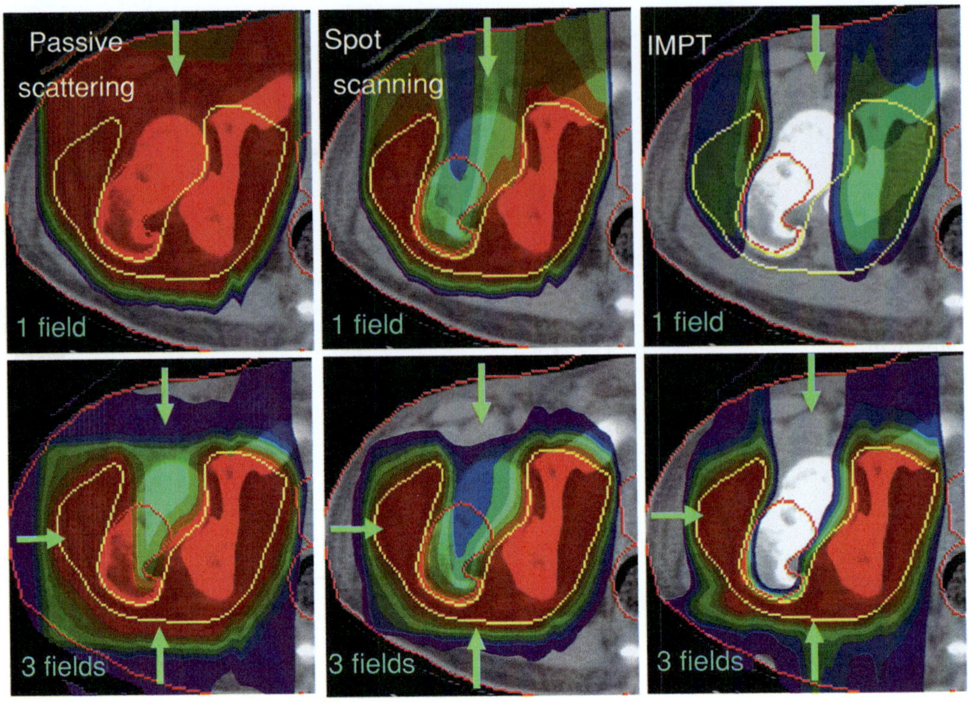

Fig. 4 Proton treatment delivery; the three "orders" of proton therapy compared (PSI 2001)

The nozzle can be moved longitudinally to reduce the air gap between nozzle and patient at the iso-center. That will give the option to mount collimators and compensators on the nozzle. Even simulation of the scattering technique with a system capable of delivering the most advanced intensity modulated proton therapy will be possible (Gantry 2, PSI).

Depending on the expected patient groups gantry layouts will be the gold standard in PT, especially for smaller facilities with 1–2 treatment rooms. Fixed beam rooms might be an optional technique if treatments are focused on, e.g., prostate cancer. Nevertheless, the freedom to deliver beam on the supine positioned patient from any direction will be important. Good access to the patient table at any time on a fixed floor should be offered by the vendors.

Finally, small treatment units are under development at the leading companies to spread out proton therapy facilities. Several radiation oncology centers are not only limited by financial resources but also by space for a large facility with cyclotron or synchrotron and beam line. Compact systems will give the option to add 1–2 treatment rooms to the existing equipment. Several companies are working on these specifications. First treatments are expected in the near future. Operation and application of beam delivery as well as quality of the beam have to be compared with established technologies. On the other hand, an ideal design for a facility has not yet been created. Customers will be still the testers of new technological solutions. To decide for the best facility layout spending a high amount of money will not be easy, because life expectancy of a proton therapy facility is calculated with 25–30 years.

6 Developmental Stages of PT for Prostate Cancer

6.1 Stage I: Safety, Feasibility

The first scientific evaluation of PT for prostate cancer was done at Harvard Cyclotron. Shipley et al. (1995) initialized a prospective dose escalation study at Massachusetts General Hospital (MGH), Boston. Photon RT with total doses of 67.2 Gy was given in 4-field box technique to arm A and B. Randomized patients in arm B also received an additional perineal PT boost to a total dose of 75.6 Gy.

The dose escalation arm was not only an innovative concept for PT but also for RT, because external beam doses in excess of 70 Gy were uncommon at the start of trial. A disadvantage of the study was the long accrual from 1982 to 1995 with a low total number of 202 patients. Due to the long accrual time, the low-dose level arm was already outdated at the time of reporting and doses in the high dose arm were already accepted routinely in many photon centers.

Apart from these limitations, results showed a significant better local tumor control rate in the high dose arm for patients with Gleason 8–10 with slightly increased low Grade rectal bleeding rates (primarily Gr. 1) in the high dose group (34 % vs. 16 %). Survival rates in both groups were similar. As a positive effect of the study it contributed to awareness of partial rectal wall tolerance (Hartford et al. 1996; Benk et al. 1993).

The worldwide first hospital-based PT facility started at Loma Linda University Medical Center (LLUMC), California, in 1992. The scientific focus of interest was prostate cancer with temporarily up to 80 % of treated PT patients. With more than 15,000 treated patients in about 20 years, LLUMC is the facility with the highest number of prostate cancer treated with protons. Some prostate studies were (co-) initiated by LLUMC. In general, all prostate patients were treated according to study protocols.

Design of the initial study was a protocol with normofractionated doses up to 74–75 Gy (Slater et al. 2004). In total 1,255 patients were recruited. Local tumor control rates were dependent on the initial PSA score before PT. Grade 3 toxicities were observed in only 0.3 % of the patients. The study showed the practicability and safety of applied homogeneous PT doses to the prostate in excess of 70 Gy (RBE) with low incidences of higher grade toxicity rates. The published results caused increased inquiries of patients regarding PT for prostate cancer.

6.2 Stage II: Introduction into Routine Clinical Use

A following randomized prospective dose escalation study was initialized by the cooperation of LLUMC with MGH. Initial treatment for all patients was photonRT with a total dose of 50.4 Gy followed by a PT boost up to 70.2 Gy versus 79.2 Gy. About 393 patients with T1b-T2b stage had been enrolled from 1996 to 1999. An update after a median follow-up time of 8.9 years showed similar results for overall survival rates as well as for high grade toxicity rates in both groups but showed increased biochemical tumor control rates for the high dose arm with 83.3 % versus 67.6 % for the lower dose arm (Zietman et al. 2010).

6.3 Stage III: Stagnation

Multiple treatment planning comparisons between photons and protons regarding treatment of the low risk prostate cancer patient have been published. Differences were mainly decreased integral doses when planning with protons. Mainly volumes of PT and IMRT were compared (Trofimov et al. 2007; Vargas et al. 2008).

6.4 Stage IV: Renaissance of Clinical Trials

Several studies were recently started in the U.S. For example, the Proton Collaborative Group (PCG) was established to organize controlled multicenter trials for protons. First results are expected during the next couple of years.

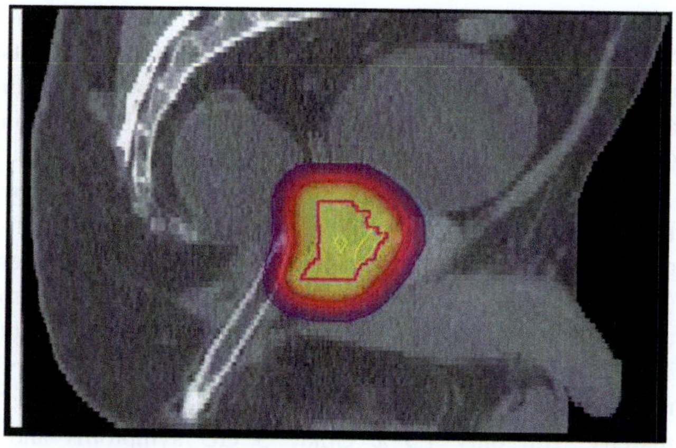

Fig. 5 Dose distribution at the prostate. Lateral opposed beam arrangement, scattered proton beams, water-filled rectal catheter, LLUMC (Courtesy of Carl Rossi)

6.4.1 Dose Escalation for Standard Fractionation-Testing the Limits

A prospective toxicity study was created by LLUMC and MGH with escalation to total doses of 82 Gy (RBE) at 2.0 Gy per fraction using opposed lateral beams. For technical reasons, dose modulation (IMPT) was not possible. First volume was treated up to 50 Gy with a safety margin of 10 mm except the posterior part (5 mm), followed by treatment of the prostate without any margin up to 82 Gy (RBE).

After a median follow-up time of 32 months, results of late GU Grade $\geq 2/\geq 3$ toxicity rates were 30 and 8 % and late GI Grade $\geq 2/\geq 3$ toxicity rates were 12 and 1 % (Coen et al. 2011). Therefore, toxicity rates were comparable to RT trials with dose escalation to the prostate. Nevertheless, Zietman et al. showed impressively the expected dose limits if applying homogeneous scattered proton radiation doses to the prostate with acceptable late morbidity.

6.4.2 Hypofractionation

LLUMC used in a following prospective phase II trial, a moderate hypofractionation scheme with daily doses of 3 Gy (RBE) for patients with low-intermediate risk (Slater 2009). With a total dose of 60 Gy (RBE) and an estimated alpha/beta ratio of 1.5, study designs took into account the biologic dose limitations of the Zietman trial. Also, in this study prescribed doses to the prostate have to be homogeneously applied. Till date there is no evidence for an increased higher grade toxicity rate (personal communication Carl Rossi) (Fig. 5).

A phase III study of mildly hypofractionated image guided PT with or without androgen suppression for intermediate risk adenocarcinoma of the prostate was designed by the PCG. Arm I consists of conformal PT alone with

2.5 Gy (RBE) 5 days a week in 28 treatments over 5.5–6.5 weeks and with a total dose of 70.0 Gy (RBE). Patients randomized to arm II receive the same PT doses but with additional androgen suppression for 6 months (Proton Collaborative Group and Vargas 2011).

Henderson at University of Florida Proton Therapy Institute (UFPTI) started a phase II study of hypofractionated PT for low and intermediate risk prostate cancer (Henderson 2011). Dose per fraction is 2.5 Gy (RBE) up to a total dose of 70 Gy (RBE) for low risk patients, but 72.5 Gy (RBE) for the intermediate risk patient. A first report of early outcomes suggest high efficacy and minimal toxicity with only 1.9 % Grade 3 GU symptoms and <0.5 % Grade 3 GI toxicities (Mendenhall et al. 2012).

There are only a few European publications on PT for prostate cancer. Johansson et al. from Uppsala University Hospital recently published the outcome of an inhomogeneous group of 278 patients with T1b to T4N0M0 disease. Patients received initial photon RT of 50 Gy, given in 25 fractions. If HDR brachytherapy boost was geometrically impossible because of a large prostate volume above 55–60 cc, patients received a PT boost of 20 Gy (RBE) in daily fractions of 5 Gy (RBE). Fifty-three percent of the patients received also neoadjuvant androgen deprivation therapy. Medium follow-up was 57 months. The 5-year PSA progression-free survival rate was 100, 95, and 74 % for low-, intermediate-, and high-risk patients, respectively. Late Grade 2, 3, and 4 GU toxicities were scored in 11, 7, and 2 % of the patients, respectively. No Grade ≥3 GI toxicity rates were observed (Johansson et al. 2012). The authors stated that a hypofractionated PT boost combined with external beam RT is associated with excellent curability of localized prostate cancer and acceptable frequencies of treatment toxicity.

6.4.3 Extreme Hypofractionation

Vargas is Principal Investigator for the PCG of a prospective randomized trial for low risk adenocarcinoma of the prostate. The control group receives treatments with a daily standard fractionation of 1.8 Gy (RBE) up to a total dose of 79.2 Gy (RBE). Patients in arm II get extreme hypofractionation with single doses of 7.6 Gy (RBE), given in 5 consecutive days of 1–2 weeks to a total dose of 38 Gy (RBE) (Proton Collaborative Group and Vargas 2010). There are no publications yet on early outcome, especially regarding toxicity rates available. But results of this trial will probably significantly influence future procedures in PT for low-risk prostate cancer patients.

6.4.4 Combined Modality Therapy

PCG also designed a phase III study of image guided PT with or without chemotherapy (Docetaxel) for high risk adenocarcinoma of the prostate. The control group gets treatment with a daily standard fractionation of 1.8 Gy (RBE) up to a total dose of 79.2 Gy (RBE) and androgen deprivation. Assessment of the number of Freedom From Failure (FFF) events comparing the chemotherapy arm to the standard treatment arm is the primary objective (Proton Collaborative Group and Vargas 2012).

UFPTI started a phase II trial for high risk prostate cancer patients. PT is given in combination with Docetaxel chemotherapy and androgen deprivation (Mendenhall 2009). The primary objective is the frequency and severity of acute and chronic toxicity after PT in combination with chemotherapy and androgen deprivation.

6.4.5 Spare Organs at Risk

An increasing number of RT centers implement injections of hyaluronic gel as a rectal-prostate spacer for treatment of prostate cancer. A first planning comparison of IMRT, VMAT, and IMPT was recently published. Only IMPT managed to decrease the rectal dose after spacer injection for all dose levels, generally with no observed increase to the bladder dose (Weber et al. 2012). Another advantage of these devices will be a reduced density uncertainty and therefore range uncertainty of protons within the treatment volume regarding the rectal filling. There is probably no need anymore for water filled rectal catheters in these patients if using these spacers.

6.4.6 Photons Versus Protons

Recently, a first intercomparison phase III trial was initiated by MGH and the University of Pennsylvania (UPENN), 461 patients were recruited. The outcome after PT versus IMRT for low or low-intermediate risk prostate cancer was evaluated. Daily doses were 1.8 Gy (RBE) or Gy per fraction, 5 days a week in 44 treatments up to total doses of 79.2 Gy (RBE) or Gy (Efstathiou and Bekelman 2012). A first publication has dealt with the issue of prospective preference assessment of patients' willingness to participate in a randomized controlled trial (Shah et al. 2012). Forty-six eligible patients were enrolled. The study group identified five major themes that impacted patients' willingness to participate in the trial: altruism/desire to compare treatments, randomization, deference to physician opinion, financial incentives, and time demands/scheduling. The authors stated that these findings would inform the recruitment efforts of a planned randomized controlled trial comparing IMRT with PT.

7 Biologic Targeting

All the above described PT trials and comparisons in general followed the same treatment planning concepts with homogeneous dose distribution to the prostate including

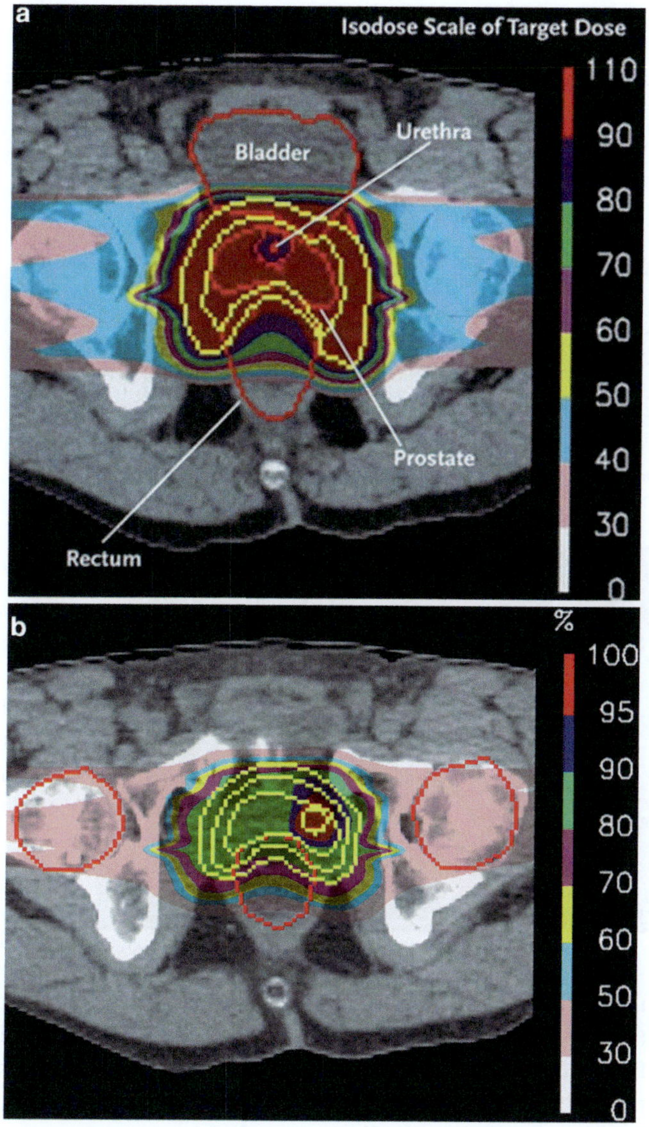

Fig. 6 **a** Selective sparing of the urethra and simultaneous dose escalation (Rutz and Lomax 2007). **b** Selective intraprostatic boost as part of biologic targeting of clonogenic centers (Rutz and Lomax 2007)

safety margins to all directions, typically using two lateral beams and a water filled rectal catheter. Biologic targeting with dose painting is not used for technical reasons. But this is a decade-old practice in brachytherapy with increased tumor control rates, but low incidences of higher grade toxicities. Especially in high risk patients, doses to the prostate gland could be modulated according to the natural behavior of prostate cancer with increased doses to the capsule and dose reduction to the urethra (Galalae et al. 2004).

Interestingly, dose distribution of IMPT fields with its inhomogeneities can be used in a relatively similar way to HDR brachytherapy. Corresponding to location and duration of a positioned radioactive source also with scanned proton beam spots, high and low doses to small volumes are possible if the size of the used pencil beam is small enough (Fig. 6a, b). In comparison to dose distribution in HDR brachytherapy, IMPT planning is independent of the manual ability of the attending physician. Rather, to estimate the robustness of an IMPT plan is decisive. This requires intensive examination of planning procedures in IMPT and knowledge of its uncertainties (Lomax 2008a, b).

A first IMPT plan imitating BT concepts and highly conformal RT was published by PSI and showed possible advantages of IMPT technology in comparison with established PT treatment concepts with scattered protons (Rutz and Lomax 2007). Nevertheless, using IMPT in this way for (extreme) hypofractionation in the moving prostate needs further scientific evaluation regarding robustness and, therefore, safety of such a treatment.

8 Pelvic and Abdominal Proton Radiotherapy

8.1 Preclinical Data

In particular, target volumes of complex shapes, such as the pelvic regional lymph nodes, can be irradiated with highly precise 3-D dose conformation. Site (the anatomical situation of a target and its relation to sensitive normal tissues), size (the extension and volume of a target as compared to neighboring healthy structures and the anatomical compartment), and shape (forms with various degrees of irregularity) of a given target challenge any radiation modality. Protons offer the highest inherent geometrical dose precision inside and the lowest dose load outside a given target volume.

Whole pelvic radiation therapy (WPRT) is commonly given in the management of intermediate to high-risk prostate cancers. However, it entails irradiation of a considerable volume of rectum, urinary bladder, small bowel, and bilateral femoral heads. Intensity-modulated radiotherapy (IMRT) has introduced novel dosimetry that often features increased dose heterogeneity to target and low to intermediate dose levels to non-target normal structures. This raises questions of the biologic effects of IMRT compared to conventional treatment in general. However, increasing the delivered radiation dose may increase the probability of local tumor control but carries a risk of greater adverse effects unless the volume of normal tissue treated along with the tumor can be reduced as it is possible by proton therapy.

The proton radiation beam possesses unique physical properties that allow its shape to be sculpted in tissue in order to achieve—especially in the particular case of large and very irregular locoregional target volumes in high risk

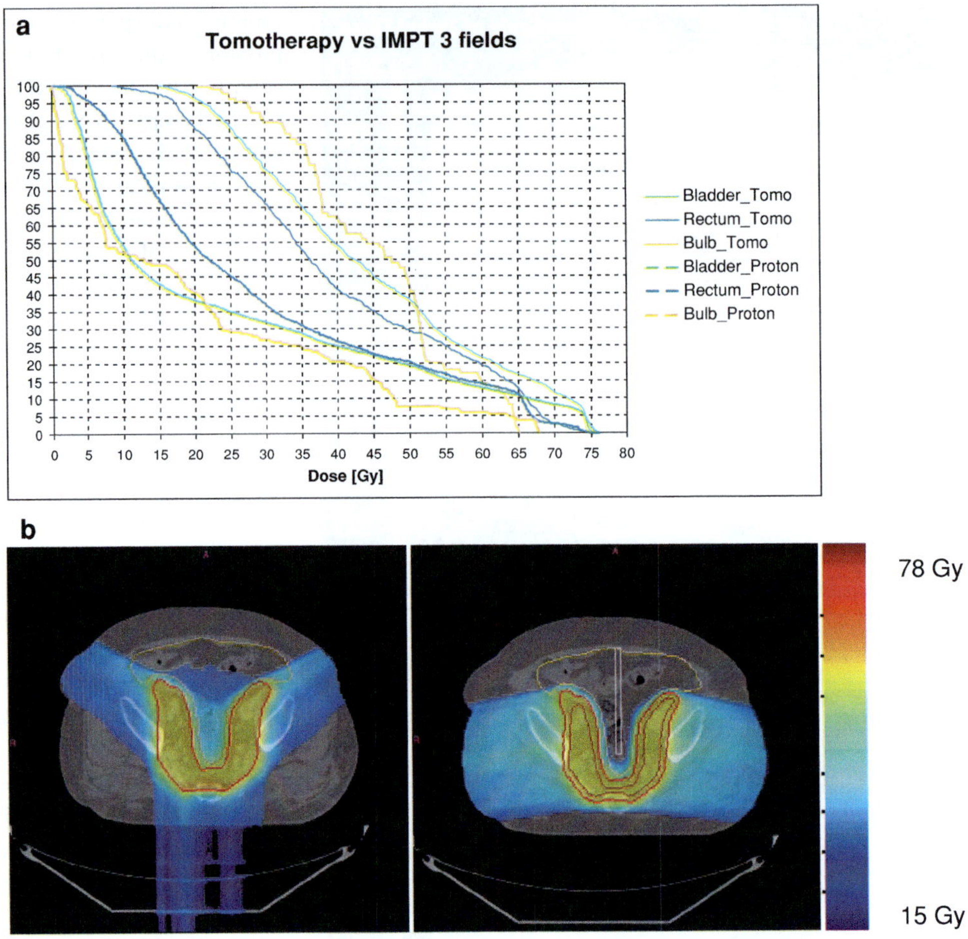

Fig. 7 **a** Dose histograms of pelvic organs; comparison tomotherapy versus IMPT (Widesott et al. 2011). **b** IMPT 3 fields versus (*left*) IMPT 2 fields and virtual block (*right*) (PSI 2009)

prostate cancer—very conformal dose depositions. It lowers also the dose in non-target healthy pelvic tissue in close vicinity to high-dose treatment areas and avoids simultaneously direct dose deposition in normal structures in target volume remote areas. Reduced dose not only applies to a reduced dose load to normal tissues adjacent to the target volume (prostate region and pelvic regional lymph nodes), but also the significant reduction of the total percentage of an anatomical compartment (e.g. the pelvis) or even of the entire body exposed to irradiation (Chera et al. 2009).

A feasibility analysis in the sense of a technical/dosimetric comparison with modern intensity modulated photon beam radiation documented a significant reduction of small bowel dose by using spot scanning-based proton radiotherapy for administration of therapeutic doses in the region of regional lymph nodes (Widesott et al. 2011). The plans of eight patients with high risk prostate cancer previously treated with Helical Tomotherapy (HT) were compared with intensity modulated proton therapy (IMPT) plans with two quasi-lateral fields (−100°; 100°). A vertical "virtual block" was designed in IMPT plans at midline of the bowel cavity (BC) to avoid field crossing (allowing no volume of the block to receive more than 10–15 Gy) and increasing the IMPT plans' robustness. PTV's and Organs at Risk (OAR's) dosimetric data were evaluated and a normal tissue complication probability (NTCP) calculation was performed for rectum using several sets of parameters (m, n, TD50) according to the literature.

This first pre-clinical study demonstrated comparable PTV coverage between HT and IMPT, improved V95 % and conformity indexes for IMPT, and lower maximum dose in the prostate with HT. The main benefit of IMPT was the decreased dose deposition at low and intermediate dose levels of healthy tissues (rectum, bladder, and small bowel). See also (Fig. 7a, b).

8.2 Potential Win–Win Situation of Protons in the Abdomen and Pelvis

Still underestimated is the potential win–win effect of proton radiation therapy in close proximity to moving organs at risk in the abdomen and pelvis. Radiation with protons will not only reduce irradiated intestine in general but will also result in unstable high dose areas to moving organs at risk at the distal edge of the beam if these organs located in close

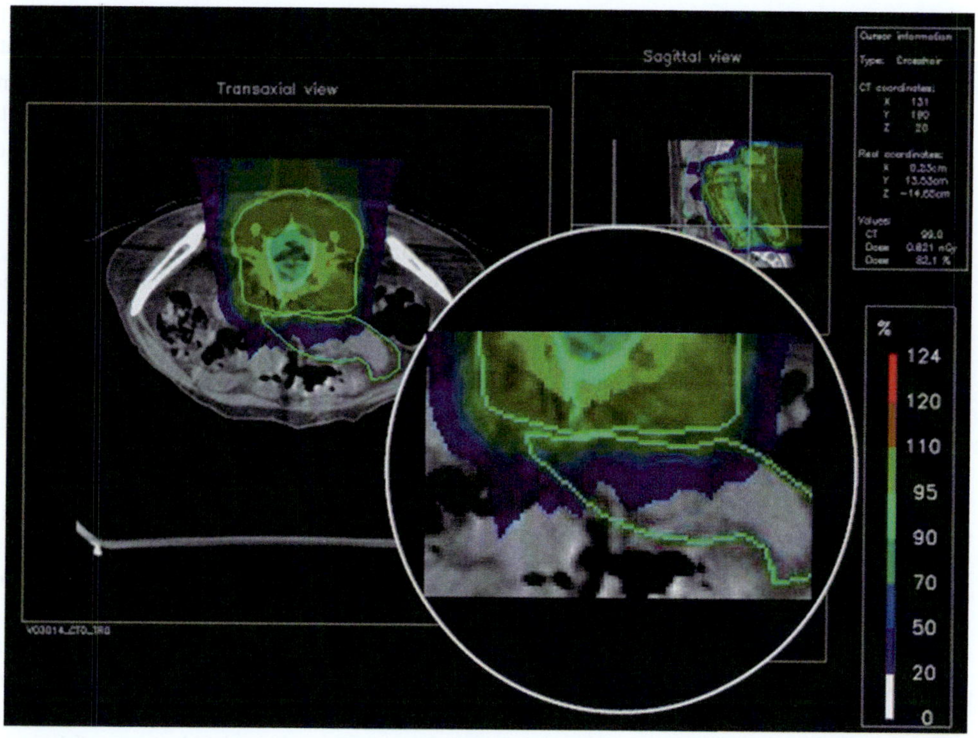

Fig. 8 Distal dose falloff of a proton treatment, non-circumferential high dose areas at small bowel loop, treatment of a sarcoma patient

proximity to the treatment volume. These two advantages could be described as the win–win effect of protons in the abdomen and pelvis (Schneider et al. 2013).

Even modern highly conformal photon irradiation techniques will not imitate this effect, because the moving organ at risk in close proximity to the target will not move outside high dose volumes because of the physical limitations of photons in comparison to protons.

Dose escalation at the high dose target by accepting higher constraints at OAR's, e.g., small bowel or rectum in selected cases may result in a higher tumor control rate without any compromising of dose to the target (Fig. 8). Especially for advanced tumors in the abdomen and pelvis with necessary lymph node involvement proton therapy could be an advantage.

8.3 Innovative Dose Escalation to Pelvic Lymph Nodes

It is still not yet solved whether pelvic lymph nodes should be included when treating high risk prostate cancer patients. The Prostate Cancer Results Study Group recently published a comparative analysis of PSA-free survival outcomes of different risk groups based on reviews of initially 18,000 papers (Grimm et al. 2012). For high-risk patients, a combination of external beam RT with brachytherapy appeared to be superior to more localized treatments.

A present, PT study at PSI for high-risk patients intends to escalate the dose loco-regionally in histological proven pelvic lymph node metastatic disease in a postoperative setting following surgery. The trial has been approved by the ethics committee. The goal will be dose escalation to infiltrated pelvic lymph nodes up to 68 Gy (RBE) delivered in 34 fractions and depending on the surgery procedure 76.5 Gy (RBE) to the prostate given as a concurrent boost. Primary objectives will be technical safety, feasibility, and reproducibility of the daily patient positioning as well as the benefit in terms of biochemical tumor control (PSA relapse-free survival).

9 Proton Radiotherapy and Secondary Malignancies

Publications from our group as well as other particle centers suggest a reduction of risk for secondary malignancies by use of protons. Several treatment planning comparisons of photons versus protons have been published showing decreased integral doses when planning with protons. The larger the planned volume the better will be the conformality of a proton beam plan. Nevertheless, first clinical data published by MGH did not yet show a significant lower rate of secondary malignancies after proton therapy in comparison to photon radiotherapy (Chung et al. 2013). The photon data (558 patients) were sampled from the claims database of the Surveillance, Epidemiology, and End Results (SEER) program and matched with 558 proton patients. The authors were unable to find matches for another 476 proton-treated patients. This retrospective study had several potential limitations. SEER patients who moved outside of SEER areas were no longer followed. Most of the proton irradiated patients received 20 % of their total dose from photon radiation. Proton therapy patients who were successfully matched with SEER patients differed from unmatched proton patients who had rare diseases with relative poor prognosis.

A third of the matched patients had prostate cancer. Nevertheless, there was no significant difference described between proton and photon radiated patients.

On the other hand, substantial reduction of risk for secondary malignancies is particularly important for postoperative adjuvant treatment of prostate cancer, because life expectancy in these patients is relatively long despite their metastatic course of disease. Thus, secondary malignancies are likely to be experienced. Further investigation with longer follow-ups and higher numbers of patients is probably needed to get valid results and to finally identify patient groups that would profit from proton beam therapy.

10 Significance of PT for Prostate Cancer

Similar to modern surgical treatment concepts, also prostate cancer technologies in radiation oncology, e.g., RT and BT have been impressively developed during the past two decades. Conformality and calculation of doses as well as improved quality of imaging lead to dose escalation to the prostate gland with increased tumor control rates and decreased toxicity rates of pelvic organs at risk.

PT, especially of the low to intermediate risk prostate cancer, competes not only with modern surgical procedures but also with established and well-tolerated radiotherapeutic modalities. Nevertheless, technical capabilities in PT have been not yet exploited. Far from it, PT is just at the beginning of rapid developments in several technological subareas.

In the U.S., surgery and all highly advanced (photon) radiation oncology methods are at a higher level of treatment costs than in European countries more comparable to PT therapy. This is often not only dependent on the technology used, but also dependent on the treating institution. Yu et al. evaluated a group of Medicare beneficiaries 66 years and older who received PT or IMRT for prostate cancer during 2008 and 2009. GU side effects were significantly reduced at 6 months or 12 months post-treatment of protons, but median Medicare reimbursement was significantly higher for PT ($32.428) than for IMRT ($18,575) (Yu et al. 2013). Early toxicity outcome is comparable to another study of Gray et al. from MGH. Outcomes of 370 patients were reviewed, 94 of them treated with PT, 123 patients treated with 3D conformal RT and 153 treated with IMRT. At 2- to 3-month follow-up, patients treated with PT reported minimal decreased GI function, whereas patients with RT reported modest bowel changes. However, at 1 and 2 years, patients in all three groups reported a decreased QOL regarding bowel function. Regarding GU toxicity all patients reported a decreased QOL. But for the PT group the adverse event also took longer to develop (Gray et al. 2013).

11 Summary

Because of its usually less complicated and fast treatment procedures, especially when using hypofractionation schemes, PT for low risk to intermediate prostate cancer is of high importance for established and upcoming PT facilities. Till date there is no publication showing a benefit for protons in comparison to other radiation oncology tools in the treatment of low risk prostate cancer patients. But there is also no evidence for a worse outcome regarding tumor control rates as well as toxicity rates when using established treatment doses for PT except for the publication of Sheets et al. (Sheets et al. 2012).

A benefit for protons might be the treatment of especially younger patients with long life expectancy with advanced prostate cancer where pelvic lymph node irradiation is indicated. Multicenter studies with higher numbers of patients should be established to objectify differences between RT and PT regarding tumor control rates and toxicity. Especially, prospective randomized controlled phase III trials comparing RT and PT are needed. UPENN and MGH started such a study. Managing of patient distribution as well as outcome of this trial will lead to further steps to this direction.

The significance of PT within the framework of modern radiation oncology in general will be dependent on the scientific elaboration of data capture of treated patients at established and upcoming facilities. Therefore, It will mainly lie in the hands of the responsible physicians and medical physicists whether the influence of the complex and cost intensive protons will increase or not in the longer term. The permanent establishment of protons in radiation therapy will also be dependent on financial resources provided by healthcare systems. That will be finally a political decision in most countries.

Nevertheless, more honesty regarding intra- and interdisciplinary discussion of PT, just in analogy to all available therapy modalities for low risk to intermediate prostate cancer, would be desirable.

References

Benk VA, Adams JA, Shipley WU et al (1993) Late rectal bleeding following combined X-ray and proton high dose irradiation for patients with stages T3-T4 prostate carcinoma. Int J Radiat Oncol Biol Phys 26(3):551–557

Chera BS, Vargas C, Morris CG et al (2009) Dosimetric study of pelvic proton radiotherapy for high-risk prostate cancer. Int J Radiat Oncol Biol Phys 75(4):994–1002

Chung CS, Yock TI, Nelson K et al (2013) Incidence of second malignancies among patients treated with proton versus photon radiation. Int J Radiat Oncol Biol Phys 87(1):46–52

Coen JJ, Bae K, Zietman AL et al (2011) Acute and late toxicity after dose escalation to 82 GyE using conformal proton radiation for localized prostate cancer: initial report of American College of Radiology Phase II study 03-12. Int J Radiat Oncol Biol Phys 81(4):1005–1009

DeLaney TF, Liebsch NJ, Pedlow FX et al (2009) Phase II study of high dose photon/proton radiotherapy in the management of spine sarcomas. Int J Radiat Oncol Biol Phys 74:732–739

Efstathiou JA, Bekelman JE (2012) Proton therapy vs. IMRT for low or low-intermediate risk prostate cancer. Phase III trial, 11-497, NCT 01617161

Galalae RM, Martinez A, Mate T et al (2004) Long-term outcome by risk factors using conformal high-dose-rate brachytherapy (HDR-BT) boost with or without neoadjuvant androgen suppression for localized prostate cancer. Int J Radiat Oncol Biol Phys 58(4):1048–1055

Gray PJ, Paly JJ, Yeap BY et al (2013) Patient-reported outcomes after 3-dimensional conformal, intensity-modulated or proton beam radiotherapy for localized prostate cancer. Cancer 2013 (in press)

Grimm P, Billiet I, Bostwick D et al (2012) Comparative analysis of prostate-specific antigen free survival outcomes for patients with low, intermediate and high risk prostate cancer treatment by radical therapy. Results from the prostate cancer results study group. BJUI 109(1):22–29

Hartford AC, Niemierko A, Adams JA et al (1996) Conformal irradiation of the prostate: estimating long-term rectal bleeding risk using dose-volume histograms. Int J Radiat Oncol Biol Phys 36(3):721–730

Henderson RH (2011) Hypofractionated proton radiation therapy for low and intermediate prostate cancer. Phase II trial, UFPTI 1103-PR07, NCT 01368055

Hug EB, Slater JD (2000) Proton radiation therapy for chordomas and chondrosarcomas of the skull base. Neurosurg Clin N Am 11(4):627–638

ICRU (2007) ICRU report 78. J ICRU 7(2)

Johansson S, Astroem L, Sandin F et al (2012) Hypofractionated proton boost combined with external beam radiotherapy for treatment of localized prostate cancer. Prostate Cancer July 8 Epub

Lomax AJ (2008a) Intensity modulated proton therapy and its sensitivity to treatment uncertainties 1: the potential effects of calculational uncertainties. Phys Med Biol 53(4):1027–1042

Lomax AJ (2008b) Intensity modulated proton therapy and its sensitivity to treatment uncertainties 2: the potential effects of inter-fraction and inter-field motions. Phys Med Biol 53(4):1043–1056

Mendenhall N (2009) Docetaxel, androgen deprivation and proton therapy for high risk prostate cancer. Phase II trial, UFPTI 0703-PR05, NCT 01040624

Mendenhall NP, Li Z, Hoppe BS et al (2012) Early outcomes from three prospective trials of image-guided proton therapy for prostate cancer. Int J Radiat Oncol Biol Phys 82(1):213–221

Paganetti H, Niemierko A, Ancukiewicz M, Gerweck LE et al (2002) Relative biological effectiveness (RBE) values for proton beam therapy. Int J Radiat Oncol Biol Phys 53(2):407–421

Paganetti H, Jiang H, Lee SY et al (2004) Accurate Monte Carlo simulations for nozzle design, commissioning and quality assurance for a proton radiation therapy facility. Med Phys 31(7):2107–2118

Proton Collaborative Group, Vargas C (2010) Study of Hypo-fractionated proton radiation for low risk prostate cancer. Phase III trial, GU 002-10, NCT 01230866

Proton Collaborative Group, Vargas C (2011) Hypo-fractionated proton radiation therapy with or without androgen suppression for intermediate risk prostate cancer. Phase III trial, GU003-10, NCT 01492972

Proton Collaborative Group, Vargas C (2012) External beam radiation with or without chemotherapy to treat high risk prostate cancer. Phase III, II trial, GU 004-11, NCT 01603420

Rutz HP, Lomax AJ (2007) Radiotherapy for prostate cancer. N Engl J Med 356:308–311

Rutz HP, Weber DC, Goitein G, Ares C, Bolsi A, Lomax AJ, Pedroni E, Coray A, Hug EB, Timmermann B (2008) Postoperative spot-scanning proton radiation therapy for chordoma and chondrosarcoma in children and adolescents: initial experience at Paul Scherrer Institute. Int J Radiat Oncol Biol Phys 71(1):220–225

Schneider RA, Vitolo V, Albertini F et al (2013) Small bowel toxicity after high dose, spot scanning-based proton therapy for paraspinal/retroperitoneal neoplasms. Strahlenther Onkol 189(12):1020–1025

Shah A, Efstathiou JA, Paly JJ et al (2012) Prospective preference assessment of patients' willingness to participate in a randomized controlled trial of intensity-modulated radiotherapy versus proton therapy for localized prostate cancer. Int J Radiat Oncol Biol Phys 83(1):e13–e19

Sheets NC, Goldin GH, Meyer AM et al (2012) Intensity-modulated radiation therapy, proton therapy, or conformal radiation therapy and morbidity and disease control in localized prostate cancer. JAMA 307(15):1611–1620

Shipley WU, Verhey LJ, Munzenrider JE et al (1995) Advanced prostate cancer: the results of a randomized comparative trial of high dose irradiation boosting with conformal protons compared with conventional dose irradiation using photons alone. Int J Radiat Oncol Biol Phys 32(1):3–12

Slater J (2009) Study of hypofractionated proton beam radiation therapy for prostate cancer. Phase II, I trial, 58116, NCT 00831623

Slater JD, Rossi CJ Jr, Yonemoto LT et al (2004) Proton therapy for prostate cancer: the initial Loma Linda University experience. Int J Radiat Oncol Biol Phys 59(2):348–352

Trofimov A, Nguyen PL, Coen JJ et al (2007) Radiotherapy treatment of early-stage prostate cancer with IMRT and protons: a treatment planning comparison. Int J Radiat Oncol Biol Phys 69(2):444–453

Vargas C, Fryer A, Mahajan C et al (2008) Dose-volume comparison of proton therapy and intensity-modulated radiotherapy for prostate cancer. Int J Radiat Oncol Biol Phys 70(3):744–751

Weber DC, Zilli T, Vallee JP et al (2012) Intensity modulated proton and photon therapy for early prostate cancer with or without transperineal injection of a polyethylen glycol spacer: a treatment planning comparison study. Int J Radiat Oncol Biol Phys 84(3):e311–e318

Widesott L, Pierelli A, Fiorino C et al (2011) Helical Tomotherapy (HT) vs. intensity-modulated proton therapy (IMPT) for whole pelvis irradiation in high risk prostate cancer patients. Dosimetric, normal tissue complication probability, and generalized equivalent uniform dose analysis. Int J Radiat Oncol Biol Phys 80(5):1589–1600

Yu JB, Soulos PR, Herrin J et al (2013) Proton versus intensity-modulated radiotherapy for prostate cancer: patterns of care and early toxicity. J Natl Cancer Inst 105(1):25–32

Zietman AL, Bae K, Slater JD et al (2010) Randomized trial comparing conventional-dose with high-dose conformal radiation therapy in early-stage adenocarcinoma of the prostate: long-term results from proton radiation oncology group/American College of Radiology 95-09. J Clin Oncol 28(7):1106–1111

There is Evidence for the Superiority of Protons and Heavy Ions, Pro

Gregor Habl and Jürgen Debus

Contents

G. Habl (✉) · J. Debus
Radiologische Universitätsklinik, Strahlenklinik,
Im Neuenheimer Feld 400, 69120 Heidelberg, Germany
e-mail: Gregor.habl@med.uni-heidelberg.de

Abstract

This chapter deals with the question of whether irradiation of the prostate with protons or other particles is superior to X-rays. The physical and biological principles of particle beam therapy are presented and the clinical aspects of proton and carbon ion therapy of the prostate are discussed. Relevant studies of particle therapies are introduced and discussed relating to differences in comparison to modern X-ray techniques.

1 Introduction

Relatively radiation "resistant" (to conventional doses of radiation) tumors such as prostate cancer require innovative radiotherapy, which produce a higher dose deposition to the tumor and a steeper dose gradient to the surrounding tissue to minimize radiogenic side effects. Both are possible through the physical advantage of the depth-dose distribution of the particles in the tissue.

Concerning ion beam therapy, the most frequently asked question remains: Is ion beam therapy superior to the current standard of care with photon treatment? This leads to fundamental questions: When is one type of radiation better than another? On the one hand if a therapy is aiming for higher cure rates, and on the other hand if therapy is better tolerated because of lower rates of side effects, should ion beam therapy be adopted as the standard of care? For this purpose, systematic reviews were performed (Allen et al. 2012; Olsen et al. 2007; Lodge et al. 2007).

In the following, the advantage of ion beam therapy is examined.

The current medical use is limited to irradiation with protons and carbon ions. In 1946, proton therapy was introduced by Robert R. Wilson at the Lawrence Berkeley Laboratory in the USA (Wilson 1946; Creutz and Wilson 1946). The first application with a patient occurred less than 10 years

H. Geinitz et al. (eds.), *Radiotherapy in Prostate Cancer*, Medical Radiology. Radiation Oncology,
DOI: 10.1007/174_2014_972, © Springer-Verlag Berlin Heidelberg 2014
Published Online: 14 May 2014

later. In 1975, the first heavy ions were used for therapy. The first proton therapy center was opened in 1990 in Loma Linda, USA. In 1994, the first heavy ion therapy center opened in Chiba, Japan. From 1997 to 2008, the department of radio-oncology at the University of Heidelberg gained clinical experience with heavy ions at the GSI (Society for Heavy Ion Research) in Darmstadt, Germany. Since 2009, patients have been treated at the Ion Beam Therapy Center (HIT) in Heidelberg, Germany. Globally, more than 70,000 patients have been treated with protons and over 7,000 patients with carbon ions. A list of current patient numbers and locations for particle therapy have been published on the website of the Particle Therapy Cooperative Group (PTCOG, http://ptcog.web.psi.ch/). Irradiation with other heavy ions aside from carbon ions has simply not been explored enough, but will certainly be of future interest.

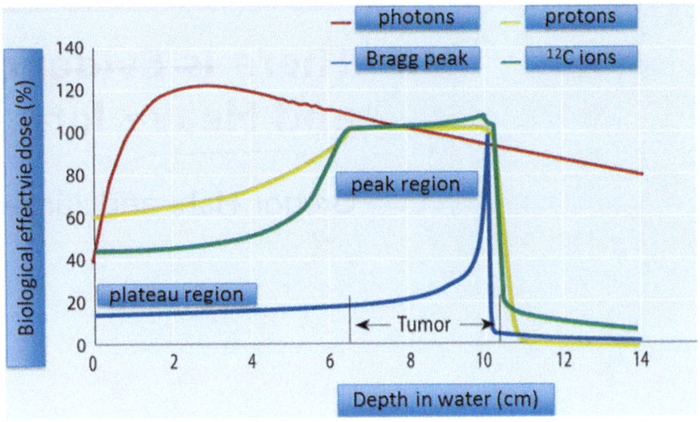

Fig. 1 Characteristic depth-dose distributions of photons, carbon ions, and protons in water

2 Physical Principles

The physical and biological characteristics of proton beams differ from those of heavier particles. Therefore, particle therapy is divided into two categories: "proton therapy" characterized by low linear energy transfer (LET) and "heavy ion therapy" with high LET characteristics. The term "heavy ions" is used for ions heavier than helium ions. The term "charged particles" contains both protons and heavy ions. In principle, "particle therapy" also covers radiation therapy with electrons, pions, and neutrons. In this context, we would like to restrict particle therapy to charged particles with masses equal to or heavier than protons.

The physical advantage of particle therapy compared to photon irradiation lies in the more favorable depth-dose distribution in the tissue (Fig. 1). Photon irradiation enters the body and reaches the maximum dose just below the skin surface. In the deeper trajectory through the body, the radiation dose decreases until it exits the body (red line). Hence, the healthy tissue is harmed in front of and behind the tumor with a certain dosage.

In contrast, protons or heavier particles such as carbon ions enter the body at very high speed. Particles pass through the tissue, slow down, and lose energy in atomic and nuclear interactions in the trajectory in front of the tumor. This reduces the energy of the particles, which in turn causes more interactions with electrons. Maximum interactions occur at the end of range causing maximum energy transfer and thus maximum dose deposition within the target area. The Bragg peak describes the sharp dose increase in a well-defined depth and the rapid dose fall-off beyond the maximum (blue line). Since the width of the Bragg peak is in the millimeter range and usually not wide enough to cover a treatment volume, several of these Bragg peaks must be superimposed to treat a tumor of a certain length and volume, respectively. These superimposed Bragg peaks are called spread-out Bragg peak (SOBP) (Fig. 1, green and yellow line). After the loss of energy at the maximum, the dose drops off abruptly to almost zero. The "residual dose" beyond the Bragg peak is referred to as fragmentation tail. It is formed by interaction of the ions with atomic nuclei in the body, and is usually $<10\,\%$. The radiation plan parameters for ion therapy must be very exact as even the slightest inaccuracy in the beam application can lead to imprecision in the range of the ion beam. Optimal treatment plans and precise patient positioning are necessary to obtain a high-dose deposition within the tumor region with maximum protection of healthy tissue surrounding the tumor.

The uncertainty of range of the ions (higher dose concentration at the end of the range of the beam) in human tissue is one of the major hurdles of radiation therapy with ions (Paganetti 2012). For various reasons, the localization of the "actual" dose deposition during treatment can differ from that of the treatment plan, for example, if patient positioning is inaccurate or if the bladder or rectal characteristics change. Therefore, several measurements should be made even during the actual dose delivery, e.g. via positron emitters (PET camera) (Frey et al. 2014) or the induced gamma radiation (Compton camera) (Mackin et al. 2012).

The ratio of Bragg peak dose to the dose in the entrance area is larger for heavy ions compared to protons. Due to their larger mass, angular and energy straggling becomes negligible for heavy ions compared to protons. Therefore, heavy ions have an improved dose conformation as opposed to photons or protons resulting in better preservation of healthy tissue surrounding the target in physical treatment planning. Additionally, heavy ions reveal a strong increase of the LET in the Bragg peak compared to the entrance region (Schulz-Ertner et al. 2006). The biological advantage of high LET radiation was already proposed in neutron therapy, in contrast however, in heavy ion radiotherapy the high LET area can be conformed to the tumor.

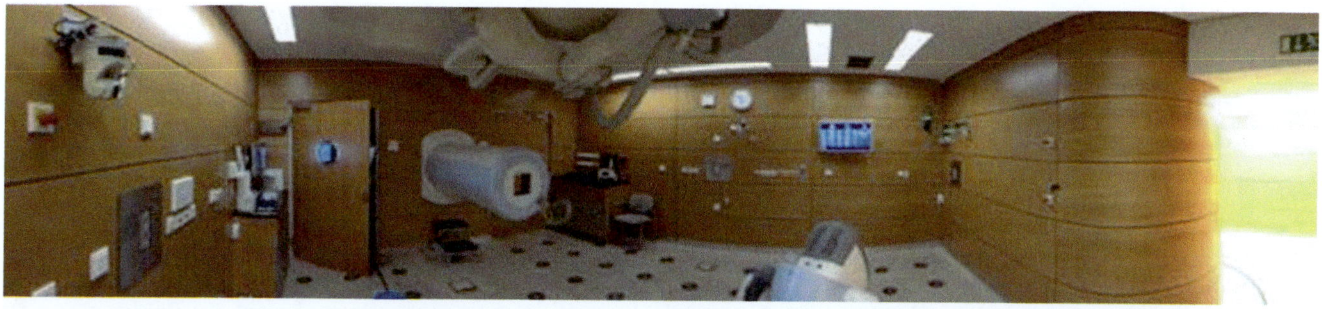

Fig. 2 The interior view of the horizontal beam line treatment room of the **H**eidelberg **I**on Beam **T**herapy Center (HIT) in Germany (*D*) in Fig. 4

2.1 Production of Charged Particles

Compared to photon beams, charged particles have the basic differences that they are slowed down while passing through tissue and thus have a finite range. The energy required to treat a tumor depends on the depth of the target in the body. Treatment with protons requires energy between 80 and 250 MeV. For these energies, cyclotrons are used to produce proton beams with sufficient energies and intensities. The energy required to treat deep-seated tumors with heavy ions is much higher compared to protons. A proton beam of 150 MeV can penetrate 16 cm in water; the same penetration depth for carbon ions can be achieved with energies of 3,000 MeV. To accelerate particles to such high energies, synchrotrons are better suited than cyclotrons. A synchrotron produces pulsed beams, and the energy can be varied from one cycle to the other with a few MeV steps. Thus, modulation of the Bragg peak can be achieved to scan a deep-seated tumor without absorbers, avoiding scattering and degradation of sharpness in energy. However, particle acceleration in synchrotrons is much more difficult and more cost-intensive than in cyclotrons.

2.2 Beam Delivery and Application Systems

2.2.1 Beam Delivery

Most experience with charged particles therapies has mainly been acquired with horizontal beam lines (Fig. 2). The success of a radiotherapy treatment is strongly increased through the possibility of applying the beam to the target using different angles (multiple field irradiation). A gantry for charged particles, however, lies in another dimension compared to photons. Although the weight of a proton gantry is around 100 tons and has a diameter of 10 m, an isocentric gantry for carbon ions has a weight of 600 tons, a length of 20 m, and a diameter of 12 m (Haberer et al. 2004). The enormous size and weight as well as the high spatial accuracy required for the beam position at the isocenter of the target volume was the reason why such a gantry was not built until 2008 in Heidelberg/Germany (Haberer et al. 2004). The first worldwide heavy ion gantry was brought online in October 2012 (Fig. 3).

The Heidelberg Ion Therapy Center (HIT) (Fig. 4) provides protons and carbon ion beams using the raster scan technique. Arbitrary particle numbers can be applied to each raster point that is defined by longitudinal range and transverse deflection of a narrow ion beam. This technique of fluence modulation allows generating almost arbitrarily shaped dose distributions in three dimensions, typically only using two beam directions. Treatment plans are usually classified by the way of dose optimization to generate the particle number distributions: single field uniform dose (SFUD: optimization of individual beams yields homogeneous dose distributions for each beam) and intensity modulated particle therapy (IMPT: simultaneous multiple beam dose optimization, may yield inhomogeneous dose distributions of the beams complementing one another). Both algorithms are driven by dose constraints for the target volume and surrounding organs at risk (Schulz-Ertner et al. 2006).

2.2.2 Beam Application

Two different principle methods for beam application exist, the passive and active beam shaping (Schulz-Ertner et al. 2006). Passive beam shaping was the first method developed and is still the most commonly used method in heavy ion therapy (Fig. 5). After the broadened beam is incoming, the variable range shifter (typically a number of homogeneous plastic plates of different thickness which can be moved into the beam) has to shift the dose into the planned depth. The compensator and collimator are patient-specific devices and adapt the dose distribution to the size and shape of the target volume.

In contrast to the passive beam shaping, in which a customized compensator compensates inhomogeneities of the tissue, in the active raster scanning method, the beam intensity and energy range can be modulated by variation. The tumor is divided into isoenergetic layers, which are sequentially scanned (Fig. 6). The advantage of the active raster scan method is the possibility to scan the target

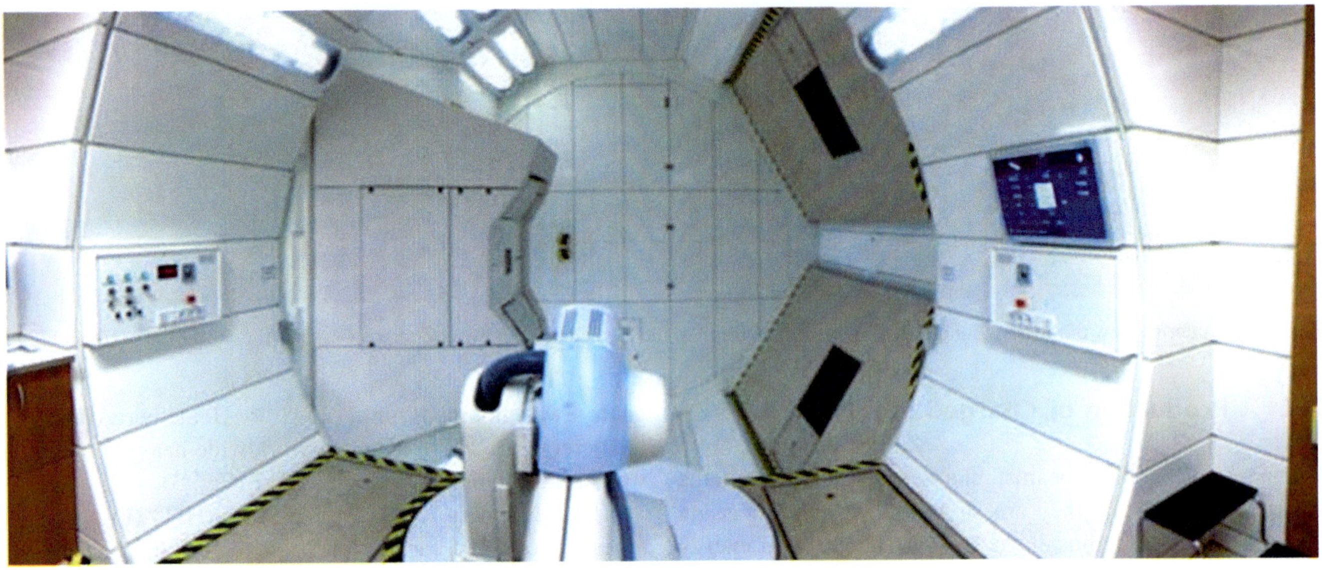

Fig. 3 The interior view of the Gantry treatment room of the **H**eidelberg **I**on Beam **T**herapy Center (HIT) in Germany, equates (*D*, *F*) in Fig. 4

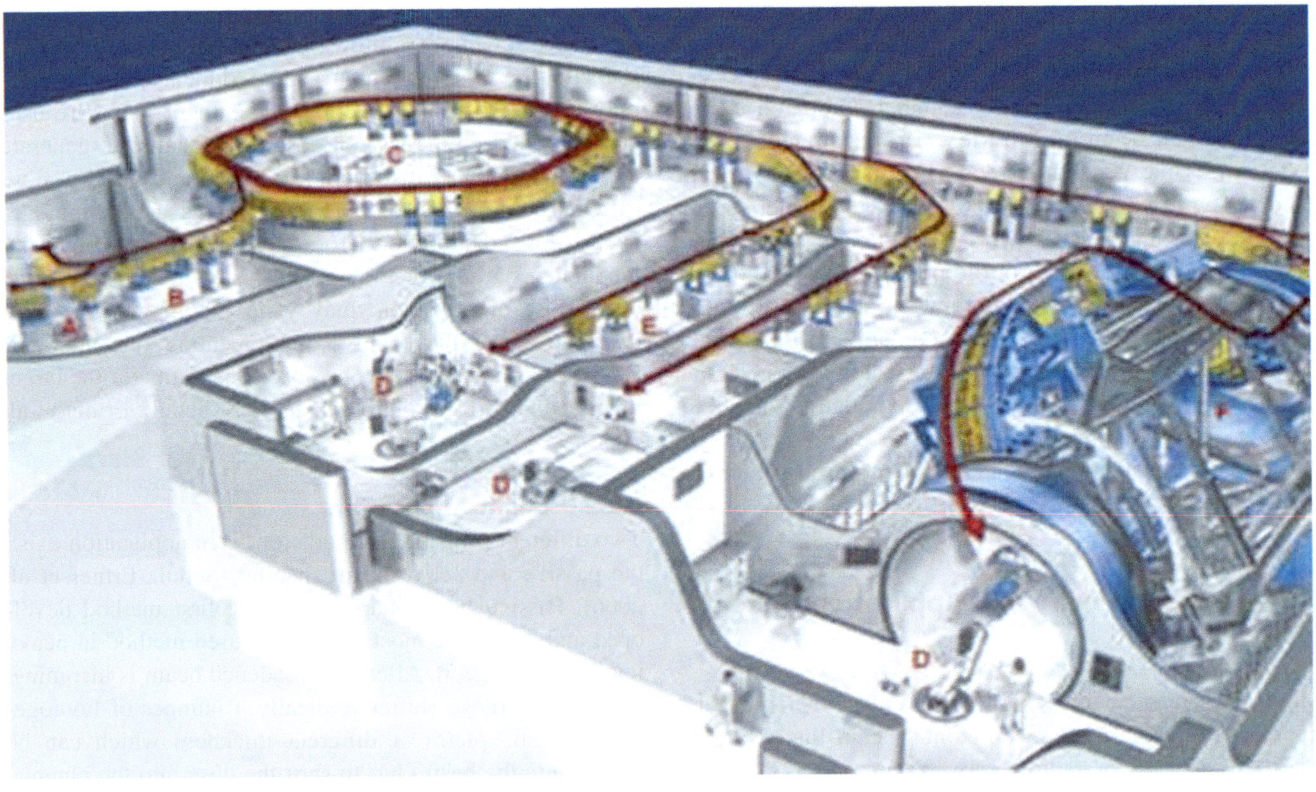

Fig. 4 The build-up of the **H**eidelberg **I**on Beam **T**herapy center (HIT). In the ion sources (*A*) ions are produced by snatching parts of the electron cloud of the atoms. The ions are bundled to a beam in electric and magnetic fields and are accelerated to high speed, approximately 10 % of the speed of light, in the linear accelerator (*B*). In the synchrotron (*C*), the ions are kept in circular orbits due to superconducting magnets. During approximately one million circulations, the high frequency powered accelerator structures increase the velocity of the ions up to 75 % of the speed of light. On the way to the treatment room (*D*), the ion beam is conducted and bundled in vacuum tubes (*E*) by magnets. The world's first ion gantry (*F*) with a length of 20 m, a diameter of 12 m, and a total weight of 600 tons, which moves around the patient, went online in October 2012

volume in three dimensions and the dose distribution can be tailored to any irregular shape without any patient-specific devices, as mentioned above. Additionally, the high-dose region can be conformed to both the proximal and distal ends, in contrast to the passive beam shaping, where only the depth dose can be tailored to the distal end of the target

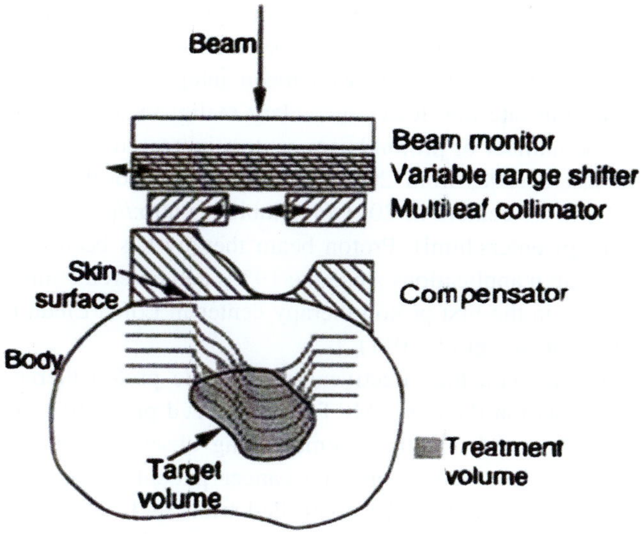

Fig. 5 Principle of passive beam shaping used for charged particle therapy, see text. The lines in the body to the treatment volume represent the distal fall-off that can be shifted to the depth by using a range shifter

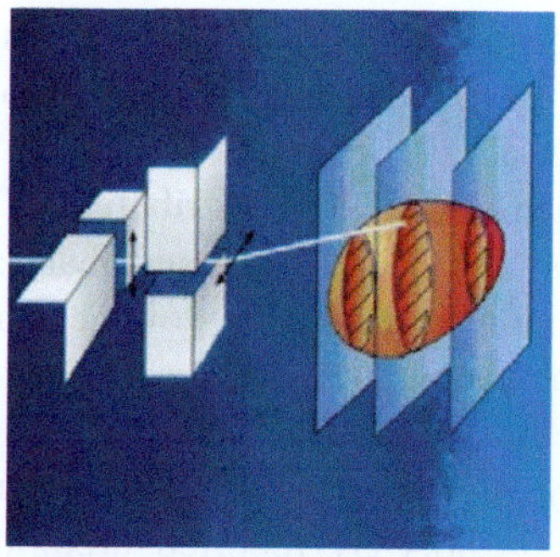

Fig. 6 Principle of active beam shaping. The beam is scanned in vertical and horizontal directions via two pairs of scanner magnets. By switching the energy of the synchrotron, the position of the Bragg peak can be changed resulting in the adaption of the scanned region to the dimension of the target in-depth

volume (Schulz-Ertner et al. 2006). The integral dose and the target volume receiving high-LET radiation are minimized in case of the active raster scan technique.

3 Biological Principles

The number of ionization events in a certain volume, the so-called ionization density, can specify the effectiveness of a certain kind of radiation. Since this quantity is difficult to measure, linear energy transfer (LET) is mostly used. The LET is a biophysical quantity and describes the number of ionizations per distance and is thus a measure of the effect of ionizing radiation on biological tissue. Sparsely ionizing radiation (low-LET <10 keV/μm) and densely ionizing radiation (high-LET >10 keV/μm) are distinguished. At a cellular level, the high-LET is characterized by a high local dose in the nucleus, thus the possibility of lethal radiation damages increases (Scholz et al. 2001). The higher the LET, the higher the relative biological effectiveness (RBE). The RBE is the ratio of biological effectiveness of one type of ionizing radiation relative to another (here the use of a photon irradiation of a conventional linear accelerator is set to equal one), given the same amount of absorbed energy. RBE can increase with increasing LET to the optimum ionization density; for high LET, however, saturation effects come into effect, which prevent a further increase in action. The RBE of SOBP protons increases with decreasing dose or dose per fraction and increasing depth in the SOBP, with the magnitude of both effects likely being dependent on the α/β ratios of the target cells or tissues (Gerweck and Kozin 1999). The increase in RBE with depth in a SOBP translates into a displacement of the distal edge of the RBE-weighted SOBP to a larger depth (Carabe et al. 2012). Clinical proton beams should always be designed to avoid risk organs at the distal drop-off of the beam. Different tumors respond differently to high-LET radiation. Especially, so-called late-reacting tissues, i.e., prostate tumors, which grow very slowly and usually are not very sensitive to radiation, react to high-LET radiation with increased RBE. The RBE is thus dependent on the tumor entity (nature of the tissue), the single-dose (different local dose distribution), the LET and the ionization density, but independent of oxygenation and cell cycle.

However, the existing experimental biological data is insufficient to define a clear correlation between RBE and dose per fraction or α/β value for in vivo endpoints (Paganetti et al. 2002). In general, it is known that RBE increases with dose-averaged linear energy transfer (LET_d), whereas it decreases with increasing dose and α/β value (Gerweck and Kozin 1999; Paganetti et al. 2002; Carabe et al. 2013). An increased RBE due to an increased LET_d and dose drop-off could cause a shift in the biologically effective range of the beam by 1–2 mm (Robertson et al. 1975; Paganetti et al. 2000). Several authors contemplated how to allow an estimation of range uncertainties by varying biological effectiveness for treatment planning purposes (Carabe et al. 2012; Bohlen et al. 2012). Biological range uncertainties are an additive to the physical range uncertainties, so treatment sites that involve very inhomogeneous tissues with low α/β values, could benefit from contemplating toward varying RBE values (Carabe et al. 2012).

The RBE value of 1.1 for protons has proven to be a good average representation across the SOBP at any dose and for all tissues (Paganetti et al. 2002), whereas the RBE of carbon ions varies from 1.4 to 5.0 (Jones 2009). If one wants to increase the accuracy of a treatment to levels below 5–10 % of uncertainty, biological effect variations must be considered. Proton RBE is known to be dependent on the α/β value of prostate tissue. The range of α/β values reported for prostate tumors (1.2–5.0) implies that the proton RBE for these tissues could vary significantly compared to the commonly used generic value of 1.1 (Carabe et al. 2013). The uncertainty in the range of the biological dose profile is smaller at higher doses, which could imply that the use of hypofractionated regimens reduces the overall range uncertainty (physical and biological) associated with protons beams (Carabe et al. 2012). Due to these considerations and the fact that proton RBE varies with fractionation, a comparison of proton and photon treatments should be made with caution.

4 Clinical Aspects

The success of irradiation in patients with localized prostate cancer correlates with the administered dose (Hall 2006; Kupelian et al. 2007; Tsuji et al. 2005; Yu et al. 2011; Zelefsky et al. 2001). This is well known for patients with an intermediate risk profile and was also recently found in patients with a low-risk profile (Gleason score <7; PSA <10 ng/ml) (Zietman et al. 2010a). Higher doses lead to higher complication rates particularly to the rectum (bleedings, fistula, and ulcer), urethra (stenosis), and bladder (chronic cystitis).

The rate of side effects is not only dependent on the dose but also on the radiation technique used. In a randomized study in the 1990s, it was noticed that the rectum toxicity was lowered significantly with the application of 3D-CT-based radiation planning compared to simulator-based planning (Dearnaley et al. 1999). In a dose escalation study by the MD Anderson, Pollack et al. described a volume dependency of the rectum toxicity (rectum volume irradiated with >70 Gy: toxicity °II or higher after 5 years 13 % or 51 % by ≤25 % or >25 % rectum volume ≥70 Gy) (Pollack et al. 2002). Due to the use of intensity modulated radiotherapy it is possible to increase the doses up to 76–81 Gy whereat the side effects in comparison to 3D-conformal radiotherapy in the same dosage could be lowered significantly to the level of radiation series with a total dose of 64–70 Gy. This monocentric historic comparison showed a significantly higher cure rate (Zelefsky et al. 2001).

5 Proton Radiotherapy

More than 2,000 prostate cancer patients treated with proton therapy were reported in the literature. Toxicity was in an acceptable range while dose escalation utilizing a proton boost had an improved outcome. Preliminary results with proton only therapy are also available and similar to combined therapy with protons and photons. Dosimetric studies suggest that the greatest benefit for conformal proton therapy lays in a reduced mean integral dose, which could translate into fewer secondary malignancies.

The number of proton beam centers increased rapidly in the last decade, from 20 centers operating worldwide in 2001, to 39 centers in 2011 (available at: http://ptcog.web.psi.ch/ptcenters.html). Proton beam therapy has been used in research applications since the 1950s and entered clinical practice in the first proton therapy center in Loma Linda in 1990 (Jarosek et al. 2011).

To compare the effectiveness of single proton therapy versus photon therapy (IMRT), randomized phase III trials would be needed with extremely long observation times, especially in low-risk prostate cancer patients. Currently, there are no randomized controlled trials and only a few well-conducted cohort studies have compared proton beam irradiation to other treatments.

Commonly mentioned refutations of the detractors of proton therapy on the one hand, say that no evidence exists for the comparative effectiveness or the harmfulness of proton therapy, and on the other hand the high costs of treatment. One report cited that the costs of providing proton therapy were twice as much as any other radiotherapy (Zietman et al. 2010b).

However, the physical dose distribution of protons argues against photons (Fig. 7). It is obvious that parts of the risk organs still remain in the target volume: base of bladder, urethra, and the facing wall of the rectum. The tolerance dose of the urethra, which is at the center of the target volume, is >85 Gy. A prospective study with a fraction scheme of 48 x 1.8 Gy = 86.4 Gy reported urethral strictures of <3 % (Cahlon et al. 2008). For both the bladder and rectum, studies found a high volume effect. The TD 5/5 for radiation of 2/3 of the bladder is 80 Gy, whereas it is 65 Gy for radiation of the whole bladder (Emami et al. 1991). For the rectum, high volume effects are known as well (Kuban et al. 2008). With proton radiation it is possible to especially preserve the posterior rectum wall in comparison to photon radiation, which leads to lesser rectal complication rates. For the proton irradiation we know the retrospective analysis data from Loma Linda (Slater et al. 2004), as well as the randomized study from Boston, in which a proton boost to a total dose of 79.2 Gy versus 70.2 Gy was used after irradiation with photons to a dose of 50.4 Gy. The study showed a significant advantage to the high-dose arm with an acceptable side effect rate (2 % acute and chronic side effects CTC grade 3 or higher) (Zietman et al. 2010a).

Concerning the survival rate data, a few major studies were conducted. One of the major dose-escalation studies was carried out at the proton center in Boston. Zietman et al. 2005, 2010a randomized 393 patients with a PSA <5 ng/ml to a low-dose arm (50.4 Gy photon therapy + 19.8 GyE

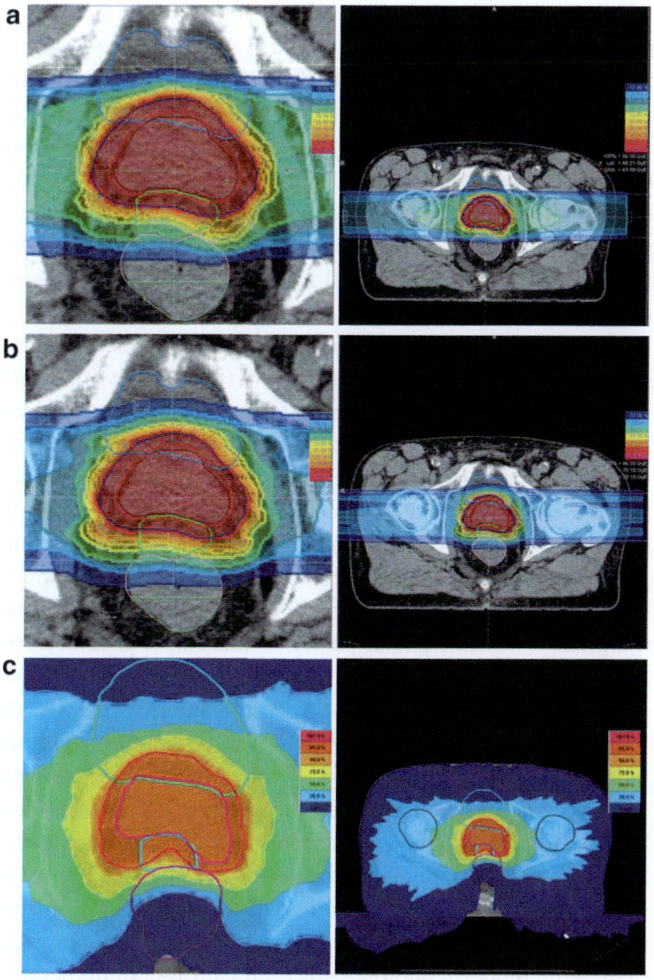

Fig. 7 Comparison of the dose distribution of **a** carbon ion, **b** proton, **c** IMRT (tomotherapy) irradiation of the prostate. To spare the rectum, a spacer gel is placed between the prostate and the rectum (in **a** + **b** the green OAR, in **c** the mint OAR), see Fig. 8. Depicted are the isodoses: *dark blue* (10 %), *light blue* (30 %), *green* (50 %), *yellow* (70 %), *orange* (90 %), *red* (95 %), and *pink* (107 %) of the applied dose

proton boost) and a high-dose arm (50.4 Gy photon + 28.8 GyE proton boost). The analysis revealed a significant difference in biochemical recurrence-free survival in favor of the high-dose arm. Subgroup analysis of low and high risk patients (depending on the Gleason score) showed a significant advantage for the high-dose group in both cases. An impact on the overall survival rate was not observed. Both acute and late toxicities were not increased in either arm compared to the incidence of comparable photon studies. A Japanese phase II study of Nihei et al. 2005 with a similar patient population and treatment approach had similar results and toxicity events.

Boston performed a further dose escalation as well as a comparative study examining photon against proton boost in patients with advanced prostate cancer (T3-4 N0-2) in 202 cases (Shipley et al. 1995). Patients were randomized in a low-dose arm (50.4 Gy photon + 16.8 Gy photons) or a high-dose arm (50.4 Gy photon + 25.2 GyE protons). A statistically significant difference in local control (84 % in the high-dose arm vs. 19 % in the low-dose arm after 8 years) was only observed in the subgroup of less differentiated carcinomas (no effect for the total study population). Regarding late toxicities, the incidence of rectal bleeding was increased significantly in the high-dose arm and the incidence of urethral strictures showed a statistical trend to an increase.

In 2007, Mayahara et al. (2007) published acute toxicity data of proton therapy of the prostate (n = 287) with a total dose of 74 GyE. No acute gastrointestinal toxicity > grade 1 was seen. Genitourinary acute toxicity grades 2 and 3 were reported in 39 and 4 % of the patients. The use of androgen deprivation therapy and a large irradiation field size were risk factors in the occurrence of genitourinary acute toxicity. The toxicity data was supported by a heavy ion study of Ishikawa et al. (2008) who found persistent GU toxicity grade 1 in 21 % and grade 2 in 2 % in patients using long–course antihormonal treatment ≥24 months.

Combination radiotherapy of pelvic lymphatics and sequential proton boost to the prostate was performed by Yonemoto et al. (1997) in a prospective study. A total of 106 patients with locally advanced prostate cancer and a high risk of recurrence were treated within this trial. Primary tumor and pelvic lymph nodes initially received 45 Gy photons followed by a proton boost of 30 GyE to the prostate. Only three patients had a local recurrence at 2 years, in another two patients a biochemical recurrence appeared without evidence of local relapse. Grade 1 and 2 late toxicities were numbered at 12 %, grade 3 and 4 toxicities were not found. Seven years later, Slater et al. 2004 published retrospective data of 1,255 patients treated according to the concept of Yonemoto. The biochemical recurrence-free survival after 5 years was 73 %. In the event of a PSA level <4 ng/ml before treatment, the biochemical recurrence-free survival was 90 %. Grade 3 or 4 gastrointestinal and genitourinary late side effects were reported with 1 %. The third major publication of Loma Linda is an evaluation of Rossi et al., who compared the prognosis of prostate cancer patients above and below 60 years (Rossi 2004). The result stated that no treatment decision should be made based on the patient's age if the prognosis is the same.

Since there are no data for hypofractionated irradiation of the prostate with protons, a study in Heidelberg was initiated in 2012 exploring the effectiveness and feasibility of this treatment. The dose concept is 20 × 3.3 GyE according to a hypofractionated irradiation schedule that is used at various institutions to treat patients with prostate cancer with carbon ions (see below).

6 Carbon Ion Radiotherapy

Due to its mass, carbon ions have a higher biological effectiveness compared to protons with comparable dose profile. In 1994, carbon ion radiotherapy started at the National Institute of Radiological Sciences (NIRS) in Chiba/Japan. Between June 1995 and March 2000, two phase I/II dose-escalation studies were carried out. Both studies were dose-escalation studies of hypofractionated carbon ion radiotherapy for both early and advanced stage prostate carcinoma patients to establish a new technique and to determine the optimal radiation dose. Akakura et al. 2004 presented the first of the two phase I /II studies after treating 96 patients in dose-escalation steps from 54 to 72 GyE in 3 GyE per fraction. The analysis revealed only one patient with "local failure" at the lowest applied dose level of 54 GyE. The toxicity data showed that 5 patients (36 %) of 14 developed grade 3 late toxicities of the rectum and bladder/urethra at dose level 72 GyE. Due to the high toxicity rate at the dose level of 72 GyE this arm was closed and the applied total dose was limited to a maximum dose of 66 GyE. The second phase I/II trial was started in January 1998 using a shrinking radiation field technique for both early and advanced prostate cancer. Patients with a T1b-T2aN0M0 (UICC TNM classification of 1997) prostate cancer were treated with a total dose of 60–66 GyE, patients with a T2b-T3b were treated with fixed doses of 66 GyE in combination with hormonal therapy. The study was completed in March 2000. No grade 3 or worse late toxicities occurred (Akakura et al. 2004). Of 96 patients who enrolled in the two phase I/II studies, 37 suffered from low-risk prostate cancer. This subgroup revealed excellent results in terms of biochemical recurrence-free survival of 96 % at 5 years, treated with a total dose of 60–66 GyE (Shimazaki et al. 2006).

To validate the feasibility and efficiency of hypofractionated carbon ion therapy, a phase II study was initiated in April 2000 using shrinking field technique and the recommended dose fractionation (66 GyE in 20 fractions over 5 weeks) obtained from the phase I/II studies, and was completed in October 2003 (Ishikawa et al. 2006a). A total of 176 patients were enrolled and local control was achieved in all but 1 patient. The 5-year biochemical recurrence-free survival was 83.2 % for all patients and 100 % for patients with low-risk prostate cancer. No late toxicity CTC grade 3 or higher was found (Tsuji et al. 2005). Grade 1 and 2 gastrointestinal (GI) and genitourinary (GU) toxicity were observed in 13 % and 2 % (GI) and 21 % and 2 % (GU) of the patients (Ishikawa et al. 2006a). Thereupon, predictive risk factors were explored for the occurrence of gastrointestinal and genitourinary side effects. The use of anticoagulation therapy and dosimetric parameters were predictive parameters for the occurrence of rectal bleeding (Ishikawa et al. 2006b). The use of long-course androgen deprivation therapy (ADT $\geq$ 24 months) increased grade 1–2 genitourinary morbidities. The use of ADT $\geq$ 24 months and acute genitourinary toxicity were associated with the occurrence of persistent toxicity (Ishikawa et al. 2008). The quality of life in men treated with carbon ion therapy for prostate cancer, in the absence of hormonal therapy, showed no significant decrease 12 months after radiotherapy (Wakatsuki et al. 2008).

The publication of Tsuji et al. (2005) describes the results of an even larger patient group (n = 201) with T1 to 3 localized prostate cancer underlining the excellent clinical results and a low incidence of side-effects highlighting the great potential of carbon ion therapy for relatively "radiation resistant" prostate cancer. In this series no patient developed grade 3 genitourinary or gastrointestinal toxicities. High-risk patients received neoadjuvant hormonal therapy for 2-6 months. Although anterior and lateral safety margins of 10 mm and a posterior margin of 5 mm were added to the CTV for the initial planning target volume, the posterior margin was reduced to fit the anterior rectal wall for the latter half of the carbon ion radiotherapy series to reduce rectal toxicity. The 5-year biochemical disease-free survival rate was 83.2 % for all patients. A 5-year biochemical disease-free survival rate of 100 % was achieved in 37 low-risk patients, whereas a rate of 80.5 % was observed in 164 high risk patients. Biochemical disease-free survival rates after carbon ion radiotherapy appear higher than with modern photon IMRT and proton radiotherapy especially for patients with high-risk prostate cancer (Ishikawa et al. 2012). However, high-risk patients at NIRS received neoadjuvant hormonal therapy. The promising results obtained with carbon ion therapy need to be confirmed in controlled clinical trials.

In an initial study in Heidelberg, Nikoghosyan et al. (Nikoghosyan et al. 2011) tested the feasibility and safety of the active beam modulation of carbon ion irradiation to the prostate. A carbon ion boost of 6 × 3 GyE in combination with an IMRT photon radiation of 30 × 2 Gy was tested. Radiotherapy was very well tolerated without any grade 3 or higher acute toxicity. Acute anal bleeding grade 2 was observed in two of 14 patients. Rectal tenesmus grade 1 was reported by three other patients. At the Heavy Ion Center in Heidelberg, since May 2012 a prospective randomized phase II trial is being carried out exploring the safety and feasibility of primary hypofractionated irradiation of the prostate with protons and carbon ions in the raster scan technique (dose concept: 20 × 3.3 GyE). 92 patients with localized prostate cancer will be enrolled. In Fig. 7, a comparison of the different dose distribution of carbon ions (a), protons (b), and photon IMRT [helical tomotherapy (c)]

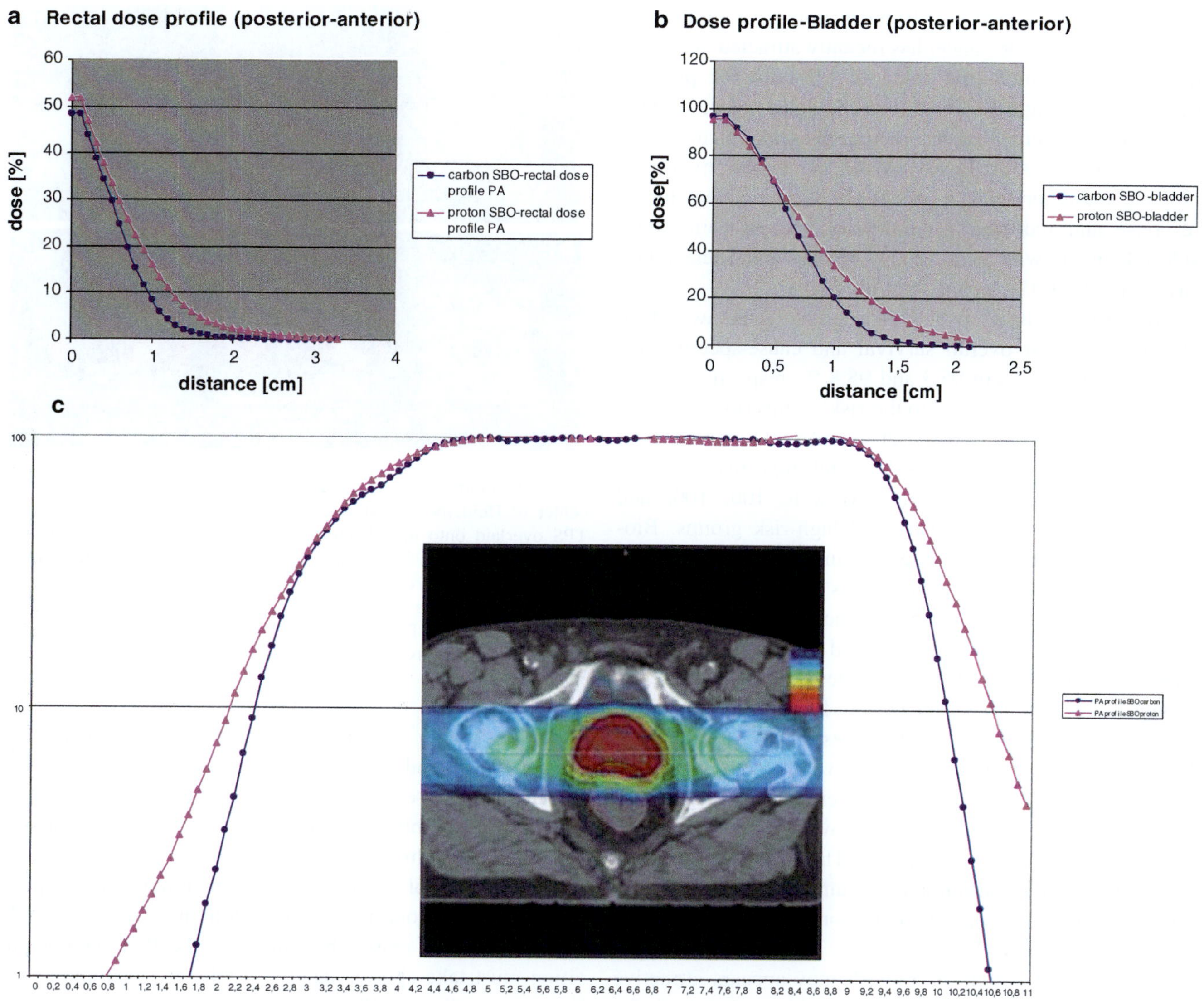

Fig. 8 Dose profiles of protons and carbon ions in comparison; **a** and **b** show the higher lateral scattering of protons due to their lower mass compared to carbon ions in the risk organs. **c** depicts the left-right dose profile in a logarithmic scale, as well a steeper dose gradient in favor of carbon ions

is displayed. In the case of carbon ions, the dose in the entrance region is possibly overestimated. Currently, the Local Effect Model (LEM) I- model has been integrated in the treatment planning system. In radiotherapy with carbon ions, the calculation of the biological effective dose during treatment planning is crucial for treating tumor patients adequately. For the modeling of the complex relationship between physical dose and relative biological effectiveness (RBE), the "Local Effect Model" (LEM) has been used for more than 1,000 patients—with excellent clinical results. At the same time, however, it is known that for the current version of the "Local Effect Model" (LEM I), there are some discrepancies between the model predictions and the experimental data. In particular, this includes the overestimation of the relative biological effectiveness in the entrance area (Elsasser et al. 2008; Karger and Jakel 2007). For this reason, the model has been constantly refined, so that today a generalized version (LEM IV) is available. Due to the lower mass of protons, the lateral scattering is higher compared to carbon ions. The lateral dose decrease is less steep compared to heavy ions (Fig. 7a, b). Figure 8a, and b shows the dose profiles of protons and carbon ions for both risk organs, rectum and bladder in comparison. The steep lateral dose gradient of carbon ions causes a steep dose decrease to the risk organs in direction of propagation of the ion beam. Figure 8c shows the left-right dose profile in a logarithmic scale in favor of carbon ions.

In Chiba/Japan, the radiooncologists completed more than 1,300 prostate treatments. The current recommended dose fractionation is 57.6 GyE in 16 fractions over 4 weeks, but a new clinical trial using further hypofractionated carbon ion radiotherapy with 12 fractions over 3 weeks is currently being carried out. Hypofractionated radiotherapy for localized prostate cancer has recently attracted attention, due to the assumed low value of α/β-ratio for prostate cancer which might be lower than the values of the organs at risk like urethra, bladder, rectum (Peschke et al. 2011; Brenner et al. 2002). Based on the LQ model, hypofractionated radiotherapy has benefits in view of local tumor response and reducing genitourinary and gastrointestinal side effects (Fowler et al. 2003; Macias and Biete 2009; Livsey et al. 2003; Arcangeli et al. 2010).

At the last follow-up of Japanese data (Ishikawa et al. 2012), the 5-year overall survival and cause-specific survival (CSS) rates were 95.3 and 98.8 %, respectively. The 5-year CSS rates according to the risk groups (low risk: T1/T2a with GS $\leq$ 6 and PSA $<$ 20 ng/ml,; intermediate risk: GS $=$ 7 with T1/2 and PSA $<$20 ng/ml; high risk: T3, PSA $>$20 ng/ml or Gleason-Score $\geq$8) were 100, 100, and 97.9 % for low, intermediate, and high-risk groups. Biochemical relapses were observed in 63 (6.8 %) of 927 patients, but local tumor control was achieved in all but 8 (0.8 %) patients. Hence, the 5-year biochemical relapse-free and local control rates were 90.6 and 98.3 %, respectively. The 5-year biological relapse-free rates according to the risk groups were 89.6, 96.8, and 88.4 % for low, intermediate, and high-risk groups. As a notable result, the 5-year rate of high-risk patients who were treated with a combination of carbon ion radiotherapy and androgen deprivation therapy was almost the same as that of the low-risk patients treated by carbon ion radiotherapy alone. This result could prove the high impact of carbon ions on tumor control for locally advanced tumors as well as the reasonable use of androgen deprivation therapy (Ishikawa et al. 2012). Further, hypofractionation of carbon ion radiotherapy appears attractive and might be realized in combination with new methods for tumor tracking.

7 Irradiation Verification in Ion Treatment

A possibility to verify the applied ion treatment, is the administration of a positron emission tomography (PET) shortly after irradiation (Enghardt et al. 2004; Parodi et al. 2007a, b; Nishio et al. 2008; Hsi et al. 2009). The PET offers an indirect three-dimensional, in vivo, noninvasive verification of the ion treatment. This kind of diagnostics is possible due to a transient β^+-activity occurring as a by-product within the therapeutic irradiation. The β^+-activity is the result of nuclear reactions between beam ions and target nuclei of irradiated tissue. By fusing the measured activity with the treatment plan as well as the patient's anatomy, given by the actual computed tomography scan, it is possible to draw conclusions about the actual dose delivery. Especially in cases in which the beam particles have to penetrate highly inhomogeneous tissue (i.e., bone, air, muscle, and metal (Jakel and Reiss 2007), the precision of the intended dose distribution could become distorted by minimal positioning errors or inaccuracies in treatment planning algorithms. The activity levels induced by the irradiation are of a much lower magnitude than typical diagnostic PET conditions known from nuclear medicine. In order to achieve reasonable statistics, the PET data acquisition must take approximately 30 min. An example of the first post-radiation PET-CT imaging of a patient with prostate cancer undergoing scanned proton irradiation is illustrated in Fig. 9. After completion of the fifth therapeutic treatment fraction of 3.3 GyE via a right and a left proton field, the patient was transferred to the PET-CT scanner, which is located in the room next to the treatment room. The patient is then, immobilized in the same position as during therapy. The signal is dominated by disintegration of ^{11}C radionuclides with a half-life of approximately 20 min. Unfortunately, the ^{15}O radionuclides with a half-life of approximately 2 min disintegrate largely during the transfer time of the patient to the PET/CT imaging. In addition to the noise of the low-statistics PET data, imaging is furthermore hampered by the quick wash-out of induced activity mainly by perfusion. First post-therapeutic measurements of prostate patients treated at HIT support the feasibility of the available imaging concept for treatment monitoring. For a conclusive verification of the applied irradiation, a more detailed quantitative analysis is needed (Bauer et al. 2013a, b).

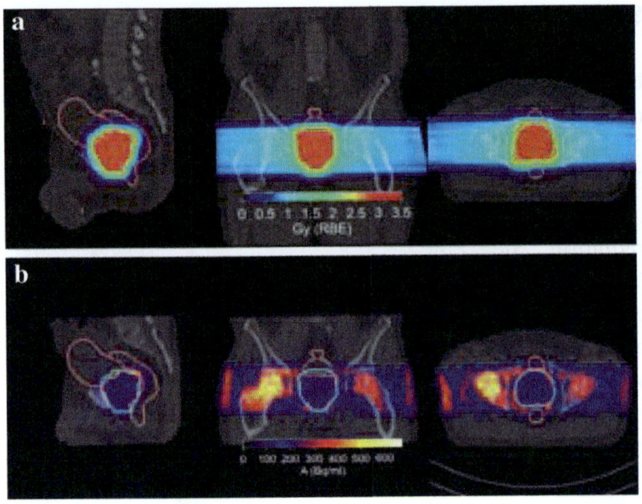

Fig. 9 Combined PET/CT scan to verify ion irradiation at the ion center of Heidelberg. **a** shows the planned dose by the commercial TPS overlaid onto the planning CT in sagittal, coronary, and axial layers. **b** shows the PET image acquired approx. 7 min after proton irradiation overlaid onto the control computed tomography, merged and visualized in the same layers as in **a**. In the prostate, the activity is already washed out. Due to progress in time, the right side of the pelvis is stronger in activity compared to the earlier irradiated left side

8 Radiation-Induced Neoplasms

Exposure to ionizing radiation may result in secondary malignancies. The period of latency is anywhere between 20 and 40 years after exposure (Schulz-Ertner et al. 2006). The incidence of radiogenic neoplasms depends on the applied dose and the dose rate of radiation, the type of radiation, the biology and volume of irradiated tissue (integral dose), and the age and sex of patient. Proton and carbon ion radiation, when compared to photon irradiation, allow delivery of increased radiation dose to the tumor while decreasing the dose to risk organs. The use of proton radiation therapy is not associated with a significantly increased risk of secondary malignancies compared to photon therapy (Chung et al. 2013).

Athar et al. (2010) assessed the comparison of lateral out-of-field doses in 6 MV IMRT and secondary neutron equivalent dose contributions in proton therapy. Close to the target, protons offer a distinct advantage due to the lower integral dose. Out-of-field, but within approximately 25 cm from the target, the scattered photon dose of IMRT turned out to be roughly a factor of 2 lower than the neutron equivalent dose from proton therapy. At further distances to the target (>25 cm), protons offer an advantage, resulting in doses that are a factor 2–3 lower.

All published studies of irradiation of the prostate with ions used a passive beam modulation. The advantage of the active beam modulation with a raster scan technique (Haberer et al. 2004) is the lower production of neutrons, therefore the risk of secondary malignancies should be lower. Despite the more exact dose application, the passive beam modulation has no advantage in developing less secondary cancer compared to IMRT irradiation (Hall 2006).

As the application of proton and carbon ion therapy have been used for treatment of prostate cancer for the past 10–15 years, and as we have perfect comparison groups, due to the rise in active surveillance groups in addition to surgery groups, useful secondary malignancy rates should be available within the next decades.

9 Outlook

In the past two decades, in nearly 40 centers worldwide, valuable clinical experience has been gained in particle therapy. The irradiation data from the prostate cancer patient groups with particles have demonstrated high rates of local and biochemical control as well as low rates of urinary and rectal toxicity. Together with the development of new technologies, especially for beam application and treatment planning, there will likely be a broader implementation of ions in clinical settings that allow for an optimal exploitation of the physical and biological potential of protons and heavy ions. Current research includes explorations of dose escalation, hypofractionation, and quality of life outcomes.

References

Akakura K, Tsujii H, Morita S, Tsuji H, Yagishita T, Isaka S, Ito H, Akaza H, Hata M, Fujime M et al (2004) Phase I/II clinical trials of carbon ion therapy for prostate cancer. Prostate 58(3):252–258

Allen AM, Pawlicki T, Dong L, Fourkal E, Buyyounouski M, Cengel K, Plastaras J, Bucci MK, Yock TI, Bonilla L et al (2012) An evidence based review of proton beam therapy: the report of ASTRO's emerging technology committee. Radiother Oncol J Eur Soc Ther Radiol Oncol 103(1):8–11

Arcangeli G, Saracino B, Gomellini S, Petrongari MG, Arcangeli S, Sentinelli S, Marzi S, Landoni V, Fowler J, Strigari L (2010) A prospective phase III randomized trial of hypofractionation versus conventional fractionation in patients with high-risk prostate cancer. Int J Radiat Oncol Biol Phys 78(1):11–18

Athar BS, Bednarz B, Seco J, Hancox C, Paganetti H (2010) Comparison of out-of-field photon doses in 6 MV IMRT and neutron doses in proton therapy for adult and pediatric patients. Phys Med Biol 55(10):2879–2891

Bauer J, Unholtz D, Kurz C, Parodi K (2013a) An experimental approach to improve the Monte Carlo modelling of offline PET/CT-imaging of positron emitters induced by scanned proton beams. Phys Med Biol 58(15):5193–5213

Bauer J, Unholtz D, Sommerer F, Kurz C, Haberer T, Herfarth K, Welzel T, Combs SE, Debus J, Parodi K (2013b) Implementation and initial clinical experience of offline PET/CT-based verification of scanned carbon ion treatment. Radiother Oncol J Eur Soc Ther Radiol Oncol 107(2):218–226

Bohlen TT, Brons S, Dosanjh M, Ferrari A, Fossati P, Haberer T, Patera V, Mairani A (2012) Investigating the robustness of ion beam therapy treatment plans to uncertainties in biological treatment parameters. Phys Med Biol 57(23):7983–8004

Brenner DJ, Martinez AA, Edmundson GK, Mitchell C, Thames HD, Armour EP (2002) Direct evidence that prostate tumors show high sensitivity to fractionation (low alpha/beta ratio), similar to late-responding normal tissue. Int J Radiat Oncol Biol Phys 52(1):6–13

Cahlon O, Zelefsky MJ, Shippy A, Chan H, Fuks Z, Yamada Y, Hunt M, Greenstein S, Amols H (2008) Ultra-high dose (86.4 Gy) IMRT for localized prostate cancer: toxicity and biochemical outcomes. Int J Radiat Oncol Biol Phys 71(2):330–337

Carabe A, Moteabbed M, Depauw N, Schuemann J, Paganetti H (2012) Range uncertainty in proton therapy due to variable biological effectiveness. Phys Med Biol 57(5):1159–1172

Carabe A, Espana S, Grassberger C, Paganetti H (2013) Clinical consequences of relative biological effectiveness variations in proton radiotherapy of the prostate, brain and liver. Phys Med Biol 58(7): 2103–2117

Chung CS, Yock TI, Nelson K, Xu Y, Keating NL, Tarbell NJ (2013) Incidence of second malignancies among patients treated with proton versus photon radiation. Int J Radiat Oncol Biol Phys 87(1):46–52

Creutz EC, Wilson RR (1946) Mono-energetic protons from a cyclotron. Rev Sci Instr 17(10):385–388

Dearnaley DP, Khoo VS, Norman AR, Meyer L, Nahum A, Tait D, Yarnold J, Horwich A (1999) Comparison of radiation side-effects of conformal and conventional radiotherapy in prostate cancer: a randomised trial. Lancet 353(9149):267–272

Elsasser T, Kramer M, Scholz M (2008) Accuracy of the local effect model for the prediction of biologic effects of carbon ion beams in vitro and in vivo. Int J Radiat Oncol Biol Phys 71(3):866–872
Emami B, Lyman J, Brown A, Coia L, Goitein M, Munzenrider JE, Shank B, Solin LJ, Wesson M (1991) Tolerance of normal tissue to therapeutic irradiation. Int J Radiat Oncol Biol Phys 21(1):109–122
Enghardt W, Parodi K, Crespo P, Fiedler F, Pawelke J, Ponisch F (2004) Dose quantification from in-beam positron emission tomography. Radiother Oncol J Eur Soc Ther Radiol Oncol 73(Suppl 2): S96–S98
Fowler JF, Ritter MA, Chappell RJ, Brenner DJ (2003) What hypofractionated protocols should be tested for prostate cancer? Int J Radiat Oncol Biol Phys 56(4):1093–1104
Frey K, Bauer J, Unholtz D, Kurz C, Kramer M, Bortfeld T, Parodi K (2014) TPSPET-A TPS-based approach for in vivo dose verification with PET in proton therapy. Phys Med Biol 59(1):1–21
Gerweck LE, Kozin SV (1999) Relative biological effectiveness of proton beams in clinical therapy. Radiother Oncol J Eur Soc Ther Radiol Oncol 50(2):135–142
Haberer T, Debus J, Eickhoff H, Jakel O, Schulz-Ertner D, Weber U (2004) The Heidelberg Ion Therapy Center. Radiother Oncol J Eur Soc Ther Radiol Oncol 73(Suppl 2):S186–S190
Hall EJ (2006) Intensity-modulated radiation therapy, protons, and the risk of second cancers. Int J Radiat Oncol Biol Phys 65(1):1–7
Hsi WC, Indelicato DJ, Vargas C, Duvvuri S, Li Z, Palta J (2009) In vivo verification of proton beam path by using post-treatment PET/CT imaging. Med Phys 36(9):4136–4146
Ishikawa H, Tsuji H, Kamada T, Yanagi T, Mizoe JE, Kanai T, Morita S, Wakatsuki M, Shimazaki J, Tsujii H (2006a) Carbon ion radiation therapy for prostate cancer: results of a prospective phase II study. Radiother Oncol J Eur Soc Ther Radiol Oncol 81(1):57–64
Ishikawa H, Tsuji H, Kamada T, Hirasawa N, Yanagi T, Mizoe JE, Akakura K, Suzuki H, Shimazaki J, Tsujii H (2006b) Risk factors of late rectal bleeding after carbon ion therapy for prostate cancer. Int J Radiat Oncol Biol Phys 66(4):1084–1091
Ishikawa H, Tsuji H, Kamada T, Hirasawa N, Yanagi T, Mizoe JE, Akakura K, Suzuki H, Shimazaki J, Nakano T et al (2008) Adverse effects of androgen deprivation therapy on persistent genitourinary complications after carbon ion radiotherapy for prostate cancer. Int J Radiat Oncol Biol Phys 72(1):78–84
Ishikawa H, Tsuji H, Kamada T, Akakura K, Suzuki H, Shimazaki J, Tsujii H (2012) Carbon-ion radiation therapy for prostate cancer. Int J Urol Off J Jpn Urol Assoc 19(4):296–305
Jakel O, Reiss P (2007) The influence of metal artefacts on the range of ion beams. Phys Med Biol 52(3):635–644
Jarosek S, Elliott S, Virnig BA (2011) Proton beam radiotherapy in the U.S. Medicare population: growth in use between 2006 and 2009: Data Points # 10. In: Data points publication series, Rockville (MD)
Jones B (2009) Joint symposium 2009 on carbon ion radiotherapy. Br J Radiol 82(983):884–889
Karger CP, Jakel O (2007) Current status and new developments in ion therapy. Strahlentherapie und Onkologie : Organ der Deutschen Rontgengesellschaft [et al] 183(6):295–300
Kuban DA, Tucker SL, Dong L, Starkschall G, Huang EH, Cheung MR, Lee AK, Pollack A (2008) Long-term results of the M. D. Anderson randomized dose-escalation trial for prostate cancer. Int J Radiat Oncol Biol Phys 70(1):67–74
Kupelian PA, Willoughby TR, Reddy CA, Klein EA, Mahadevan A (2007) Hypofractionated intensity-modulated radiotherapy (70 Gy at 2.5 Gy per fraction) for localized prostate cancer: Cleveland clinic experience. Int J Radiat Oncol Biol Phys 68(5):1424–1430
Livsey JE, Cowan RA, Wylie JP, Swindell R, Read G, Khoo VS, Logue JP (2003) Hypofractionated conformal radiotherapy in carcinoma of the prostate: five-year outcome analysis. Int J Radiat Oncol Biol Phys 57(5):1254–1259
Lodge M, Pijls-Johannesma M, Stirk L, Munro AJ, De Ruysscher D, Jefferson T (2007) A systematic literature review of the clinical and cost-effectiveness of hadron therapy in cancer. Radiother Oncol J Eur Soc Ther Radiol and Oncol 83(2):110–122
Macias V, Biete A (2009) Hypofractionated radiotherapy for localised prostate cancer. Review of clinical trials. In: Clinical & translational oncology : official publication of the federation of Spanish oncology societies and of the national cancer institute of Mexico, vol 11(7), pp 437-445
Mackin D, Peterson S, Beddar S, Polf J (2012) Evaluation of a stochastic reconstruction algorithm for use in Compton camera imaging and beam range verification from secondary gamma emission during proton therapy. Phys Med Biol 57(11):3537–3553
Mayahara H, Murakami M, Kagawa K, Kawaguchi A, Oda Y, Miyawaki D, Sasaki R, Sugimura K, Hishikawa Y (2007) Acute morbidity of proton therapy for prostate cancer: the Hyogo Ion Beam Medical Center experience. Int J Radiat Oncol Biol Phys 69(2):434–443
Nihei K, Ogino T, Ishikura S, Kawashima M, Nishimura H, Arahira S, Onozawa M (2005) Phase II feasibility study of high-dose radiotherapy for prostate cancer using proton boost therapy: first clinical trial of proton beam therapy for prostate cancer in Japan. Jpn J Clin Oncol 35(12):745–752
Nikoghosyan AV, Schulz-Ertner D, Herfarth K, Didinger B, Munter MW, Jensen AD, Jakel O, Hoess A, Haberer T, Debus J (2011) Acute toxicity of combined photon IMRT and carbon ion boost for intermediate-risk prostate cancer—acute toxicity of 12C for PC. Acta Oncol 50(6):784–790
Nishio T, Miyatake A, Inoue K, Gomi-Miyagishi T, Kohno R, Kameoka S, Nakagawa K, Ogino T (2008) Experimental verification of proton beam monitoring in a human body by use of activity image of positron-emitting nuclei generated by nuclear fragmentation reaction. Radiol Phys Technol 1(1):44–54
Olsen DR, Bruland OS, Frykholm G, Norderhaug IN (2007) Proton therapy—a systematic review of clinical effectiveness. Radiother Oncol J Eur Soc Ther Radiol Oncology 83(2):123–132
Paganetti H (2012) Range uncertainties in proton therapy and the role of Monte Carlo simulations. Phys Med Biol 57(11):R99–R117
Paganetti H, Gerweck LE, Goitein M (2000) The general relation between tissue response to x-radiation (alpha/beta-values) and the relative biological effectiveness (RBE) of protons: prediction by the Katz track-structure model. Int J Radiat Biol 76(7):985–998
Paganetti H, Niemierko A, Ancukiewicz M, Gerweck LE, Goitein M, Loeffler JS, Suit HD (2002) Relative biological effectiveness (RBE) values for proton beam therapy. Int J Radiat Oncol Biol Phys 53(2):407–421
Parodi K, Paganetti H, Shih HA, Michaud S, Loeffler JS, DeLaney TF, Liebsch NJ, Munzenrider JE, Fischman AJ, Knopf A et al (2007a) Patient study of in vivo verification of beam delivery and range, using positron emission tomography and computed tomography imaging after proton therapy. Int J Radiat Oncol Biol Phys 68(3):920–934
Parodi K, Ferrari A, Sommerer F, Paganetti H (2007b) Clinical CT-based calculations of dose and positron emitter distributions in proton therapy using the FLUKA Monte Carlo code. Phys Med Biol 52(12):3369–3387
Peschke P, Karger CP, Scholz M, Debus J, Huber PE (2011) Relative biological effectiveness of carbon ions for local tumor control of a radioresistant prostate carcinoma in the rat. Int J Radiat Oncol Biol Phys 79(1):239–246
Pollack A, Zagars GK, Starkschall G, Antolak JA, Lee JJ, Huang E, von Eschenbach AC, Kuban DA, Rosen I (2002) Prostate cancer radiation dose response: results of the M. D. Anderson phase III randomized trial. Int J Radiat Oncol Biol Phys 53(5):1097–1105
Robertson JB, Williams JR, Schmidt RA, Little JB, Flynn DF, Suit HD (1975) Radiobiological studies of a high-energy modulated proton beam utilizing cultured mammalian cells. Cancer 35(6):1664–1677

Rossi CJ Jr, Slater JD, Yonemoto LT, Jabola BR, Bush DA, Levy RP, Grove R, Slater JM (2004) Influence of patient age on biochemical freedom from disease in patients undergoing conformal proton radiotherapy of organ-confined prostate cancer. Urology 64(4): 729–732

Scholz M, Jakob B, Taucher-Scholz G (2001) Direct evidence for the spatial correlation between individual particle traversals and localized CDKN1A (p21) response induced by high-LET radiation. Radiat Res 156(5 Pt 1):558–563

Schulz-Ertner D, Jakel O, Schlegel W (2006) Radiation therapy with charged particles. Seminars in radiation oncology 16(4):249–259

Shimazaki J, Akakura K, Suzuki H, Ichikawa T, Tsuji H, Ishikawa H, Harada M, Tsujii H (2006) Monotherapy with carbon ion radiation for localized prostate cancer. Jpn J Clin Oncol 36(5):290–294

Shipley WU, Verhey LJ, Munzenrider JE, Suit HD, Urie MM, McManus PL, Young RH, Shipley JW, Zietman AL, Biggs PJ et al (1995) Advanced prostate cancer: the results of a randomized comparative trial of high dose irradiation boosting with conformal protons compared with conventional dose irradiation using photons alone. Int J Radiat Oncol Biol Phys 32(1):3–12

Slater JD, Rossi CJ Jr, Yonemoto LT, Bush DA, Jabola BR, Levy RP, Grove RI, Preston W, Slater JM (2004) Proton therapy for prostate cancer: the initial Loma Linda University experience. Int J Radiat Oncol Biol Phys 59(2):348–352

Tsuji H, Yanagi T, Ishikawa H, Kamada T, Mizoe JE, Kanai T, Morita S, Tsujii H (2005) Hypofractionated radiotherapy with carbon ion beams for prostate cancer. Int J Radiat Oncol Biol Phys 63(4): 1153–1160

Wakatsuki M, Tsuji H, Ishikawa H, Yanagi T, Kamada T, Nakano T, Suzuki H, Akakura K, Shimazaki J, Tsujii H (2008) Quality of life in men treated with carbon ion therapy for prostate cancer. Int J Radiat Oncol Biol Phys 72(4):1010–1015

Wilson RR (1946) Radiological use of fast protons. Radiology 47(5): 487–491

Yonemoto LT, Slater JD, Rossi CJ Jr, Antoine JE, Loredo L, Archambeau JO, Schulte RW, Miller DW, Teichman SL, Slater JM (1997) Combined proton and photon conformal radiation therapy for locally advanced carcinoma of the prostate: preliminary results of a phase I/II study. Int J Radiat Oncol Biol Phys 37(1):21–29

Yu JB, Makarov DV, Gross C (2011) A new formula for prostate cancer lymph node risk. Int J Radiat Oncol Biol Phys 80(1):69–75

Zelefsky MJ, Fuks Z, Hunt M, Lee HJ, Lombardi D, Ling CC, Reuter VE, Venkatraman ES, Leibel SA (2001) High dose radiation delivered by intensity modulated conformal radiotherapy improves the outcome of localized prostate cancer. J Urol 166(3):876–881

Zietman AL, DeSilvio ML, Slater JD, Rossi CJ Jr, Miller DW, Adams JA, Shipley WU (2005) Comparison of conventional-dose vs high-dose conformal radiation therapy in clinically localized adenocarcinoma of the prostate: a randomized controlled trial. JAMA 294(10):1233–1239

Zietman AL, Bae K, Slater JD, Shipley WU, Efstathiou JA, Coen JJ, Bush DA, Lunt M, Spiegel DY, Skowronski R et al (2010a) Randomized trial comparing conventional-dose with high-dose conformal radiation therapy in early-stage adenocarcinoma of the prostate: long-term results from proton radiation oncology group/ american college of radiology 95-09. J Clin Oncol Off J Am Soc Clin Oncol 28(7):1106–1111

Zietman A, Goitein M, Tepper JE (2010b) Technology evolution: is it survival of the fittest? J Clin Oncol Off J Am Soc Clin Oncol 28(27):4275–4279

There is Evidence for the Superiority of Protons or Heavy Ions, Contra

Daniel Robert Henderson and Nicholas van As

Contents

Abstract

Photon therapy is a safe and effective treatment for localised prostate cancer. It is used widely and has a strong evidence base. For three decades, proponents of proton and heavy ion therapy have claimed that these modalities have theoretical advantages which will translate into clinical benefit. However, there is no current evidence to support this. In this chapter we will assess the theoretical and clinical evidence for proton and heavy ion therapy and compare this with that for photon therapy. The health economic perspective will also be examined. We will show that there is no evidence for the superiority of protons or heavy ions over photon therapy.

1 Introduction

In this chapter we will show that, in the treatment of localised prostate cancer, there is no evidence for the superiority of protons or heavy ions over photon therapy. To set the scene, photon therapy has been successfully used by radiation departments for decades and the evolution from fixed fields to conformal radiotherapy and IMRT (intensity modulated radiotherapy) has resulted in progressive improvements in biochemical control and reduced toxicity (Dearnaley et al. 1999, 2007; Cahlon et al. 2008). Long-term follow-up of patients treated with IMRT has demonstrated excellent biochemical control and acceptable late toxicity (Spratt et al. 2012). Additionally, newer techniques such as image guidance and stereotactic body radiotherapy (SBRT) have the potential to further improve the therapeutic ratio of photon treatments, and produce better outcomes for patients (King et al. 2012). In view of this, photon treatment for localised prostate cancer has set a high standard for alternative modalities to beat.

Those in favour of proton and heavy ion therapy claim that their theoretical advantages (particularly regarding dose distribution) will translate into superior benefit for

D. R. Henderson
Clinical Oncology Royal Marsden Hospital London, London, SW3 6JJ, UK

N. van As (✉)
The Royal Marsden Hospital, Fulham Road, London, SW3 6JJ, UK
e-mail: Nicholas.VanAs@rmh.nhs.uk

H. Geinitz et al. (eds.), *Radiotherapy in Prostate Cancer*, Medical Radiology. Radiation Oncology,
DOI: 10.1007/174_2013_915,

Published Online: 29 October 2013

patients—for example, with reduced late normal tissue toxicity allowing dose escalation. However, notwithstanding over 30 years of research with proton therapy for localised prostate cancer, there is no clinical data to support this assertion and, as is clear from the title of this chapter, we are concerned with *evidence* for the *superiority* of proton or heavy ion therapy.

There remains a significant lack of evidence in this field, in that no phase III trials comparing proton or heavy ion therapy with photon therapy exist. As we shall see, there is a good quality phase III trial comparing photons with a higher- and lower-dose proton boost, but this provides little information with regard to the current discussion. Ultimately, phase II studies and retrospective comparisons make up the majority of the data available. Pro-proton groups have argued that a phase III trial of protons versus photons is unnecessary, as the advantages of proton therapy are self-evident (Goitein and Cox 2008). We disagree with this, as will be seen in the coming discussion.

Health economics is also a significant factor here. The setup and running costs of a proton or heavy ion facility are far in excess of even the most advanced photon facility. As such, evidence for superiority of these therapies must be strong before the allocation of resources toward proton or heavy ion therapy can be justified.

In this chapter we will discuss the current theoretical and clinical evidence for proton and heavy ion therapy. Our contention is that these therapies are at very best equivalent to current photon therapy, but at a much greater cost.

2 Theoretical and Planning Considerations

2.1 Physical Properties

The physical properties of proton and heavy ion beams produce steep dose fall-off at depth and at beam margins. Dose can drop from 90 to 10 % over a distance of a few millimetres. Protons and heavy ions are much more sensitive to tissue inhomogeneities than photons and Hounsfield units on computed tomography planning scans must be converted to relative stopping power of each tissue (Joiner and Kogel 2009). A relative biological effectiveness (RBE) of 1.1 is quoted for protons and this value is used by treatment planning programs and when comparing doses to photon therapy (Paganetti et al. 2002). However, RBE may be significantly higher in the terminal part of the proton beam and as much as two to four times higher in the final 2 cm of a heavy ion beam (Kramer et al. 2003). There is therefore significant uncertainty and complexity in planning, compared with photon treatments.

2.2 Organ Motion

It is well established that there is significant variability in the intra- and inter-fraction position of the prostate during radiotherapy treatment. This variability is introduced due to day-to-day differences in rectal, and to a lesser extent bladder, filling. It is also established that this movement can compromise planning target volume (PTV) coverage in photon and proton therapy (Wang et al. 2011). The PTV margin required to account for this motion in photon therapy has been estimated as 6–7 mm in the anterioposterior direction (Wu et al. 2001). Image-guided therapy systems (using implanted fiducial markers) are now in routine use for photon treatments and have had success in reducing PTV and associated rectal and urinary toxicity (Zelefsky et al. 2012b). With regard to proton and heavy ion therapy, given the uncertainties around dose distribution close to the treatment volume (see Sect. 2.1) and the fact that image guidance is not routine, there are significant theoretical concerns regarding toxicity to surrounding tissues. This is particularly the case for patients where the rectal wall is very closely applied to the posterior aspect of the prostate.

2.3 Planning Studies

In an important planning study, Trofimov et al. compared dose distributions for IMRT (using seven equally spaced coplanar fields) and conformal proton therapy (two parallel opposed lateral fields). A dose of 79.2 Gy/GyE was used (Trofimov et al. 2007). This study found that IMRT demonstrated better conformity to the target volume and equivalent rectal dose when compared with conformal proton therapy. Furthermore, the volume of bladder receiving 70 Gy or above was reduced by 34 % with IMRT. Another group compared IMRT with intensity modulated proton therapy (IMPT) (Cella et al. 2001). Both IMRT and IMPT plans used five coplanar fields. For dose up to 99 Gy/GyE conformity to the target volume and organ at risk sparing were equivalent. Thus, in theory, clinical toxicity should be equivalent for IMRT and photon treatments at equivalent doses. If this is the case, there is no scope for dose escalation with proton therapy and no clear theoretical ration for its use.

2.4 Second Malignancy Risk

One advantage of proton therapy and heavy ion therapy over IMRT regularly cited by those advocating these treatments is the theoretical reduction in radiation-induced malignancy risk. IMRT treatments irradiate a significantly larger volume to a low dose (under 30 Gy) when compared with proton treatments. This is the so-called "low dose bath" (Miralbell et al. 2002). Although this increases the theoretical risk of second malignancy, the uncertainty in these calculations may be up to 30 % (Fontenot et al. 2010). A recently published study looking at second malignancy after high-dose IMRT showed an in-field second malignancy risk of 4.8 % at 10 years with a mortality rate of 0.7 % also at 10 years. Just under 900 patients were included. As such, second malignancy may be less relevant to the majority of patients treated for prostate cancer, who are over the age of 70. Additionally, it appears from this data that many second malignancies are treatable or curable (Zelefsky et al. 2012a). There is no clinical evidence comparing second malignancy after photon treatment with that after proton or heavy ion treatment.

3 Review of Clinical Evidence

3.1 Photons Versus Protons or Heavy Ions Alone

3.1.1 Phase III Data and Systematic Reviews

There are currently no reported randomised clinical trials comparing photon treatments with proton or heavy ion therapy alone (De Ruysscher et al. 2012). In localised prostate cancer, multiple systematic reviews of the available clinical data have concluded that, at present, there is no evidence of benefit for proton or heavy ion therapy over photon therapy, with regard to toxicity or tumour control (Brada et al. 2007, 2009; Lodge et al. 2007; Olsen et al. 2007; Allen et al. 2012). In the light of these facts alone it is clear that strong evidence for the superiority of proton or heavy ion therapy to photon therapy is lacking.

3.1.2 Phase II Data

Proponents of proton therapy feel that its potential theoretical advantages, particularly with regard to dose distribution, will translate into a reduction in treatment-related toxicity (Goitein and Cox 2008). If dose-limiting late rectal and urinary toxicity can be reduced with proton therapy, it is claimed that dose escalation could then be undertaken. There is abundant evidence from photon therapy that higher doses of radiation reduce biochemical relapse in the treatment of localised prostate cancer—although a survival benefit has not yet been demonstrated (Viani et al. 2009). Naturally, this improvement comes at the cost of increased late (urinary and rectal) toxicity, and this has limited escalation of dose above 80–90 Gy in 2 Gy fractions, although further clinical benefit is predicted.

However, from the available phase II data, there is no clinical evidence that late toxicity is reduced with proton therapy compared with photon therapy. In fact, in a recent report on the American College of Radiology 03–12 study, 26 % of patients receiving conformal proton monotherapy to a dose of 82 GyE experienced RTOG (Radiation Therapy Oncology Group) grade two or above late toxicity (Coen et al. 2011). This study looked at a cohort of 85 men with a median follow-up of just under 3 years who were treated with a parallel opposed lateral beam technique. It concluded that further proton dose escalation with a conformal technique risked unacceptable late toxicity. A collaborative phase II study by three Japanese proton institutions enrolled 151 patients to be treated with the lower dose of 74 GyE using a conformal parallel opposed beam technique. At 2 years, CTC late grade two or above toxicity was 4.1 and 2.0 % for genitourinary and gastrointestinal symptoms, respectively. These studies can be compared with the Memorial Sloane-Kettering Cancer Centre (MSKCC) review of 170 patients treated with a dose of 81 Gy using a five field IMRT technique (Alicikus et al. 2011). At 10 years of follow-up actuarial prostate-specific antigen (PSA) relapse-free survival was 81, 78, and 62 % for low-, intermediate-, and high-risk disease. Grade two or greater late genitourinary and rectal toxicity was 16 and 3 %, respectively. A further review by the same group of over 1000 patients treated with 86.4 Gy photon IMRT with a median follow-up of 7 years found that grade two or above late genitourinary and rectal toxicity was 21.1 and 4.4 %, respectively (Spratt et al. 2012). The Fox Chase Cancer Centre have also produced published results for IMRT with doses of 74–78 Gy (Eade et al. 2008). A 3 year actuarial grade two and above genitourinary and gastrointestinal toxicities were 3.5 and 2.4 %, respectively.

Turning to therapy with carbon ions, a Japanese group at Chiba University have recently reported on over 700 patients treated with hypofractionated carbon ion therapy for localised prostate cancer (Okada et al. 2012). Doses of 66–57.6 GyE in 20–16 fractions were used. Late toxicities of grade two or above for the 664 patients with at least 1 year of follow-up were 8.0 and 2.4 %, respectively, for genitourinary and gastrointestinal symptoms. A comparison can be made with patients treated in the hypofractionated arms of the multi-centre United Kingdom CHHiP study (Dearnaley et al. 2012). Patients in these arms (150 patients each) received 60 Gy in 20 fractions or 57 Gy in 19 fractions using IMRT. At 2 years RTOG grade two and above toxicity was under 3 % for bladder toxicity and less than 4 % for bowel toxicity.

In summary, although with the caveat that we are comparing between series, it must be concluded that the available phase II evidence does not show an advantage for proton or heavy ion treatments over photon therapy with regard to toxicity. Furthermore, although there are not a large quantity of mature phase II data on proton and heavy ion therapy, it appears that these treatments are at best equivalent to photon therapy in terms of tumour control (Jensen et al. 2011). These factors argue against the possibility of significant dose escalation with protons or heavy ions.

3.1.3 Population-Based Retrospective Studies

Although no prospective comparative studies exist, a recent, large retrospective study has yielded some important results (Sheets et al. 2012). This study used the United States SEER (Surveillance, Epidemiology and End Results) database to identify patients treated with radiotherapy for localised prostate cancer. The SEER database links to several population-based cancer registries and includes around a quarter of the United States (US) population. The investigators identified 684 men treated with proton therapy and these were propensity-matched to the same number of patients treated with IMRT. Patients were treated between 2002 and 2007. The investigators found that diagnoses of urinary incontinence, erectile dysfunction and need for additional cancer therapy (a surrogate for disease relapse) were equal between the groups. However, diagnoses of gastrointestinal morbidity and the need for related procedures, such as colonoscopy, were significantly higher in the group treated with proton therapy. Acknowledging the limitations of this retrospective study, it provides the best long-term comparative evidence of photon and proton therapy. Not only does it show no difference in cancer outcome, but it also shows a potential increase in gastrointestinal toxicity, which is consistent with theoretical concerns about the uncertainty of proton therapy dose distributions, particularly without image guidance. In a similar population-based retrospective cohort study Kim et al. identified 4645 patients treated with IMRT and 337 treated with proton therapy alone or as a boost to photon therapy (Kim et al. 2011). This study found a hazard ratio of 0.30 (0.19–0.47) for any gastrointestinal toxicity, in favour of IMRT (compared with proton therapy).

3.2 Photons With a Proton or Heavy Ion Boost

As discussed above, no phase III trials comparing photons with proton or heavy ion therapy have been reported. However, there is mature outcome data from a phase III trial comparing two proton boost doses in addition to conformal photon therapy in patients with localised prostate cancer (Zietman et al. 2005). This study was undertaken by two US institutions—Massachusetts General Hospital (MGH) and Loma Linda University Medical Centre (LLUMC)—who recruited 393 patients with low and intermediate risk disease between 1996 and 1999. All patients received 50.4 Gy of conformal photon therapy to the prostate. Patients were randomised to receive either a 19.8 or 28.8 GyE boost with conformal proton therapy. Patients were treated with a single perineal proton beam (MGH) or lateral opposed beam pair (LLUMC). At a median follow-up of 8.9 years, rates of biochemical control were 68 and 83 %, respectively for the low (70.2 GyE) and high (79.2 GyE) dose arms. In the high-dose arm, late genitourinary toxicity of grade two and above was seen in 27 % and late gastrointestinal toxicity in 24 % (Zietman et al. 2010).

However, a number of conformal photon-only dose-escalation trials have also been performed comparing 68–70 Gy doses with 78–80 Gy doses (Pollack et al. 2002; Peeters et al. 2006; Michalski et al. 2012). A meta-analysis of these studies, and others, including over 2500 patients, found an improvement in biochemical control of between 14 and 20 %, dependent on disease risk, when escalating from 70 to 80 Gy (Viani et al. 2009). Grade two late genitourinary toxicity in those treated with high-dose conformal radiotherapy is around 10 % and late gastrointestinal toxicity approximately 15 %, at 5 years (Zelefsky et al. 1999).

Thus, dose escalation can be achieved with conformal photon therapy alone with similar outcomes to using a proton boost. The MGH/LLUMC study only tells us that a higher dose of radiation improves outcomes in localised prostate cancer. It is not informative on the question of whether protons are superior to photons. Furthermore, data from IMRT photon studies indicate that 80 Gy and higher can be delivered to the prostate with late toxicity much lower than that seen with conformal photon or proton therapy (Eade et al. 2008; Alicikus et al. 2011; Spratt et al. 2012).

With regard to heavy ion therapy, the University of Heidelberg group in Germany have published early results delivering 78 GyE with a combination of IMRT photons and a carbon ion boost (Nikoghosyan et al. 2011). Only a small number of patients (14) had been recruited to this phase II trial and equivalent acute toxicity to IMRT alone has been reported.

3.3 Image-Guided Therapy

Much of the outcome data available for proton therapy are for conformal techniques. These techniques have been superseded in photon therapy by the advent of intensity modulated radiotherapy, increasingly given with image guidance. There is good evidence that these techniques reduce toxicity and therefore allow dose escalation in excess of 80 Gy (Spratt et al. 2012). Intensity modulation and image guidance have more latterly been adopted in proton therapy. Again, only phase II data are available, but evidence that proton therapy is superior is lacking. A recent phase II study reported by the University of Florida Proton Therapy Institute investigated 211 patients treated with image-guided proton therapy (Mendenhall et al. 2012). An intraprostatic fiducial marker technique was used for image guidance. Patients were treated with 78–82 GyE, dependent on risk group, with systemic therapy being given in high-risk cases. A 2 year prevalence of grade two and above late toxicity was 24 % for genitourinary and 4 % for gastrointestinal. Compare this with an MSKCC series of 186 patients treated with image-guided IMRT photons to a dose of 86.4 Gy (Zelefsky et al. 2012b). At 3 years, grade two and above late genitourinary toxicity was 10 % and late rectal toxicity 1 %. A similar study by the Tohoku University group using image-guided IMRT to a dose of 80 Gy found 5-year rates of late genitourinary toxicity of 6.0 % and with 6.3 % for late gastrointestinal toxicity (Takeda et al. 2012). Similar outcomes for disease control were reported in these studies. Clearly it is not optimal to compare across series, but these data are difficult to construe as evidence for the superiority of proton therapy.

Newer and more advanced techniques such as stereotactic body radiotherapy (SBRT) give an indication that the maximum therapeutic ratio for photon treatments has yet to be reached. A recently reported phase II trial using CyberKnife technology to deliver 36.25 Gy in five fractions provides encouraging results (King et al. 2012). This technology uses real-time tracking of intraprostatic fiducial markers, allowing reduction in planning target volume. Due to increased geometrical accuracy, there is potential to deliver hypofractionated doses with reduced normal tissue toxicity. SBRT has been used to treat prostate cancer for more than 5 years although, as yet, there is no randomised evidence demonstrating equivalence with standard fractionation. Freeman et al. were the first to report 5-year outcomes in a small cohort of 41 patients with low-risk disease (Freeman and King 2011). Biochemical control was 93.7 % at 5 years and only one grade 3 toxicity (GU) occurred during follow-up. Most series in the literature have used the Cyberknife® system to deliver these hypofractionated regimens. However, there is one series which delivered SBRT on a conventional linear accelerator. Madsen et al. treated 40 low-risk patients with 33.5 Gy in 5 fractions and showed a 48 month bRFS of 90 % (Madsen et al. 2007).

A large pooled analysis of SBRT was presented at ASTRO 2012. Katz et al. presented the results of 1101 patients with organ confined disease (30 % intermediate risk, 11 % high risk) treated at 9 different institutions. Most received 35–36.25 Gy in five fractions and 14 % received hormonal therapy. Biochemical relapse-free survival was 95 % for low risk, 90 % for intermediate risk and 80 % for high risk at 5 years (although the median follow-up in the whole cohort was 36 months) (Katz 2012). No data exist for similar fractionation regimens delivered with protons.

4 Health Economic Perspective

Proton and heavy ion treatments are expensive. The setup cost of a charged particle facility has been estimated at between €138 and 94 million depending on whether the unit is able to deliver protons alone or protons and heavy ions. Compare this with €23 million for a modern photon facility. Furthermore, the cost per fraction is increased by three to five times for proton and heavy ion therapy compared with photon therapy (Peeters et al. 2010). In a study from the United States, Konski et al. calculated the cost per quality adjusted life year (QALY) of proton therapy compared with IMRT. Making the assumption that proton therapy would allow a 10 GyE dose escalation above IMRT with the predicted clinical benefit, at 15 years the cost per QALY was $64,000 (Konski et al. 2007). Even with the generous assumption that protons could produce such a benefit, the cost per QALY is well above the $50,000 usually considered to indicate health economic viability. Newer photon-based technologies such as SBRT techniques (see Sect. 3.3), by allowing hypofractionation and reducing late toxicity, are likely to produce a much greater health economic benefit by reducing treatment time and also the need for additional medical treatments (Hodges et al. 2012).

5 Conclusion

We conclude that there is no evidence for the superiority of protons and heavy ions over current photon therapy. In view of the available evidence, at best, protons and heavy ions are equivalent to IMRT photon treatment. They are however, vastly more expensive. We believe this cost is not justified given that the same outcome can be achieved with a less expensive and more widely used technology. Furthermore, newer photon technologies are beginning to show potential in reducing treatment time and late toxicity without compromising efficacy and with a potential reduction in cost.

The question of whether a phase III trial of protons versus photons is appropriate is difficult. The high cost of proton therapy, its potentially significant late gastrointestinal toxicity and the possible increase in late malignancy risk with IMRT mean that there is potential equipoise between these treatments (Glatstein et al. 2008; Tepper 2008). However, given the rapid development of delivery technologies (such as SBRT and IGRT) for both protons and photons it would be difficult to select which to compare, especially with the timescales involved in phase III trials. Ultimately, it is difficult to justify the continued use of costly charged particle treatment without a good evidence base where a proven (and more cost effective) alternative exits.

References

Alicikus ZA, Yamada Y et al (2011) Ten-year outcomes of high-dose, intensity-modulated radiotherapy for localized prostate cancer. Cancer 117(7):1429–1437

Allen AM, Pawlicki T et al (2012) An evidence based review of proton beam therapy: the report of ASTRO's emerging technology committee. Radiother Oncol 103(1):8–11

Brada M, Pijls-Johannesma M et al (2007) Proton therapy in clinical practice: current clinical evidence. J Clin Oncol 25(8):965–970

Brada M, Pijls-Johannesma M et al (2009) Current clinical evidence for proton therapy. Cancer J 15(4):319–324

Cahlon O, Hunt M et al (2008) Intensity-modulated radiation therapy: supportive data for prostate cancer. Semin Radiat Oncol 18(1):48–57

Cella L, Lomax A et al (2001) Potential role of intensity modulated proton beams in prostate cancer radiotherapy. Int J Radiat Oncol Biol Phys 49(1):217–223

Coen JJ, Bae K et al (2011) Acute and late toxicity after dose escalation to 82 GyE using conformal proton radiation for localized prostate cancer: initial report of American College of Radiology Phase II study 03–12. Int J Radiat Oncol Biol Phys 81(4):1005–1009

De Ruysscher D, Mark Lodge M et al (2012) Charged particles in radiotherapy: a five-year update of a systematic review. Radiother Oncol 103(1):5–7

Dearnaley D, Syndikus I et al (2012) Conventional versus hypofractionated high-dose intensity-modulated radiotherapy for prostate cancer: preliminary safety results from the CHHiP randomised controlled trial. Lancet Oncol 13(1):43–54

Dearnaley DP, Khoo VS et al (1999) Comparison of radiation side-effects of conformal and conventional radiotherapy in prostate cancer: a randomised trial. Lancet 353(9149):267–272

Dearnaley DP, Sydes MR et al (2007) Escalated-dose versus standard-dose conformal radiotherapy in prostate cancer: first results from the MRC RT01 randomised controlled trial. Lancet Oncol 8(6):475–487

Eade TN, Horwitz EM et al (2008) A comparison of acute and chronic toxicity for men with low-risk prostate cancer treated with intensity-modulated radiation therapy or (125)I permanent implant. Int J Radiat Oncol Biol Phys 71(2):338–345

Fontenot JD, Bloch C et al (2010) Estimate of the uncertainties in the relative risk of secondary malignant neoplasms following proton therapy and intensity-modulated photon therapy. Phys Med Biol 55(23):6987–6998

Freeman DE, King CR (2011) Stereotactic body radiotherapy for low-risk prostate cancer: five-year outcomes. Radiat Oncol 6:3

Glatstein E, Glick J et al (2008) Should randomized clinical trials be required for proton radiotherapy? An alternative view. J Clin Oncol 26(15):2438–2439

Goitein M, Cox JD (2008) Should randomized clinical trials be required for proton radiotherapy? J Clin Oncol 26(2):175–176

Hodges JC, Lotan Y et al (2012) Cost-effectiveness analysis of stereotactic body radiation therapy versus intensity-modulated radiation therapy: an emerging initial radiation treatment option for organ-confined prostate cancer. J Oncol Pract 8(3 Suppl):e31s–e37s

Jensen A.D, Munter, MW et al (2011). Review of clinical experience with ion beam radiotherapy. Br J Radiol 84 Spec No 1: S35–47

Joiner M, Kogel Avd (2009). Basic clinical radiobiology. London, Hodder Arnold

Katz A (2012). Five-year biochemical control rates for stereotactic body radiotherapy for organ confined prostate cancer: a multi-institutional pooled analysis.Oral presentation at ASTRO annual meeting 2012

Kim S, Shen S et al (2011) Late gastrointestinal toxicities following radiation therapy for prostate cancer. Eur Urol 60(5):908–916

King CR, Brooks JD et al (2012) Long-term outcomes from a prospective trial of stereotactic body radiotherapy for low-risk prostate cancer. Int J Radiat Oncol Biol Phys 82(2):877–882

Konski A, Speier W et al (2007) Is proton beam therapy cost effective in the treatment of adenocarcinoma of the prostate? J Clin Oncol 25(24):3603–3608

Kramer M, Weyrather WK et al (2003) The increased biological effectiveness of heavy charged particles: from radiobiology to treatment planning. Technol Cancer Res Treat 2(5):427–436

Lodge M, Pijls-Johannesma M et al (2007) A systematic literature review of the clinical and cost-effectiveness of hadron therapy in cancer. Radiother Oncol 83(2):110–122

Madsen BL, Hsi RA et al (2007) Stereotactic hypofractionated accurate radiotherapy of the prostate (SHARP), 33.5 Gy in five fractions for localized disease: first clinical trial results. Int J Radiat Oncol Biol Phys 67(4):1099–1105

Mendenhall NP, Li Z et al (2012) Early outcomes from three prospective trials of image-guided proton therapy for prostate cancer. Int J Radiat Oncol Biol Phys 82(1):213–221

Michalski J, Winter K et al (2012) Clinical outcome of patients treated with 3D conformal radiation therapy (3D-CRT) for prostate cancer on RTOG 9406. Int J Radiat Oncol Biol Phys 83(3):e363–e370

Miralbell R, Lomax A et al (2002) Potential reduction of the incidence of radiation-induced second cancers by using proton beams in the treatment of pediatric tumors. Int J Radiat Oncol Biol Phys 54(3):824–829

Nikoghosyan AV, Schulz-Ertner D et al (2011) Acute toxicity of combined photon IMRT and carbon ion boost for intermediate-risk prostate cancer—acute toxicity of 12C for PC. Acta Oncol 50(6):784–790

Okada T, Tsuji H et al (2012) Carbon ion radiotherapy in advanced hypofractionated regimens for prostate cancer: from 20 to 16 fractions. Int J Radiat Oncol Biol Phys 84(4):968–972

Olsen DR, Bruland OS et al (2007) Proton therapy—a systematic review of clinical effectiveness. Radiother Oncol 83(2):123–132

Paganetti H, Niemierko A et al (2002) Relative biological effectiveness (RBE) values for proton beam therapy. Int J Radiat Oncol Biol Phys 53(2):407–421

Peeters A, Grutters JP et al (2010) How costly is particle therapy? Cost analysis of external beam radiotherapy with carbon-ions, protons and photons. Radiother Oncol 95(1):45–53

Peeters ST, Heemsbergen WD et al (2006) Dose-response in radiotherapy for localized prostate cancer: results of the Dutch multicenter randomized phase III trial comparing 68 Gy of radiotherapy with 78 Gy. J Clin Oncol 24(13):1990–1996

Pollack A, Zagars GK et al (2002) Prostate cancer radiation dose response: results of the M. D. Anderson phase III randomized trial. Int J Radiat Oncol Biol Phys 53(5):1097–1105

Sheets NC, Goldin GH et al (2012) Intensity-modulated radiation therapy, proton therapy, or conformal radiation therapy and morbidity and disease control in localized prostate cancer. JAMA 307(15):1611–1620

Spratt DE, Pei X et al (2012). Long-term survival and toxicity in patients treated with high-dose intensity modulated radiation therapy for localized prostate cancer. Int J Radiat Oncol Biol Phys

Takeda K, Takai Y et al (2012) Treatment outcome of high-dose image-guided intensity-modulated radiotherapy using intra-prostate fiducial markers for localized prostate cancer at a single institute in Japan. Radiat Oncol 7:105

Tepper JE (2008) Protons and parachutes. J Clin Oncol 26(15): 2436–2437

Trofimov A, Nguyen PL et al (2007) Radiotherapy treatment of early-stage prostate cancer with IMRT and protons: a treatment planning comparison. Int J Radiat Oncol Biol Phys 69(2):444–453

Viani GA, Stefano EJ et al (2009) Higher-than-conventional radiation doses in localized prostate cancer treatment: a meta-analysis of randomized, controlled trials. Int J Radiat Oncol Biol Phys 74(5):1405–1418

Wang Y, Efstathiou JA et al (2011) Evaluation of the dosimetric impact of interfractional anatomical variations on prostate proton therapy using daily in-room CT images. Med Phys 38(8):4623–4633

Wu J, Haycocks T et al (2001) Positioning errors and prostate motion during conformal prostate radiotherapy using on-line isocentre set-up verification and implanted prostate markers. Radiother Oncol 61(2):127–133

Zelefsky MJ, Cowen D et al (1999) Long term tolerance of high dose three-dimensional conformal radiotherapy in patients with localized prostate carcinoma. Cancer 85(11):2460–2468

Zelefsky MJ, Housman DM et al (2012a) Incidence of secondary cancer development after high-dose intensity-modulated radiotherapy and image-guided brachytherapy for the treatment of localized prostate cancer. Int J Radiat Oncol Biol Phys 83(3):953–959

Zelefsky MJ, Kollmeier M et al (2012b) Improved clinical outcomes with high-dose image guided radiotherapy compared with non-IGRT for the treatment of clinically localized prostate cancer. Int J Radiat Oncol Biol Phys 84(1):125–129

Zietman AL, Bae K et al (2010) Randomized trial comparing conventional-dose with high-dose conformal radiation therapy in early-stage adenocarcinoma of the prostate: long-term results from proton radiation oncology group/american college of radiology 95–09. J Clin Oncol 28(7):1106–1111

Zietman AL, DeSilvio ML et al (2005) Comparison of conventional-dose vs high-dose conformal radiation therapy in clinically localized adenocarcinoma of the prostate: a randomized controlled trial. JAMA 294(10):1233–1239

The manufacturer's authorised representative in the EU is Springer Nature Customer Service Centre GmbH, Europaplatz 3, 69115 Heidelberg, Germany. If you have any concerns regarding our products, please contact ProductSafety@springernature.com

Printed and bound by CPI Group (UK) Ltd, Croydon, CR0 4YY
23/07/2026
02175041-0001